1982

Neuroendocrine Perspectives
Volume 1

Neuroendocrine Perspectives

edited by

Eugenio E. Müller
Department of Pharmacology, University of Milan, School of Medicine,
20129, Milan, Italy

and

Robert M. MacLeod
Department of Internal Medicine, University of Virginia, School of Medicine,
Charlottesville, VA 22908, USA

Volume 1

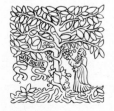

1982

Elsevier Biomedical Press
Amsterdam · New York · Oxford

ISBN (vol.) 0-444-80365-3
ISBN (set) 0-444-80364-5

Published by:
Elsevier Biomedical Press
PO Box 211
1000 AZ Amsterdam
The Netherlands

Sole distributors for the USA and Canada:
Elsevier North-Holland Inc.
52 Vanderbilt Avenue
New York, NY 10017
USA

Library of Congress Cataloguing in Publication Data

Neuroendocrine Perspectives

   Bibliography: p.
   Includes index.
   1. Neuroendocrinology. I. Müller, E.E.
II. MacLeod, R.M. (Robert Meredith) [DNLM:
1. Endocrinology, Period.   2. Neurophysiology–Period.
W1 NE328C]
QP356.4.N477   612'.8   81-17445
ISBN 0-444-80365-3 (v.1)   AACR2
ISBN 0-444-80364-5 (set)

Printed in Belgium by N.V. Drukkerij Erasmus, Ghent

Foreword

When Ernst Scharrer in 1928 reported his discovery of hypothalamic neurosecretory cells and proposed the then revolutionary concept of their endocrine nature as well as their possible relationship with hypophysial function, he could not have foreseen in his wildest dreams the spectacular developments in this area of research. This postulate foreshadowed the growing realization of the close interdependence between the two systems of integration which much later found expression in the emergence of a new discipline, neuroendocrinology. Over the years major new insights have been gained into the rationale for this interaction and the diverse modes of communication by which the nervous system governs the endocrine apparatus and, in turn, receives and responds to afferent hormonal signals.

The solution of the old enigma of the hypothalamic origin of the 'posterior lobe hormones' established the existence of a new class of peptide hormones of neuronal origin and thus earned the brain the status of an endocrine organ in its own right. The search for a second group of neurohormones, the hypophysiotropins (releasing or regulating factors) providing the long-awaited link to the adenohypophysis, captured the interest of investigators in several camps, and their heroic efforts resulted in the chemical identification and synthesis of some of these bioactive peptides. Additional major breakthroughs followed in rapid succession. One of these was the demonstration of an impressive number of neuropeptides other than those provided by the classical neurosecretory neurons and their wide distribution in extrahypothalamic areas of the central nervous system of vertebrates and in the ganglia of virtually all invertebrates. Some of these substances were shown to be shared by the brain and some non-neural tissues, e.g., the adenohypophysis and the diffuse neuroendocrine system of the digestive tract.

It is now known that not all of these neuron-derived principles enter the circulation. The mapping of their distribution by light and electron microscopy, in combination with immunocytochemical methodology, has revealed peptidergic terminals in close vicinity to, or even in synaptoid contact with, adenohypophysial cells suggesting a mode of neuroendocrine control other than that mediated by the hypophysial portal system. The further observation that such junctional relationships occur between peptidergic neurons and other nerve cells speaks for a role of peptides as neurotransmitters. What seems even more remarkable is that this role can apparently be carried out even by peptides such as vasopressin primarily known for their neurohormonal capacity. These new developments, as well as the remarkable demonstration that peptides may coexist in the same neuron together with traditional neurotransmitters such as noradrenaline, have drastically changed some basic concepts of long standing. Evidently, the nerve cell can no longer be set apart from other cellular species as readily as in the past when the traditional tenets of the neuron doctrine prevailed. The new vistas, reflecting an impressive versatility in neurochemical communication, are clearly an outgrowth of research in neuroendocrinology that reaches beyond the confines of this discipline.

The contributions of this first volume of *Neuroendocrine Perspectives* are focussed primarily on neurohormonal activities effecting control over adenohypophysial function. Among the topics treated in depth and accompanied by comprehensive bibliographic documentation are the following:

– The demonstration of the direct or indirect participation of 'new' neuropeptides as well as nonpeptidergic neuroregulators (catecholamine, 5HT in the operation of the neuroendocrine axis;

– The detailed tracing of the pathways conveying afferent, including exteroceptive, directives to cells that provide endocrine factors (prolactin, oxytocin) which exert complex multiphase control over the mammary gland during lactation;

– An exploration of the use of hypothalamic in vitro systems as models for the study of the dynamics of peptidergic neurons;

– The elucidation of the biosynthetic mechanism giving rise to several neuropeptides (ACTH, β-LPH, β-endorphin) by cleavage of a large common precursor, pro-opiomelanocortin;

– The search for the ultrastructural correlates of the functional states of anterior pituitary cells under conditions of stimulation and rest;

– An exploration of the still uncertain regulation of the renin-angiotensin-aldosterone system; and lastly

– A discussion of the clinical implications of this newly acquired information for the control of fertility, hypertension, and certain forms of depression.

Berta Scharrer

Introduction to Volume 1

During the past decade, we have seen the field of neuroendocrinology expand far beyond its classically defined parameters. With increased awareness of the contributions made by neuroendocrine research to the solution of numerous problems in fundamental and clinical science has come the need for an annual discussion of important trends and new data, as well as for the reinterpretation of concepts involved in the neuroendocrine system. The object of this series is to provide a forum for the presentation of new data within the critical perspective of a comprehensive review of the topic.

Hypophysiotrophic hormones, although recognized not to be produced solely by the brain, have been most thoroughly studied in nervous tissue. The complex morphologic and chemical interrelationships among aminergic and peptidergic mechanisms in the median eminence are beginning to emerge as a network responsive to central and peripheral stimuli. Neuroendocrinologists originally recognized that functional changes in pituitary hormone secretory patterns result from electrical and chemical modifiers produced by endogenous environmental messages. This elementary perception of brain–endocrine relationships must now be modified by the realization that some pituitary hormones may also be synthesized by specific brain cells. This complexity is compounded by studies indicating that pro-opiocortin and ACTH synthesis have common points of control. The recognition that certain prolactin and MSH-secreting cells are controlled by dopaminergic mechanisms previously reserved for nervous cells requires that these anatomically separate systems be considered as a more integrated entity.

This initial volume of *Neuroendocrine Perspectives* addresses these fundamentally important concepts and discusses their application in related fields of hypertension, behavior and reproduction. It should therefore be of particular interest to neuroendocrinologists, cell biologists, neurochemists, pharmacologists and clinical scientists interested in endocrine-related topics of hypertension, psychology, psychiatry and neurology.

Eugenio E. Müller
Robert M. MacLeod

Contributors

Carey, R.M.
  Division of Endocrinology and Metabolism, Department of Internal Medicine,
  University of Virginia School of Medicine, Charlottesville, VA 22908
  USA

Cronin, M.J.
  Department of Physiology,
  University of Virginia School of Medicine, Charlottesville, VA 22908,
  USA

Dufy, B.
  Unité de Recherches de Neurobiologie du Comportement,
  INSERM U. 176,
  33077 Bordeaux, Cedex,
  France

Grosvenor, C.E.
  Department of Physiology and Biophysics,
  University of Tennessee Center for the Health Sciences,
  894 Union Avenue,
  Memphis, TN 38163,
  USA

Imura, H.
  Department of Medicine, Kyoto University Faculty of Medicine,
  54 Kawaharacho, Shogoin, Sakyo-ku, Kyoto 606,
  Japan

Johnston, C.A.
  Department of Pharmacology and Toxicology, Michigan State University,
  East Lansing, MI 48824,
  USA

McCann, S.M.
  Department of Physiology,
  University of Texas, Health Science Center at Dallas,
  5323 Harry Hines Boulevard,
  Dallas, TX 75235,
  USA

Mena, F.
  Instituto de Investigaciones Biomedicas, University of Mexico,
  Mexico City,
  Mexico

Moore, K.E.
  Department of Pharmacology and Toxicology, Michigan State University,
  East Lansing, MI 48824,
  USA

Nakai, Y.
  Department of Medicine, Kyoto University Faculty of Medicine,
  54 Kawaharacho, Shogoin, Sakyo-ku, Kyoto 606,
  Japan

Nakao, K.
  Department of Medicine, Kyoto University Faculty of Medicine,
  54 Kawaharacho, Shogoin, Sakyo-ku, Kyoto 606,
  Japan

Oki, S.
  Department of Medicine, Kyoto University Faculty of Medicine,
  54 Kawaharacho, Shogoin, Sakyo-ku, Kyoto 606,
  Japan

Poland, R.E.
  Department of Psychiatry, Harbor-UCLA Medical Center,
  Torrance, CA 90509,
  USA

Reichlin, S.
  Endocrine Division, Tufts-New England Medical Center Hospital,
  Boston, MA 02111,
  USA

Robbins, R.
  Department of Medicine, University of Colorado,
  School of Medicine,
  Denver, CO 80262,
  USA

Rubin, R.T.
  Department of Psychiatry, Harbor-UCLA Medical Center,
  Torrance, CA 90509,
  USA

Sandow, J.
  Hoechst AG, Pharmacology H 821,
  D-6230, Frankfurt 80,
  FRG

Tanaka, I.
  Department of Medicine, Kyoto University Faculty of Medicine,
  54 Kawaharacho, Shogoin, Sakyo-ku, Kyoto 606,
  Japan

Tixier-Vidal, A.
  Groupe de Neuroendocrinologie Cellulaire, Collège de France,
  75231-Paris 05,
  France

Tougard, C.
  Groupe de Neuroendocrinologie Cellulaire, Collège de France,
  75231-Paris 05,
  France

Vincent, J.D.
  Unité de Recherches de Neurobiologie du Comportement, INSERM U. 176,
  33077 Bordeaux, Cedex,
  France

Contents

Chapter 3
Regulating mechanisms for oxytocin and prolactin secretion during lactation
Clark E. Grosvenor and Flavio Mena

Chapter 4
In vitro systems for the study of secretion and
synthesis of hypothalamic peptides
Richard Robbins and Seymour Reichlin

Chapter 5
Control of biosynthesis and secretion of ACTH,
endorphins and related peptides
Hiroo Imura, Yoshikatsu Nakai, Kazuwa Nakao,
Shogo Oki and Issei Tanaka

Chapter 6
The role and direct measurement of the dopamine receptor(s)
in the anterior pituitary
Michael J. Cronin

Chapter 7
Morphological, functional and electrical correlates in anterior pituitary cells
A. Tixier-Vidal, C. Tougard, B. Dufy and J.D. Vincent

Chapter 8
Neuroendocrine regulation of the renin–angiotensin–aldosterone system
Robert M. Carey

Chapter 9
The chronoendocrinology of endogenous depression
Robert T. Rubin and Russell E. Poland

Chapter 10
Gonadotropic and antigonadotropic actions of LH-RH analogues
J. Sandow

E.E. Müller and R.M. MacLeod (eds) Neuroendocrine Perspectives Vol. 1
© Elsevier Biomedical Press, 1982

Chapter 1

The role of brain peptides in the control of anterior pituitary hormone secretion

S.M. McCann

INTRODUCTION

Oxytocin and vasopressin were the first naturally occurring hypothalamic peptides to be isolated and synthesized (Share and Grosvenor 1974). In the late 1950s and through the 1960s, a number of hypothalamic releasing and inhibiting hormones which affect pituitary hormone secretion were identified and attempts were made to isolate and characterize them (McCann et al. 1974a). TRH, a tripeptide, was characterized in 1969 (Böler et al. 1969; Burgus et al. 1969), LH-RH, a decapeptide, in 1971 (Matsuo et al. 1971), and the growth hormone inhibiting factor (Krulich et al. 1968), a tetradecapeptide, in 1973 (Brazeau et al. 1973). This factor was renamed somatostatin.

Leeman and her colleagues, while attempting to purify corticotrophin-releasing factor (CRF), noticed that some of the hypothalamic fractions induced salivation. She named the factor sialogen and used this salivation assay to elucidate the structure and synthesize sialogen which was later identified to be substance P (Chang and Leeman 1970). She also noted that blood pressure decreased following injection of certain hypothalamic fractions and on the basis of this activity, a new peptide, named neurotensin, was isolated and characterized (Carraway and Leeman 1973). Thus, five peptides were isolated from hypothalamic tissue, three on the basis of their effects on pituitary hormone secretion and two as byproducts of attempts to purify CRF.

There are a number of additional hypothalamic activities which are thought to regulate pituitary hormone release, i.e. prolactin inhibiting factor (PIF), prolactin releasing factor, growth hormone releasing factor, FSH releasing factor and factors reported to both stimulate and inhibit MSH release. Structures of the latter two have been reported but have not been universally accepted (Krulich and Fawcett 1977). The PIF activity in hypothalamus may be at least partially accounted for by dopamine (MacLeod 1969; Gibbs and Neill 1978), but none of the other presumed peptidergic factors have yet been isolated. There is little doubt that the major direct control of anterior pituitary hormone secretion is accomplished by this constellation of brain peptides. In this review we will not discuss in detail the action of the various releasing and inhibiting hormones but instead will concern ourselves with the effects of a variety of peptides not thought to be primarily hypo-physiotrophic which have now been shown to affect pituitary hormone secretion.

Great excitement developed following the discovery of the endogenous opioid receptors (Goldstein et al. 1971; Pert and Snyder 1973), and this culminated in the isolation and determination of structure of the enkephalins (Hughes et al. 1975) and endorphins (Li and Chung 1976). Even more recently it has become apparent that a pro-opiocortin molecule is synthesized not only in anterior and intermediate lobes of the pituitary but also in neurons whose cell bodies lie in the arcuate nucleus (Krieger et al. in press). Cleavage of the prohormone results in production of ACTH, α-MSH, γ-MSH, β-endorphin, and associated molecules such as corticotropin-like intermediary peptide (CLIP). It now appears that the arcuate system can release fragments of this molecule, but it is not clear whether the same cells release all of these peptides, or certain specialized cells release one or another fragment of the pro-opiocortin molecule. Evidence is now accruing for the existence of other anterior lobe hormones within the brain. A central system of prolactinergic neurons has been described (Toubeau et al. 1979) and there is some evidence to suggest the existence of growth hormone (Pacold et al. 1978), and gonadotropin and TSH cells (Lawrence et al. in press) in the brain as well. Evidence for a central angiotensin system had begun to accrue by the early 1970s (Phillips et al. 1979) and by the late 1970s evidence developed for the existence within the brain of a number of gastrointestinal peptides (Straus and Yalow 1979). All of these findings have led to the suggestion that all biologically active peptides may eventually be found to reside in the brain (McCann et al. 1979).

Considerable literature has grown up concerning the effects of these various peptides on pituitary hormone secretion. The earliest studies involved the opioid peptides because an abundant literature had developed on the effects of morphine which accurately mimics the effects of the opioid peptides. The discovery of these peptides produced a tremendous expansion of activity in this area of research. Data gathered about other peptides are more limited but in this review we will attempt to describe our current understanding of the actions of all these peptides on the pituitary and attempt to assess their physiological significance.

THE OPIOID PEPTIDES

Prior to the discovery of the endogenous opioid peptides, the actions of morphine on pituitary hormone secretion had been described. We will first discuss these effects and then relate them to the new knowledge of the opioid peptides. It was shown early that morphine would block ovulation (Barraclough and Sawyer 1955), evoke prolactin release, as determined by mammary gland changes and induction of pseudopregnancy (Meites 1962), and stimulate ACTH secretion as indicated by an elevation in plasma adrenal steroid levels (George 1971). More recent work using primarily immunoassay of pituitary hormone changes indicates that morphine evokes a spectrum of changes in pituitary hormone secretion as follows: it stimulates ACTH (Munson 1973), growth hormone (Kokka and George 1974; Bruni et al. 1977); and prolactin (McCann et al. 1974b) release and inhibits FSH, LH (Pang et al. 1977; Muraki et al. 1977) and TSH (Lomax et al. 1970) release.

The site of morphine's action to evoke ACTH release is located in the medial basal hypothalamus, apparently near the rostral end of the arcuate nucleus (George and Way 1959). Injection of morphine into more rostral regions, however, while evoking changes in temperature regulation had little or no effect on corticoid output (VanRee et al. 1976). Similarly, microinjection of opioid peptides into the rostral parts of the medial basal tuberal region evokes prolactin release (Grandison and Guidotti 1980).

Although it was originally thought that these were pharmacological actions of morphine, it now appears likely that morphine was interacting with opioid receptors in the brain to evoke these hormonal changes. Following the synthesis of the enkephalins and endorphins, a number of workers administered these systemically or microinjected them into the brain ventricles and evoked a similar pattern of hormonal responses (DuPont et al. 1977; Cusan et al. 1977; Cocchi et al. 1977). Met-enkephalin, the major opioid pentapeptide found in hypothalamus, is more effective than Leu-enkephalin to release prolactin. The potency of enkephalin analogues parallels their potency in other indices of enkephalin action (Meltzer et al. 1978). That the actions of morphine, enkephalins and endorphins are specific is suggested by the fact that they are blocked by the opiate antagonist, naloxone.

Since the enkephalins have a hypothalamic distribution different from the endorphins (Elde and Hökfelt 1979), the site of action of the various opioid peptides following their injection into the brain ventricle is not established. It appears that one site of action is probably in the region of the arcuate nucleus. This is the site of neuronal perykaria which synthesize proopiocortin and whose projections extend into various other regions of the brain. The fact that microinjection of morphine or endorphin into this site provoked changes in ACTH and prolactin similar to those obtained with intraventricular or systemic injection of the opioid peptides certainly suggests that this is one site of action (George and Way 1959; Grandison and Guidotti 1980). On the other hand, the enkephalinergic neurons seem to be located more in the periventricular region and in the rostral hypothalamus. Some of these neurons have cell bodies in the paraventricular nucleus and axons which extend to the neurohypophysis (Elde and Hökfelt 1979). It is possible that some of the actions of intraventricularly administered morphine or opioid peptides may be exerted on receptors in the vicinity of these neurons or their projections.

The evidence indicates that opioid peptides act on the hypothalamus to inhibit LH release, and not on the pituitary, since the response to LH-RH is not blocked in vivo (Cicero et al. 1977) and LH release by pituitary cells incubated in vitro is unaffected (Shaar et al. 1977). The prolactin-releasing action is also probably exerted at the hypothalamic level either via an action to stimulate prolactin-releasing factor discharge or to inhibit the release of prolactin inhibiting factor. However, Kordon's group has reported that morphine will antagonize the inhibitory action of dopamine on prolactin release in vitro (Enjalbert 1979); however, others have found no effect on prolactin release at the pituitary level even in the presence of the inhibitory action of apomorphine, a dopaminergic agonist (Login and MacLeod 1979; Grandison et al. 1980). The weight of evidence would indicate that the principal action is at the hypothalamic level.

The mechanism of action at the hypothalamic level may involve monoaminergic systems. It appears that morphine or opioid peptides inhibit dopaminergic turnover in the tuberoinfundibular dopaminergic system (Ferland et al. 1977; Gudelsky and Porter 1979), and augment serotoninergic turnover (Yarbrough et al. 1971); they may possibly increase noradrenergic turnover as well (Smith et al. 1970). There is decreased dopamine in portal blood after administration of opiates (Gudelsky and Porter 1979) and since dopamine appears to be a physiologically important prolactin inhibiting factor (MacLeod 1969; Gibbs and Neill 1978), removal of this dopaminergic inhibition may account in part for the prolactin-releasing action of opiates. On the other hand, injection of serotonin receptor blockers, inhibition of serotonin biosynthesis by *para*-chlorophenylalanine, or destruction of central serotoninergic systems by intraventricular injection of 5,7-dihydroxytryptamine has been associated with a blunting of the prolactin release in response to morphine (Koenig et al. 1979; Spampinato et al. 1979). These results suggest that the serotoninergic system is important in mediating this response either by stimulating release of prolactin-releasing factor or by inhibiting release of a peptidergic prolactin inhibiting factor. Since blockade of dopamine synthesis with alpha-methyltyrosine did not block the response to morphine in these experiments, the participation of the dopaminergic system did not seem to be critical.

In the case of growth hormone, considerable evidence indicates that the increase in serum growth hormone induced by opiates may be mediated by central noradrenergic neurons acting via alpha receptors, since a variety of inhibitors of norepinephrine synthesis and alpha, but not beta receptor blockers blocked the growth hormone-releasing action of morphine (Koenig et al. 1980). Very recently, Casanueva et al. (1980; 1981) have reported that opioid-induced GH release may be mediated by acetylcholine and histamine release.

Part of the action of opiates to elevate growth hormone may occur via inhibition of somatostatin release, since this effect has been seen with hypothalamic incubations (Pimstone et al. 1979). The inhibition of gonadotropin release may occur via blockade of dopaminergic stimulation of LH-RH release, since in an in vitro incubation system morphine blocked the dopamine-induced release of LH-RH from the incubates (Rotsztejn et al. 1978).

The possible physiological significance of the endogenous opioid peptides in control of pituitary hormone secretion is indicated by the fact that naloxone, the opiate receptor blocking drug, can decrease serum prolactin levels (Shaar et al. 1977) and interfere with stress-induced prolactin release (VanVoogt et al. 1978; Okajima et al. 1980). Furthermore, naloxone administration results in elevated gonadotropin levels in developing female rats at a variety of ages and in males at 30 days (Ieiri et al. 1979), but to a lesser extent also in aging animals (Steger et al. 1980). Injection of naloxone augments not only the preovulatory type of LH release (Sylvester et al. 1980), but also LH release in the castrate (Meites et al. 1979). This suggests that inhibitory opioid tone moderates gonadotropin release under most circumstances. One caveat which must be kept in mind is the possibility that the doses of naloxone might have been sufficiently high to exert effects other than those related only to blockade of opiate receptors (Sawynok et al. 1979).

Using an immunoassay for enkephalins, one report states that the content of immunoassayable enkephalin in the preoptic-anterior hypothalamic area declines during the afternoon of proestrus at the time of the preovulatory surge of gonadotropins (Kumar et al. 1979). This suggests that removal of inhibitory opioid tone may be involved in initiation of the preovulatory release of gonadotropins. Prolonged hyperprolactinemia has been found to reduce β-endorphin but not Met-enkephalin levels in most brain areas and the anterior lobe, whereas lactation was accompanied by declines in brain contents of both peptides (Panerai et al. 1980).

Stress-induced ACTH release is apparently associated with concomitant release of β-endorphin from the pituitary, a process associated with a decline in β-endorphin in anterior but not intermediate lobe, whereas the content in the hypothalamus was unchanged (Rossier et al. 1979). This suggests that similar mechanisms may govern the release of ACTH, β-endorphin and prolactin. These decreases could be reversed by treatment with dexamethasone.

Taken as a whole there is convincing evidence for a capability of the opioid peptides, mimicked by morphine, to modify the release of anterior pituitary hormones and evidence suggesting that this may be of physiological significance.

CHOLECYSTOKININ

Because growth hormone release increases in response to meals or administration of amino acids (Daughaday 1974), it occurred to us that blood-borne gastrointestinal hormones might influence pituitary hormone release. In the meantime, evidence for the central nervous system location of a variety of gut peptides accrued (Straus and Yalow 1979). Since cholecystokinin (CCK) had been reported to evoke satiety (Smith 1980) and had been found in brain (Straus and Yalow 1979), we decided to evaluate this peptide first. It is found in the hypothalamus, including the external layer of the median eminence, but the cerebral cortex contains the highest concentration.

In the ovariectomized rat, intraventricular injection of CCK lowered plasma LH; the minimal effective dose being less than 4 ng (Vijayan et al. 1979a). At the same time a dose-related increase in growth hormone occurred, but serum TSH levels decreased with doses of 40 or 500 ng of CCK. In the case of prolactin, results were ambiguous because an increase was found only with the 40 ng dose. The effects were observed within 5 min and lasted for up to an hour after injection. These results were obtained in cannulated animals who were freely moving around the cage. It is important to point out here that the use of anesthetized animals may result in enhancement or elimination of effects, yielding ambiguous results.

To determine whether the actions of intraventricular CCK were mediated centrally, the peptide was injected intravenously, causing a dose-related increase in plasma prolactin levels within 5 min, but only the highest dose of 1000 ng produced a significant decrease in plasma LH. No significant changes in values for the other hormones were observed. Thus, it would appear that CCK acts after intraventricular injection to inhibit TRH and LH-RH release, producing the lower plasma levels of TSH and LH, and to raise GH levels, either by stimulating GH-releasing factor or by inhibiting somatostatin release, or both. We postulate a site of action on the hypothalamus; however, since CCK is also located at other brain sites, an action at these more distant sites cannot be ruled out.

Action at the pituitary level appeared to be negated in our studies by the failure of a variety of doses up to a maximum of 2500 ng per ml to affect the release of pituitary hormones from hemipituitaries of male rats incubated in vitro. One group (Morley et al. 1979) has reported that relatively high doses of CCK (10^{-6} M) can release growth hormone. At this dose they also reported a decrease in TSH and an increase in LH release from pituitary cells in vitro, suggesting a possible action of CCK directly on the pituitary gland.

Recently, intraventricular cholecystokinin has been found to increase plasma corticosterone in the rat. Peripheral injections produced the same results, even in vagotomized rats, suggesting a central action. Since there was little action on the pituitary itself, it was postulated that the effect occurred via a release of CRF from the brain (Itoh et al. 1979). In these experiments a possible contaminant of the CCK preparation, motilin, was without effect.

Thus, it would appear that cholecystokinin in quite small doses has profound effects on pituitary hormone secretion, probably mediated largely through hypothalamic releasing and inhibiting hormones. In the absence of a convenient antagonist of CCK, it is impossible to determine whether these results have physiological significance, even though the location of CCK at hypothalamic sites suggests that this is likely. CCK may play a role not only in satiety but also in producing changes in pituitary hormone secretion related to food intake.

VASOACTIVE INTESTINAL PEPTIDE (VIP)

This gastrointestinal peptide has been located at various brain sites by both radioimmunoassay (Samson et al. 1979a; 1979b) and immunocytochemistry (Sims et al. 1980). Cell bodies of neurons containing VIP are located in the suprachiasmatic nucleus and their axons extend to various hypothalamic loci including, particularly, the dorsal hypothalamus with some projections to the median eminence. These loci are more easily seen in man than in rats. VIP has been detected in high concentrations in portal blood (Said and Porter 1979) and also has been localized to the pituitary itself (Samson et al. 1979a; 1979b), which suggests that significant amounts may be released from terminals in juxtaposition to portal vessels to perfuse the pituitary.

We demonstrated that intraventricular injection of VIP in ovariectomized, conscious rats produced a significant elevation in plasma LH within 5 min, while prolactin levels were elevated only by 4 and 100 ng doses; however, the highest dose of 500 ng had no effect on plasma LH or prolactin levels (Vijayan et al. 1979b). Plasma GH levels increased significantly 15 min after the injection of each dose and remained elevated for the 60 min duration of the experiment. Following intravenous injection at doses of 40 and 1000 ng there was no effect on plasma LH, but prolactin levels were elevated by the higher dose. Plasma GH was not modified by i.v. injection of 40 ng, while the 1000 ng dose induced a significant reduction. No changes in FSH or TSH were observed following injections of VIP. Injection into the third ventricle of 100 ng had no effect on blood pressure, whereas intravenous injection of 1000 ng significantly lowered it. In a correlative study, in vitro incubation of hemipituitaries with doses of VIP ranging 10 ng to 10 µg had no effect on pituitary hormone release into the medium. The results were interpreted to mean that VIP can alter pituitary hormone release by a hypothalamic site of action and are certainly consistent with the concept that the peptide might act as a transmitter or modulator of neuronal activity controlling pituitary hormone release.

Kordon's group reported that VIP enhanced release of prolactin from pituitaries incubated in vitro in the presence of bacitracin to inhibit peptide degradation (Ruberg et al. 1978). This result was confirmed by Shaar et al. (1979) and we were able to demonstrate that, indeed, under these conditions VIP would release prolactin (Samson et al. 1980). The effect was relatively small and the dose-response curve was flat, but prolactin release was demonstrated not only from pituitaries incubated in vitro but also from dispersed pituitary cell preparations (Fig. 1.1). Therefore, it is clear that VIP could act as a prolactin-releasing factor, particularly since it is present in high concentrations in portal blood (Said and Porter 1979) and can even be demonstrated in the anterior pituitary (Samson et al. 1979a; 1979b). The action of VIP to release prolactin may be mediated via cyclic AMP (cAMP) since there was an increase in cAMP in the cells after addition of VIP. The further increase in cAMP with 10^{-5} M VIP, which occurred without further increase in prolactin release, is unexplained. LH-RH elevated cAMP, presumably associated with its LH-releasing action, but did not alter prolactin release.

VIP acts at a hypothalamic level to release LH-RH, which in turn raises LH levels, since VIP released significant LH-RH in a hypothalamic synaptosome preparation (Fig. 1.2) (Samson et al. submitted). This tissue preparation was viable, since release was also induced by high potassium medium, blocked by chelation of calcium and also induced by dopamine. Similarly, VIP acts at the hypothalamic level to elevate GH release since it inhibits somatostatin release in vitro (Epelbaum et al. 1979).

Interestingly, recent experiments indicate that dexamethasone can block the prolactin-releasing action of VIP (Rotsztejn et al. 1980). Since prolactin is released in response to stress and this release can also be blocked by dexamethasone, these results suggest the possibility that VIP is involved in stress-induced prolactin release. Additionally, adrenalectomy was found to decrease VIP concentrations in the hippocampus and increase them in

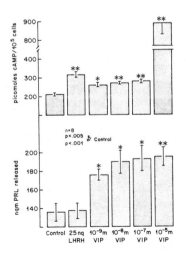

Fig. 1.1. Effect of VIP and LH-RH on cAMP accumulation in (upper panel) and PRL release from (lower panel) dispersed male rat anterior pituitary cells (7.0×10^5 cells per tube). (From W.K. Samson et al. Peptides 1, 325-332, 1980).

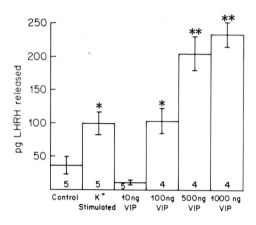

Fig. 1.2. Effects of 60 mM K^+ or VIP on LH-RH release from crude median eminence (ME) synaptosomes incubated in 2 ml of media (0.5 ME equivalents per flask). Number of flasks per group is indicated within each bar. Values presented are mean ± SEM. Significance levels compared to controls determined by t test. (From Samson et al. Reg. Peptides 2, 253-264, 1981).

the adenohypophysis, whereas corticosterone restored VIP levels to control values only in the dorsal hippocampus. In contrast dexamethasone counteracted the decrease and increase of VIP following adrenalectomy in hippocampus and adenohypophysis, respectively. This suggests that corticosteroids are involved in the regulation of VIP release.

The problem is complicated by the lack of VIP antagonists, which makes it difficult to assess the physiological significance of the peptide. Experiments utilizing passive immunization with antisera to VIP may clarify this matter. At present it appears likely that VIP functions as a synaptic transmitter or modulator of synaptic function to alter releasing factor release at the hypothalamic level and that it may also have a physiologically significant prolactin-releasing action.

It has been possible to demonstrate that both cholecystokinin and VIP release in vitro are calcium dependent and increased by depolarization of membranes by high potassium (Emson et al. 1980). This suggests that both peptides are released from nerve endings as a result of depolarization from nerve impulses and may act as synaptic transmitters or neuromodulators.

GASTRIN

Gastrin has been localized in various brain areas by radioimmunoassay (Rehfeld et al. 1979). Although there has been some controversy concerning the specificity of the antisera employed, it appears clear that gastrin is localized in the median eminence and in portions of the neurohypophysis. Consequently, it could play a role in control of anterior pituitary function.

In ovariectomized rats intraventricular injection of 1 and 5 μg of gastrin pentapeptide produced significant suppression of plasma LH and prolactin levels within 5 min of injection (Vijayan et al. 1978). The lower dose had no effect on plasma GH, but 5 μg induced a progressive elevation which reached a peak at 60 min. In contrast, TSH titers were lowered by both doses of gastrin within 5 min and remained low for 60 min. Intravenous gastrin did not affect plasma gonadotropins, GH and TSH, but produced an elevation in prolactin levels.

Incubations of pituitaries in vitro with gastrin failed to modify release of gonadotropins, growth hormone or prolactin but slightly inhibited TSH release at the highest dose of 5 μg. These results indicate that synthetic gastrin can alter pituitary hormone release and suggest a hypothalamic site of action for the peptide, since pituitary hormone secretion was not directly affected. The inhibitory effect on TSH may be mediated by both hypothalamic and direct action in view of the fact that TSH release by glands in vitro was suppressed. The physiological significance of these observations remains to be established.

SUBSTANCE P

Several studies have evaluated the effect of this peptide on pituitary hormone release. In our own experiments, again employing conscious, ovariectomized rats, intraventricular injection of substance P (0.5 or 2.0 μg) induced a significant, dose-related elevation in plasma LH within 5 min of injection (Vijayan and McCann 1979). The levels returned toward preinjection level by 60 min with either 0.5 or 2 μg doses. Substance P injected intravenously at a 1 μg dose produced a slight but significant decline of plasma LH at 15 and 30 min, an effect opposite to that obtained with intraventricular injection. Substance P failed to alter release of LH in vitro. Thus, it appears that substance P can act at the hypothalamic level to stimulate LH release. Of the peptides tested so far, only VIP shares this LH-releasing action, and it appears to be by far the more potent of the two.

Intraventricular injection of the lower dose of substance P had no effect on plasma prolactin, but it was elevated within 5 min by the 2 μg dose. Plasma prolactin was elevated by intravenous substance P even more than by the 2 μg dose injected into the ventricle. Incubation of pituitaries with substance P resulted in increased prolactin release into the medium with doses of 50 or more ng per ml. The elevation of prolactin following intraventricular injection of substance P may be via direct stimulation of the pituitary after its uptake by portal vessels and delivery to the gland, since it was active in vitro.

Plasma growth hormone was elevated after 5 min by either dose of substance P injected intraventricularly, and the values remained elevated for 60 min (Vijayan and McCann 1980). There was no effect on plasma TSH. Intravenous substance P had no effect on plasma GH or TSH and it did not alter release of either GH or TSH when incubated with pituitaries in vitro. Thus, it appears that substance P also has a capacity to release growth hormone, probably via a hypothalamic action.

Earlier, Rivier et al. (1977) had reported that systemic administration of substance P elevated prolactin and GH levels and they attributed the actions to an effect on the CNS. On the other hand our own experiments show a direct effect on prolactin release by the pituitary. It is difficult to evaluate results with systemic administration of peptides since these could induce changes in blood pressure or other effects, provoking a stress response. Stress is known to elevate prolactin in many species and it also lowers growth hormone in the rat (Krulich et al. 1974). Kato et al. (1976) obtained a dose-related increase in both growth hormone and prolactin after intravenous injection of substance P at the high doses of 5–50 μg 100 g^{-1} body weight. Again the effect on prolactin could be a stress response or mediated by direct stimulation of lactotrophs.

Chihara et al. (1978) recently obtained significant suppression of serum GH after lateral ventricular injection of substance P in urethane-anesthetized male rats, a result opposite to the elevation observed in our experiments. This discrepancy may be related to the use of lateral instead of third ventricular injections; to the use of anesthetized instead of conscious rats or to the use of males rather than ovariectomized females which were employed in our experiments. In other situations anesthetics have been clearly shown to modify the response to intraventricularly injected drugs. An example of this is GABA (Pass and Ondo 1977). Consequently, it is unwise to use anesthetized animals for this type of study. Interestingly, substance P potentiated the elevation in GH observed after injection of β-endorphin in the experiments of Chihara et al. (1978), which is consistent with our results. The inhibition of GH release by substance P in their experiment was completely abolished by prior injection of antisera to somatostatin, suggesting that it was mediated by somatostatin release.

Kato et al. (1976) found that plasma prolactin was elevated by large doses of substance P given intravenously in rats with large hypothalamic lesions, which presumably removed the gland from hypothalamic influences. This result agrees with our findings that suggest a direct action of substance P to stimulate release of prolactin from lactotrophs.

In the only experiment employing antiserum directed against substance P, Kerdelhue et al. (1978) observed that administration of these antisera at noon on proestrus provoked a significant increase in plasma LH and FSH just before or after the preovulatory surges, but had no effect on their occurrence or magnitude. They suggested that substance P had an inhibitory role in gonadotropin regulation.

NEUROTENSIN

Several studies have implicated a role for neurotensin in control of pituitary hormone secretion. In ovariectomized, conscious rats the injection of neurotensin into the third ventricle lowered plasma LH concentrations within 5 min and they remained low for 60 min after either 0.5 or 2 μg doses (Vijayan and McCann 1979). These doses similarly lowered prolactin. The intermediate dose of 1 μg of neurotensin intravenously had no effect on LH but elevated prolactin, an effect opposite to that following intraventricular injection. Incubation of hemipituitaries from the animals with various doses of neurotensin did not alter gonadotropin release but prolactin release was enhanced with doses of 50 or more ng per ml of medium. These results suggest that neurotensin acts centrally to inhibit LH-RH release and to bring about an inhibition of prolactin release, and that it can act directly on the pituitary to stimulate release of prolactin. Rivier et al. (1977) had earlier shown an increase in plasma prolactin following intravenous administration of neurotensin which may be due to this action on the pituitary.

The intraventricular injection of neurotensin at 0.5 or 2 μg doses elevated plasma GH concentrations within 5 min and they remained elevated for 60 min (Vijayan and McCann 1980). There was no effect on plasma TSH. The intermediate dose of 1 μg intravenously had no effect on GH but elevated plasma TSH. When the peptide was incubated with hemipituitaries in vitro there was no effect on GH release but TSH release was enhanced at doses greater than 100 ng per ml medium. Neurotensin may act centrally to stimulate GH release and also directly on the pituitary to stimulate TSH release. The elevation in GH we observed is similar to that previously observed by Rivier et al. (1977) following systemic administration of this peptide.

Recently Maeda and Frohman (1978) obtained significant elevation in plasma TSH following systemic injection of a considerably larger dose of neurotensin than that employed in our experiments, whereas a lowering of TSH followed the intraventricular injection of the peptide in estrogen-primed male rats, anesthetized with urethane. They also found that intraventricular neurotensin blunted the TRH-stimulated TSH release in these circumstances. The discrepancy between their results and those obtained by us may be related to the use of the lateral ventricular rather than the third ventricular route of injection, which could have led to actions on other sites in the brain or to the use of anesthetized, estrogen-primed males in their study, instead of the unanesthetized, ovariectomized animals used in our experiments. Maeda and Frohman (1978) further reported (without presentation of data) that neurotensin did not affect TSH secretion by dispersed adenohypophyseal cells, a result different from the stimulation observed in our experiments utilizing hemipituitaries from ovariectomized females. The explanation for the discrepancy is not apparent but could be related to their use of dispersed cells in which receptors for neurotensin could have been removed by the dispersion procedure.

Some light has been thrown on the possible mechanism of action of substance P, neurotensin and enkephalins to stimulate growth hormone release by studies in which the peptides were added to hypothalami incubated in vitro. Substance P (Sheppard et al. 1979) and neurotensin (Maeda and Frohman 1980) both provoked a rise in immunoreactive somatostatin release from the incubated hypothalami and the minimal effective dose was 100 ng per ml of peptide. On the other hand, Met- and Leu-enkephalin had no effect (Sheppard et al. 1979*). Since both substance P and neurotensin elevate growth hormone release it may be that this action is accomplished by discharge of growth hormone-releasing factor which overcomes the inhibitory effect of the somatostatin released. The elevation of growth hormone induced by the enkephalins would then also be attributable to growth hormone releasing factor discharge, since no effect was seen on somatostatin release.

It is possible that some of the actions of neurotensin may be mediated via its effect on the hypothalamic temperature regulating centers, since intracerebroventricular administration of the tridecapeptide lowered body temperature (Nemeroff et al. 1980). This action was not blocked by anti-muscarinic, anti-noradrenergic, or anti-opiate agents. Similarly, depletion of brain serotonin via *para*-chlorophenylalanine did not alter the neurotensin-induced hypothermia. Depletion of brain catecholamines by 6-hydroxydopamine instead resulted in significant potentiation of the hypothermia as did pretreatment with haloperidol to block dopamine receptors. Furthermore, in rats with selective depletion of brain dopamine but not norepinephrine, neurotensin-induced hypothermia was augmented. This suggests an interaction between dopamine and neurotensin on the hypothalamic temperature-regulating centers. Interestingly, neurotensin-induced hypothermia was antagonized by TRH. Intrahypothalamic administration of neurotensin reduced TSH levels in thyroidectomized animals. Thus, there appears to be interaction between neurotensin and TRH.

* But see Pimstone et al. (1979).

BRADYKININ

Bradykinin, a nonapeptide, has recently been located within the central nervous system (Correa et al. 1979). Consequently, we have tested this peptide, particularly since the bradykinin-like immunoreactivity is highest within the hypophysiotrophic area of the rat brain. In conscious, ovariectomized female rats, intraventricular injection of bradykinin significantly suppressed plasma prolactin at 15 and 30 min post-injection, with levels returning to control by 60 min (Steele et al. 1980). Pretreatment of the rats with bradykinin-potentiating factor (BPF) prolonged the prolactin suppression for up to 2 h. Levels of other hormones (i.e. LH, FSH, TSH and GH) were not significantly altered; however, bradykinin plus BPF resulted in a lowering of FSH concentration at 75 min post-BPF while BPF alone appeared to increase GH levels at 45 min. Although there was no effect on most hormones, incubation of pituitaries with bradykinin caused suppression of GH and FSH release by the lowest dose only of bradykinin tested (0.083 ng per ml). The results suggest that bradykinin may have an inhibitory role in the control of prolactin secretion. The effects appear to be specific since they are augmented by preventing the degradation of the peptide by BPF. Since there was no effect on in vitro secretion of prolactin or after intravenous injection of bradykinin, the suppressive effect on prolactin release appears to be mediated via the hypothalamus.

ANGIOTENSIN II

Considerable evidence indicates that there is a central angiotensin II system with angiotensin II-producing neurons localized around the rostral hypothalamus (Phillips et al. 1979) and some angiotensin found in the region of the median eminence (Elde and Hökfelt 1979). We have also evaluated this peptide and found that it can inhibit prolactin release by a direct action on the brain and may also inhibit growth hormone release (Steele et al. submitted). It has previously been shown to stimulate ACTH release. High doses of angiotensin II have stimulated release of prolactin, GH, TSH and LH by pituitaries incubated in vitro (Steele et al. submitted).

BOMBESIN

Although bombesin has not been conclusively demonstrated in the brain, it is clear that acid extracts of brain contain substances that cross react in radioimmunoassays for this amphibian peptide (Walsh et al. 1979). The highest concentration of bombesin-like activity in the brain is in the hypothalamus.

Brown and Vale have tested the effects of bombesin and related peptides on pituitary hormone release (Brown et al. 1978). They reported elevated prolactin and growth hormone release from intravenous administration of ng doses of bombesin. The activity was less after intracisternal injection. The growth hormone-releasing but not the prolactin-releasing action was antagonized by somatostatin and by naloxone. Since there was no action on pituitaries in vitro, the action may be mediated centrally.

Recently it has been shown that bombesin-like activity is released by elevated potassium in a calcium-dependent manner from rat hypothalamic slices (Moody et al. 1980). These findings suggest that this peptide also may be released by nerve impulses and could serve as a synaptic transmitter or neuromodulator.

EFFECT OF SOMATOSTATIN ON RELEASE OF HYPOPHYSIOTROPIC HORMONES

A number of years ago Martini and co-workers postulated ultrashort loop feedback of releasing hormones to alter their own release (Piva et al. 1979). We injected somatostatin intraventricularly to determine its effect on plasma growth hormone levels (Lumpkin et al. 1981). There was a paradoxical elevation of growth hormone evoked by 1 or 5 μg doses of the peptide into the third ventricle in conscious, ovariectomized rats (Fig. 1.3). The effect was greater but more short lived with the 1 μg dose. The elevation of growth hormone could be blocked by intravenous injection of somatostatin. Consequently, intraventricular soma-tostatin appears to exert a hypothalamic action either to suppress somatostatin release and thereby relieve the pituitary of inhibitory somatostatinergic control or to stimulate the

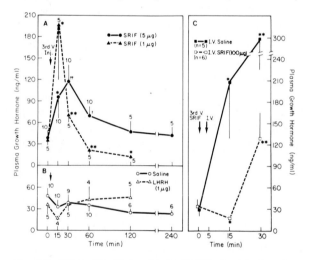

Fig. 1.3. Effect of the third ventricular (3rd V) microinjection of somatostatin (SRIF), LH-RH, or saline on the plasma levels of GH in OVX rats. (A) Effect of 1- and 5-μg doses of SRIF on plasma GH after 3rd V injection. (B) Effect of saline or LH-RH (1 μg) on plasma GH after 3rd V injection. Points represent the means of hormone values and vertical bars represent the standard errors. Serial blood samples were taken at zero (0) time, immediately before intraventricular administration, and at 15, 30, 60, 120, and in some instances, at 240 min after microinjection. The sample size for each point is indicated above or below the vertical standard error bar. Levels of significance were determined by the paired-sample t test, comparing hormone values before and after a particular treatment and are denoted as *P< .05, **P< .025, †P< .01, and ††P< .0025. (C) In this experiment, 1 μg of SRIF was microinjected into 3rd V of 2 groups of OVX rats. In one group (broken line), a bolus of 100 μg of SRIF was injected intravenously (i.v.) 5 min after 3rd V injection. In the other group (solid line), a corresponding volume of saline was injected i.v. 5 min after 3rd V injection. Blood samples were taken at zero (0) time and at 15 and 30 min after 3rd V injection to determine plasma GH levels. Levels of significance were determined and are denoted as above. (Taken from M.D. Lumpkin et al. Science 211, 1072-1074, 1981).

release of growth hormone-releasing factor, or both actions may have been manifest. We favor the latter possibility. At the same time somatostatin lowered gonadotropin and TSH levels, suggesting that it also inhibited the release of LH-RH and TRH. The effect of somatostatin intraventricularly on TSH release is probably via a direct inhibition of TRH release since somatostatin has been found to inhibit release of TRH from organ cultures of rat hypothalamus (Hirooka et al. 1978).

ARGININE VASOTOCIN

Although arginine vasotocin (AVT) has been claimed to be localized to the pineal gland using bioassay (Pavel et al. 1973–74), recent evidence using specific antisera appears to indicate that the substance is not found in rats after all (Negro-Vilar et al. 1979). A variety of studies have been carried out to determine the effects of this peptide on pituitary hormone secretion. Arginine vasotocin appears to inhibit gonadal and uterine growth both in PMS-treated mice and in rats when administered systemically (Johnson et al. 1978). AVT can also inhibit compensatory ovarian hypertrophy (Berkowitz et al. 1979). Intravenous or intraventricular injection also eliminated the preovulatory LH and prolactin surge in the experiments of Cheesman et al. (1977a). On the other hand, arginine vasotocin failed to inhibit the rise in LH induced by PGE_2 or by electrochemical stimulation to the medial preoptic area of proestrous female rats (Osland et al. 1977). Thus, AVT appears to inhibit LH release at a higher level than the prostaglandin-induced release of LH-RH. Similarly, AVT will block the anticipated surge of gonadotropins in ovariectomized estrogen-primed animals (Blask et al. 1978). Vaughan and colleagues (1979a) report that AVT inhibits binding of [^{3}H]estradiol to estrogen receptors in the cystosol fraction of uteri. It is possible that its action in the brain may be mediated similarly. Surprisingly, several injections of AVT through the afternoon of the expected FSH surge on proestrus failed to inhibit the FSH rise (Cheesman et al. 1977b). Since the LH rise is blocked this would fit with the idea of a separate FSH–RF (Blask et al. 1978). Because these effects could not be evoked by similar doses of vasopressin or oxytocin, they appear to be specific for AVT.

In contrast to its inhibitory hypothalamic action, incubation of AVT with pituitaries in vitro stimulates LH secretion from male rat pituitaries and potentiates LH-RH-induced LH secretion in ovariectomized estrogen-primed rats (Vaughan et al. 1975). Similar effects of AVT were found in in vivo studies of urethane-anesthetized males (Vaughan et al. 1979b). Vasopressin but not oxytocin induced similar effects. Others have found neither stimulation nor inhibition of the LH-RH-induced surge of LH by vasotocin (Cheesman et al. 1977).

AVT can release prolactin from pituitaries incubated in vitro, from prolactin-producing pituitary clonal strains and from bovine pituitary cell cultures (Vaughan 1981). Propranolol has been found to inhibit the AVT-induced prolactin release but haloperidol had no effect, suggesting participation of beta-adrenergic receptors in the releasing mechanism (Blask et al. 1977). In vivo, AVT also stimulates prolactin release in a dose-related manner in several types of test rat (Vaughan et al. 1976). The action is not mediated via the pineal, but arginine vasopressin also has this effect whereas oxytocin is inactive (Vaughan et al. 1978a).

Castration blocks the stimulatory action of AVT on prolactin release, which can be restored by administration of estrogen, progesterone, testosterone and androsterone, but not by dihydrotestosterone or androstenedione (Vaughan et al. 1978b). Since aromatizable and non-aromatizable steroids were effective, the ability to restore the prolactin-releasing effect of AVT was not dependent on aromatization.

It is clear that arginine vasotocin has effects on pituitary hormone secretion, but the physiological significance of these actions is open to question, in view of the possibility that AVT is not present in mammals.

INHIBIN

Inhibin is a peptidic substance, apparently secreted by the Sertoli cells in the male and by the follicular cells in the female, which has been demonstrated to have a selective inhibitory effect on the release of FSH both in vivo and in vitro (Franchimont et al. 1979). A direct inhibition of FSH and to a lesser extent LH occurs upon incubation of pituitaries in vitro with inhibin. We have recently evaluated the possible actions of inhibin on the hypothalamus to inhibit FSH release. Intraventricular injection of a purified inhibin preparation supplied by Franchimont selectively inhibited FSH release in ovariectomized rats (Lumpkin et al. 1981). That the action was exerted on the brain and not the pituitary was verified by the fact that there was no suppression of the LH-RH-induced release of FSH or LH in these animals. Thus, these data support the concept that inhibin may act both at the hypothalamic and pituitary level to suppress FSH release. The selective inhibition of FSH release following intraventricular inhibin is explained most readily by postulating that inhibin suppresses release of an FSH–RF.

CALCITONIN

Recently, calcitonin-like immunoreactive molecules and calcitonin receptors have been localized in the brain (Galan Galan et al. 1981; Rizzo and Goltzman 1981). It is therefore understandable that calcitonin injected into the lateral ventricle has been shown to induce a significant and dose-related increase of plasma prolactin in urethane-anesthesized male rats (Iwasaki et al. 1979). The effect was not blocked by naloxone. Salmon, porcine and human calcitonin were similarly effective. Intravenous injection of the peptide had no effect but there was a small stimulation of prolactin release from anterior pituitary cells cultured in vitro. These results suggest that calcitonin may also be involved in pituitary hormone release.

CONCLUSIONS

In general most of the above peptides appear to act at a hypothalamic site to alter pituitary hormone release. They appear to be synthesized and released from neurons within the hypothalamus and in many cases can be shown to be released from hypothalamic slices or synaptosomal preparations. Their release is usually stimulated by depolarizing concentra-

Table 1.1

BRAIN PEPTIDES AND PITUITARY HORMONE RELEASE. CNS ACTION

Peptide	Dosage	ACTH	Prolactin	GH	TSH	FSH	LH
CCK	ng	+	+	+	−	0	−
Gastrin	µg	nt[A]	−	+	−	0	−
VIP	ng	nt	+	+	0	0	+
SP	µg	nt	?+	+	0	0	+
NT	µg	nt	−	+	0	0	−
Opioids	µg	+	+	+	−	−	−
Bradykinin	µg	nt	−	0	0	−	0
Angiotensin II	µg	+	−	−	0	−	0
Bombesin	ng	nt	+	+	nt	nt	nt
Somatostatin	µg	nt	0	+	−	−	−
Vasotocin	µg	nt	−	nt	nt	−	0
Inhibin	µg	nt	nt	nt	nt	−	0

[A] nt = not tested. Abbreviations: CCK = cholecystokinin; VIP = vasoactive intestinal peptide; SP = substance P; NT = neurotensin.

Table 1.2

BRAIN PEPTIDES AND PITUITARY HORMONE RELEASE. PITUITARY ACTION

Peptide	Dosage	ACTH	Prolactin	GH	TSH	FSH	LH
CCK	µg	nt[A]	0	0	0	0	0
Gastrin	µg	nt	0	0	−	0	0
VIP	µg	nt	+	0	0	0	0
SP	ng	nt	+	0	0	0	0
NT	ng	nt	+	0	+	0	0
Opioids	µg	nt	0	0	0	0	0
Bradykinin	µg	nt	0	?−	0	?−	0
Angiotensin II	µg	nt	+[B]	+[B]	+[B]	0	+[B]
Bombesin	ng	nt	0	0	nt	nt	nt
Vasotocin	µg	nt	+	nt	nt	+	+
Inhibin	µg	nt	nt	nt	nt	−	0[C]

[A] Not tested.   [B] Only high doses effective (2–25 µg ml⁻¹).   [C] Higher doses also suppress LH.

tions of potassium and appears to be calcium dependent. In some cases the peptides may act directly on the releasing factor neuron by interaction with specific receptors on the neuronal surface; in other cases, as for example the opioid peptides, they may act via interneurons which in turn alter the discharge of releasing factor neurons by small molecular weight transmitters, such as dopamine, norepinephrine or serotonin.

The actions on the hypothalamus of the peptides so far evaluated are summarized in Table 1.1. Two peptides, CCK and VIP, are extremely potent and are active at ng doses following their intraventricular injection. The remainder require µg doses to induce their effects. A pattern of responses is beginning to emerge. Only two of the peptides stimulate

LH-RH discharge, namely VIP and substance P. The others usually inhibit it, but angiotensin and bradykinin failed to alter it. Effects on FSH secretion were seldom seen. Growth hormone release was stimulated by most peptides tested; bradykinin was an exception and inhibited it. Angiotensin may also inhibit growth hormone release.

Some of the peptides alter pituitary hormone release in vitro and thus become candidates as the remaining uncharacterized releasing and inhibiting hormones (Table 1.2). The stimulatory action of VIP on prolactin release is established and since it has been found in portal blood and in the anterior lobe itself, it could be a significant prolactin releasing factor. Neurotensin and substance P similarly stimulated prolactin release and neurotensin inhibited TSH release.

Although the physiological significance of many of the peptides in pituitary hormone secretion is yet to be established, their action at low doses and their presence in the hypothalamus and other areas of the brain known to be concerned with pituitary function suggest that they may be of considerable importance. The ability of naloxone to elevate gonadotropin release suggests that the opioid peptides may have an important inhibitory influence on LH-RH release. The ability of the angiotensin II antagonist, saralasin, to elevate prolactin supports the concept of a tonic inhibitory action of angiotensin on prolactin release. Further studies in the next few years should clarify the physiological significance of these many peptides in pituitary hormone secretion.

ACKNOWLEDGEMENTS

Supported by NIH grants HD-09988 and AM-10073.

REFERENCES

Barraclough, C.A. and Sawyer, C.H. (1955) Inhibition of the release of pituitary ovulatory hormone in the rat by morphine. Endocrinology 57, 329-337.

Berkowitz, A., Jackson, F.L., Philo, R.C. Lloyd, J.A. and Preslock, J.P. (1979) The effects of melatonin and arginine vasotocin on compensatory ovarian hypertrophy in two strains of *Mus musculus*. Proc. Soc. Exp. Biol. Med. 1, 40.

Blask, D.E., Vaughan, M.K. and Reiter, R.J. (1977) Modification by adrenergic blocking agents of arginine vasotocin-induced prolactin secretion in vitro. Neuroscience Lett. 6, 91-93.

Blask, D.E., Vaughan, M.K., Reiter, R.J. and Johnson, L.Y. (1978) Influence of arginine vasotocin on the estrogen-induced surge of LH and FSH in adult ovariectomized rats. Life Sci. 23, 1035-1040.

Böler, J., Enzmann, F., Folkers, K., Bowers, C.Y. and Schally, A.V. (1969) The identity of chemical and hormonal properties of thyrotropin releasing hormone and pyroglutamyl-histidyl-prolineamide. Biochem. Biophys. Res. Commun. 37, 705-710.

Brazeau, P., Vale, W., Burgus, R., Ling, N., Butcher, M., Rivier, J. and Guillemin, R. (1973) Hypothalamic polypeptide that inhibits the secretion of immunoreactive pituitary growth hormone. Science 179, 77-79.

Brown, M., Rivier, J., Kobiashi, J. and Vale, W. (1978) Neurotensin like and bombesin like peptides: CNS distribution and actions. In: Colon and Gut Hormones (Bloom, S.R. ed.), pp. 550-558, Churchill Livingston, Edinburgh.

Bruni, J.F., Van Vugt, D., Marshall, S. and Meites, J. (1977) Effects of naloxone, morphine and methionine enkephalin on serum prolactin, luteinizing hormone, follicle stimulating hormone, thyroid stimulating hormone and growth hormone. Life Sci. 21, 461-466.

Burgus, R., Dunn, T.F., Desiderio, D. and Guillemin, R. (1969) Structure moleculaire du facteur hypothalamique hypophysiotropique TRF d'origine ovine: mise en évidence par spectrométrie de masse de la séquence PCA-His-Pro-NH₂. C. R. Hebd. Séance. Acad. Sci. (Paris) 269, 1870-1873.

Carraway, R. and Leeman, S.E. (1973) The isolation of a new hypotensive peptide, neurotensin, from bovine hypothalami. J. Biol. Chem. 248, 6854-6861.

Casanueva, F., Betti, R., Frigerio, C., Cocchi, D., Mantegazza, P. and Müller, E.E. (1980) Growth hormone-releasing effect of an enkephalin analog in the dog: evidence for cholinergic mediation. Endocrinology 106, 1239-1245.

Casanueva, F., Betti, R., Cocchi, D., Chieli, T., Mantegazza, P. and Müller, E.E. (1981) Proof for histaminergic but not for adrenergic involvement in the growth hormone-releasing effect of an enkephalin analog in the dog. Endocrinology 108, 157-163.

Chang, M.C. and Leeman, S.E. (1970) Isolation of a sialogogic peptide from bovine hypothalamic tissue and its characterization as substance P. J. Biol. Chem. 245, 4784-4790.

Cheesman, D.W., Osland, R.B. and Forsham, P.H. (1977a) Suppression of the preovulatory surge of luteinizing hormone and subsequent ovulation in the rat by arginine vasotocin. Endocrinology 101, 1194-1202.

Cheesman, D.W., Osland, R.B. and Forsham, P.H. (1977b) Effects of 8-arginine vasotocin on plasma prolactin and follicle-stimulating hormone surges in the proestrus rat. Proc. Soc. Biol. Med. 156, 369-372.

Chihara, K., Arimura, A., Coy, D.H. and Schally, A.V. (1978) Studies on the interaction of endorphins, substance P, and endogenous somatostatin in growth hormone and prolactin release in rats. Endocrinology 102, 281-290.

Cicero, T.J., Badger, T.M., Wilcox, C.E., Bell, R.D. and Myer, E.R. (1977) Morphine decreases luteinizing hormone by an action on the hypothalamic pituitary axis. J. Pharmacol. Exp. Ther. 203, 548-554.

Cocchi, D., Santagostino, A., Gil-Ad, I., Ferri, S. and Müller, E.E. (1977) Leu- and Met-enkephalin-stimulated growth hormone and prolactin release in the rat: Comparison with the effect of morphine. Life Sci. 20, 2041-2046.

Correa, F.M., Innis, R.B., Uhl, G.R. and Snyder, S. (1979) Bradykinin-like immunoreactive neuronal systems localized systematically in rat brain. Proc. Natl. Acad. Sci. USA 76, 1489-1493.

Cusan, L., DuPont, A., Kledzik, G.S., Labrie, F., Coy, D.H. and Schally, A.V. (1977) Potent prolactin and growth hormone-releasing activity of more analogues of Met-enkephalin. Nature 268, 544-547.

Daughaday, W.H. (1974) The Adenohypophysis. In: Textbook of Endocrinology (Williams, R.H. ed.), pp. 31-79, W.B. Saunders Company, Philadelphia.

DuPont, A., Cusan, L., Labrie, F., Coy, D.H. and Li, C.H. (1977) Stimulation of prolactin release in the rat by intraventricular injection of β-endorphin and methionine-enkephalin. Biochem. Biophys. Res. Commun. 75, 76-82.

Elde, R. and Hökfelt, T. (1979) Localization of hypophysial tropic peptides and other biologically active peptides within the brain. Annu. Rev. Physiol. 41, 587-602.

Emson, P.C., Lee, C.M. and Rehfeld, J.F. (1980) Cholecystokinin octapeptide: vesicular localization and calcium dependent release from rat brain in vitro. Life Sci. 26, 2157-2163.

Enjalbert, A., Ruberg, M., Fiore, L., Arancibia, S., Priam, M. and Kordon, C. (1979) Effect of morphine on dopamine inhibition of pituitary prolactin release in vitro. Eur. J. Pharmacol. 53, 211-212.

Ferland, L., Fuxe, K., Eneroth, T., Gustafsson, J.A. and Skett, P. (1977) Effects of methionine-enkephalin on prolactin release and catecholamine levels and turnover in the median eminence. Eur. J. Pharmacol. 43, 89-90.

Franchimont, P., Verstraelen-Proyard, J., Hazee-Hagelstein, M.T., Renard, Ch., Demoulin, A., Bourguignon, J.P. and Hustin, J. (1979) Inhibin: From Concept to Reality. Vitamins and Hormones 37, 243-302.

Galan Galan, F., Rogers, R.M., Girgis, S.L. and MacIntyre, I. (1981) Immunoreactive calcitonin in the central nervous system of the pigeon. Brain Res. 212, 59-66.

George, R. and Way, E.L. (1959) The role of hypothalamus in pituitary-adrenal activation and antidiuresis by morphine. J. Pharmacol. Exp. Ther. 125, 111-115.

George, R. (1971) In: Narcotics, Biochemical Pharmacology (Kluit, D.H. ed.), pp. 283-299, Plenum Press, New York.

Gibbs, D.M. and Neill, J.D. (1978) Dopamine levels in hypophysial stalk blood in the rat are sufficient to inhibit prolactin secretion in vivo. Endocrinology 102, 1895-1900.

Goldstein, A., Lowney, L.I. and Pal, B.K. (1971) Stereospecific and nonspecific interactions of the morphine congener levorphanol in subcellular fractions of the mouse brain. Proc. Natl. Acad. Sci. USA 68, 1742-1747.

Grandison, L. and Guidotti, A. (1980) Endorphin stimulation of prolactin release: its relationship to median eminence DA neurons. In: Catecholamines: Basic and Clinical Frontiers (Usdin, E., Kopin, I.J. and Barchas, J. eds.), Proc. 4th Intl. Catecholamine Symposium, pp. 1242-1244, Pergamon Press, New York.

Grandison, L., Fratta, W. and Guidotti, A. (1980) Location and characterization of opiate receptors regulating pituitary secretion. Life Sci. 26, 1633-1642.

Gudelsky, G.A. and Porter, J.C. (1979) Morphine and opioid peptide-induced inhibition of the release of dopamine from tuberoinfundibular neurons. Life Sci. 25, 1697-1702.

Hirooka, Y., Holander, C.S., Susuki, S., Ferdinand, P. and Wan, S.I. (1978) Somatostatin inhibits release of thyrotropin releasing factor from organ cultures of rat hypothalamus. Proc. Natl. Acad. Sci. USA 75, 4509-4513.

Hughes, J., Smith, T.W., Kosterlitz, H.W., Fothergill, L.A., Morgan, B.A. and Morris, H.R. (1975) Identification of two related pentapeptides from the brain with potent opiate agonist activity. Nature (London) 258, 577-579.

Ieiri, T., Chen, H.T. and Meites, J. (1979) Effects of morphine and naloxone on serum levels of LH and prolactin in prepubertal male and female rats. Neuroendocrinology 29, 288-292.

Itoh, S., Hirota, R., Katsuruura, G. and Otaguchi, A. (1979) Adrenal cortical stimulation by cholecystokinin preparation in the rat. Life Sci. 25, 1725-1730.

Iwasaki, Y., Chihara, K., Ilisaki, J., Abe, H. and Fugita, T. (1979) Effect of calcitonin on prolactin release in rats. Life Sci. 25, 1243-1248.

Johnson, L.Y., Vaughan, M.K., Reiter, R.J., Blask, D.E. and Rudeen, P.K. (1978) The effects of arginine vasotocin on pregnant mare's serum-induced ovulation in the immature female rat. Acta Endocrinol. (Copenhagen) 87, 367-376.

Kato, Y., Chihara, K., Ohgo, S., Iwasaki, Y., Abe, H. and Imura, H. (1976) Growth hormone and prolactin release by substance P in rats. Life Sci. 19, 441-446.

Kerdelhué, B., Valens, M. and Langlois, Y. (1978) Stimulation de la secretion de la LH et de la FSH hypophysaires après immunoneutralisation de la substance P endogene, chez le ratte cyclique. C. R. Acad. Sci. (Paris) 286, 977-979.

Koenig, J.A., Mayfield, M.A., McCann, S.M. and Krulich, L. (1979) Stimulation of prolactin secretion by morphine: role of the central serotonergic system. Life Sci. 25, 853-864.

Koenig, J., Mayfield, M.A., Coppings, R.J., McCann, S.M. and Krulich, L. (1980) Role of central nervous system neurotransmitters in mediating the effects of morphine on growth hormone- and prolactin-secretion in the rat. Brain Res. 197, 453-468.

Kokka, N. and George, R. (1974) Effects of narcotic analgesics, anesthetics, and hypothalamic lesions on growth hormone and adrenocorticotropic hormone secretion in rats. In: Narcotics and the Hypothalamus (Zimmerman, E. and George, R. eds), pp. 137-159, Raven Press, New York.

Krieger, D.T., Liotta, A.S., Brownstein, M.J. and Zimmerman, E.A. ACTH, β-lipotropin and related peptide in brain, pituitary and blood. Recent Prog. Horm. Res. 36, 277-344.

Krulich, L., Dhariwal, A.P.S. and McCann, S.M. (1968) Stimulatory and inhibitory effects of purified hypothalamic extract on growth hormone release from rat pituitary in vitro. Endocrinology 83, 783-790.

Krulich, L., Hefco, E., Illner, P. and Read, C.B. (1974) Effects of acute stress on the secretion of LH, FSH, prolactin and GH in the male rat. Neuroendocrinology 16, 293-311.

Krulich, L. and Fawcett, C.P. (1977) The hypothalamic hypophysiotropic hormones. In: Endocrine Physiology (McCann, S.M. ed.) Vol. 2, pp. 35-92, University Park Press, Baltimore.

Kumar, M.S.A., Chen, C.L. and Muther, T.F. (1979) Changes in pituitary and hypothalamic content of Met- and Leu-enkephalin during the estrous cycle of rats. Life Sci. 25, 1687-1696.

Lawrence, A.M., Hojvat, S. and Kirsteins, L. (1979) Pituitary hormones of brain origin. In: Abstract Book International Symposium on Neuroactive Drugs in Endocrinology (Müller, E.E. ed.), p. 23, Ricerca Scientifica ed Educazione Permanente.

Li, C.H. and Chung, D. (1976) Isolation and structure of an untriakontapeptide with opiate activity from camel pituitary glands. Proc. Natl. Acad. Sci. USA 73, 1145-1148.

Login, I.S. and MacLeod, R.M. (1979) Failure of opiates to reverse dopamine inhibition of prolactin secretion in vitro. Eur. J. Pharmacol. 60, 253-255.

Lomax, P., Kokka, N. and George, R (1970) Thyroid activity following intracerebral injection of morphine in the rat. Neuroendocrinology 6, 146-152.

20

Lumpkin, M.D., Negro-Vilar, A. and McCann, S.M. (1981) Paradoxical elevation of growth hormone by intraventricular somatostatin: possible ultrashort-loop feedback. Science 211, 1072-1074.

Lumpkin, M., Negro-Vilar, A., Franchimont, P. and McCann, S.M. (1981) Evidence for a hypothalamic site of action of inhibin to suppress FSH release. Endocrinology 108, 1101-1104.

MacLeod, R.M. (1969) Influence of norepinephrine and catecholamine depleting agents on synthesis and release of prolactin and growth hormone. Endocrinology 85, 916-923.

Maeda, K. and Frohman, L.A. (1978) Dissociation of systemic and central effects of neurotensin on secretion of growth hormone, prolactin and TSH. Endocrinology 103, 1903-1909.

Maeda, K. and Frohman, L.A. (1980) Release of somatostatin and thyrotropin-releasing hormone from rat hypothalamic fragments in vitro. Endocrinology 106, 1837-1842.

Matsuo, H., Baba, Y., Nair, R.M.G., Arimura, A. and Schally, A.V. (1971) Structure of porcine LH- and FSH-releasing hormone. I. The proposed amino acid sequence. Biochem. Biophys. Res. Commun. 43, 1334-1339.

McCann, S.M., Fawcett, C.P. and Krulich, L. (1974a) Hypothalamic hypophysial releasing and inhibiting hormones. In: Endocrine Physiology (McCann, S.M. ed.), Vol. 1, pp. 31-66, University Park Press, Baltimore.

McCann, S.M., Ojeda, S.R., Libertun, C., Harms, P.G. and Krulich, L. (1974b) Drug-induced alterations in gonadotropin and prolactin release in the rat. In: Narcotics and the Hypothalamus (Zimmerman, E. and George, R. eds), pp. 121-136, Raven Press, New York.

McCann, S.M., Vijayan, E., Koenig, J. and Krulich, L. (1979) Role of brain peptides in control of pituitary hormone release. In: Brain and Pituitary Peptides (Wuttke, W., Weindl, A., Voight, K.H. and Dries, R.R. eds), pp. 223-233, Karger, Basel.

Meites, J. (1962) In: Pharmacological Control of Release of Hormones Including Diabetic Drugs (Guillemin, R. ed.), pp. 151-180, Pergamon Press, London.

Meites, J., Bruni, J.F., VanVugt, D.A. and Smith, A.F. (1979) Relation of endogenous opioid peptides and morphine to neuroendocrine function. Life Sci. 24, 1325-1336.

Meltzer, H.Y., Miller, R.J., Fessler, R.G., Simonovic, M. and Fang, V.S. (1978) Effects of enkephalin analogs on prolactin release in the rat. Life Sci. 22, 1931-1938.

Moody, T.W., Thoa, N.B., O'Donohue, T.L. and Pert, C.B. (1980) Bombesin-like peptides in rat brain: localization in synaptosomes and release from hypothalamic slices. Life Sci. 26, 1707-1712.

Morley, J.E., Melmed, S., Briggs, J., Carlson, H.E., Hershman, J.M., Soloman, T.E., Lammers, C. and Damasa, D.A. (1979) Cholecystokinin octapeptide releases growth hormone from the pituitary in vitro. Life Sci. 25, 1201-1206.

Munson, P.L. (1973) Effects of morphine and related drugs in the ACTH-stress reaction. Prog. Brain. Res. 39, 361-372.

Muraki, T., Tokunaga, Y. and Makino, T. (1977) Effects of morphine and naloxone on serum LH, FSH and prolactin levels and on hypothalamic content of LH-RF in proestrous rats. Endocrinol. Jpn 24, 313-315.

Negro-Vilar, A., Sanchez-Franco, F., Kwiatkowski, M. and Samson, W.K. (1979) Failure to detect arginine vasotocin in mammalian pineals by radioimmunoassay. Brain Res. Bull. 4, 789-792.

Nemeroff, C.B., Bissette, G., Manberg, P.J., Osbahr, A.J., Breese, G.R. and Prange, A.J. (1980) Neurotensin-induced hypothermia: evidence for interaction with dopaminergic systems and the hypothalamic pituitary thyroid axis. Brain Res. 195, 69-84.

Okajima, T., Motomatso, T., Kato, K. and Ibayashi, H. (1980) Naloxone inhibits prolactin and growth hormone release by intracellular glucopenia in rats. Life Sci. 27, 755-760.

Osland, R.B., Cheesman, D.W. and Forsham, P.H. (1977) Studies on the mechanism of the suppression of the preovulatory surge of luteinizing hormone in the rat by arginine vasotocin. Endocrinology 101, 1203-1209.

Pacold, S.T., Kirsteins, L., Hojvat, S., Lawrence, A.M. and Hagen, T.C. (1978) Biologically active pituitary hormones in the rat brain amygdaloid nucleus. Science 199, 804-805.

Panerai, A.E., Sawynok, J., LaBella, F.S. and Friesen, H.G. (1980) Prolonged hyperprolactinemia influences β-endorphin and Met-enkephalin in the brain. Endocrinology 106, 1804-1808.

Pang, C.N., Zimmerman, E. and Sawyer, C.H. (1977) Morphine inhibition of the preovulatory surges of plasma luteinizing hormone and follicle stimulating hormone in the rat. Endocrinology 101, 1726-1732.

Pass, K.A. and Ondo, J.G. (1977) The effects of γ-aminobutyric acid on prolactin and gonadotropin secretion in the unanesthetized rat. Endocrinology 100, 1437-1442, 1977.

Pavel, S., Dimitru, I., Klepsh, I. and Dorcescu, M. (1973-74) Gonadotropin inhibiting principle in the pineal of human fetuses. Evidence for its identity with arginine vasotocin. Neuroendocrinology 13, 41-46.

Pert, C.B. and Snyder, S.H. (1973) Opiate receptor: demonstration in nervous tissue. Science 179, 1011-1014.

Phillips, M.I., Weyhenmeyer, J., Felix, D., Ganton, D. and Hoffman, W.E. (1979) Evidence for an endogenous brain renin-angiotensin system. Fed. Proc. 38, 2260-2266.

Pimstone, B.L., Sheppard, M., Shapiro, B., Kronheim, S., Hudson, A., Hendricks, S. and Walegora, K. (1979) Localization in and release of somatostatin from brain and gut. Fed. Proc. 38, 2330-2332.

Piva, F., Motta, M. and Martini, L. (1979) Regulation of hypothalamic and pituitary function: long, short, and ultrashort feedback loops. In: Endocrinology (deGroot, J. ed.), Vol. I, pp. 21-33, Grune and Stratton, New York.

Rehfeld, J.F., Goltermann, N., Larsson, L.I., Emson, P.M. and Lee, C.M. (1979) Gastrin and cholecystokinin in central and peripheral neurons. Fed. Proc. 38, 2325-2329.

Rivier, C., Brown, M. and Vale, M. (1977) Effect of neurotensin, substance P and morphine sulfate on secretion of prolactin and growth hormone in the rat. Endocrinology 100, 751-754.

Rizzo, A.J. and Goltzman, D. (1981) Calcitonin receptors in the central nervous system of the rat. Endocrinology 108, 1662-1677.

Rossier, J., French, E., Gros, C., Minick, S., Guillemin, R. and Bloom, F.E. (1979) Adrenalectomy, dexamethasone or stress alters opioid peptide levels in rat anterior pituitary but not intermediate lobe of brain. Life Sci. 25, 2105-2112.

Rotsztejn, W.H., Drouva, S.V., Pattou, E. and Kordon, C. (1978) Effect of morphine on basal and dopamine-induced release of LHRH from medial basal hypothalamic fragments in vitro. Eur. J. Pharmacol. 50, 285-286.

Rotsztejn, W.H., Benoist, L., Besson, J., Beraud, G., Bluet-Pajot, M.T., Kordon, C., Rosselin, G. and Duval, J. (1980) Effect of vasoactive intestinal peptide on release of adenohypophysial hormones from purified cells obtained by unit gravity sedimentation. Neuroendocrinology 31, 282-286.

Ruberg, M., Rotsztejn, W.H., Arancibia, S., Besson, J. and Enjalbert, A. (1978) Stimulation of prolactin release by vasoactive intestinal peptide. Eur. J. Pharmacol. 51, 319-320.

Said, S.I. and Porter, J.C. (1979) Vasoactive intestinal polypeptide: release into hypophyseal portal blood. Life Sci. 24, 227-230.

Samson, W.K., Said, S.I. and McCann, S.M. (1979a) Radioimmunologic localization of vasoactive intestinal polypeptide in extra hypothalamic sites in the rat brain. Neurosci. Lett. 12, 265-296.

Samson, W.K., Said, S.I., Gramm, J.W. and McCann, S.M. (1979b) Localization of vasoactive intestinal peptide in human brain. IRCS Med. Sci. 7, 13.

Samson, W.K., Said, S.I., Snyder, G. and McCann, S.M. (1980) In vitro stimulation of prolactin release by vasoactive intestinal peptide. Peptides 1, 325-332.

Samson, W.K., Burton, K.P., Reeves, J.P. and McCann, S.M. (1981) Vasoactive intestinal peptide stimulates LHRH release from median eminence synaptosomes. Regulatory Peptides 2, 253-264.

Sawynok, J., Pinsky, C. and LaBella, F.S. (1979) Minireview: Specificity of naloxone as an opiate antagonist. Life Sci. 25, 1621-1632.

Shaar, C.J., Fredrickson, R.C.A., Dininger, N.B. and Jackson, L. (1977) Enkephalin analogs and naloxone modulate the release of growth hormone and prolactin-evidence of regulation by endogenous opioid peptides in brain. Life Sci. 21, 853-860.

Shaar, C.J., Clemens, J.A. and Dininger, N.B. (1979) Effect of vasoactive intestinal polypeptide on prolactin release in vitro. Life Sci. 25, 2071-2074.

Share, L. and Grosvenor, C.E. (1974) The Neurohypophysis. In: Endocrine Physiology (McCann, S.M. ed.), Vol. 1, pp. 1-30, University Park Press, Baltimore.

Sheppard, M.C., Kronheims, S. and Pimstone, B.L. (1979) Effect of substance P, neurotensin and enkephalins on somatostatin release from rat hypothalamus in vitro. J. Neurochem. 32, 647-649.

Sims, K.B., Hoffman, D.L., Said, S.I. and Zimmerman, E.A. (1980) Vasoactive intestinal polypeptide (VIP) in mouse and rat brain: an immunohistochemical study. Brain Res. 186, 165-183.

Smith, C.B., Villareal, J.E., Bednarczk, J.H. and Sheldon, M.I. (1970) Tolerance to morphine-induced increases in [^{14}C]catecholamine synthesis in mouse brain. Science 170, 1106-1108.

Smith, G.P. (1980) Satiety effect of gastrointestinal hormones. In: Polypeptide Hormones (Beers, R.F. and Bassett, E.G. eds), pp. 413-420, Raven Press, New York.

Spampinato, S., Locatelli, V., Cocchi, D., Vicentini, S., Bajusz, S., Ferri, S. and Müller, E.E. (1979) Involvement of brain serotonin in prolactin-releasing effect of opioid peptides. Endocrinology 105, 163-170.

Steele, M.K., Negro-Vilar, A. and McCann, S.M. (1980) Effect of central injection of bradykinin and bradyki-nin-potentiating factor upon release of anterior pituitary hormones in ovariectomized female rats. Peptides 1, 201-205.

Steele, M., Negro-Vilar, A. and McCann, S.M. (1981) Effect of angiotensin II on in vivo and in vitro release of anterior pituitary hormones in the female rat. Endocrinology 109, 893-899.

Steger, R.W., Sonntag, W.E., VanVoogt, D.A., Foreman, L.J. and Meites, J. (1980) Reduced ability of naloxone to stimulate LH and testosterone release in aging male rats: possible relation to increase in hypothalamic Met-enkephalin. Life Sci. 27, 747-753.

Straus, E. and Yalow, R.S. (1979) Gastrointestinal peptides in the brain. Fed. Proc. 38, 2320.

Sylvester, P.W., Chen, H.T. and Meites, J. (1980) Effects of morphine and naloxone on phasic release of LH and FSH. Proc. Soc. Exp. Biol. Med. 164, 207-211.

Toubeau, G., Desclin, G., Parmentier, M. and Pasteels, J.L. (1979) Cellular localization of a prolactin like antigen in the rat brain. J. Endocrinol. 83, 261-266.

Van Ree, J.M., Spaapen-Kok, W.B. and De Wied, D. (1976) Differential localization of pituitary adrenal activation and temperature changes following intrahypothalamic microinjection of morphine in rats. Neuroendocrinology 22, 318-324.

Van Vugt, D.A., Bruni, J.F. and Meites, J. (1978) Naloxone inhibition of stress-induced increase in prolactin secretion. Life Sci. 21, 85-90.

Vaughan, M.K. (1981) The pineal gland – A survey of its antigonadotrophic substances and their actions. In: Endocrine Physiology III (McCann, S.M. ed.), Vol. 24, pp. 41-95, University Park Press, Baltimore.

Vaughan, M.K., Blask, D.E., Johnson, L.Y. and Reiter, R.J. (1975) Prolactin-releasing activity of arginine vasotocin in vitro. Hormone Res. 6, 342-350.

Vaughan, M.K., Blask, D.E., Vaughan, D.M. and Reiter, R.J. (1976) Dose-dependent prolactin releasing activity of arginine vasotocin in intact and pinealectomized estrogen-progesterone treated adult male rats. Endocrinology 99, 1319-1322.

Vaughan, M.K., Little, J.C., Johnson, L.Y., Blask, D.E., Vaughan, D.M. and Reiter, R.J. (1978a) Effects of melatonin and natural and synthetic analogues or arginine vasotocin on plasma prolactin levels in adult male rats. Hormone Res. 9, 236-246.

Vaughan, M.K., Blask, D.E., Johnson, L.Y., Trakulrungsi, C. and Reiter, R.J. (1978b) Effect of several androgens, cyproterone acetate or estrogen-progesterone on the prolactin-releasing activity of arginine vasoto-cin in castrated male rats. Mol. Cell. Endocrinol. 12, 309-318.

Vaughan, M.K., Buchanan, J., Blask, D.E. and Reiter, R.J. (1979a) Diurnal variation in uterine estrogen receptors in immature female rats – inhibition by arginine vasotocin. Endocrinol. Res. Commun. 6, 191-201.

Vaughan, M.K., Blask, D.E., Johnson, L.Y. and Reiter, R.J. (1979b) The effect of subcutaneous injections of melatonin, arginine vasotocin, and related peptides on pituitary and plasma levels of luteinizing hormone, follicle-stimulating hormone, and prolactin in castrated adult male rats. Endocrinology 104, 212-217.

Vijayan, E., Samson, W.K. and McCann, S.M. (1978) Effects of intraventricular injection of gastrin on release of LH, prolactin, TSH and GH in conscious ovariectomized rats. Life Sci. 23, 2225-2232.

Vijayan, E., Samson, W.K. and McCann, S.M. (1979a) In vivo and in vitro effects of cholecystokinin on gonadotropin, prolactin, growth hormone and thyrotropin release in the rat. Brain Res. 172, 295-302.

Vijayan, E., Samson, W.K., Said, S.I. and McCann, S.M. (1979b) Vasoactive intestinal peptide (VIP): evidence for a hypothalamic site of action to release growth hormone, luteinizing hormone, and prolactin in conscious ovariectomized rats. Endocrinology 104, 53-57.

Vijayan, E. and McCann, S.M. (1979) In vivo and in vitro effect of substance P and neurotensin on gonadotropin and prolactin release. Endocrinology 105, 64-68.

Vijayan, E. and McCann, S.M. (1980) Effects of substance P and neurotensin on growth hormone and TSH release in vivo and in vitro. Life Sci. 26, 321-327.

Walsh, J.H., Wong, H.C. and Dockray, G.J. (1979) Bombesin-like peptides in mammals. Fed. Proc. 38, 2315-2319.

Yarbrough, G.G., Buxbaum, D.M. and Sanders-Bush, E. (1971) Increased serotonin turnover in the acutely morphine-treated rat. Life Sci. 10, 977-983.

E.E. Müller and R.M. MacLeod (eds) Neuroendocrine Perspectives Vol. 1

Chapter 2

The median eminence: aminergic control mechanisms

K.E. Moore and C.A. Johnston

INTRODUCTION

The median eminence (ME) is the most ventral region of the medial hypothalamus; in most mammalian species it forms the floor of the third ventricle and its caudal end is contiguous with the pituitary stalk. It contains a dense network of many different types of neuronal terminals intermingled with glial cells (tanycytes). The ventral surface of the ME is invaginated by capillary loops which make up the proximal portion (primary plexus) of the hypothalamic-hypophyseal portal system. Neurohormones which are released from neuro-secretory neurons terminating in the ME are transported in the blood of this portal system to the anterior pituitary. In this way the central nervous system exerts regulatory control over the release of hormones from the anterior pituitary. Several excellent reviews on the anatomy and physiology of the median eminence have been prepared (Knigge et al. 1972; Müller et al. 1977; Schiebler et al. 1978).

The ME is a storehouse of putative neurotransmitter substances and of hormones which regulate anterior pituitary hormonal release (Palkovits 1980). This review will consider only aminergic neurotransmitters in the ME of the rat. It will focus on those neurons containing catecholamines (epinephrine (E), norepinephrine (NE) and dopamine (DA)) and 5-hydroxytryptamine (5HT, serotonin), and will not consider other putative aminergic neurotransmitters such as histamine, acetylcholine, or γ-aminobutyric acid. Emphasis will be on the ME per se, but some consideration will also be given to those medial hypothala-mic regions (e.g., arcuate and periventricular nuclei) which contain cell bodies of DA and possibly 5HT neurons which terminate in the ME.

There are numerous reviews and monographs dealing with the influence of hypothalamic catecholamines and 5HT on the release of hormones from the anterior and posterior pituitaries (e.g., Wilson 1974; Knowles and Vollrath 1974; McCann and Ojeda 1976; Müller et al. 1977; Weiner and Ganong 1978; Sawyer 1979). Some of these actions will be discussed briefly, but the major focus will be on the mechanisms by which those aminergic neurons terminating in the ME are regulated. Since these appear to be concerned primarily with endocrine regulatory processes it seems reasonable that their activities, in turn, are

24

influenced by alterations in endocrine status. The primary emphasis, therefore, will be on the aminergic neuronal responses to endocrine changes which accompany various physiological states or which result from environmental or pharmacological manipulations.

DISTRIBUTION

Anatomical

The development of histofluorescent methods (Falck et al. 1962; Lindvall and Björklund 1974) for visualizing catecholamines and 5HT in tissues has made it possible to map the projections of neurons containing these amines throughout the central nervous system. These techniques have been complemented by the development of immunocytochemical procedures for visualizing neurons containing specific enzymes (e.g. tyrosine hydroxylase for catecholamine neurons; Pickel et al. 1975, 1976). Among these neurons it has been possible to identify those containing NE (and E) by staining for dopamine β-hydroxylase

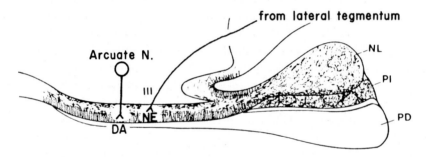

Fig. 2.1. Schematic distribution of catecholaminergic neurons in the median eminence–pituitary region. Abbreviations: NL, neural lobe; PI, intermediate lobe (pars intermedia); PD, anterior lobe (pars distalis); III, third ventricle. Modified from Björklund et al. 1973a.

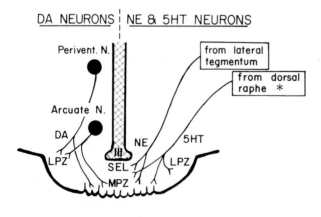

Fig. 2.2. Schematic diagram of frontal section of a central region of the mediobasal hypothalamus depicting innervation by dopaminergic (DA), noradrenergic (NE) and 5-hydroxytryptaminergic (5HT) neurons. Abbreviations: III, third ventricle; LPZ, lateral palisade zone; MPZ, medial palisade zone; SEL, subependymal layer. (Modified from Löfström et al. 1976a); *, There are reports of 5HT-containing cell bodies in the hypothalamus (Smith and Kappers, 1975; Kent and Sladek, 1978; Beaudet and Descarries, 1979).

(DBH; Swanson and Hartman 1975) and those containing E by staining for phenylethano-lamine-*N*-methyltransferase (PNMT; Hökfelt et al. 1974).

Catecholaminergic innervation

Since the initial observations by Carlsson et al. (1962) and Fuxe (1963) it has been known that the ME is richly innervated by catecholamine-containing neurons (see Fig. 2.1). For descriptive purposes the ME has been divided into several different regions. From the third ventricle in a ventral direction the regions are the: ependyma, subependymal layer, internal zone, external zone. The latter region has been divided into the reticular zone and the most ventral palisade zone (Schiebler et al. 1978). In the present discussion reference will be made only to the subependymal layer (SEL), the region lying between the surface of the third ventricle and the dorsal projections of the capillary loops, and the external layer. The external layer is divided (see Fig. 2.2 and Löfström et al. 1976a) into the medial palisade zone (MPZ), which is the region containing capillary loops on either side of the midline, and the lateral palisade zone (LPZ), which is the region on either side of the MPZ. Fluorescent catecholamine-containing axons and varicosities (axonal dilations) are observed throughout the ME with the most dense concentration in the external layer. It has been estimated that from 10 to 30% of the terminals in the latter region are monoaminergic (Ajika and Hökfelt 1973).

Studies employing selective lesioning and pharmacological manipulations, in combination with microspectrofluorometry and immunocytochemistry have demonstrated that DA neurons make up a rich system of delicate varicose fibers which distribute to the MPZ and LPZ, and possibly to the SEL as well. NE neurons appear as coarse varicose fibers in the SEL with some distribution to the MPZ. Details of the catecholaminergic innervation of the ME can be found in a number of research and review publications; these include descriptions of studies employing histofluorescent (Smith and Simpson 1970; Björklund et al. 1970, 1973a; Löfström et al. 1976a; Lindvall and Björklund 1978; Moore and Bloom 1978, 1979) and electron microscopic techniques (Ajika and Hökfelt 1973; Daikoku et al. 1978).

Lesions which separate the mediobasal hypothalamus (including the ME) from the rest of the brain cause the loss of coarse varicose fibers and of NE from the SEL. This indicates that the perikarya of NE neurons terminating in this region lie outside the medial basal hypothalamus. On the other hand, fine fibers distributing to the external layer (and the DA concentrations) remain intact (Jonsson et al. 1972; Björklund et al. 1973b), indicating that cell bodies of DA neurons terminating in the ME are within the medial basal hypothalamus. Complete hypothalamic deafferentations cause the 5HT concentration within the island to fall to only 30–40% of control, suggesting the presence of structures within this region capable of synthesizing or storing 5HT (Vermes et al. 1973a).

Noradrenergic innervation. The anatomical distribution of NE and E neuronal systems in the rat brain have been recently reviewed (Lindvall and Björklund 1978; Moore and Bloom 1979). Virtually all NE cell bodies are located in the medullary and pontine reticular formation. Neuronal systems originating from these cells have been divided into two major subdivisions based on the origin of the cells, those in the locus coeruleus (A_4 and A_6

according to the designation of Dahlström and Fuxe, 1964) and those located in the lateral tegmental regions (A_1, A_2, A_5, A_7) ranging from the caudal medulla to the caudal mesencephalon. Most hypothalamic nuclei, and the ME, appear to be innervated by the lateral tegmental system (Olson and Fuxe 1972; Jones and Moore 1977) although the periventricular nucleus may receive as much as 40% of its NE innervation from cells in the locus coeruleus. Axons from NE cell bodies in the lateral tegmental region ascend in the medial forebrain bundle to the level of the hypothalamus and then turn medially along the ventral surface of the brain to terminate in the SEL and MPZ; these neurons have been referred to as the reticuloinfundibular NE system. It is not known whether NE neurons in the lateral tegmental system project specifically to the ME, or whether the terminals are collaterals of neurons passing through the hypothalamus on the way to forebrain regions. With the extensive collateralization of NE neurons throughout the brain it is conceptually difficult to relate to them a specific endocrine function, but some cell bodies of NE neurons do specifically bind estradiol so they might be targets for the actions of this hormone (Sar and Stumpf 1981). NE neurons may serve a coordinating function in the hypothalamus.

It has been possible to confirm and extend observations made by the Falck-Hillarp histofluorescent procedure by developing antibodies to catecholamine synthesizing enzymes and employing them in immunohistofluorescent techniques. In general, the distribution of NE- and DBH-containing neurons parallel one another. Axons containing DBH have been identified in the SEL and in the MPZ lying close to the pericapillary spaces (Fuxe et al. 1973a).

Adrenergic innervation. Using an immunohistochemical technique, Hökfelt et al. (1974) identified two groups of PNMT-containing cell bodies in the medulla. One group, designated C_1, was located in the ventrolateral reticular formation (corresponding to region A_1) and the other, C_2, was located near the medial part of the ventral surface of the fourth ventricle (corresponding to area A_2). PNMT-positive terminals have been identified in various hypothalamic nuclei including the ventrolateral region of the arcuate nucleus and in the SEL (Fuxe et al. 1976). Biochemical measurements have also revealed PNMT activity in the ME. Thus, current evidence suggests that E-containing neurons project directly to the ME and also onto other neurons (e.g. in arcuate nucleus) that, in turn, project to the ME.

Dopaminergic innervation. The anatomical distribution of DA neurons within the rat brain has been reviewed by Moore and Bloom (1978) and by Lindvall and Björklund (1978). DA neurons which terminate in the ME belong to the tuberoinfundibular neuronal system. Cell bodies of these neurons are located in the arcuate nucleus and in the regions of the anterior periventricular nucleus lying just dorsal to the former nucleus (A_{12}, according to Dahlström and Fuxe 1964). The perikarya of these hypothalamic DA neurons are not as densely packed as those catecholamine-containing neurons in the locus coeruleus (NE neurons) or substantia nigra (DA neurons).

There is one report (Kizer et al. 1976b) that some DA neurons which terminate in the ME originate in the ventral tegmental region. Most results, however, obtained using both histofluorescent (Jonsson et al. 1972; Löfström et al. 1976a) and biochemical techniques Weiner et al. 1972; Björklund et al. 1973b; Brownstein et al. 1976a; Gudelsky et al. 1978; Gallardo et al. 1978) reveal no loss of DA concentrations in the ME following complete hypothalamic deafferentation with a Halasz knife. Thus, DA terminals in the ME appear to originate from perikarya that are within the medial basal hypothalamus (i.e. arcuate and periventricular nuclei).

The tuberoinfundibular DA neurons have short axons which project ventrally to terminate in all regions of the ME, but they are more abundant in the external layer where they are densely packed in a palisade-like manner close to the capillaries of the hypothalamic-hypophyseal portal system. DA released from these neurons is transported via the hypophyseal portal system to activate receptors on lactotrophs (prolactin-secreting cells) in the anterior pituitary. This activation results in the inhibition of prolactin release. In addition, some DA neurons, particularly in the LPZ (Hökfelt et al. 1976) appear to terminate in close proximity to luteinizing hormone releasing hormone (LH-RH)-containing nerve terminals. Sladek et al. (1978), employing formaldehyde or glyoxylic acid histofluorescent techniques in conjunction with immunocytochemical techniques, have identified DA terminals making contact with gonadotropin releasing hormone (GnRH)-containing terminals in the LPZ. These same investigators have also observed terminals of DA neurons in juxtaposition with tanycytes (Sladek and Sladek 1978). Thus, DA released from terminals of tuberoinfundibular neurons may act as a releasing hormone (i.e. prolactin-inhibitory factor), alter the release of other releasing hormones (e.g. LH-RH, GnRH) and/or influence glial (tanycyte) functions.

5-Hydroxytryptaminergic innervation

The distribution of 5HT neurons in the brain has been thoroughly reviewed by Azmitia (1978). Dahlström and Fuxe (1964) originally described nine major groups of 5HT-containing cells in the rat brainstem, which were designated B_1–B_9. Perikarya in at least four of these nuclear groups project to the forebrain. Most evidence suggests that projections to the medial hypothalamus, including the arcuate and periventricular nuclei and the ME, originate from perikarya in the dorsal raphe nucleus (B_7). It is, however, difficult to identify 5HT neurons in the ME using the Falck-Hillarp procedure because the formaldehyde-induced fluorescence of 5HT is relatively low and evanescent when compared to that of DA and NE. Using an antiserum to 5HT Hökfelt et al. (1979) noted a moderately dense network of 5HT-immunoreactive fibers in the LPZ.

Taking advantage of the specific 5HT uptake system (Shaskan and Snyder 1970), Calas et al. (1974) were able to identify ^{3}H-labelled, 5HT-containing neurons in the ME, although the silver grains were found in less than 1% of axons in this region. These were small unmyelinated fibers distributed throughout the ME, becoming more abundant in the external layer. Belenky et al. (1979) employed radioautographic techniques following ^{3}H-labelled 5HTP administration in an effort to characterize 5HT neurons in the ME, but since this synthetic precursor does not accumulate exclusively in 5HT neurons, their results must be interpreted with caution.

Since 5HT-containing axons within the ME contain no regions of synaptic specialization it has been proposed that 5HT is released by extrasynaptic diffusion and possibly transported to remote receptors. In most brain regions 5HT causes a long-lasting inhibition of postsynaptic cells; it is not known what actions this putative neurotransmitter has in the

ME. Since some 5HT-containing neurons appear to make contact with tanycytes and with the basement membrane close to portal vessels, 5HT has been proposed to be involved with glial transport processes, and/or be released into the hypophyseal portal system (Calas et al. 1974).

Although 5HT neurons terminating in the ME are generally considered to originate in the dorsal midbrain raphe the results of some experiments indicate that there may also be another source. The relatively high concentrations of 5HT and its synthetic enzyme tryptophan hydroxylase found in the ME following lesions to the raphe or surgical isolation of the medial basal hypothalamus (Brownstein et al. 1976b; Palkovits et al. 1977) suggest the presence of 5HT neurons in the latter brain region. 5HT-containing perikarya have been identified in the rat medial hypothalamus using a combination of pharmacological, microspectrofluorometric and radioautographic techniques (Smith and Kappers 1975; Kent and Sladek 1978; Beaudet and Descarries 1979). Microspectrofluorimetric techniques have also revealed the presence of 5HT within tanycytes in the ME (Sladek and Sladek 1978). The functional role of 5HT within these cells, which have been postulated to play a role in the transport of neurohormones from the third ventricle to the hypophyseal portal system, is currently unknown.

Biochemical

Prior to the development of sensitive microanalytical techniques it was technically impossible to measure the concentrations of catecholamines and 5HT in the rat ME unless tissues from many animals were pooled. For example, in 1970 Björklund et al. pooled ME from 100 rats in order to measure the concentration of NE and DA using a fluorimetric procedure. Several years later Kavanaugh and Weisz (1974), using a more sensitive fluorimetric assay, were able to measure DA and NE in ME pooled from 6 or 7 rats. With the development of radioenzymatic, high performance liquid chromatographic (HPLC) and mass fragmentographic techniques it became possible to analyze the concentrations of catecholamines and 5HT, and many of their metabolites, in a single rat ME (Johnston and Moore 1981).

The concentrations of DA and NE reported for the rat ME vary depending on the size of the piece of medial basal hypothalamus analyzed. Kavanaugh and Weisz (1974) analyzed superficial, intermediate and deep sections of the medial basal hypothalamus for NE and DA. The superficial layer, which was essentially the ME, contained approximately 10 μg g^{-1} DA and 2 μg g^{-1} NE. In the deeper sections the concentration of DA fell while that of NE remained essentially the same. Providing that the dissection of ME weighs less than 0.5 mg the concentration of DA is greater than that of NE; ratios of DA/NE of approximately 2–8 have been reported (see Table 2.1).

A variety of techniques have been employed to dissect the ME. Many investigators merely cut this region free from fresh tissue with iris scissors while viewing the medial basal hypothalamus under a dissecting microscope (Cuello et al. 1973). Chiocchio et al. (1976a) employed a similar technique with frozen brain, making initial cuts with a razor blade and then removing the ME from the base of the brain with a 22 gauge needle. The weight of the

Table 2.1

CONCENTRATIONS OF DA AND NE IN RAT MEDIAN EMINENCE

Reference	Sex of rat	DA	NE	Weight (mg)
A. *Based on wet weight of median eminence ($\mu g\ g^{-1}$)*				
1. Bacopoulos et al. 1975	male	3.5	3.4	1.08
2. Versteeg et al. 1975	male	7.6	3.6	0.51
3. Kavanagh and Weisz 1974	female	12.5	1.8	0.45
4. Cuello et al. 1973	male	10.3	4.1	0.30
5. Gudelsky and Moore 1976	male	12.0	—	0.17
6. Chiocchio et al. 1976	male	29.0	4.5	0.07
B. *Based on protein content of median eminence (ng mg^{-1} protein)*				
1. Versteeg et al. 1976	male	58	24	
2. Palkovits et al. 1974	male	65	30	
3. Nicholson et al. 1978	male	128	38	
	female	67	12	
4. Selmanoff et al. 1976	female	132	17	
5. Moore et al. 1978	female	150	45	

All values were quantified by radioenzymatic assays, except those reported by Kavanagh and Weisz who employed a fluorometric procedure.

ME (0.07 mg) reported by these investigators is less than that reported by others, probably because they carefully removed the pituitary stalk; part of the stalk is generally included with the ME when dissected from fresh brain. In most reports the ME weighs 0.2–0.3 mg and contains a total of 2–4 ng DA and generally less than 1 ng NE. Palkovits (1973) devised a procedure in which appropriate brain regions can be punched out of frozen slices of brain; with this technique semicircular punches of ME are pooled from appropriate frontal brain slices (Brownstein et al. 1976a). Most investigators report amine concentrations in the ME on the basis of the protein content; a range of 60–150 ng DA mg^{-1} protein and 15–50 ng NE mg^{-1} protein have been reported. Values from some early reports are listed in Table 2.1.

Recently developed radioenzymatic assays for dihydroxyphenylacetic acid (DOPAC) have allowed the measurement of concentrations of this metabolite of DA in the ME; values range from 6 to 10 ng mg^{-1} protein (Umezu and Moore 1979; Fekete et al. 1978, 1980). Similar values for DOPAC have been obtained using HPLC with electrochemical detection (Johnston and Moore, unpublished).

There are relatively few reports on the concentrations of 5HT and its major metabolite, 5-hydroxyindole acetic acid (5HIAA) in the ME. Using a radioenzymatic assay Saavedra et al. (1974) reported 15 ng 5HT per mg protein; similar values (13–20 ng mg^{-1} protein) have been obtained using HPLC with electrochemical detection (Johnston and Moore, unpublished). Using the same procedure the ME was found to contain 10–13 ng 5HIAA per mg protein.

The activities of enzymes which synthesize catecholamines and 5HT have been measured in the ME (for review see Brownstein et al. 1976a). Activities of tyrosine hydroxylase and DBH have been measured in this region. It has not been possible to unequivocally demonstrate the presence of E in the ME, but this region does contain PNMT activity, suggesting the presence of E nerve terminals. Koslow and Schlumpf (1974) have identified small amounts of E (6 ng mg^{-1} protein) in the arcuate nucleus-infundibulum. In addition, the ME contains tryptophan hydroxylase activity (Kizer et al. 1976c) supporting the existence of 5HT nerve terminals in this region.

ESTIMATIONS OF ACTIVITY

Impulse traffic in aminergic neurons in the CNS can be recorded using electrophysiological techniques. For example, the activity of central NE and 5HT neurons has been estimated by recording from cell bodies in the pons-medulla and raphe nuclei, respectively. It is difficult, however, to determine whether the recorded cells project to the ME. Extracellular recordings have also been made from cells in the arcuate nucleus and other medial hypothalamic regions which have been found via antidromic stimulation techniques to project to the ME (i.e., tuberoinfundibular neurons; Moss 1976; Renaud 1980). It has not been possible, however, to determine whether the recorded tuberoinfundibular neurons are dopaminergic. Unlike perikarya of nigrostriatal DA neurons, which are tightly packed within the substantia nigra pars compacta, the cell bodies of tuberoinfundibular DA neurons are diffusely distributed throughout the arcuate and periventricular nuclei, making it difficult to record from identifiable DA neurons.

In most of the experiments discussed in this review the activities of aminergic neurons which terminate in the ME have been estimated biochemically. One important advantage of using biochemical techniques is that they can be employed in unanesthetized animals. In order to understand these techniques, neurochemical events occurring at the terminals of DA, NE and 5HT nerve terminals will be briefly reviewed.

Neurochemistry of catecholaminergic neurons

Most information on the neurochemical events occurring in DA nerve terminals has been obtained from studies on nigrostriatal DA neurons (see review Moore and Wuerthele 1979). Although many of the properties of tuberoinfundibular DA neurons resemble those in the nigrostriatal system, there are several important differences (see Moore et al. 1980a).

The neurochemical events believed to occur at terminals of tuberoinfundibular DA neurons are depicted schematically in Fig. 2.3A. Tyrosine is transported into the neuron and converted to L-dihydroxyphenylalanine (DOPA) by the rate-limiting synthesizing enzyme, tyrosine hydroxylase. This enzyme is regulated, in part, by an end-product inhibitory process so that decreases in intraneuronal DA concentrations result in increased DA synthesis, and vice versa. By this mechanism concentrations of DA within the nerve terminal remain fairly constant despite alterations in the amount of transmitter released. DOPA, which is synthesized from tyrosine, is rapidly decarboxylated to DA by L-aromatic amino acid decarboxylase (AAD). The newly synthesized DA can be stored in vesicles or released from the nerve terminal in response to action potentials. In the LPZ the released

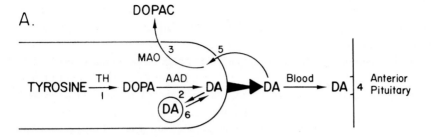

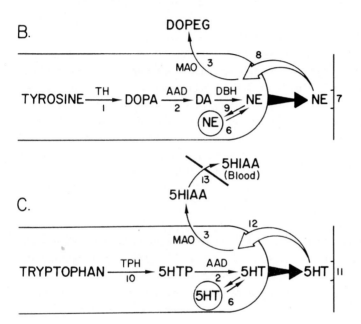

Fig. 2.3. Schematic diagram of (A) dopaminergic, (B) noradrenergic and (C) 5-hydroxytryptaminergic nerve terminals and receptors depicting sites of drug action. Abbreviations: TH, tyrosine hydroxylase; TPH, tryptophan hydroxylase; AAD, aromatic L-amino acid decarboxylase; DBH, dopamine-β-hydroxylase; MAO, monoamine oxidase; DOPA, dihydroxyphenylalanine; DA, dopamine; DOPAC, dihydroxyphenylacetic acid; DOPEG, dihydroxyphenylglycol; NE, norepinephrine; 5HTP, 5-hydroxytryptophan; 5HT, 5-hydroxytryptamine; 5HIAA, 5-hydroxyindoleacetic acid. Numbers represent the sites of drug action: 1, tyrosine hydroxylase inhibitors (α-methyltyrosine); 2, aromatic L-amino acid decarboxylase inhibitors (Ro-4-4602; NSD 1015); 3, monoamine oxidase inhibitors (pargyline); 4, dopamine agonists (bromocriptine, apomorphine) and antagonists (haloperidol); 5, dopamine uptake inhibitors (cocaine, d-amphetamine); 6, amine depletors (reserpine); 7, norepinephrine agonists (clonidine) and antagonists (phenoxybenzamine); 8, norepinephrine uptake inhibitors (desmethylimipramine); 9, dopamine-β-hydroxylase inhibitors (disulfiram, diethyldithiocarbamate); 10, tryptophan hydroxylase inhibitors (p-chlorophenylalanine); 11, 5-hydroxytryptamine agonists (quipazine) and antagonists (cyproheptadine, metergoline, methysergide); 12, 5-hydroxytryptamine uptake inhibitors (fluoxetine, chlorimipramine); 13, acid transport inhibitors (probenecid).

DA may activate receptors on axon terminals of other neurons (e.g. those containing LH-RH), but most DA terminals in the external layer of the ME are believed to release DA into the primary plexus of the hypophyseal portal blood.

Terminals of DA neurons in forebrain regions have a high affinity uptake mechanism which transports released DA back into the nerve terminal. In this way the actions of DA at pre- and postsynaptic receptors are terminated. Such a high affinity DA uptake system appears to be absent from tuberoinfundibular neurons (Demarest and Moore 1979a; Annunziato et al. 1980). An uptake mechanism is probably not needed by these neurons since DA is rapidly removed from the region of the terminals by the blood. Tuberoinfundibular DA neurons also differ from nigrostriatal and other major ascending DA neurons in that they lack presynaptic autoreceptors which regulate the synthesis (and possibly release) of DA in the latter neurons (Demarest and Moore 1979b).

The ME contains DOPAC, the oxidatively deaminated product of DA, but the concentration of this metabolite is relatively lower here than it is in other brain regions rich in DA nerve terminals (Moore et al. 1979). Since the concentration of DOPAC in the striatum appears to represent the amount of DA released and then recaptured by the neuron it has been used as a biochemical index of nigrostriatal DA neuronal activity (Roth et al. 1976). Because DA which is released from tuberoinfundibular neurons is not efficiently recaptured by the nerve terminal and converted by intraneuronal monoamine oxidase (MAO) to DOPAC, the concentration of this metabolite in the ME cannot be used to estimate the activity of tuberoinfundibular neurons (Umezu and Moore 1979; Moore et al. 1980a).

There are, however, several biochemical techniques that can be employed to estimate the activity of tuberoinfundibular DA neurons. Biochemical estimates of DA neuronal activity are based primarily upon measurements of DA turnover. Some of these techniques also measure NE neuronal activity, so they will be discussed together. It is appropriate, therefore, also to consider neurochemical dynamics at NE nerve terminals (Fig. 2.3B). In these neurons the synthesized DA is taken up by storage vesicles and converted to NE by DBH, which is contained within these vesicles. NE is then released in response to the arrival of nerve action potentials or to the actions of drugs. Within the synaptic cleft NE is free to interact with putative pre- or postsynaptic receptors. The action of this neurotransmitter at these receptors is terminated when the amine is actively transported back into the NE nerve terminal and oxidatively deaminated by intraneuronal MAO. The deaminated products (3,4-dihydroxyphenylglycol is the main metabolite in the brain) can then be further metabolized by catechol-o-methyltransferase which is localized in glial cells. 3-Methoxy,4-hydroxyphenylglycol (MHPG), is the metabolite that has generally been regarded to reflect NE neuronal activity (e.g. Adér et al. 1978). That is, increased concentrations of MHPG reflect increased activity of NE neurons, and vice versa. To date, however, this technique has not been employed to estimate the activity of NE neurons in the ME.

The concentrations of DA and NE in the nerve terminals do not change appreciably when impulse traffic increases or decreases. An exception to this generalization, peculiar only to the major ascending DA neurons, is that following acute cessation of neuronal impulse traffic (e.g. after sectioning the neurons or administration of drugs such as γ-butyrolactone) there is a brief increase in the rate of synthesis and accumulation of DA in the nerve terminal. This is due to an absence of autoreceptor activation (for discussion see Nowycky and Roth 1978; Moore and Wuerthele 1979). Because the tuberoinfundibular DA neurons lack autoreceptors these changes do not occur in the ME (Demarest and Moore 1979b).

Except as indicated above, the concentrations of catecholamines in nerve terminals do not change during periods of increased or decreased neuronal activity. It is believed, therefore, that synthesis of these amines keeps pace with release, and that degradation of amine transmitters occurs primarily after they have been released. Thus, synthesis, release and degradation are related in such a way that a change in one process is associated with similar changes in the other processes. Accordingly, changes in any of these processes can be used to estimate the activities of aminergic neuronal systems. Despite the assumptions that have to be made in order to measure amine turnover rates (Weiner 1974) valuable information has been obtained from such investigations. Those biochemical procedures which have been employed to estimate catecholamine neuronal activity within the ME are described briefly below.

Rates of catecholamine synthesis

Since the rates of synthesis of catecholamines are regulated at the step catalyzed by tyrosine hydroxylase, many estimations of catecholamine turnover are based upon in vitro and in vivo measures of the activity of this enzyme. Tyrosine hydroxylase catalyzes the synthesis of both NE and DA, but in the ME the activity of this enzyme primarily reflects DA synthesis (Kizer et al. 1976a; Demarest et al. 1979b).

In vitro. Electrical stimulation of nigrostriatal DA neurons causes an allosteric activation of tyrosine hydroxylase which persists for approximately 10–15 min following termination of the stimulus (Roth et al. 1975). Although a similar study has not been done with the tuberoinfundibular neurons, the activity of tyrosine hydroxylase has been measured in homogenates of the ME following a variety of endocrinological manipulations (Kizer et al. 1974, 1976a, 1978). Because of limitations in the sensitivity of the assay, measurements of the kinetic properties of this enzyme have required the pooling of several ME for each determination.

In vivo. In whole brain and in selected brain regions tyrosine hydroxylase can be estimated in vivo by quantifying the rate of conversion of intravenously injected radioactive tyrosine to radioactive products, DOPA, DA and NE. Unfortunately, radioactive tracer techniques are not sensitive enough to quantify the small amounts of catecholamines that are synthesized in the ME. A non-radioactive tracer technique has been employed to estimate the rate of catecholamine synthesis in vivo (Carlsson et al. 1972a). This technique involves the measurement of the rate of accumulation of DOPA in brain regions following the systemic administration of centrally active decarboxylase inhibitors such as benserazide (Ro4-4602) or 3-hydroxybenzylhydrazine (NSD 1015). The development of sensitive radioenzymatic and HPLC techniques for assaying picogram quantities of DOPA (Hefti and Lichtensteiger 1976; Crombeen et al. 1978; Nagatsu et al. 1979; Wagner et al. 1979; Demarest and Moore 1980) has made it possible to quantify the rate of catecholamine synthesis in the ME. The rate of DOPA accumulation in the striatum during the 10–30 min period after the administration of a decarboxylase inhibitor is related to the activity of nigrostriatal DA neurons (Roth et al. 1975). The rate of accumulation of DOPA in the ME reflects primarily the activity of tuberoinfundibular DA neurons, since under most conditions the rate of synthesis of NE represents only approximately 10% of the total catecholamine synthesis in this region (Demarest et al. 1979).

Decline of catecholamine concentrations after inhibition of synthesis

Under steady state conditions the rate of synthesis of catecholamines equals the rate of release so that the concentrations of these amines do not change despite marked changes in neuronal activity. Some pharmacological and endocrinological manipulations do alter brain catecholamine concentrations, but it is difficult to relate these changes to neuronal activity. Following administration of α-methyltyrosine (αMT), an inhibitor of tyrosine hydroxylase, the concentrations of these amines in the brain fall in an exponential manner; the rate of fall is proportional to impulse activity in the neurons. The advantage of this technique is that it permits the estimation of both NE and DA turnover. With the recent development of quantitative microfluorimetric procedures it has been possible to estimate the αMT-induced decline of NE and DA in various anatomical subdivisions of the ME (Bacopoulous et al. 1975; Löfström et al. 1976a).

Release of catecholamines

The release of catecholamines from the ME has been detected using both in vitro (Perkins and Westfall 1978; Perkins et al. 1979) and in vivo techniques (Ben-Jonathan et al. 1977; Gibbs and Neill 1978). In the latter procedure, the DA and NE concentrations are quantified in the hypophyseal portal blood of anesthetized animals permitting a direct measure of impulse flow in aminergic neurons which terminate in the ME. One problem associated with this technique is that anesthesia per se appears to alter the activity of tuberoinfundibular DA neurons (Pilotte et al. 1980).

Evaluation of methods

In summary, several biochemical and histochemical methods can be employed to estimate the activities of catecholaminergic neurons which terminate in the ME. In vitro and in vivo measures of tyrosine hydroxylase activity can be performed relatively quickly (the rate of DOPA accumulation in the ME can be measured within 10 min after intravenous administration of a decarboxylase inhibitor (Alper et al. unpublished) and when there are changes in steady state concentrations of catecholamines (e.g. after administration of reserpine). Furthermore, unlike the αMT method the DOPA accumulation procedure does not require 'zero time' values to be obtained since in the absence of a decarboxylase inhibitor the concentration of DOPA in brain is essentially zero (Demarest and Moore 1979a, 1980). On the other hand, the DOPA accumulation technique estimates synthesis of total catecholamines so that it is difficult to determine whether pharmacological or endocrinological manipulations selectively influence NE or DA neurons. Changes in the activity of NE neurons in the ME may be missed because DOPA accumulation in these neurons represents such a small fraction of that in DA neurons.

The relative activities of NE and DA neurons in the ME can be estimated by the αMT technique. Biochemical measurements of these amines permit the quantification of the rate of decline of NE and DA, but only in the whole ME. Histochemical procedures, on the other hand, make it possible to determine changes in catecholamine turnover in different regions of the ME, and the development of microspectrofluorimetric techniques has allowed the quantification of these changes. Since the spectra of the fluorophors of NE and DA are the same, concentrations of these amines have been estimated on the basis of their regional distribution – DA in LPZ and NE in SEL. Where these amines are present together (e.g. MPZ) it is difficult to relate the fluorescence to NE or DA, although the major amine in this region is DA. The αMT technique has several shortcomings. First, it cannot provide unequivocal results when steady state concentrations of the amines are altered by pharmacological (e.g. reserpine), endocrinological (e.g. long-term ovariectomy) or environmental (e.g. stress) manipulations per se. Secondly, the high doses of αMT needed to inhibit catecholamine synthesis can cause toxic effects (Moore et al. 1967). It is imperative, therefore, to measure catecholamine concentrations as soon as possible (30–60 min) after the administration of αMT in order to minimize toxic effects of the drug (Moore et al. 1967) and also those effects which may be secondary to synthesis inhibition (Hökfelt and Fuxe 1972b).

Procedures for measuring DA concentrations in hypophyseal portal blood have been extremely useful for estimating the activity of tuberoinfundibular DA neurons. A disadvantage of this technique is that it must be performed in anesthetized animals. There have been recent efforts to employ electrochemical detection procedures (implanted carbon electrodes) to estimate DA release in conscious freely moving animals (Clemens et al. 1980).

Since all these methods have shortcomings and some of them provide only comparative rather than absolute estimates of neuronal activity it is advisable to confirm the results of experiments by more than one method whenever possible. For the most part, however, the results of studies on the effects of various manipulations on catecholaminergic neurons which terminate in the ME have been remarkably consistent despite the fact that they have been carried out in different laboratories using different techniques.

Neurochemistry of 5HT neurons

A schematic representation of the events thought to occur at the terminals of a 5HT neuron is depicted in Fig. 2.3C. Tryptophan is actively transported into 5HT neurons where it is hydroxylated to form 5-hydroxytryptophan (5HTP) by tryptophan hydroxylase. This enzyme controls the rate-limiting step in the synthesis of 5HT but the precise manner by which it is regulated is not completely understood. Tryptophan hydroxylase, unlike tyrosine hydroxylase in catecholaminergic neurons, is not tightly regulated by an end-product inhibitory mechanism. Furthermore, tryptophan hydroxylase is not saturated by concentrations of tryptophan that are normally found in the brain so that raising or lowering brain concentrations of tryptophan can alter the saturation of the enzyme, and thus the rate of 5HT synthesis (Fernström and Wurtman 1971). Thus, alterations in the availability of 'free' tryptophan in the brain induced by dietary, hormonal, environmental, and/or pharmacological manipulations can influence brain 5HT synthesis (Curzon et al. 1972; Curzon and Knott 1977; Pardridge 1977; Fernström and Faller 1978). 5HTP synthesized in 5HT neurons is rapidly decarboxylated by AAD (thought to be the same enzyme that converts DOPA to DA) to 5HT. Newly synthesized 5HT, in turn, may be stored in vesicles or released from the nerve terminals in response to the arrival of nerve impulses, electrical stimulation or drugs (Müller et al. 1977). Following its release, 5HT is free to interact with postsynaptic 5HT receptors. Activation of these receptors is terminated when 5HT is either metabolized by extraneuronal MAO or is transported back into the nerve terminal by a stereospecific active uptake mechanism. Within the neuron 5HT is oxidatively deaminated to form the end-product of 5HT degradation, 5HIAA. This acid metabolite is then removed from the brain by a probenecid-sensitive acid transport mechanism.

Methods for estimating 5HT neuronal activity

Although a relation between nerve impulse flow and turnover of 5HT has been demonstrated (Carlsson et al. 1972b), synthesis and degradation of 5HT in the CNS may not be exclusively linked to 5HT neuronal activity. Nevertheless, changes in the rates of synthesis and metabolism of this amine have been used to estimate the activity of 5HT neurons (e.g. Héry et al. 1972; Neckers and Meek 1976). Some of the methods that have been employed include measurements of the following.

The relative concentrations of 5HT and 5HIAA. 5HIAA concentrations alone, or 5HIAA/5HT ratios, have been related to turnover and used as an estimate of 5HT neuronal activity (Tagliamonte et al. 1971; Héry et al. 1972).

Rates of accumulation of labelled 5HT and 5HIAA following systemic or intracerebroventricular (icv) administration of radioactive tryptophan (Neff et al. 1971).

Rates of accumulation of 5HT (Neff et al. 1967; Lin et al. 1969) or disappearance of 5HIAA (Tozer et al. 1966) after the administration of an inhibitor of MAO such as pargyline.

Rates of accumulation of 5HIAA after administration of the acid transport inhibitor, probenecid (Neff et al. 1967).

The activity of tryptophan hydroxylase. This has been measured in vitro following treatment of the animals (Kizer et al. 1976c; Palkovits et al. 1976) or in vivo by measuring the rate of accumulation of 5HTP after the administration of an AAD inhibitor (NSD 1015; Ro4-4602). In the absence of an AAD inhibitor the concentration of 5HTP in brain is essentially zero, but it increases linearly with time once the decarboxylating enzyme is inhibited (Carlsson et al. 1972a, b).

Until recently it has not been possible to carry out these procedures in small brain regions because the analytical techniques have not been sensitive enough to measure the amounts of 5HT, 5HIAA or 5HTP present in these regions. The development of sensitive radioenzymatic (Tappaz and Pujol 1980) and HPLC (Meek and Lofstrandh 1976; Krstulovic and Matzura 1979) assays for 5HTP, and assays employing HPLC in combination with electrochemical detection for measuring 5HT, 5HIAA and 5HTP (Loullis et al 1979) now make it possible to employ biochemical techniques to estimate 5HT neuronal activity in the medial basal hypothalamus and ME.

Results of studies in which biochemical techniques have been used to estimate 5HT neuronal activity must be viewed with caution. 5HT continues to be synthesized and metabolized to 5HIAA even after impulse traffic in 5HT neurons ceases (Carlsson and Lindqvist 1973). Furthermore, 5HT synthesis can be influenced by tryptophan concentrations and 5HT can be metabolized by MAO without first being released. Thus, it is difficult to know what proportion of synthesized 5HT is actually released and what proportion is merely metabolized within the neuron. Nevertheless, despite the fact that 5HT synthesis is not precisely linked to release, there does appear to be a relationship between 5HT neuronal activity and 5HT synthesis and metabolism (Carlsson et al. 1972b; Neckers and Meek 1976).

Not only is the regulation of 5HT synthesis and turnover not well understood, but many of the pharmacological tools used to study 5HT synthesis and activity exhibit questionable specificity. High doses of the 5HT precursor, 5HTP, can displace endogenous catecholamines from catecholaminergic terminals following its uptake into these neurons and subsequent decarboxylation to 5HT (Ng et al. 1972). The tryptophan hydroxylase inhibitor, p-chlorophenylalanine (pCPA) is a neutral amino acid and as such competes with tryptophan for uptake into the brain as well as monoaminergic neurons. Lastly, many of the putative 5HT receptor-antagonists may not be active in the central nervous system, and many possess agonistic and antagonistic effects towards other aminergic neuronal systems (Lamberts and MacLeod 1978; Besser et al. 1980).

EFFECTS OF PHARMACOLOGICAL MANIPULATIONS

Drugs which alter the dynamics of catecholaminergic systems

Drugs which characteristically alter the synthesis and storage of amines in the major catecholaminergic neurons in the brain have similar effects in those aminergic neurons which terminate in the ME. Reserpine, which disrupts the catecholamine binding capabilities of synaptic vesicles and thereby exposes the amines to intraneuronal MAO, depletes the ME of DA and NE (Gudelsky and Porter 1979a; Umezu and Moore 1979; Fekete et al. 1980) and increases the rate of synthesis of these amines (Demarest and Moore 1979b). MAO inhibitors act in the ME as they do in other brain regions to increase the concentrations of NE and DA and decrease the concentration of DOPAC (Fekete et al. 1979; Umezu and Moore 1979). Furthermore, increased intraneuronal amine concentrations induced by MAO inhibitors are accompanied by corresponding decreases in catecholamine synthesis, as evidenced in vivo by the reduced rate of DOPA accumulation (Demarest and Moore 1979b). Thus, synthesis of catecholamines in the ME, as in other brain regions, is regulated, in part, by end-product inhibition. Studies with the relatively specific MAO inhibitors, clorgyline and deprenyl, reveal that DA and NE neurons in the ME contain type

A MAO (Demarest and Moore, unpublished). In the ME, as in other brain regions except the striatum, administration of probenecid, an acid transport inhibitor, blocks the transport of DOPAC out of the brain, thereby causing the concentration of this acidic metabolite of DA to increase (Umezu and Moore 1979).

Inhibitors of catecholaminergic synthetic enzymes produce the same biochemical effects in the ME as they do in other brain regions. αMT, an inhibitor of tyrosine hydroxylase, and NSD 1015, an inhibitor of AAD, inhibit the synthesis of catecholamines at the steps catalyzed by these enzymes. It is possible, therefore, to employ these drugs as tools to disrupt catecholamine synthesis and thereby obtain a biochemical estimate of the activity of NE and DA neurons which terminate in the ME. αMT also significantly reduces the DA content in hypophyseal portal blood (Gudelsky and Porter 1979a).

6-Hydroxydopamine (6-OHDA) has been employed as a tool to examine the functional consequences of destroying catecholaminergic neurons in the central nervous system (Breese 1975). The selectivity of this drug relates to the ability of catecholaminergic neurons to actively accumulate the neurotoxin. Tuberoinfundibular DA neurons are relatively resistant to the destructive actions of 6-OHDA (Jonsson et al 1972; Cuello et al 1974; Smith and Helme 1974), probably because they lack a high affinity active amine transport system and therefore cannot accumulate the neurotoxin (Demarest and Moore 1979a). Relatively high doses of 6-OHDA administered icv (Demarest et al. 1979) or iv (Day and Willoughby 1980) do destroy some DA neurons in ME, but this loss is not accompanied by an increased serum concentration of prolactin.

Unlike DA neurons, NE nerve terminals in the ME are destroyed by 6-OHDA (Jonsson et al. 1972; Cuello et al. 1974; Day and Willoughby 1980). Depending on the route of administration, 6-OHDA may cause only a transitory loss of NE (1–2 weeks) which is accompanied by alterations in the plasma concentrations of corticosterone and growth hormone.

Catecholaminergic agonists and antagonists

Direct-acting DA receptor agonists (e.g. apomorphine) reduce the activity of major ascending DA neurons, while DA receptor antagonists (e.g. haloperidol) increase the activity of these neurons. These actions are believed to result from the activation of: (1) postsynaptic DA receptors which, in turn, regulate long neuronal feedback loops and/or (2) short autoreceptor (presynaptic receptor) – mediated feedback loops (for discussion see recent reviews by Nowycky and Roth 1978; Moore and Wuerthele 1979). Tuberoinfundibular neurons are unique among DA neurons in that they are unresponsive to the acute effects of these drugs. Injections of a variety of DA agonists (apomorphine, piribedil, bromocriptine) do not alter the αMT-induced decline of DA in the ME when measured histochemically (Fuxe and Hökfelt 1974) or biochemically (Gudelsky and Moore 1976), and do not influence the rate of DOPA accumulation in the brain region after the administration of a decarboxylase inhibitor (Demarest and Moore 1979b). Similarly, acute administration of DA antagonists (haloperidol, pimozide, sulpiride, thioridazine, clozapine, spiroperidol), increased the αMT-induced decline of DA and the rate of DOPA accumulation in terminals of DA neurons in all brain regions except the ME (Hökfelt and Fuxe 1972b; Fuxe and Hökfelt 1974; Fuxe et al. 1975a, b; Gudelsky and Moore 1977). While acutely administered DA receptor agonists are without effect on tuberoinfundibular DA neurons there are reports that a high dose of clonidine, a NE agonist, reduces and phenoxybenzamine and phentolamine, NE antagonists, increase the αMT-induced decline of DA in the ME (Fuxe and Hökfelt 1974).

Although administration of DA agonists and antagonists has no major acute actions on tuberoinfundibular DA neurons, repeated administration of these drugs does alter the biochemical measures of activity of these neurons. Repeated injections of a variety of neuroleptics enhance the αMT-induced decline of histofluorescence in the ME (Hökfelt and Fuxe 1972b; Fuxe et al. 1975a, b) and a single large dose of haloperidol, thioridazine and clozapine increases the αMT-induced decline of DA (Gudelsky and Moore 1977) and the accumulation of DOPA in the ME (Demarest and Moore 1980), and increases the concentration of DA in hypophyseal portal blood (Gudelsky and Porter 1980) some 12–16 h after injection. These delayed actions of neuroleptics are peculiar to DA neurons in the tuberoinfundibular system and are not seen in hypophysectomized animals. This suggests that the action of neuroleptics on these neurons is mediated indirectly as a result of their ability to increase serum concentrations of prolactin (Gudelsky and Moore 1977). Total hypothalamic deafferentation fails to prevent the haloperidol-induced activation of tuberoinfundibular DA neurons, indicating that the elevated serum concentrations of prolactin resulting from the administration of the neuroleptic are acting within the mediobasal hypothalamus, possibly on the tuberoinfundibular DA neurons themselves (Gudelsky et al. 1978). There is one report, however, which suggests that haloperidol may have a direct action on tuberoinfundibular DA neurons. Kizer et al. (1978) reported that repeated injections of haloperidol enhanced the αMT-induced decline of DA and increased the V_{max} of tyrosine hydroxylase for substrate and cofactor in the ME of hypophysectomized rats. These authors maintain that the difference between their studies and those of others who report that hypophysectomy blocks the effects of haloperidol on tuberoinfundibular DA neurons is related to the fact that they replace thyroid hormone in their hypophysectomized animals. It should be noted, however, that these researchers have not reported an acute effect of haloperidol on tuberoinfundibular neuronal activity, and that thyroxine per se reduces the activity of these neurons.

An acute injection of a long-acting DA agonist (bromocriptine) is reported to increase DA turnover in the ME, but when tuberoinfundibular DA neuronal activity is high repeated injections of bromocriptine reduce DA turnover (Hökfelt and Fuxe 1972a; Fuxe and Hökfelt 1974). More recently it has been reported that repeated injections of bromocriptine over a 24 h period significantly reduced the higher rate of DOPA accumulation in the ME of the female rat, but was without marked effect on the lower basal activity of tuberoinfundibular DA neurons in males (Moore et al. 1980b). This reduction in neuronal activity is believed to be secondary to the ability of bromocriptine to chronically reduce circulating levels of prolactin.

Several drugs which influence the activities of central and peripheral catecholaminergic neurons have been reported to influence tuberoinfundibular DA neurons. For example, an injection of a large dose of d-amphetamine increases the DA content of hypophyseal portal blood (Gudelsky and Porter 1979a). On the other hand, repeated large doses of meth-amphetamine reduce the concentration of DA and tyrosine hydroxylase in the striatum, but not in the ME (Morgan and Gibb 1980). Antimuscarinic drugs (atropine and benztropine) have no effect on tuberoinfundibular DA neurons (Hökfelt and Fuxe 1972b), while an acute injection of nicotine increases the turnover of DA in the ME (Fuxe et al. 1976).

Drugs which inhibit impulse flow in dopaminergic neurons

γ-Butyrolactone and baclofen inhibit impulse traffic in the major ascending DA neurons and increase the synthesis and concentration of DA in the terminal regions of these neurons (see Nowycky and Roth 1978; Moore and Demarest 1980). It is believed that by stopping impulse flow these drugs reduce the release of DA into the synaptic cleft, thereby removing the inhibitory influence of presynaptic autoreceptors on DA synthesis. γ-Butyrolactone and baclofen reduce activity of tuberoinfundibular DA neurons, as evidenced by the reduced rate of decline of DA in ME after αMT, but they do not alter the concentration or rate of synthesis of DA in this region (Moore et al. 1978; Fekete et al. 1978; Demarest and Moore 1979b; Moore and Demarest 1980). This suggests that tuberoinfundibular DA nerve terminals lack autoreceptors, a proposal supported by the inability to identify DA receptors by means of radiolabelled ligand binding in the ME (Brown et al. 1976). The results of studies employing DA agonists and antagonists and γ-butyrolactone and baclofen indicate that DA synthesis (and possibly release) in tuberoinfundibular DA neurons, unlike that of other DA neurons in the CNS, is not regulated by DA-receptor mediated mechanisms. Instead, these neurons appear to be regulated in a sluggish manner by endocrinological factors (see below).

Morphine and opiate peptides

There has been a long-standing interest in the actions of narcotic analgesics (primarily morphine), and more recently of opioid peptides, on aminergic neurons in the CNS (see reviews, Way 1971; Iwamoto and Way 1979). These drugs also have marked effects on neuroendocrine systems (see reviews, Bruni et al. 1977; Meites et al. 1979; Holaday and Loh 1979; Van Vugt and Meites 1980). It is not surprising, therefore, that efforts have been made to relate causally the neuroendocrine actions of opioids with their actions on aminergic neurons terminating in the medial basal hypothalamus.

Both β-endorphin and the less potent enkephalins are believed to have neurotransmitter or neuromodulatory roles. In the rat, icv or intrahypothalamic injections of β-endorphin and synthetic enkephalins act like systemically administered morphine to increase circulating concentrations of ACTH, GH and prolactin, decrease LH and possibly TSH, and are without effect on FSH (see Holaday and Loh 1979; Meites et al. 1979). Most of these actions are blocked by the narcotic antagonists, naloxone or naltrexone. In addition, most reports indicate that narcotic antagonists have endocrinological effects per se; they have been reported to alter basal and stress-induced concentrations of circulating levels of prolactin, GH and LH (Shaar et al. 1977; Bruni et al. 1977; Van Vugt et al. 1978; Koenig et al. 1979; Meites et al. 1979). On the other hand, Martin et al. (1979) report that naloxone does not alter the physiological release of prolactin or GH.

Morphine and opioid peptides do not have a direct effect on the anterior pituitary (Rivier et al. 1977; Login and MacLeod 1979; Grandison et al. 1980) so it is generally believed that their abilities to alter the release of anterior pituitary hormones are mediated via hypothalamic mechanisms. From a neurochemical-neuroendocrinological standpoint, results of studies on the interactions of opioids with prolactin and tuberoinfundibular DA neurons are the most unequivocal. Morphine and some of the opioid peptides interact with DA neurons differentially. For example, they increase the activity of nigrostriatal DA neurons but depress the activity of tuberoinfundibular DA neurons. This latter effect has been demonstrated in vivo by measuring the αMT-induced decline of DA in the ME using histofluorescent (Ferland et al. 1977; Fuxe et al. 1979) and biochemical techniques (Van Vugt et al. 1979; Deyo et al. 1979; Van Loon et al. 1980), by quantifying the rate of DOPA accumulation (Alper et al. 1980) and by measuring the DA concentration in hypophyseal portal blood (Gudelsky and Porter 1979b). Similar results have been obtained in vitro. Using a superfused hypothalamic preparation Wilkes and Yen (1980) reported that the efflux of DA and DOPAC was reduced by the addition of β-endorphin to the perfusing fluid. It would appear, therefore, that the morphine-induced increase of prolactin secretion results from the depression of the tonic DA inhibitory action on prolactin-secreting cells in the anterior pituitary. The opioid-induced increase of serum prolactin and the decrease of tuberoinfundibular DA neuronal activity are blocked by naloxone or naltrexone (Deyo et al. 1979; Gudelsky and Porter 1979b; Grandison et al. 1980; Alper et al. 1980), although there is a report that the effects of β-endorphin are not (Fuxe et al. 1979). Tolerance develops to both the morphine-induced decrease of DA turnover in the ME and the increase of serum prolactin concentrations (Deyo et al. 1980).

There have been relatively few studies attempting to relate the opioid-induced changes in the secretion of ACTH, LH, TSH or GH specifically to the ability of these compounds to depress tuberoinfundibular DA neurons. A decrease of tuberoinfundibular DA activity should reduce GH release since DA stimulates the release of this hormone. In fact, opioids increase GH release. If one believes that DA stimulates LH release, then the depression of these neurons by morphine may be important for the reduction of circulating concentrations of this hormone. Evidence suggests, however, that DA depresses rather than stimulates LH release (see below); the effect may be dependent on the endocrine status of the animal (Vijayan and McCann 1978).

The mechanisms by which narcotic antagonists alter basal circulating concentrations of anterior pituitary hormones are unknown. Most reports agree, however, that although naloxone and naltrexone block the depressant effects of opiates on tuberoinfundibular DA neurons, these antagonists have little effect on these neurons per se. In the ME naloxone did not alter the αMT-induced decline of DA (Deyo et al. 1979, 1980; Fuxe et al. 1979) or DOPA accumulation (Alper et al. 1980), and did not alter the release of DA into hypophyseal portal blood (Gudelsky and Porter 1979b). Thus, if naloxone or naltrexone alters basal or stress-induced changes in anterior pituitary hormone release, this action does not appear to result from a direct action on tuberoinfundibular DA neurons. Morphine and opioid peptides may exert some of their effects on tuberoinfundibular DA neurons and on anterior pituitary hormone secretion indirectly by interacting with 5HT neuronal systems. (See Chapter 1).

Morphine causes a transient increase in serum levels of GH, which can be prevented by naloxone or by disrupting NE transmission by pretreatment with diethyldithiocarbamate (a DBH inhibitor) or with phenoxybenzamine (an α-NE receptor blocker); DA receptor blocking drugs are without effect (Koenig et al. 1980). β-Endorphin also increases GH, but this effect is reportedly enhanced rather than blocked by naloxone (Fuxe et al. 1979). Morphine is known to increase NE concentrations in the hypothalamus (Roffman et al. 1970; van Ree et al. 1976); more recently it has been demonstrated that systemic morphine or icv β-endorphin increases the αMT-induced decline of NE in the ME and periventricular regions of the hypothalamus (Fuxe et al. 1979). Thus, the ability of morphine and opiate peptides to cause the secretion of GH may be due to their abilities to activate NE neuronal systems.

Gastrointestinal peptides

Most pharmacological and endocrinological manipulations which alter the activity of tuberoinfundibular DA neurons do so only after a pronounced latent period (see subsequent sections). The exceptions are the narcotic analgesics and opioid peptides discussed above, and several other peptides which also have acute effects on tuberoinfundibular DA neurons.

The hypothalamus is richly innervated with neurons that are immunoreactive to a number of different peptides, including those that are thought of as 'gastrointestinal hormones' (vasoactive intestinal polypeptide (VIP), secretin, glucagon; Fuxe et al. 1980). Some of these neurons appear to influence the activity of catecholaminergic neurons which terminate in the ME, and may have endocrine regulatory roles. It has been suggested, for example, that VIP is a PRF (Clemens and Shaar 1980). (See also Chapter 1). Intracerebroventricular injections of high doses of VIP, secretin and glucagon caused acute changes in the turnover of NE and DA in the ME (Fuxe et al. 1979, 1980). NE turnover in SEL was increased by VIP but not influenced by secretin or glucagon; DA turnover in MPZ and LPZ was decreased by glucagon, increased by secretin and not altered by VIP. The same effects were observed when the latter two hormones were infused intravenously.

EFFECTS OF ENDOCRINOLOGICAL MANIPULATIONS

Fuxe and Hökfelt and their collaborators pioneered the study of endocrine manipulations on the characteristics of aminergic neuronal systems in the ME. They initially made semiquantitative estimations of the αMT-induced decline of histofluorescence in the ME (e.g. Fuxe and Hökfelt 1967, 1969). Subsequently, they developed and employed microfluorimetric techniques to quantify these changes (Löfström et al. 1976a, b). The development of sensitive microchemical techniques has now permitted similar studies to be carried out using quantifiable analytical procedures. The results of the histochemical and biochemical studies are remarkably similar. The most pronounced and consistent endocrinologically-induced change in tuberoinfundibular DA neuronal activity is that produced by alterations in serum concentrations of prolactin.

Prolactin

Systemic injections of rat or ovine prolactin increase the αMT-induced decline of catecholamine histofluorescence in the ME. The effect is observed in the MPZ and LPZ, but not in SEL, suggesting that the activity of DA but not NE neurons is increased (Wiesel et al. 1978). There was a marked latent period before this effect could be observed; for example, it occurred 24 h after a single iv injection of ovine prolactin (Hökfelt and Fuxe 1972a) and was maintained if the hormone was administered twice daily for 7 days, although the effect tolerated out by 14 days (Fuxe et al. 1977). The characteristic delay in the prolactin-induced increase of DA turnover in the ME was reduced if the hormone was injected into hypophysectomized animals (Hökfelt and Fuxe 1972a).

The results of these histochemical studies have been confirmed biochemically. Repeated systemic injections of ovine prolactin significantly enhanced the αMT-induced decline of DA in the ME at 26 but not at 10 h after the start of the injections (Gudelsky et al. 1976). Injections of ovine or rat prolactin into the cerebroventricular system increased the αMT-induced decline of DA (Annunziato and Moore 1978), the accumulation of DOPA (Johnston et al. 1980) and the activity of tyrosine hydroxylase (Nicholson et al. 1980) in the ME. Again, these changes were not seen until at least 12–16 h after the injections of prolactin, at a time when the hormone had probably disappeared from the cerebroventricular system (Login and MacLeod 1977). Thus, prolactin appears to trigger a neuronal event which ultimately leads to a sustained activation of the tuberoinfundibular DA neurons. Results of recent studies with cycloheximide reveal that this inhibitor of protein synthesis prevents the ability of icv administered prolactin to increase DOPA accumulation in the ME (Johnston et al. 1980). Thus, the latent period for the prolactin-induced acceleration of DA synthesis in the ME may be due to the time required for prolactin to induce tyrosine hydroxylase in the soma of tuberoinfundibular DA neurons and the subsequent transport of this newly synthesized enzyme down the axons of these neurons to their terminals in the ME.

The increased turnover of DA in the ME which follows a variety of pharmacological or endocrinological manipulations also appears to be related to the ability of these treatments to elevate circulating concentrations of prolactin. The consequences of the neuroleptic-induced increase of prolactin levels have been described. The actions of estrogens are described in the next section. Rats with prolactin-secreting tumors release increased amounts of DA into pituitary stalk blood (Cramer et al. 1979b) and transplantation of the anterior pituitary under the renal capsule increases serum concentrations of prolactin and increases the αMT-induced decline of DA and the activity of tyrosine hydroxylase in the ME-arcuate nucleus (Olson et al. 1972; Krieger and Wuttke 1980; Morgan and Herbert 1980; Nicholson et al. 1980). In these animals the serum LH concentration is low and it has been suggested that the increased activity of DA neurons, particularly in the LPZ, inhibits LH-RH secreting cells (Löfström et al. 1977; Hohn and Wuttke 1978). This may be the mechanism for the inverse relationship between serum concentrations of LH and prolactin.

Gonadotropins and gonadal hormones

Catecholaminergic neuronal systems have been implicated in the regulation of LH secretion. It is generally agreed that NE neurons facilitate LH release from the anterior pituitary, but there is some controversy regarding the role of DA neurons. It has been suggested that DA neurons both inhibit and facilitate LH release (Schneider and McCann 1970; Hökfelt and Fuxe 1972b; Hökfelt et al. 1976; Weiner and Ganong 1978; Sawyer 1979). Without commenting directly on this controversy, a summary of the effects of changing blood levels of gonadal steroids on aminergic neuronal systems in the ME is presented below.

Castration has been reported to alter the dynamics of catecholamines in the ME in a variety of ways. Acute castration (4–24 h) is reported to increase the concentration of NE but not of DA in the ME (Chiocchio et al. 1976b). Long-term ovariectomy is reported not to alter catecholamine concentrations in the mediobasal hypothalamus (Honma and Wuttke 1980) or ME (Kizer et al. 1978). Other researchers (Gudelsky et al. 1977; Löfström 1979) have reported an increased concentration of DA but not NE in the ME of ovariectomized rats and that the increase in DA can be reversed by estrogen administration.

Tyrosine hydroxylase in the ME reflects primarily activity of DA neurons since the activity of this enzyme does not change appreciably when NE neurons in this region are destroyed (Kizer et al. 1976a; Demarest et al. 1979). Castration is reported not to alter (Krieger and Wuttke 1980), to decrease (Nakahara et al. 1976), and to increase (Kizer et al. 1974, 1976c) the activity of tyrosine hydroxylase in the ME. The increase noted by the latter workers represented an increase in V_{max} without a change in the K_m of the enzyme for its substrate or cofactor (tetrahydrobiopterin). They subsequently reported (Kizer et al. 1978) that αMT-induced decline of DA in the ME was reduced 10 days after castration, but in contrast to most other reports, the decline of catecholamines did not follow first order kinetics. Using histofluorescent techniques, Fuxe et al. (1969a) reported that castration did not alter the αMT-induced decline of catecholamines in ME of males, but eliminated changes associated with the estrous cycle in females.

Injections of androgens and estrogens selectively enhance DA turnover in the ME. In castrated male and female rats, three daily injections of estradiol or testosterone and other androgens increased the αMT-induced decline of catecholamines in the ME, while progesterone and glucocorticoids were without effect (Fuxe et al. 1969a; Fuxe and Hökfelt 1974; Fuxe et al. 1978). In subsequent studies using quantitative microfluorimetry it was noted that repeated injections of estrogen into ovariectomized rats increased serum concentrations of prolactin and the αMT-induced decline of fluorescence in the LPZ and MPZ, and reduced the serum concentration of LH and the decline of fluorescence in SEL (Löfström et al. 1977; Wiesel et al. 1978).

Using the same techniques it was noted that repeated injections of androgens increased

DA turnover in LPZ and MPZ but did not alter NE turnover in SEL (Fuxe et al. 1978). These authors postulated that the estrogen-induced reduction of LH secretion is related to the ability of estrogen to activate DA neurons in LPZ, and thereby inhibit LH-RH neurosecretory cells.

Biochemical studies have generally confirmed the results of these histochemical studies. Three daily injections of estradiol increased the αMT-induced decline of DA and the rate of DOPA accumulation in the ME of male rats (Eikenburg et al. 1977; Demarest and Moore 1980). Since these effects were not observed in hypophysectomized rats it was postulated that the estrogen-induced activation of tuberoinfundibular DA neurons was not due to the direct effect of this hormone on the neurons per se, but rather to the ability of estrogens to increase circulating concentrations of prolactin. Gudelsky et al. (1981) have recently reported that repeated injections of estrogens into ovariectomized rats increase serum concentrations of prolactin and the concentration of DA in pituitary stalk blood.

Progesterone is reported to be without effect on the turnover of catecholamines in the ME (Fuxe et al. 1969a, b), but a recent report by Cramer et al. (1979c) indicates that injection of progesterone into ovariectomized-adrenalectomized rats increased the concentration of DA in the pituitary stalk blood. It was suggested that the increased activity of tuberoinfundibular DA neurons during pregnancy may result, in part, from the actions of progesterone.

LH per se does not appear to influence tuberoinfundibular DA neurons. Intravenous administration of this hormone did not alter the αMT-induced decline of catecholamine histofluorescence (Hökfelt and Fuxe 1972b) and icv LH did not alter the rate of DOPA accumulation in the ME (Moore et al. 1980a); these negative results should be interpreted cautiously since they may have been obtained at inappropriate times or after inadequate doses of LH.

ACTH and adrenocortical steroids

There have been numerous studies concerned with the role of catecholamines on the regulation of the pituitary-adrenal axis (see recent reviews by Müller et al. 1977; Ganong 1977; Weiner and Ganong 1978). Most evidence supports the existence of a coordinating and inhibiting action of NE neurons on the release of corticotropin-releasing hormone (CRH). In keeping with the theme of this chapter, one might suspect that if NE neurons participate in the regulation of CRH, and thus ACTH secretion, these neurons, in turn, may be responsive to alterations in circulating concentrations of ACTH or adrenocortical hormones. The results of studies dealing directly with this possibility, however, are rather confusing.

There are many reports on the effects of adrenalectomy and corticosteroids on the concentrations and rates of turnover of catecholamines in whole brain or hypothalamus, but relatively few of these deal with the dynamics of these amines specifically in the ME. Neither adrenalectomy nor administration of ACTH or corticosteroids have marked effects on the concentrations of NE in the whole hypothalamus (Shen and Ganong 1976a; Telegdy and Kovacs 1979). In the median eminence adrenalectomy did not alter the concentrations of NE in SEL or DA in LPZ, but caused a slight decrease in catecholamine histofluorescence in the MPZ (Löfström 1979). Fekete et al. (1976) observed an increased DA concentration in the ME following glucocorticoid administration.

The NE turnover in the ME is reported to increase following adrenalectomy, and this effect can be reversed in a dose-dependent fashion by corticosteroids; in intact animals, however, glucocorticoids were without effect (Fuxe et al. 1973a). Shen and Ganong (1976b) also reported an increased turnover of NE in the hypothalamus of adrenalectomized rats. Acute adrenalectomy and ovariectomy did not alter the concentration of DA in hypophyseal portal blood (Cramer et al. 1979c). Hökfelt and Fuxe (1972b) reported that several injections of ACTH did not alter the αMT-induced decline of catecholamine fluorescence in the ME but in a subsequent report it was noted that intravenously administered ACTH increased NE but not DA turnover in the ME (Fuxe et al. 1978).

Adrenalectomy is reported to reduce tyrosine hydroxylase but not DBH in the ME (Kizer et al. 1974), while the activity of the latter enzyme is reported to decrease in the whole hypothalamus (Shen and Ganong 1976b). Glucocorticoids reversed the effect on tyrosine hydroxylase but not on DBH.

The administration of high doses of dexamethasone to newborn or adult rats increases the activity of PNMT and the concentration of epinephrine in the hypothalamus, but the significance of the effect of glucocorticoids on E-containing hypothalamic neurons is not currently understood (Moore and Phillipson 1975).

Other hormones

Hypothyroidism induced either by thyroidectomy for 7–10 days or by administration of propylthiouracil in the drinking water for 3 weeks increased tyrosine hydroxylase in the ME; this was demonstrated to be related to an increase in V_{max} and the affinity of tyrosine hydroxylase for the cofactor, tetrahydrobiopterin (Kizer et al. 1974, 1976c, 1978; Nakahara et al. 1976). It has also been reported that the DA and NE concentrations in the ME were not altered 10 days after thyroidectomy, but that the αMT-induced decline of DA, but not NE, was enhanced in these animals (Kizer et al. 1978). On the other hand, injections of thyroxine reduced tyrosine hydroxylase activity in the ME (Kizer et al. 1974). These results suggest that a deficiency of thyroid hormone increases the activity of tuberoinfundibular DA neurons. This may be the mechanism by which thyroidectomy reduces serum concentrations of prolactin (Jahnke et al. 1980).

The role of catecholamines in regulating release of growth hormone has been recently reviewed (Weiner and Ganong 1978); the results are somewhat controversial, possibly related to the pulsatile release of this hormone in the rat. DA agonists increase serum levels of growth hormone in rats, and this effect is blocked by DA antagonists (Mueller et al. 1976a), although a biphasic effect has been reported after administration of apomorphine (Cocchi et al. 1979). Clonidine, an α-adrenergic agonist, also increases the secretion of growth hormone. Thus, both DA and NE neuronal systems may play a role in the regulation of growth hormone secretion. Is the reverse also true? Intravenous injections of growth hormone into hypophysectomized rats caused a reduction in the concentration of NE in SEL of the ME, but did not alter its rate of turnover (Andersson et al. 1977). On the other hand, these same investigators noted that growth hormone reduced DA turnover in the MPZ and LPZ. Since somatostatin-containing neurosecretory neurons have been identified in the LPZ, and to a lesser extent in the MPZ (Hökfelt et al. 1975b), it was suggested that DA neurons in these regions exert an inhibitory action on the somatostatin neurons (Fuxe et al. 1978).

PHYSIOLOGICALLY INDUCED CHANGES OF ACTIVITY

Estrous cycle

There is general agreement among the various researchers on the changes in activities of catecholaminergic neurons in the ME during the estrous cycle. In an early study utilizing the histofluorescent technique it was noted that the turnover of DA was lower during proestrus–estrus than during metestrus–diestrus (Ahren et al. 1971). It was proposed at this time that the reduction of DA inhibitory input to LH-RH secretory neurons was responsible for the LH surge on the afternoon of proestrus. In a subsequent study employing the microfluorimetric technique, Löfström (1977) noted that NE turnover in SEL was higher and DA turnover in LPZ was lower on proestrus than at any other time during the estrous cycle. A similar pattern was observed when the αMT-induced decline of catecholamines was analyzed biochemically in the whole ME; that is, the turnover of NE was increased while that of DA was decreased on the early afternoon of proestrus (Demarest et al. 1981). It had been reported previously that the concentration of catecholamines in the ME does not change during the estrous cycle (Selmanoff et al. 1976; Gudelsky et al. 1977). It was more difficult to see a pattern of change in catecholamine synthesis when it was estimated in vivo by measuring the accumulation of DOPA in the ME, probably because the increase in NE turnover and the decrease in DA turnover cancel each other. Nevertheless, the accumulation of DOPA in the ME was lower on the morning and afternoon of proestrus than it was on the morning of estrus (Demarest et al. 1981). Consistent with these findings is the report that tyrosine hydroxylase in the mediobasal hypothalamus was reduced on the afternoon of proestrus, while the activity of DBH was increased at this time (Carr and Voogt 1980). Furthermore, the concentration of DA in pituitary stalk blood is lowest on proestrus, while the NE content is too low to be measured accurately (Ben-Jonathan et al. 1977; Cramer et al. 1979a). These results suggest, but do not prove, that the surges of prolactin and LH on the afternoon of proestrus are due, in part, to alterations in the activities of catecholaminergic neurons which terminate in the ME.

Pregnancy and lactation

Initial reports indicated that there was an increase in the number and intensity of DA cell bodies in the arcuate nucleus and that the rate of decline of catecholamine histofluorescence in the ME after αMT was increased in pregnant and lactating rats when compared to ovariectomized controls (Fuxe et al. 1969a, b; Hökfelt and Fuxe 1972b). It was suggested that the high circulating concentrations of prolactin were responsible for the increased activity of the tuberoinfundibular DA neurons during these physiological states. It should be noted, however, that in rat plasma the concentration of prolactin is low during gestation and increases only on the day of parturition and during lactation (Ben-Jonathan et al. 1980).

The apparent increase in activity of tuberoinfundibular DA neurons during pregnancy has been confirmed using different techniques. The turnover of catecholamines in the ME, as determined by the microfluorimetric procedure, was reported to 'show a tendency to increase' in rats that were pregnant for 15–21 days (Löfström et la. 1976b). The rate of DOPA accumulation in the ME exhibited two daily peaks in pregnant rats, and the mean rate was much higher than that in diestrous control rats (McKay et al. unpublished). Furthermore, the DA concentration in the hypophyseal portal blood is markedly elevated during pregnancy (Ben-Jonathan et al. 1977).

The reports of tuberoinfundibular DA neuronal activity are not as consistent in lactating rats as they are in pregnant rats. Early reports (e.g. Fuxe et al. 1969b) indicated that catecholamine turnover was increased in the ME of lactating rats, although details of how the animals were manipulated prior to sacrifice (e.g., were they pup-deprived?) are not described. In a report by Mena et al. (1976) lactating rats on day 6–8 postpartum were separated from their pups for 24 h and then allowed to nurse for 5–60 min prior to sacrifice. They noted that the whole hypothalamic content of DA was lower and NE was higher than in ovariectomized controls, and that suckling caused a further lowering of DA but was without effect on NE. Chiocchio et al. (1979) also reported that suckling reduces the DA content in the ME. Moyer et al. (1979) examined the dynamics of catecholamines in the ME of lactating rats on day 5 postpartum. These animals were deprived of their pups for 6 h and then allowed to suckle for 1 h prior to sacrifice. Suckling altered neither the steady state concentration nor the αMT-induced decline of NE or DA in the ME or arcuate nucleus. On the other hand, the rate of DOPA accumulation in the ME of lactating rats which were pup-deprived for 4 h was markedly lower than that of diestrous controls, and suckling further reduced the DOPA accumulation (McKay et al. 1980). These results suggest that tuberoinfundibular DA neuronal activity is reduced in lactating animals, a conclusion that is just opposite to that of previous workers (Fuxe et al. 1969a, b; Hökfelt and Fuxe 1972b). Reduced tuberoinfundibular DA neuronal activity during lactation is consistent with the recent report by Ben-Jonathan et al. (1980) who noted that the DA content of pituitary stalk blood from lactating animals was lower than that in pregnant rats (the values were also lower than those reported previously for diestrous or estrous rats, Ben-Jonathan et al. 1977). Separation of the pups from their mothers for 24 h caused a significant increase in the DA content in the stalk blood. The authors concluded from their studies that under physiological conditions of low prolactin release, hypothalamic DA secretion is elevated, and vice versa.

Stress

Results of early studies revealed that a variety of stressful procedures (e.g. immobilization, heat, electric foot shock) causes a generalized decrease in the concentration of NE and an increase in NE turnover in the brain (e.g. Thierry et al. 1968; Corrodi et al. 1971).

Subsequent experiments have indicated that similar stressful situations increase DA neuronal activity in selected brain regions such as the nucleus accumbens and frontal cortex (Thierry et al. 1976; Fadda et al. 1978). There have been relatively few reports on the effects of stress on catecholaminergic neuronal systems which terminate in the ME.

Acute stressful procedures (immobilization, formalin injections) reduced the DA and NE concentrations in the arcuate nucleus but had no effect in the ME, while repeated immobilization over several days caused an increase in tyrosine hydroxylase in the arcuate nucleus (Palkovits et al. 1975) and an increase in the concentration of NE in the ME (Kvetňansky et al. 1977). Fuxe and Hökfelt (1967) reported that a variety of stressful procedures (heat, cold, ether) did not alter the αMT-induced decline of DA histofluorescence in the ME. Immobilization is reported to increase the αMT-induced decline of NE in the hypothalamus and reduce the decline of DA in the ME (Lidbrink et al. 1972). A causal relationship between stress-induced changes in catecholaminergic neuronal dynamics in the mediobasal hypothalamus and alterations in endocrine status (e.g. increased secretion of ACTH, prolactin, etc.) remains to be established.

EFFECTS OF PHARMACOLOGICAL MANIPULATIONS OF 5HT NEURONS

Drugs which alter the dynamics of 5HT systems

There are relatively few reports of studies designed specifically to characterize 5HT neurons in the ME. This is due primarily to technical problems associated with the relatively poor histochemical procedures for this amine, and the lack of sensitivity of analytical techniques for analyzing 5HT, its precursor, 5HTP, and its major metabolite, 5HIAA. Unlike tuberoinfundibular DA neurons, which originate and terminate within the mediobasal hypothalamus, many 5HT neurons which end in the ME may be merely branches of neurons which terminate throughout the hypothalamus. Accordingly, in the following sections an effort has been made to review the dynamics of 5HT neurons which innervate not only the ME, but also those that terminate throughout the basal hypothalamus. Results of future studies, however, may reveal important differences in the properties of 5HT neurons in these two brain regions. To date, most pharmacological manipulations appear to cause similar changes in neurochemical characteristics of 5HT neurons in the ME and hypothalamus.

Analytical assays employing HPLC with electrochemical detection (Loullis et al. 1979) are sensitive enough to quantify concentrations of 5HT, its major deaminated metabolite, 5HIAA, and its immediate precursor, 5HTP in a single rat ME. The results of recent studies (discussed below) employing this technique (Johnston and Moore 1981) reveal that 5HT neurons terminating in the ME respond to drugs in a manner similar to 5HT neurons in other brain regions. For example, following the administration of a decarboxylase inhibitor the 5HTP concentration in the ME increases progressively with time for up to 1 h. Reserpine causes a marked decline in the concentration of 5HT and an increase in 5HTP accumulation in the ME. This is consistent with previous reports that reserpine increases tryptophan hydroxylase activity in the brain (Zivkovic et al. 1973; Sze et al. 1976). The concentration of 5HIAA in the ME is reduced by treatment with a monoamine oxidase inhibitor and increased by probenecid, a blocker of acid transport mechanisms. The potent 5HT uptake inhibitor, chlorimipramine, caused a decrease in the conversion of 5HT to 5HIAA and in the synthesis of 5HT in the ME. The specific 5HT uptake blocker, fluoxetine, also decreased the conversion of 5HT to 5HIAA.

Morphine and opiate peptides

Morphine appears to exert some of its neuroendocrinological effects via central 5HT neuronal systems. For example, low doses of morphine that are ineffective in increasing serum concentrations of prolactin per se, are effective following pretreatment with fluoxetine, a 5HT uptake blocker (Meites et al. 1979). The morphine-induced increase of serum concentrations of prolactin is reduced by procedures which disrupt 5HT transmission. For example, pretreatment with putative 5HT antagonists (cyproheptadine, metergoline, methysergide) or with 5,7-dihydroxytryptamine (5,7DHT) which destroys 5HT neurons, greatly reduces the increase in serum concentrations of prolactin induced by morphine and opiate peptides (Koenig et al. 1979, 1980; Spampinato et al. 1979). Caution should be exercised when interpreting the results of 5HT antagonists since these compounds also have dopaminergic and histaminergic properties (Cocchi et al. 1978; Lamberts and MacLeod 1978; Besser et al. 1980). Studies with *para*-chlorophenylalanine have yielded equivocal results (Dupont et al. 1979; Spampinato et al. 1979; Taché et al. 1979; Koenig et al. 1980). Although there is some evidence that 5HT neurons stimulate the release of growth hormone, disruption of 5HT neurons with the above treatments did not alter the morphine-induced increases in release of this hormone (Koenig et al. 1980; Taché et al. 1979).

Acute administration of morphine increases the turnover of 5HT in whole brain (Neff et al. 1967; Yarbrough et al. 1971, 1973) and in hypothalamus (Roffman et al. 1970; Haubrich and Blake 1973). Acute administration of morphine did not alter the concentration of 5HT in the medial basal hypothalamus (less ME) or the ME, but did increase the rate of 5HTP accumulation in the former region (Johnston and Moore 1981). There are recent reports that the administration of synthetic enkephalins (Algeri et al. 1978) and β-endorphin (Van Loon and De Souza 1978; Garcia-Sepilla et al. 1978) increase 5HT turnover in the hypothalamus.

The ability of morphine to influence 5HT neurons, tuberoinfundibular DA neurons, and serum prolactin levels may be related. Results of recent studies (Demarest and Moore 1981) reveal that disruption of 5HT transmission processes with metergoline or 5,7DHT pretreatments had no effect on basal serum prolactin concentrations or the activity of tuberoinfundibular DA neurons per se, indicating a lack of a tonic 5-hydroxytryptaminergic regulatory influence. On the other hand, these treatments blocked the effects of morphine, suggesting that the morphine-induced depression of tuberoinfundibular DA neurons and the consequent secretion of prolactin result from the stimulation of 5HT neurons which terminate in the mediobasal hypothalamus. This conclusion must be tempered, however, by the report that morphine increases serum prolactin levels in the rat following hypothalamic deafferentation (Grandison et al. 1980), which should eliminate extrahypothalamic afferent input to the tuberoinfundibular DA neurons. Morphine may, however, exert its neuroendocrinological effects by interacting with putative intrahypothalamic 5HT neurons.

EFFECTS OF ENDOCRINOLOGICAL MANIPULATIONS OF 5HT NEURONS

The following sections review the effects of endocrine manipulations on the dynamics of 5HT neuronal systems in the hypothalamus and ME; these include effects on concentrations of 5HT and 5HIAA, the rate of 5HT turnover, and the activity of tryptophan hydroxylase.

Prolactin

5HT neuronal systems are believed to exert a modulatory role in the regulation of prolactin release from the anterior pituitary. Although 5HT has no effect on the pituitary per se (Birge et al. 1970), pharmacological evidence suggests that 5HT neurons play a stimulatory role in situations where dynamic changes in prolactin secretion are occurring (see reviews, Müller et al. 1977; Weiner and Ganong 1978). Inhibition of 5HT synthesis with PCPA prevents the estrogen-progesterone-induced increase of prolactin in ovariectomized rats (Caligaris and Taleisnik 1974). 5HT agonists (quipazine), precursors (5HTP, tryptophan) and releasers (fenfluramine) all increase serum prolactin concentrations in rats (Müller et al. 1977; Weiner and Ganong 1978; Schettini et al. 1980). Fluoxetine, an inhibitor of neuronal uptake of 5HT does not alter resting concentrations of prolactin, but enhances the prolactin releasing actions of 5HTP (Krulich 1975; Clemens et al. 1977). Several putative 5HT antagonists are reported to attenuate or abolish the increases in serum prolactin concentrations resulting from a variety of pharmacological and endocrinological treatments.

There have been no reports on the effects of exogenously administered prolactin on the dynamics of 5HT neurons in the ME. On the other hand, there have been numerous efforts to relate physiologically-induced changes (e.g. stress, lactation, estrous cycle) in prolactin secretion to changes in the activity of hypothalamic 5HT neurons. These studies are discussed in the next section.

Luteinizing hormone and gonadal steroids

The role of 5HT neurons in controlling LH secretion is controversial. Administration of 5HT into the cerebral ventricles, inhibition of 5HT synthesis with PCPA, or destruction of 5HT neurons with 5,6- or 5,7-DHT have been reported to increase, decrease and produce no change in the basal secretion of LH. Nevertheless, the marked increases in serum LH concentrations that occur on the afternoon of proestrus or in estradiol-pretreated ovariectomized rats can be prevented by drugs which disrupt 5HT neurotransmission (Weiner and Ganong 1978; Baumgarten et al. 1978). In addition, there appears to be a correlation between the 5HT antagonistic properties of a number of tricyclic and ergot-derivative compounds with their ability to inhibit the pre-ovulatory surges of LH (Markó and Flückiger, 1980).

Unfortunately, there have been relatively few reports of experiments dealing with possible relationships between altered serum concentrations of LH and the activity of 5HT neurons in the mediobasal hypothalamus. The administration of melatonin is reported to suppress the ability of pinealectomy to induce ovulation in constant estrous-anovulatory rats and to increase the hypothalamic content of 5HT (Anton-Tay et al. 1968; Mess et al. 1971). It has been suggested that pinealectomy may induce ovulation by removing a melatonin-mediated stimulation of 5HT synthesis which normally inhibits LH secretion (Trentini et al. 1974).

Electrical stimulation of 5HT neurons in the dorsal raphe inhibits LH secretion in ovariectomized rats (Arendash and Gallo 1978) and the inhibition of LH and LH-RH release caused by stimulating the arcuate nucleus can be reversed by pretreating animals with PCPA (Gallo and Moberg 1977).

5HT neurons may play a role in the feedback regulation of LH secretion by gonadal steroids. The castration-induced increases of serum LH concentrations and 5HT concentrations in the ventromedial hypothalamic nucleus were reversed by the administration of testosterone (Van de Kar et al. 1978). In ovariectomized rats a single injection of estradiol reduced the serum concentration of LH without altering the 5HT content in the ME; the administration of progesterone caused a surge of LH and a marked increase in the concentration of 5HT (Crowley et al. 1979). Wirz-Justice and Hackman (1972) have reported a decreased ^{3}H-labelled 5HT uptake into hypothalamic slices of ovariectomized rats 2 h after a subcutaneous injection of estradiol. Ladisich (1974) demonstrated that progesterone administration in a dosage regimen producing plasma progesterone concentrations in a physiological range increased hypothalamic 5HT concentrations in ovariectomized rats 24 h following the last injection. On the other hand, neither LH-RH, pregnant mare serum gonadotropin, nor human chorionic gonadotropin caused any change in 5HT concentrations in the hypothalamus (Telegdy and Szontágh 1979). There have been no reports of changes in 5HT turnover in the ME following LH-RH or gonadotropin administration, but Fuxe et al. (1973b) reported that the inhibitory feedback exerted by estrogen on LH secretion was associated with an increase of 5HT turnover in the hypothalamus (as estimated by the rate of decline of 5HT after the administration of a tryptophan hydroxylase inhibitor). Kizer et al. (1976c) noted that tryptophan hydroxylase activity in the ME did not change following castration or the administration of testosterone.

ACTH and adrenocortical steroids

Results of a number of pharmacological experiments suggest that 5HT neurons exert a stimulatory effect on ACTH secretion (Fuller 1981). In general, administration of 5HT precursors or agonists increases serum concentrations of corticosterone, and these effects are blocked by pretreatment with putative 5HT antagonists. Presumably the increased circulating corticosteroids result from the ability of 5HT to release corticotropin-releasing hormone from the hypothalamus, and the subsequent release of ACTH from the anterior pituitary.

There are relatively few reports on the effects of ACTH or adrenal corticoids on the activity of central 5HT neurons and, unfortunately, most of these do not focus on the ME or hypothalamus. The administration of hydrocortisone to neonatal rats increased 5HT concentrations in the mediobasal hypothalamus when examined 30 days later (Ulrich et al. 1975). Sze et al. (1976) induced tryptophan hydroxylase in neonatal but not adult rat brains with multiple injections of cortisone. Neckers and Sze (1975) observed an increased uptake of tryptophan (and thus an increased 5HT synthesis) within hours after the administration of large doses of hydrocortisone to mice. On the other hand, dramatic decreases of 5HT have been observed in the brains of rats following the administration of glucocorticoids (Curzon and Green 1968, 1971; Nisticò and Preziosi 1969; Scapagnini et al. 1969). The different results may be related to the dose of glucocorticoid administered, since Kovacs et al. (1975) found that low doses (1 mg kg^{-1}) of corticosterone increased while a higher dose (10 mg kg^{-1}) reduced the brain concentration of 5HT.

Adrenalectomy is reported to reduce the concentration and uptake of 5HT (Vermes et al. 1973b; Telegdy and Vermes 1975) and the activity of tryptophan hydroxylase (Azmitia and McEwen 1969) in the hypothalamus; some of these effects are reversed by corticosteroid replacement. Sze et al. (1976) noted that adrenalectomy blocked the normal increase of tryptophan hydroxylase in the developing brain. On the other hand, Kizer et al. (1976c) failed to observe any change in tryptophan hydroxylase activity in the ME following adrenalectomy or dexamethasone administration.

In general, results of studies carried out to date suggest that release of CRH from the ME is under a dual feedback control by corticoids and ACTH and that part of this feedback control is mediated by a 5HT neuronal system.

Other hormones

There is no consistency in reports relating central 5HT neuronal systems with the regulation of the thyroid gland. It has been reported that 5HTP administration increases (Shopsin et al. 1974) and tryptophan administration decreases (Mueller et al. 1976b) TSH secretion. Inhibition of 5HT synthesis with PCPA is reported to decrease TSH secretion (Shopsin et al. 1974) but not alter the thyrotropin releasing hormone content in the hypothalamus of rats (Kardon et al. 1977). Rastogi and Singhal (1974) noted that the 5HT content and tryptophan hydroxylase activity in the hypothalamus were reduced in hypothyroid rats, and that these effects were reversed by triiodothyronine administration. Similarly, Jacoby et al. (1975) reported that thyroidectomy decreased and thyroxine pretreatment increased the rate of 5HTP accumulation in the brain (an in vivo estimate of tryptophan hydroxylase activity). On the other hand, Kizer et al. (1976c) found no change in tryptophan hydroxylase activity in the ME or arcuate nucleus of thyroidectomized or thyroxine-pretreated rats.

Growth hormone, like prolactin, does not appear to act on a specific target organ, which prompts the speculation that, like prolactin, growth hormone may act in the hypothalamus to regulate its own secretion. The mechanism of such a postulated feedback loop has not been elucidated but indirect experiments suggest that 5HT neurons may play a role in such a mechanism. Brain concentrations of 5HT were unchanged in hypophysectomized rats while the concentrations of tryptophan and 5HIAA were increased, suggesting an increased activity of 5HT neurons (Cocchi et al. 1975). The administration of growth hormone reversed the elevated concentrations of tryptophan and 5HIAA in the hypophysectomized animals suggesting that it is the lack of this hormone which is responsible for the apparent increased 5HT neuronal activity in the brains of hypophysectomized rats. Finally, pre-treatment with growth hormone, implantations of bovine or human growth hormone into central nervous system sites, or implantation of a growth hormone-secreting tumor have been shown to prevent the increased growth hormone release induced by insulin injection in rats, suggesting that growth hormone may feedback to inhibit its own secretion (Müller 1973).

PHYSIOLOGICALLY INDUCED CHANGES IN THE DYNAMICS OF 5HT NEURONS IN THE MEDIAN EMINENCE–HYPOTHALAMUS

Cyclical changes

The concentrations of 5HT and 5HIAA and rate of turnover of 5HT (rate of decline of 5HIAA after MAO inhibition) in the anterior hypothalamus of ovariectomized rats are lower in the afternoon than they are in the morning (Munaro 1978). Estradiol treatment for three days reduced the values in the morning and thus abolished the morning-afternoon differences. Progesterone treatment of the ovariectomized, estrogen-primed rats reinstated the cyclical patterns to those observed in ovariectomized animals. It is not obvious why estrogens alter the dynamics of 5HT neurons only in the mornings.

The turnover of 5HT in the hypothalamus of female rats is reported to be greater at the time of the proestrous preovulatory surge of LH than it is at the end of the surge (Walker 1980). Furthermore, when the LH surge was prolonged by exposing the rats to light on the evening of proestrus the hypothalamic 5HT turnover remained high. 5HT antagonists and agonists also altered the preovulatory surge of LH in a temporally dependent manner. These results suggest that the proestrous surge of LH is accompanied by and may be partially dependent upon 5HT neuronal activity.

Lactation

Results of studies in the lactating rat suggest that 5HT neuronal systems are involved in the suckling-induced release of prolactin. The dramatic increase in serum prolactin concentrations observed 5–10 min after the onset of the suckling stimulus is maintained until the suckling stimulus is removed (Kordon et al. 1973). This response can be abolished by pretreatment with PCPA, and re-established by administering 5HTP (Kordon et al. 1973; Héry et al. 1976). Mena et al. (1976) observed a decrease in hypothalamic 5HT and an increase in 5HIAA within 5 min of the suckling stimulus, and this effect was maintained as long as suckling was continued. These results suggest that hypothalamic 5HT neurons are activated during suckling.

Stress

Pharmacological studies suggest that the stress-induced increase of serum concentrations of prolactin, ACTH and corticosteroids are associated with an activation of hypothalamic 5HT neuronal systems. For example, putative 5HT antagonists block while 5HT uptake inhibitors enhance the stress-induced release of prolactin (Krulich 1975) and ACTH and corticosteroids (Fuller 1981). Accordingly, efforts have been made to relate the stress-induced endocrine changes to alterations in the activity of 5HT neurons in the hypothalamus. Palkovits et al. (1976) reported a decreased content of 5HT and activity of tryptophan hydroxylase in the ME 3 h after immobilization (restraint) or formaldehyde injections. On the other hand, Čulman et al. (1980) noted an increased concentration of 5HT in the ME after 5 and 15 min of restraint. Technical problems have made it difficult to perform 5HT turnover studies in the ME, but Mueller et al. (1976b) noted an increase in 5HT turnover in the hypothalamus after immobilization stress, while Morgan et al. (1975) reported no change in 5HT turnover in the diencephalon (hypothalamus plus thalamus). With results reported to date, it is difficult to know whether 5HT neurons are activated during stressful situations in the rat.

ACKNOWLEDGEMENTS

The authors acknowledge the excellent assistance of Diane Hummel in the preparation of the manuscript. Craig A. Johnston is a predoctoral student at Michigan State University supported by USPHS grant NS9174; unpublished observations cited in the manuscript are the result of experiments supported by this grant.

REFERENCES

Adér, J.P., Mukiet, F.A.J., Jeuring, H.J. and Korf, J. (1978) On the origin of vanillylmandelic acid and 3-methoxy-4-hydroxyphenylglycol in the rat brain. J. Neurochem. 30, 1213-1216.

Ahrén, K., Fuxe, K., Hamberger, L. and Hökfelt, T. (1971) Turnover changes in the tubero-infundibular dopamine neurons during the ovarian cycle of the rat. Endocrinology 88, 1415-1424.

Ajika, K. and Hökfelt, T. (1973) Ultrastructural identification of catecholamine neurones in the hypothalamic periventricular-arcuate nucleus-median eminence complex with special reference to quantitative aspects. Brain Res. 57, 97-117.

Algeri, S., Consolazione, A., Calderini, G., Achilli, G., Puche-Canas, E. and Garattini, S. (1978) Effect of the administration of (D-Ala)^2-methionine-enkephalin on the serotonin metabolism in rat brain. Experientia 34, 1488-1489.

Alper, R.H., Demarest, K.T. and Moore, K.E. (1980) Morphine differentially alters synthesis and turnover of dopamine in central neuronal systems. J. Neural Transmission 48, 157-165.

Andersson, K., Fuxe, K., Eneroth, P., Gustafsson, J.A. and Skett, P. (1977) On catecholamine control of growth hormone regulation. Evidence for discrete changes in dopamine and noradrenaline turnover following growth hormone administration. Neurosci. Lett. 5, 83-89.

Annunziato, L. and Moore, K.E. (1978) Prolactin in CSF selectively increases dopamine turnover in the median eminence. Life Sci. 22, 2037-2042.

Annunziato, L., Leblanc, P., Kordon, C. and Weiner, R.I. (1980) Differences in the kinetics of dopamine uptake in synaptosome preparations of the median eminence relative to other dopaminergically innervated brain regions. Neuroendocrinology 31, 316-320.

Anton-Tay, F., Chou, C., Anton, S. and Wurtman, R.J. (1968) Brain serotonin concentration: Elevation following intraperitoneal administration of melatonin. Science 162, 277-278.

Arendash, G.W. and Gallo, R.V. (1978) Serotonin involvement in the inhibition of episodic luteinizing hormone release during electrical stimulation of the midbrain dorsal raphe nucleus in ovariectomized rats. Endocrinology 102, 1199-1206.

Azmitia, E.C. (1978) The serotonin-producing neurons of the midbrain median and dorsal raphe nuclei. Handbook of Psychopharmacology (Iversen, LL., Iversen, S.D. and Snyder, S.H. eds), Vol. 9, pp. 233-314, Plenum Press, New York.

Azmitia, E.C., Jr. and McEwen, B.S. (1969) Corticosterone regulation of tryptophan hydroxylase in midbrain of the rat. Science 166, 1274-1276.

Bacopoulos, N.G., Bhatnagar, R.K., Schnute, W.J. and Van Orden, L.S., III (1975) On the use of the fluorescence histochemical method to estimate catecholamine content in brain. Neuropharmacology 14, 291-299.

Baumgarten, H.G., Björklund, A. and Wuttke, W. (1978) Neural control of pituitary LH, FSH and prolactin secretion: The role of serotonin. In: Brain-Endocrine Interaction. III. Neural Hormones and Reproduction, 3rd International Symposium Würzburg 1977, pp. 327-343, Karger Press, Basel.

Beaudet, A. and Descarries, L. (1979) Radioautographic characterization of a serotonin-accumulating nerve cell group in adult rat hypothalamus. Brain Res. 160, 231-243.

Belenky, M.A., Chetverukhin, V.K. and Polenov, A.L. (1979) Quantitative radioautographic light and electron microscopic analysis of the localization of monoamines in the median eminence of the rat. II. Serotonin. Cell Tissue Res. 204, 305-317.

Ben-Jonathan, N., Oliver, C., Weiner, H.J., Mical, R.S. and Porter, J.C. (1977) Dopamine in hypophysial portal blood of the rat during the estrous cycle and throughout pregnancy. Endocrinology 100, 452-458.

Ben-Jonathan, N., Neill, M.A., Arbogast, L.A., Peters, L.L. and Hoefer, M.T. (1980) Dopamine in hypophysial portal blood – Relationship to circulating prolactin in pregnant and lactating rats. Endocrinology 106, 690-697.

Besser, G.M., Delitala, G., Grossman, A. and Yeo, T. (1980) Metergoline and cyproheptadine suppress prolactin release by a non-5-hydroxytryptaminergic, non-dopaminergic mechanism. Brit. J. Pharmacol. 70, 5-7.

Birge, C.A., Jacobs, L.S., Hammer, C.T. and Daughaday, W.H. (1970) Catecholamine inhibition of prolactin secretion by isolated rat adenohypophyses. Endocrinology 86, 120-130.

Björklund, A., Falck, B., Hromek, F., Owman, C. and West, K.A. (1970) Identification and terminal distribution of the tubero-hypophyseal monoamine fiber system in the rat by means of stereotaxic and microspectrofluorimetric techniques. Brain Res. 17, 1-24.

Björklund, A., Falck, B., Nobin, A. and Stenevi, U. (1973a) Organization of the dopamine and noradrenaline innervations of the median eminence-pituitary regions in the rat. In: Neurosecretion – The Final Neuroendocrine Pathway (Knowles, F. and Vollrath, L. eds), pp. 209-222, Springer-Verlag, New York.

Björklund, A., Moore, R.Y., Nobin, A. and Stenevi, U. (1973b) The organization of tubero-hypophyseal and reticulo-infundibular catecholamine neuron systems in the rat brain. Brain Res. 51, 171-191.

Breese, G.R. (1975) Chemical and immunochemical lesions by specific neurotoxic substances and antisera. Handbook of Psychopharmacology (Iversen, L.L., Iversen, S.D. and Snyder, S.H. eds), Vol. 1, pp. 137-189, Plenum Press, New York.

Brown, G.M., Seeman, P. and Lee, T. (1976) Dopamine-neuroleptic receptors in basal hypothalamus and pituitary. Endocrinology 99, 1407-1410.

Brownstein, M.J., Palkovits, M., Saavedra, J.M. and Kizer, J.S. (1976a) Distribution of hypothalamic hormones and neurotransmitters within the diencephalon. In: Frontiers in Neuroendocrinology (Ganong, W.F. and Martini, L. eds), Vol. 4, pp. 1-23, Raven Press, New York.

Brownstein, M.J., Palkovits, M., Tappaz, M.L., Saavedra, J.M. and Kizer, J.S. (1976b) Effect of surgical isolation of the hypothalamus on its neurotransmitter content. Brain Res. 117, 287-295.

Bruni, J.F., Van Vugt, D., Marshall, S. and Meites, J. (1977) Effects of naloxone, morphine and methionine enkephalin on serum prolactin, luteinizing hormone, follicle stimulating hormone, thyroid stimulating hormone, and growth hormone. Life Sci. 21, 461-466.

Calas, A., Alonso, G., Arnauld, E. and Vincent, J.D. (1974) Demonstration of indoleaminergic fibers in the median eminence of the duck, rat and monkey. Nature 250, 241-243.

Caligaris, L. and Taleisnik, S. (1974) Involvement of neurons containing 5-hydroxytryptamine in the mechanism of prolactin release induced by oestrogen. J. Endocrinol. 62, 25-33.

Carlsson, A. and Lindqvist, M. (1973) In vivo measurements of tryptophan and tyrosine hydroxylase activities in mouse brain. J. Neural Transmission 34, 79-91.

Carlsson, A., Falck, B. and Hillarp, N.-A. (1962) Cellular localization of brain monoamines. Acta Physiol. Scand. 56, Suppl. 196.

Carlsson, A., Davis, J.N., Kehr, W., Lindqvist, M. and Atack, C.V. (1972a) Simultaneous measurement of tyrosine and tryptophan hydroxylase activities in brain in vivo using an inhibitor of the aromatic amino acid decarboxylase. Naunyn-Schmiedeberg's Arch. Pharmacol. 275, 153-168.

Carlsson, A., Kehr, W., Lindqvist, M., Magnusson, T. and Atack, C.V. (1972b) Regulation of monoamine metabolism in the central nervous system. Pharmacol. Rev. 24, 371-384.

Carr, L.A. and Voogt, J.L. (1980) Catecholamine synthesizing enzymes in the hypothalamus during the estrous cycle. Brain Res. 196, 437-446.

Chiocchio, S.R., Cannata, M.A. and Tramezzani, J.H. (1976a) The size, weight and catecholamine content of the median eminence of the rat. Brain Res. 110, 612-618.

Chiocchio, S.R., Negro-Vilar, A. and Tramezzani, J.H. (1976b) Acute changes in norepinephrine content in median eminence induced by orchidectomy or testosterone replacement. Endocrinology 99, 629-635.

Chiocchio, S.R., Cannata, M.A., Cordero-Funes, J.R. and Tramezzani, J.H. (1979) Involvement of adenohypophysial dopamine in the regulation of prolactin release during suckling. Endocrinology 105, 544-547.

Clemens, J.A. and Shaar, C.J. (1980) Control of prolactin secretion in mammals. Fed. Proc. 39, 2588-2592.

Clemens, J.A., Sawyer, B.D. and Cerimele, B. (1977) Further evidence that serotonin is a neurotransmitter involved in the control of prolactin secretion. Endocrinology 100, 692-698.

Clemens, J.A., Smalstig, E.B., Shaar, C.J., Kornfeld, E.C. and Bach, N. (1980) Effects of drugs that alter dopaminergic neurotransmission on prolactin release: A pituitary or CNS site of action. In: Neuroactive Drugs in Endocrinology (Müller, E.E. ed.), pp. 201-212, Elsevier/North-Holland, Amsterdam.

Cocchi, D., Di Giulio, A., Groppetti, A., Mantegazza, P., Müller, E.E. and Spano, P.F. (1975) Hormonal inputs and brain tryptophan metabolism: The effect of growth hormone. Experientia 31, 384-386.

Cocchi, D., Locatelli, V., Carminati, R. and Müller, E.E. (1978) Mechanisms underlying the prolactin-lowering effect of metergoline in the rat. Life Sci. 23, 927-936.

Cocchi, D., Locatelli, V., Gil-Ad, I., Mantegazza, P. and Müller, E.E. (1979) Control of growth hormone and prolactin secretion: Neuropharmacological aspects. In: Neuroendocrinology: Biological and Clinical Aspects (Polleri, A. and MacLeod, R.M. eds), pp. 27-46, Academic Press, New York.

Corrodi, H., Fuxe, K., Lidbrink, P. and Olson, L. (1971) Minor tranquilizers, stress and central catecholamine neurons, Brain Res. 29, 1-16.

Cramer, O.M., Parker, C.R. and Porter, J.C. (1979a) Estrogen inhibition of dopamine release into hypophysial portal blood. Endocrinology 104, 419-422.

Cramer, O.M., Parker, C.R. and Porter, J.C. (1979b) Secretion of dopamine into hypophysial portal blood by rats bearing prolactin-secreting tumors or ectopic pituitary glands. Endocrinology 105, 636-640.

Cramer, O.M., Parker, C.R. and Porter, J.C. (1979c) Stimulation of dopamine release into hypophysial portal blood by administration of progesterone. Endocrinology 105, 929-933.

Crombeen, J.P., Kraak, J.C. and Poppe, H. (1978) Reversed-phase systems for the analysis of catecholamines and related compounds by high-performance liquid chromatography. J. Chromatogr. 167, 219-230.

Crowley, W.R., O'Donohue, T.L., Muth, E.A. and Jacobowitz, D.M. (1979) Effects of ovarian hormones on levels of luteinizing hormone in plasma and on serotonin concentrations in discrete brain nuclei. Brain Res. Bull. 4, 571-574.

Cuello, A.C., Horn, A.S., Mackay, A.V.P. and Iversen, L.L. (1973) Catecholamines in the median eminence: New evidence for a major noradrenergic input. Nature (London) 243, 465-467.

Cuello, A.C., Shoemaker, W.J. and Ganong, W.F. (1974) Effect of 6-hydroxydopamine on hypothalamic norepinephrine and dopamine content, ultrastructure of the median eminence and plasma corticosterone. Brain Res. 78, 57-69.

Čulman, J., Kvetňanský, R., Torda, T. and Murgaš, K. (1980) Serotonin concentration in individual hypothalamic nuclei of rats exposed to acute immobilization stress. Neuroscience 5, 1503-1506.

Curzon, G. and Green, A.R. (1968) Effect of hydrocortisone on rat brain 5-hydroxytryptamine. Life Sci. 7, 657-663.

Curzon, G. and Green, A.R. (1971) Regional and subcellular changes in the concentrations of 5-hydroxytrypta-mine and 5-hydroxyindoleacetic acid in the rat brain caused by hydrocortisone, DL-α-methyltryptophan, l-kynurenine and immobilization. Brit. J. Pharmacol. 43, 39-52.

Curzon, G. and Knott, P.J. (1977) Environmental, toxicological, and related aspects of tryptophan metabolism with particular reference to the central nervous system. CRC Crit. Rev. Toxicol. 5, 145-187.

Curzon, G., Joseph, M.H. and Knott, P.J. (1972) Effects of immobilization and food deprivation on rat brain tryptophan metabolism. J. Neurochem. 19, 1963-1974.

Dahlström, A. and Fuxé, K. (1964) Evidence for the existence of monoamine-containing neurons in the central nervous system. Acta Physiol. Scand. 62, Suppl. 232, 1-55.

Daikoku, S., Ozaki, Y. and Yamamoto, Y. (1978) Aminergic innervation of the subependymal neurons in the median eminence. Brain Res. 142, 353-357.

Day, T.A. and Willoughby, J.O. (1980) Noradrenergic afferents to median eminence: Inhibitory role in rhythmic growth hormone secretion. Brain Res. 202, 335-346.

Demarest, K.T. and Moore, K.E. (1979a) Lack of a high affinity transport system for dopamine in the median eminence and posterior pituitary. Brain Res. 171, 545-551.

Demarest, K.T. and Moore, K.E. (1979b) Comparison of dopamine synthesis regulation in terminals of nigrostriatal, mesolimbic, tuberoinfundibular and tuberohypophyseal neurons. J. Neural Transmission 46, 263-277.

Demarest, K.T. and Moore, K.E. (1980) Accumulation of L-dopa in the median eminence: An index of tuberoinfundibular dopaminergic nerve activity. Endocrinology 106, 463-468.

Demarest, K.T. and Moore, K.E. (1981) Disruption of 5-hydroxytryptaminergic neuronal function blocks the action of morphine on tuberoinfundibular dopaminergic neurons. Life Sci. 28, 1345-1351.

Demarest, K.T. Alper, R.A. and Moore, K.E. (1979) DOPA accumulation is a measure of dopamine synthesis in the median eminence and posterior pituitary. J. Neural Transmission 46, 183-193.

Demarest, K.T., Johnston, C.A. and Moore, K.E. (1981) Biochemical indices of catecholaminergic neuronal activity in the median eminence during the estrous cycle of the rat. Neuroendocrinology 32, 24-27.

Deyo, S.N., Swift, R.M. and Miller, R.J. (1979) Morphine and endorphins modulate dopamine turnover in rat median eminence. Proc. Natl. Acad. Sci. USA 76, 3006-3009.

Deyo, S.N., Swift, R.H., Miller, R.J. and Fang, V.S. (1980) Development of tolerance to the prolactin-releasing action of morphine and its modulation by hypothalamic dopamine. Endocrinology 106, 1469-1474.

DuPont, A., Cusan, L., Ferland, L., Lemay, A. and Labrie, F. (1979) Evidence for a role of endorphins in the control of prolactin secretion. In: Central Nervous System Effects of Hypothalamic Hormones and Other Peptides (Collu, R., Barbeau, A., Ducharme, J.R. and Rochefort, J.G. eds), pp. 283-300, Raven Press, New York.

Eikenburg, D.C., Ravitz, A.J., Gudelsky, G.A. and Moore, K.E. (1977) Effects of estrogen on prolactin and tuberoinfundibular dopaminergic neurons. J. Neural Transmission 45, 235-244.

Fadda, F., Argiolas, A., Melis, M.R., Tissari, H.A., Onali, P.L. and Gessa, G.L. (1978) Stress-induced increase in 3,4-dihydroxyphenylacetic acid (DOPAC) levels in the cerebral cortex and in nucleus accumbens: Reversal by diazepam. Life Sci. 23, 2219-2224.

Falck, B., Hillarp, N.-A., Thieme, G. and Torp, A. (1962) Fluorescence of catecholamines and related compounds condensed with formaldehyde. J. Histochem. Cytochem. 10, 348-354.

Fekete, M., Herman, J., Palkovits, M. and Stark, E. (1976) ACTH-induced changes in the transmitter amine concentrations of individual brain nuclei of the rat. In: Catecholamines and Stress (Usdin, E., Kvetňanský, and Kopin, I.J. eds), pp. 69-75, Pergamon Press, Oxford.

Fekete, M.I.K., Kanyicska, B. and Herman, J.P. (1978) Simultaneous radioenzymatic assay of catecholamines and dihydroxyphenylacetic acid (DOPAC). Comparison of effects of drugs on tuberoinfundibular and striatal dopamine metabolism and on plasma prolactin level. Life Sci. 23, 1549-1556.

Fekete, M.I.K., Herman, J.P., Kanyicska, B. and Palkovits, M. (1979) Dopamine, noradrenaline and 3,4-di-hydroxyphenylacetic acid (DOPAC) levels of individual brain nuclei, effects of haloperidol and pargyline. J. Neural. Transmission 45, 207-218.

Fekete, M.I.K., Szentendrei, T., Herman, J.P. and Kanyicska, B. (1980) Effects of reserpine and antidepressants on dopamine and DOPAC (3,4-dihydroxyphenylacetic acid) concentrations in the striatum, olfactory tubercle and median eminence of rats. Eur. J. Pharmacol. 64, 231-238.

Ferland, L., Fuxe, K., Eneroth, P., Gustafsson, J.A. and Skett, P. (1977) Effects of methionine-enkephalin on prolactin release and catecholamine levels and turnover on the median eminence. Eur. J. Pharmacol. 43, 89-90.

Fernstrom, J.D. and Faller, D.V. (1978) Neutral amino acids in the brain: Changes in response to food ingestion. J. Neurochem. 30, 1531-1538.

Fernstrom, J.D. and Wurtman, R.J. (1971) Brain serotonin content: Physiological dependence on plasma tryptophan levels. Science 173, 149-152.

Fuller, R.W. (1981) Serotonergic stimulation of pituitary-adrenocortical function in rats. Neuroendocrinology 32, 118-127.

Fuxe, K. (1963) Cellular localization of monoamines in the median eminence and infundibular stem of some mammals. Acta Physiol. Scand. 58, 383-384.

Fuxe, K. and Hökfelt, T. (1967) The influence of central catecholamine neurons on the hormone secretion from the anterior and posterior pituitary. Neurosecretion. IV International Symposium on Neurosecretion (Stutinsky, F. ed.), pp. 165-177, Springer-Verlag, New York.

Fuxe, K. and Hökfelt, T. (1969) Monoamine afferent input to the hypothalamus and the dopamine afferent input to the median eminence. Progress Endocrinol. 184, 495-502.

Fuxe, K. and Hökfelt, T. (1974) The effects of hormones and psychoactive drugs on the tuberoinfundibular neurons. In: Some Aspects of Hypothalamic Regulation of Endocrine Functions, pp. 51-61, F.K. Schattaver Verlag, Stuttgart.

Fuxe, K., Hökfelt, T. and Nilsson, O. (1969a) Castration, sex hormones and tuberoinfundibular dopamine neurons. Neuroendocrinology 5, 107-120.

Fuxe, K., Hökfelt, T. and Nilsson, O. (1969b) Factors involved in the control of the activity of tubero-infundibular dopamine neurons during pregnancy and lactation. Neuroendocrinology 5, 257-270.

Fuxe, K., Hökfelt, T., Jonsson, G., Levine, S., Lidbrink, P. and Löfström, A. (1973a) Brain and pituitary–adrenal interactions: Studies on central monoamine neurones. In: Brain-Pituitary-Adrenal Interrelationships (Brodish, A. and Redgate, E.S. eds), pp. 239-269, Karger Press, Basel.

Fuxe, K., Hökfelt, T., Jonsson, G. and Löfström, A. (1973b) Recent morphological and functional studies on hypothalamic dopaminergic and noradrenergic mechanisms. In: Frontiers in Catecholamine Research (Usdin, E. and Snyder, S.H. eds), pp. 787-794, Pergamon, Oxford.

Fuxe, K., Agnati, L., Tsuchiya, K., Hökfelt, T., Johansson, O., Jonsson, G., Lidbrink, P. and Löfström, A. (1975a) Effect of antipsychotic drugs on central catecholamine neurons of rat brain. In: Antipsychotic Drugs, Pharmacodynamics and Pharmacokinetics (Sedvall, G. ed.), pp. 117-132, Pergamon, New York.

Fuxe, K., Agnati, L.F., Hökfelt, T., Jonsson, G., Lidbrink, P., Ljungdahl, A., Löfström, A. and Ungerstedt, U. (1975b) The effect of dopamine receptor stimulating and blocking agents on the activity of supersensitive dopamine receptors and on the amine turnover in various dopamine nerve terminals in the rat brain. J. Pharmacol. (Paris) 6, 117-129.

Fuxe, K., Hökfelt, T., Agnati, L., Löfström, A., Everitt, B., Johansson, O., Jonsson, G., Wuttke, W. and Goldstein, M. (1976) Role of monoamines in the control of gonadotropin secretion. In: Neuroendocrine Regulation of Fertility (Kumar, A. ed.), pp. 124-140, Karger, Basel.

Fuxe, K., Ferland, L., Eneroth, P. and Gustafsson, J.A. (1977) Neurotransmitter-neuropeptide interactions: Effects of opioid peptides and prolactin on central dopamine pathways. Exp. Brain Res. 28, R53-R54.

Fuxe, K., Ferland, L., Andersson, K., Eneroth, P., Gustafsson, J.A. and Skett, P. (1978) On the functional role of hypothalamic catecholamine neurons in the control of the secretion of hormones from the anterior pituitary, particularly in the control of LH and prolactin secretion. In: Brain-Endocrine Interaction. Neural Hormones and Reproduction (Scott, D.E., Kozlowski, G.P. and Weindl, A. eds), pp. 172-182, Karger, Basel.

Fuxe, K., Andersson, K., Hökfelt, T., Mutt, V., Ferland, L., Agnati, L.F., Ganten, D., Said, S., Eneroth, P. and Gustafsson, J.A. (1979) Localization and possible function of peptidergic neurons and their interactions with central catecholamine neurons, and the central actions of gut hormones. Fed. Proc. 38, 2333-2340.

Fuxe, K., Andersson, K., Locatelli, V., Mutt, V., Lundberg, J., Hökfelt, T., Agnati, L.F., Eneroth, P. and Bolme, P. (1980) Neuropeptides and central catecholamine systems: Interactions in neuroendocrine and central cardiovascular regulation. In: Neural Peptides and Neuronal Communication (Costa, E. and Trabucchi, M. eds), Adv. Biochem. Psychopharmacol. 22, 37-50.

Gallardo, E.A., Voloschin, L.M. and Negro-Vilar, A. (1978) Effect of independent deafferentation of each border of the medial basal hypothalamus on catecholamine content of the median eminence and on serum LH and prolactin levels in ovariectomized rats. Brain Res. 148, 121-128.

Gallo, R.V. and Moberg, G.P. (1977) Serotonin mediated inhibition of episodic luteinizing hormone release during electrical stimulation of the arcuate nucleus in ovariectomized rats. Endocrinology 100, 945-954.

Ganong, W.F. (1977) Neurotransmitters involved in ACTH secretion: Catecholamines. Ann. N.Y. Acad. Sci. 297, 509-517.

Garcia-Sepilla, J.A., Ahtee, L., Magnusson, T. and Carlsson, A. (1978) Opiate-receptor mediated changes in monoamine synthesis in rat brain. J. Pharm. Pharmacol. 30, 613-621.

Gibbs, D.M. and Neill, J.B. (1978) Dopamine levels in hypophysial stalk blood in rat are sufficient to inhibit prolactin secretion in vivo. Endocrinology 102, 1895-1900.

Grandison, L., Fratta, W. and Guidotti, A. (1980) Location and characterization of opiate receptors regulating pituitary secretion. Life Sci. 26, 1633-1642.

Gudelsky, G.A. and Moore, K.E. (1976) Differential drug effects on dopamine concentrations and rates of turnover in the median eminence, olfactory tubercle and corpus striatum. J. Neural Transmission 38, 95-105.

Gudelsky, G.A. and Moore, K.E. (1977) A comparison of the effects of haloperidol on dopamine turnover in the striatum, olfactory tubercle and median eminence. J. Pharmacol. Exp. Ther. 202, 149-156.

Gudelsky, G.A. and Porter, J.C. (1979a) Release of newly synthesized dopamine into the hypophysial portal vasculature of the rat. Endocrinology 104, 583-587.

Gudelsky, G.A. and Porter, J.C. (1979b) Morphine- and opioid peptide-induced inhibition of the release of dopamine from tuberoinfundibular neurons. Life Sci. 25, 1697-1702.

Gudelsky, G.A. and Porter, J.C. (1980) Release of dopamine from tuberoinfundibular neurons into pituitary stalk blood after prolactin or haloperidol administration. Endocrinology 106, 526-529.

Gudelsky, G.A., Simpkins, J., Mueller, G.P., Meites, J. and Moore, K.E. (1976) Selective actions of prolactin on catecholamine turnover in the hypothalamus and on serum LH and FSH. Neuroendocrinology 22, 206-215.

Gudelsky, G.A., Annunziato, L. and Moore, K.E. (1977) Increase in dopamine content of the rat median eminence after long-term ovariectomy and its reversal by estrogen replacement. Endocrinology 101, 1894-1897.

Gudelsky, G.A., Annunziato, L. and Moore, K.E. (1978) Localization of the site of the haloperidol-induced, prolactin-mediated increase of dopamine turnover in the median eminence: Studies in rats with complete hypothalamic deafferentation. J. Neural Transmission 42, 181-192.

Gudelsky, G.A., Nansel, D.D. and Porter, J.C. (1981) Role of estrogen in the dopaminergic control of prolactin secretion. Endocrinology 108, 440-444.

Haubrich, D.R. and Blake, D.E. (1973) Modification of serotonin metabolism in rat brain after acute or chronic administration of morphine. Biochem. Pharmacol. 22, 2753-2795.

Hefti, F. and Lichtensteiger, W. (1976) An enzymatic-isotopic method for DOPA and its use for the measurement of dopamine synthesis in rat substantia nigra. J. Neurochem. 27, 647-649.

Héry, F., Rouer, E. and Glowinski, J. (1972) Daily variation of serotonin metabolism in the rat brain. Brain Res. 43, 445-465.

Héry, M., LaPlante, E. and Kordon, C. (1976) Participation of serotonin in the plasma release of LH. I. Evidence from pharmacological experiments. Endocrinology 99, 496-503.

Hohn, K.G. and Wuttke, W.O. (1978) Changes in catecholamine turnover in the anterior part of the mediobasal hypothalamus and the medial preoptic area in response to hyperprolactinemia in ovariectomized rats. Brain Res. 156, 241-252.

Hökfelt, T. and Fuxe, K. (1972a) Effects of prolactin and ergot alkaloids on the tuberoinfundibular dopamine neurons. Neuroendocrinology 9, 100-122.

Hökfelt, T. and Fuxe, K. (1972b) On the morphology and the neuroendocrine role of the hypothalamic catecholamine neurons. In: Brain-Endocrine Interaction. Median Eminence: Structure and Function (Knigge, K.M., Scott, D.E. and Weindl, A. eds), pp. 181-223, Karger, Basel.

Hökfelt, T., Fuxe, K., Goldstein, M. and Johansson, O. (1974) Immunohistochemical evidence for the existence of adrenaline neurons in the rat brain. Brain Res. 66, 235-251.

Hökfelt, T., Johansson, O., Fuxe, K., Löfström, A., Goldstein, M., Park, D., Ebstein, R., Fraser, H., Jeffcoate, S., Efendic, S., Luft, R. and Arimura, A. (1976) Mapping and relationship of hypothalamic neurotransmitters and hypothalamic hormones. Proc. 6th Int. Cong. Pharmacol. 3, 93-110.

Hökfelt, T., Johansson, O., Ljungdall, A., Lundberg, J., Schultzberg, M., Fuxe, K., Goldstein, M., Steinbusch, H., Verhofstad, A. and Edde, R.P. (1979) Neurotransmitters and neuropeptides: Distribution patterns and cellular localization as revealed by immunocytochemistry. In: Central Regulation of the Endocrine System (Fuxe, K., Hökfelt, T. and Luft, R. eds), pp. 31-48, Plenum, New York.

Holaday, J.W. and Loh, H.H. (1979) Endorphin-opiate interactions with neuroendocrine systems. In: Neurochemical Mechanisms of Opiates and Endorphins (Loh, H.H. and Ross, D.H. eds), Adv. Biochem. Psychopharmacol. 20, 227-258.

Honma, K. and Wuttke, W. (1980) Norepinephrine and dopamine turnover rates in the medial preoptic area and the mediobasal hypothalamus in the rat brain after various endocrinological manipulations. Endocrinology 106, 1848-1853.

Iwamoto, E.T. and Way, E.L. (1979) Opiate actions and catecholamines. In: Neurochemical Mechanisms of Opiates and Endorphins (Loh, H.H. and Ross, D.H. eds). Adv. Biochem. Psychopharmacol. 20, 357-407.

Jacoby, J.H., Mueller, G. and Wurtman, R.J. (1975) Thyroid state and brain monoamine metabolism. Endocrinology 97, 1332-1335.

Jahnke, G., Nicholson, G., Greeley, G.H., Youngblood, W.W., Prange Jr, A.G. and Kizer, J.S. (1980) Studies of the neural mechanisms by which hypothyroidism decreases prolactin secretion in the rat. Brain Res. 191, 429-442.

Johnston, C.A. and Moore, K.E. (1981) Characteristics of 5-hydroxytryptaminergic neurons in discrete regions of the rat hypothalamus. Fed. Proc. 40, 266.

Johnston, C.A., Demarest, K.T. and Moore, K.E. (1980) Cycloheximide disrupts the prolactin-mediated stimulation of dopamine synthesis in tuberoinfundibular neurons. Brain Res. 195, 236-240.

Jones, B.E. and Moore, R.Y. (1977) Ascending projections of the locus coeruleus in the rat. II. Autoradiographic study. Brain Res. 127, 23-53.

Jonsson, G., Fuxe, K. and Hökfelt, T. (1972) On the catecholamine innervation of the hypothalamus, with special reference to the median eminence. Brain Res. 40, 271-281.

Kardon, F., Marcus, R.J., Winokur, A. and Utiger, R.D. (1977) Thyrotropin-releasing hormone content of rat brain and hypothalamus: Results of endocrine and pharmacologic treatments. Endocrinology 100, 1604-1609.

Kavanagh, A. and Weisz, J. (1974) Localization of dopamine and norepinephrine in the medial basal hypothalamus of the rat. Neuroendocrinology 13, 201-217.

Kent, D.L. and Sladek, J.R. (1978) Histochemical, pharmacological and microspectrofluorometric analysis of new sites of serotonin localization with rat hypothalamus. J. Comp. Neurol. 180, 221-236.

Kizer, J.S., Palkovits, M., Zivin, J. and Brownstein, M. (1974) The effect of endocrinological manipulations on tyrosine hydroxylase and dopamine–β-hydroxylase activities in individual hypothalamic nuclei of the adult male rat. Endocrinology 95, 799-812.

Kizer, J.S., Muth, E. and Jacobowitz, D.M. (1976a) The effect of bilateral lesions of the ventral noradrenergic bundle on endocrine-induced changes of tyrosine hydroxylase in the rat median eminence. Endocrinology 98, 886-893.

Kizer, J.S., Palkovits, M. and Brownstein, M.J. (1976b) The projections of the A8, A9 and A10 dopaminergic cell bodies: Evidence for a nigral-hypothalamic median eminence dopaminergic pathway. Brain Res. 108, 363-370.

Kizer, J.S., Palkovits, M., Kopin, I.J., Saavedra, J.M. and Brownstein, M.J. (1976c) Lack of effect of various endocrine manipulations on tryptophan hydroxylase activity of individual nuclei of the hypothalamus, limbic system and midbrain of the rat. Endocrinology 98, 743-747.

Kizer, J.S., Humm, J., Nicholson, G., Greeley, G. and Youngblood, W. (1978) The effect of castration, thyroidectomy and haloperidol upon the turnover rates of dopamine and norepinephrine and the kinetic properties of tyrosine hydroxylase in discrete hypothalamic nuclei of the male rat. Brain Res. 146, 95-108.

Knigge, K.M., Scott, D.E. and Weindl, A. (eds) (1972) Brain-Endocrine Interaction. Median Eminence: Structure and Function, Karger, Basel.

Knowles, F. and Vollrath, L. (eds) (1974) Neurosecretion – The Final Neuroendocrine Pathway, Springer-Verlag, New York.

Koenig, J.I., Mayfield, M.A., McCann, S.M. and Krulich, L. (1979) Stimulation of prolactin secretion by morphine: Role of the central serotonergic system. Life Sci. 25, 853-864.

Koenig, J., Mayfield, M.A., Coppings, R.J., McCann, S.M. and Krulich, L. (1980) Role of central nervous system neurotransmitters in mediating the effects of morphine on growth hormone- and prolactin-secretion in the rat. Brain Res. 197, 453-468.

Kordon, C., Blake, C.A., Terkel, J. and Sawyer, C. (1973) Participation of serotonin-containing neurons in the suckling induced rise in plasma prolactin levels in lactating rats. Neuroendocrinology 13, 213-233.

Koslow, S. and Schlumpf, M. (1974) Quantitation of adrenaline in rat brain nuclei and areas by mass fragmento-graphy. Nature 251, 530-531.

Kovacs, G.L., Telegdy, G. and Lisśak, K. (1975) Dose-related dual action of corticosterone on hypothalamic serotonin content in rats. Acta Physiol. Acad. Sci. Hung. 46, 79-81.

Krieger, A. and Wuttke, W. (1980) Effects of ovariectomy and hyperprolactinemia on tyrosine hydroxylase and dopamine-β-hydroxylase activity in various limbic and hypothalamic structures. Brain Res. 193, 173-180.

Krstulovic, A.M. and Matzura, C. (1979) Rapid analysis of tryptophan metabolites using reversed-phase high-performance liquid chromatography with fluorometric detection. J. Chromatogr. 163, 72-76.

Krulich, L. (1975) The effect of a serotonin uptake inhibitor (Lilly 110 140) on the secretion of prolactin in the rat. Life Sci. 17, 1141-1144.

Kvetňanský, R., Palkovits, M., Mitro, A., Torda, T. and Mikulaj, L. (1977) Catecholamines in individual hypothalamic nuclei of acutely and repeatedly stressed rats. Neuroendocrinology, 23, 257-267.

Ladisich, W. (1974) Effect of progesterone on regional 5-hydroxytryptamine metabolism in the rat brain. Neuropharmacology 13, 877-883.

Lamberts, S.W.J. and MacLeod, R.M. (1978) The interaction of the serotonergic and dopaminergic systems on prolactin secretion in the rat. Endocrinology 103, 287-295.

Lidbrink, P., Corrodi, H., Fuxe, K. and Olson, L. (1972) Barbiturates and meprobamate: Decreases in catecholamine turnover of central dopamine and noradrenaline neuronal systems and the influence of immobilization stress. Brain Res. 45, 507-524.

Lin, R.C., Costa, E., Neff, N.H., Wang, C.T. and Ngai, S.H. (1969) In vivo measurement of 5-hydroxytryptamine turnover rate in the rat brain from the conversion of C^{14}-tryptophan to C^{14}-5-hydroxytryptamine. J. Pharmacol. Exp. Ther. 170, 232-238.

Lindvall, O. and Björklund, A. (1974) The glyoxylic acid fluorescence histochemical method: A detailed account of the methodology for the visualization of central catecholamine neurons. Histochemistry 39, 97-127.

Lindvall, O. and Björklund, A. (1978) Organization of catecholamine neurons in the rat central nervous system. In: Handbook of Psychopharmacology (Iversen, L.L., Iversen, S.D. and Snyder, S.H. eds), Vol. 9, pp. 139-231, Plenum Press, New York.

Löfström, A. (1977) Catecholamine turnover alterations in discrete areas of the median eminence of the 4 and 5 day cyclic rat. Brain Res. 120, 113-132.

Löfström, A. (1979) Catecholamine content of the rat median eminence following removal of endocrine glands. Psychoneuroendocrinology 4, 57-65.

Löfström, A., Jonsson, G. and Fuxe, K. (1976a) Microfluorimetric quantitation of catecholamine fluorescence in rat median eminence. I. Aspects on the distribution of dopamine and noradrenaline nerve terminals. J. Histochem. Cytochem. 24, 415-429.

Löfström, A., Jonsson, G., Wiesel, F.A. and Fuxe, K. (1976b) Microfluorimetric quantitation of catecholamine fluorescence in rat median eminence. II. Turnover changes in hormonal states. J. Histochem. Cytochem. 24, 430-442.

Löfström, A., Eneroth, P., Gustafsson, J.A. and Skett, P. (1977) Effects of estradiol benzoate on catecholamine levels and turnover in discrete areas of the median eminence and limbic forebrain, and on serum luteinizing hormone, follicle stimulating hormone and prolactin concentrations in the ovariectomized female rat. Endocrinology, 10, 1559-1569.

Login, I.S. and MacLeod, R.M. (1977) Prolactin in human and rat brain serum and CSF. Brain Res. 132, 477-485.

Login, I.S. and MacLeod, R.M. (1979) Failure of opiates to reverse dopamine inhibition of prolactin secretion in vitro. Eur. J. Pharmacol. 60, 253-255.

Loullis, C.C., Felten, D.L. and Shea, P.A. (1979) HPLC determination of biogenic amines in discrete brain areas in food deprived rats. Pharmacol. Biochem. Behav. 11, 87-93.

Markó, M. and Flückiger, E. (1980) Role of serotonin in the regulation of ovulation – Evidence from pharmacological studies. Neuroendocrinology 30, 228-231.

Martin, J.B., Tolis, G., Woods, I. and Guyda, H. (1979) Failure of naloxone to influence physiological growth hormone and prolactin secretion. Brain Res. 168, 210-216.

McCann, S.M. and Ojeda, S.R. (1976) Synaptic transmitters involved in the release of hypothalamic releasing and inhibiting hormones. Rev. Neurosci. 2, 91-110.

McKay, D.W., Demarest, K.T., Riegle, G.D. and Moore, K.E. (1980) Lactation alters the activity of tuberoinfundibular dopaminergic neurons. Soc. Neurosci. Abstract 6, 455.

Meek, J.L. and Lofstrandh, S. (1976) Tryptophan hydroxylase in discrete brain nuclei: Comparison of activity in vitro and in vivo. Eur. J. Pharmacol. 37, 377-380.

Meites, J., Bruni, J.F. and Van Vugt, D.A. (1979) Effects of endogenous opiate peptides on release of anterior pituitary hormones. In: Central Nervous System Effects of Hypothalamic Hormones and Other Peptides (Collu, R., Ducharme, J.R., Barbeau, A. and Rochefort, J.G. eds), pp. 261-271, Raven Press, New York.

Mena, F., Enjalbert, A., Carbonell, L., Priam, M. and Kordon, C. (1976) Effect of suckling on plasma prolactin and hypothalamic monoamine levels in rat. Endocrinology 99, 445-451.

Mess, B., Heizer, A., Tóth, A. and Tima, L. (1971) Luteinization induced by pinealectomy in the polyfollicular ovaries of rats bearing anterior hypothalamic lesions. In: The Pineal Gland, 1970, CIBA Foundation Symposium (Wolstenholme, G.E.W. and Knight, J. eds), pp. 229-240, Churchill Livingston, Edinburgh and London.

Moore, K.E. and Demarest, K.T. (1980) Effects of baclofen on different dopaminergic neuronal systems. Brain Res. Bull. 5 (Suppl. 2), 531-536.

Moore, K.E. and Phillipson, O.T. (1975) Effects of dexamethasone on phenylethanolamine N-methyltransferase and adrenaline in brain and superior cervical ganglia of adult and neonatal rats. J. Neurochem. 25, 289-294.

Moore, K.E. and Wuerthele, S.M. (1979) Regulation of nigrostriatal and tuberoinfundibular-hypophyseal dopaminergic neurons. Progress in Neurobiology 13, 325-359.

Moore, K.E., Wright, P.F. and Bert, J.K. (1967) Toxicological studies with α-methyltyrosine, an inhibitor of tyrosine hydroxylase. J. Pharmacol. Exp. Ther. 155, 506-515.

Moore, K.E., Annunziato, L. and Gudelsky, G.A. (1978) Studies on tuberoinfundibular dopamine neurons. In: Dopamine (Roberts, P.J., Woodruff, G.N. and Iversen, L.L. eds), Adv. Biochem. Psychopharmacol. 19, 193-204.

Moore, K.E., Umezu, K. and Demarest, K.T. (1979) Regulation of tuberoinfundibular dopamine neurons. In: Catecholamines: Basic and Clinical Frontiers (Usdin, E., Kopin, I.J. and Barchas, J. eds), pp. 1230-1232, Pergamon, New York.

Moore, K.E., Demarest, K.T., Johnston, C.A. and Alper, R.H. (1980a) Pharmacological and endocrinological manipulations of tuberoinfundibular and tuberohypophyseal dopaminergic neurons. In: Neuroactive Drugs in Endocrinology (Müller, E.E. ed.), pp. 109-121, Elsevier/North-Holland, Amsterdam.

Moore, K.E., Demarest, K.T. and Johnston, C.A. (1980b) The actions of prolactin on tuberoinfundibular dopaminergic neurons in male and female rats. In: Progress in Psychoneuroendocrinology (Brambilla, F., Racagni, G. and deWied, D. eds), pp. 359-366, Elsevier/North-Holland, Amsterdam.

Moore, R.Y. and Bloom, F.E. (1978) Central catecholamine neuron systems: Anatomy and physiology of the dopamine systems. Annu. Rev. Neurosci. 1, 129-169.

Moore, R.Y. and Bloom, F.E. (1979) Central catecholamine neuron systems: Anatomy and physiology of the norepinephrine and epinephrine systems. Annu. Rev. Neurosci. 2, 113-168.

Morgan, M.E. and Gibb, J.W. (1980) Short-term and long-term effects of methamphetamine on biogenic amine metabolism in extra-striatal dopaminergic nuclei. Neuropharmacology 19, 989-995.

Morgan, W.W. and Herbert, D.C. (1980) Early responses of the dopaminergic tuberoinfundibular neurons to anterior pituitary homographs. Neuroendocrinology 31, 215-221.

Morgan, W.W., Rudeen, P.K. and Pfeil, K.A. (1975) Effect of immobilization stress on serotonin content and turnover in regions of the rat brain. Life Sci. 17, 143-150.

Moss, R.L. (1976) Unit responses in preoptic and arcuate neurons related to anterior pituitary function. In: Frontiers in Neuroendocrinology (Ganong, W.F. and Martini, L. eds), Vol. 4, pp. 95-128, Raven Press, New York.

Moyer, J.A., O'Donahue, T.L., Herrenkohl, L.R., Gala, R.R. and Jacobowitz, D.M. (1979) Effects of suckling on serum prolactin levels and catecholamine concentrations and turnover in discrete brain regions. Brain Res. 176, 125-134.

Mueller, G.P., Simpkins, J., Meites, J. and Moore, K.E. (1976a) Differential effects of dopamine agonists and haloperidol on release of prolactin, thyroid stimulating hormone, growth hormone and luteinizing hormone in rats. Neuroendocrinology 20, 121-135.

Mueller, G.P., Twohy, C.P., Chen, H.T., Advis, J.P. and Meites, J. (1976b) Effects of L-tryptophan and restraint stress on hypothalamic and brain serotonin turnover, and pituitary TSH and prolactin release in rats. Life Sci. 18, 715-724.

Müller, E.E. (1973) Nervous control of growth hormone secretion. Neuroendocrinology 11, 338-369.

Müller, E.E., Nisticò, G. and Scapagnini, U. (1977) Neurotransmitters and Anterior Pituitary Function, Academic Press, New York.

Munaro, N.I. (1978) The effect of ovarian steroids on hypothalamic 5-hydroxytryptamine neuronal activity. Neuroendocrinology 26, 270-276.

Nagatsu, T., Oka, K. and Kato, T. (1979) Highly sensitive assay for tyrosine hydroxylase activity by high-performance liquid chromatography. J. Chromatogr. 163, 247-252.

Nakahara, T., Uchimura, H., Hirano, M., Saito, M. and Ito, M. (1976) Effects of gonadectomy and thyroidectomy on the tyrosine hydroxylase activity in individual hypothalamic nuclei and lower brain stem catecholaminergic cell groups in the rat. Brain Res. 117, 351-356.

Neckers, L.M. and Meek, J.L. (1976) Measurement of 5-HT turnover in discrete nuclei of rat brain. Life Sci. 19, 1579-1584.

Neckers, L. and Sze, P.Y. (1975) Regulation of 5-hydroxytryptamine metabolism in mouse brain by adrenal glucocorticoids. Brain Res. 93, 123-132.

Neff, N.H., Tozer, T.N. and Brodie, B.B. (1967) Application of steady-state kinetics to studies of the transfer of 5-hydroxyindoleacetic acid from brain to plasma. J. Pharmacol. Exp. Ther. 158, 214-218.

Neff, N.H., Spano, P.F., Groppetti, A., Wang, C.T. and Costa, E. (1971) A simple procedure for calculating the synthesis rate of norepinephrine, dopamine and serotonin in rat brain. J. Pharmacol. Exp. Ther. 176, 701-710.

Ng, L.K.Y., Chase, T.N., Colburn, R.W. and Kopin, I.J. (1972) Release of ^{3}H-dopamine by L-5-hydroxytryptophan. Brain Res. 45, 499-505.

Nicholson, G., Greeley, G., Humm, J., Youngblood, W. and Kizer, J.S. (1978) Lack of effect of noradrenergic denervation of hypothalamus and medial preoptic area on feedback regulation of gonadotropin secretion and estrous cycle of rat. Endocrinology 103, 559-566.

Nicholson, G., Greeley, G.H., Humm, J., Youngblood, W.W. and Kizer, J.S. (1980) Prolactin in cerebrospinal fluid: A probable site of prolactin autoregulation. Brain Res. 190, 447-458.

Nisticò, G. and Preziosi, P. (1969) Brain and liver tryptophan pathways and adrenocortical activation during restraint stress. Pharmacol. Res. Commun. 1, 363-368.

Nowycky, M.C. and Roth, R.H. (1978) Dopaminergic neurons: Role of presynaptic receptors in the regulation of transmitter biosynthesis. Progress in Neuropsychopharmacology 2, 139-160.

Olson, L. and Fuxe, K. (1972) Further mapping out of central noradrenaline systems. Projections of the 'subcoeruleus' area. Brain Res. 43, 289-295.

Olson, L., Fuxe, K. and Hökfelt, T. (1972) The effect of pituitary transplants on the tubero-infundibular dopamine neurons in various endocrine states. Acta Endocrinol. (Copenhagen) 71, 233-244.

Palkovits, M. (1973) Isolated removal of hypothalamic or other brain nuclei of the rat. Brain Res. 59, 449-450.

Palkovits, M. (1980) Mapping of neurotransmitters and hypothalamic hormones. In: Neuroactive Drugs in Endocrinology (Müller, E.E. ed.), pp. 35-48, Elsevier/North-Holland, Amsterdam.

Palkovits, M., Brownstein, M., Saavedra, J.M. and Axelrod, J. (1974) Norepinephrine and dopamine content of hypothalamic nuclei of the rat. Brain Res. 77, 137-150.

Palkovits, M., Kobayashi, R.M., Kizer, J.S., Jacobowitz, D.M. and Kopin, I.J. (1975) Effects of stress on catecholamines and tyrosine hydroxylase activity of individual hypothalamic nuclei. Neuroendocrinology 18,

144-153.

Palkovits, M., Brownstein, M., Kizer, J.S., Saavedra, J.M. and Kopin, I.J. (1976) Effect of stress on serotonin concentration and tryptophan hydroxylase activity of brain nuclei. Neuroendocrinology 22, 298-304.

Palkovits, M., Saavedra, J.M., Jacobowitz, D.M., Kizer, J.S., Zaborszky, L. and Brownstein, M.J. (1977) Serotoninergic innervation of the forebrain: Effect of lesions on serotonin and tryptophan hydroxylase levels. Brain Res. 130, 121-134.

Pardridge, W.M. (1977) Regulation of amino acid availability to the brain. In: Nutrition and the Brain (Wurtman, R.J. and Wurtman, J.J. eds), Vol. 1, pp. 141-204, Raven Press, New York.

Perkins, N.A. and Westfall, T.C. (1978) The effect of prolactin on dopamine release from rat striatum and medial basal hypothalamus. Neuroscience 3, 59-63.

Perkins, N.A., Westfall, T.C., Paul, C.V., MacLeod, R. and Rogol, A.D. (1979) Effect of prolactin on dopamine synthesis in medial basal hypothalamus: Evidence for a short loop feedback. Brain Res. 160, 431-444.

Pickel, V.M., Joh, T. and Reis, D. (1975) Ultrastructural localization of tyrosine hydroxylase in noradrenergic neurons of brain. Proc. Natl. Acad. Sci. USA 72, 659-663.

Pickel, V.M., Joh, T.H. and Reis, D.J. (1976) Monoamine-synthesizing enzymes in central dopaminergic, noradrenergic and serotonergic neurons. Immunocytochemical localization by light and electron microscopy. J. Histochem. Cytochem. 24, 792-806.

Pilotte, N.S., Gudelsky, G.A. and Porter, J.C. (1980) Relationship of prolactin secretion to dopamine release into hypophysial portal blood and dopamine turnover in the median eminence. Brain Res. 193, 284-288.

Rastogi, R.B. and Singhal, R.L. (1974) Thyroid hormone control of 5-hydroxytryptamine metabolism in developing rat brain. J. Pharmacol. Exp. Ther. 191, 72-81.

Renaud, L.P. (1980) The endocrine hypothalamus: Neurophysiological organization. In: Neuroactive Drugs in Endocrinology (Müller, E.E. ed.), pp. 49-67, Elsevier/North-Holland, Amsterdam.

Rivier, C., Vale, W., Ling, N., Brown, M. and Guillemin, R. (1977) Stimulation in vivo of the secretion of prolactin and growth hormone by β-endorphin. Endocrinology 100, 238-241.

Roffman, M., Casseus, G. and Schildkraut, J.J. (1970) The effects of acute and chronic administration of morphine on norepinephrine turnover in rat brain regions. Biochem. Pharmacol. 26, 2355-2358.

Roth, R.H., Walters, J.R., Murrin, L.C. and Morgenroth, V.H. (1975) Dopamine neurons: Role of impulse flow and pre-synaptic receptors in the regulation of tyrosine hydroxylase. In: Pre- and Postsynaptic Receptors (Usdin, E. and Bunney, W.E. eds), pp. 5-46, Dekker, New York.

Roth, R.H., Murrin, L.C. and Walters, J.R. (1976) Central dopaminergic neurons: Effects of alterations in impulse flow on the accumulation of dihydroxyphenylacetic acid. Eur. J. Pharmacol. 36, 163-171.

Saavedra, J.M., Palkovits, M., Brownstein, M.J. and Axelrod, J. (1974) Serotonin distribution in the nuclei of the rat hypothalamus and preoptic region. Brain Res. 77, 157-165.

Sar, M. and Stumpf, W.E. (1981) Central noradrenergic neurons concentrate ^{3}H-oestradiol. Nature 289, 500-501.

Sawyer, C.H. (1979) The Seventh Stevenson Lecture. Brain amines and pituitary gonadotrophin secretion. Can. J. Physiol. Pharmacol. 57, 667-680.

Scapagnini, U., Preziosi, P. and De Schaepdryver, A. (1969) Influence of restraint stress, corticosterone and betamethasone on brain amine levels. Pharmacol. Res. Commun. 1, 63-69.

Schettini, G., Quattrone, A., Di Renzo, G. and Preziosi, P. (1980) Serotonergic involvement in neuroendocrine function. Pharmacol. Res. Commun. 12, 249-254.

Schiebler, T.H., Leranth, C., Zaborszky, L., Bitsch, P. and Rutgel, H. (1978) On the glia of the median eminence. In: Neural Hormones and Reproduction (Scott, D.E., Koszlowski, G.P. and Weindl, A. eds), pp. 46-56, Karger, Basel.

Schneider, H.P.G. and McCann, S.M. (1970) Mono- and indoleamines and control of LH secretion. Endocrinology 86, 1127-1133.

Selmanoff, M.K., Pramik-Holdaway, M.J. and Weiner, R.I. (1976) Concentrations of dopamine and norepinephrine in discrete hypothalamic nuclei during the rat estrous cycle. Endocrinology 99, 326-329.

Shaar, C.J., Frederickson, R.C.A., Dininger, N.B. and Jackson, L. (1977) Enkephalin analogues and naloxone modulate the release of growth hormone and prolactin. Evidence for regulation by an endogenous opioid peptide in brain. Life Sci. 21, 853-860.

Shaskan, E.G. and Snyder, S.H. (1970) Kinetics of serotonin accumulation into slices from rat brain: Relationship to catecholamine uptake. J. Pharmacol. Exp. Ther. 175, 404-418.

Shen, J.T. and Ganong, W.F. (1976a) Effect of variations in pituitary-adrenal activity on dopamine-β-hydroxylase activity in various regions of rat brain. Neuroendocrinology 20, 311-318.

Shen, J.T. and Ganong, W.F. (1976b) Effect of variations in adrenocortical function on dopamine-β-hydroxylase and norepinephrine in the brain of the rat. J. Pharmacol. Exp. Ther. 199, 639-648.

Shopsin, B., Shenkman, L., Sanghui, I. and Hollander, C.S. (1974) Toward a relationship between the hypothalamic-pituitary-thyroid axis and the synthesis of serotonin. In: Serotonin: New Vistas (Costa, E., Gessa, G.L. and Sandler, M. eds), Adv. Biochem. Psychopharmacol. 10, 279-286.

Sladek, J.R. and Sladek, C.D. (1978) Localization of serotonin within tanycytes of the rat median eminence. Cell Tiss. Res. 186, 465-474.

Sladek, J.R., Sladek, C.D., McNeill, T.H. and Wood, J.G. (1978) New sites of monoamine localization in the endocrine hypothalamus as revealed by new methodological approaches. In: Brain-Endocrine Interactions. III Neural Hormones and Reproduction (Scott, D.E., Weindl, A. and Kozslowski, G.P. eds), pp. 154-171, Karger, Basel.

Smith, A.R. and Kappers, J.A. (1975) Effect of pinealectomy, gonadectomy, pCPA and pineal extracts on the rat parvocellular neurosecretory hypothalamic system; a fluorescence histochemical investigation. Brain Res. 86, 353-371.

Smith, G.C. and Helme, R.D. (1974) Ultrastructural and fluorescence histochemical studies on the effects of 6-hydroxydopamine on the rat median eminence. Cell Tissue Res. 152, 493-512.

Smith, G.C. and Simpson, R.W. (1970) Monoamine fluorescence in the median eminence of foetal, neonatal and adult rats. Z. Zellforsch. 104, 541-556.

Spampinato, S., Locatelli, V., Cocchi, D., Vicentini, L., Bajusz, S., Ferri, S. and Müller, E.E. (1979) Involvement of brain serotonin in the prolactin-releasing effect of opioid peptides. Endocrinology 105, 163-170.

Swanson, L.W. and Hartman, B.K. (1975) The central adrenergic system. An immunofluorescence study of the localization of cell bodies and their efferent connections in the rat utilizing dopamine-beta-hydroxylase as a marker. J. Comp. Neurol. 163, 467-505.

Sze, P.Y., Neckers, L. and Towle, A.C. (1976) Glucocorticoids as a regulatory factor for brain tryptophan hydroxylase. J. Neurochem. 26, 169-173.

Taché, Y., Charpenet, G., Chrétien, M. and Collu, R. (1979) Role of serotonergic pathways in hormonal changes induced by opioid peptides. In: Central Nervous System Effects of Hypothalamic Hormones and Other Peptides (Collu, R., Barbeau, A., Ducharme, J.R. and Rochefort, J.G. eds), pp. 301-313, Raven Press, New York.

Tagliamonte, A., Tagliamonte, P., Perez-Cruet, J., Stern, S. and Gessa, G.L. (1971) Effect of psychotropic drugs on tryptophan concentration in the rat brain. J. Pharmacol. Exp. Ther. 177, 475-480.

Tappaz, M.L. and Pujol, J-F. (1980) Estimation of the rate of tryptophan hydroxylation in vivo: A sensitive microassay in discrete rat brain nuclei. J. Neurochem. 34, 933-940.

Telegdy, G. and Kovacs, G.L. (1979) Role of monoamines in mediating the action of ACTH, vasopressin, and oxytocin. In: Central Nervous System Effects of Hypothalamic Hormones and Other Peptides (Collu, R., Ducharme, J.R., Barbeau, A. and Rochefort, J.G. eds), pp. 189-205, Raven Press, New York.

Telegdy, G. and Szontágh, L. (1979) Effects of LH-RH and gonadotropins on brain neurotransmitter metabolism. In: Psychoneuroendocrinology in Reproduction (Zichella, L. and Pancheri, P. eds), pp. 81-86, Elsevier/North-Holland, Amsterdam.

Telegdy, G. and Vermes, I. (1975) Effect of adrenocortical hormones on activity of the serotoninergic system in limbic structures in rats. Neuroendocrinology 18, 16-26.

Thierry, A., Javoy, F., Glowinski, J. and Kety, S.S. (1968) Effects of stress on the metabolism of norepinephrine, dopamine and serotonin in the central nervous system of the rat. 1. Modification of norepinephrine turnover. J. Pharmacol. Exp. Ther. 163, 163-171.

Thierry, A.M., Tassin, J.P., Blanc, G. and Glowinski, J. (1976) Selective activation of the mesocortical dopamine system by stress. Nature (London) 263, 242-244.

Tozer, T.N., Neff, N.H. and Brodie, B.B. (1966) Application of steady state kinetics to the synthesis rate and turnover time of serotonin in the brain of normal and reserpine-treated rats. J. Pharmacol. Exp. Ther. 153,

177-182.

Trentini, G.P., Tima, L., DeGaetani, C.F. and Mess, B. (1974) Luteinization induced by p-chlorophenylalanine treatment in constant oestrous anovulatory rats. Steroids Lipids Res. 5, 262-267.

Ulrich, R.S., Yuwiler, A. and Geller, A. (1975) Effects of hydrocortisone on biogenic amine levels in the hypothalamus. Neuroendocrinology 19, 259-268.

Umezu, K. and Moore, K.E. (1979) Effects of drugs on regional brain concentrations of dopamine and dihydroxyphenylacetic acid. J. Pharmacol. Exp. Ther. 208, 49-56.

van de Kar, L., Levine, J. and Van Orden III, L.S. (1978) Serotonin in hypothalamic nuclei: Increased content after castration of male rats. Neuroendocrinology 27, 186-192.

van Loon, G.R. and De Souza, E.B. (1978) Effect of β-endorphin on brain serotonin metabolism. Life Sci. 23, 971-978.

van Loon, G.R., De Souza, E.B. and Shin, S.H. (1980) Dopaminergic mediation of β-endorphin-induced prolactin secretion. Neuroendocrinology 31, 292-296.

van Ree, J.M., Versteeg, D.H.G., Spaaken-Kek, W.B., deWied, D. (1976) Effects of morphine on hypothalamic noradrenaline and on pituitary-adrenal activity in rats. Neuroendocrinology 22, 305-317.

Van Vugt, D.A. and Meites, J. (1980) Influence of endogenous opiates on anterior pituitary function. Fed. Proc. 39, 2533-2538.

Van Vugt, D.A., Bruni, J.F. and Meites, J. (1978) Naloxone inhibition of stress-induced increase in prolactin secretion. Life Sci. 22, 85-90.

Van Vugt, D.A., Bruni, J.F., Sylvester, P.W., Chen, H.T., Ieri, T. and Meites, J. (1979) Interaction between opiates and hypothalamic dopamine on prolactin release. Life Sci. 24, 2361-2368.

Vermes, I., Molnas, D. and Telegdy, G. (1973a) Hypothalamic serotonin content and pituitary-adrenal function following hypothalamic deafferentation. Acta Physiol. Acad. Sci. Hung. 43, 239-245.

Vermes, I., Telegdy, G. and Lissak, K. (1973b) Correlation between hypothalamic serotonin content and adrenal function during acute stress. Effect of adrenal corticosteroids on hypothalamic serotonin content. Acta Physiol. Acad. Sci. Hung. 43, 33-42.

Versteeg, D.H.G., van der Gugten, J. and van Ree, J.M. (1975) Regional turnover and synthesis of catecholamines in rat hypothalamus. Nature 256, 502-503.

Versteeg, D.H.G., van der Gugten, J., de Jong, W. and Palkovits, M. (1976) Regional concentrations of noradrenaline and dopamine in rat brain. Brain Res. 113, 563-574.

Vijayan, E. and McCann, S.M. (1978) The effect of systemic administration of dopamine and apomorphine on plasma LH and prolactin concentrations in conscious rats. Neuroendocrinology 25, 221-235.

Wagner, J., Palfreyman, M. and Zraika, M. (1979) Determination of dopa, dopamine, dopac, epinephrine, norepinephrine, α-monofluoromethyldopa and α-difluoromethyldopa in various tissues of mice and rats using reverse-phase ion-pair liquid chromatography with electrochemical detection. J. Chromatogr. 164, 41-54.

Walker, R.F. (1980) Serotonin neuroleptics change patterns of preovulatory secretion of luteinizing hormone in rats. Life Sci. 27, 1063-1068.

Way, E.L. (1971) Role of serotonin in morphine effects. Fed. Proc. 31, 113-120.

Weiner, N. (1974) A critical assessment of methods for the determination of monoamine synthesis turnover rates in vivo. In: Neuropsychopharmacology of Monoamines and Their Regulatory Enzymes (Usdin, E. ed.), Adv. Biochem. Psychopharm. 12, 143-159.

Weiner, R.I. and Ganong, W.F. (1978) Role of brain monoamines and histamine in regulation of anterior pituitary secretion. Physiol. Rev. 58, 905-976.

Weiner, R.I., Shryne, J.E., Gorski, R.A. and Sawyer, C.H. (1972) Changes in the catecholamine content of the rat hypothalamus following deafferentation. Endocrinology 90, 867-873.

Wiesel, F.A., Fuxe, K., Hökfelt, T. and Agnati, L.F. (1978) Studies on dopamine turnover in ovariectomized or hypophysectomized female rats. Effects of 17β-estradiol benzoate, ethynodioldiacetate and ovine prolactin. Brain Res. 148, 399-412.

Wilkes, M.M. and Yen, S.S.C. (1980) Reduction by β-endorphin of efflux of dopamine and DOPAC from superfused medial basal hypothalamus. Life Sci. 27, 1387-1391.

Wilson, C.A. (1974) Hypothalamic amines and the release of gonadotrophins and other anterior pituitary hormones. Adv. Drug Res. 8, 119-204.

68

Wirz-Justice, A. and Hackmann, E. (1972) Effect of oestradiol propionate and progesterone on monoamine uptake in the rat brain. Experientia 28, 736.

Yarbrough, G.G., Buxbaum, D.M. and Sanders-Bush, E. (1971) Increased serotonin turnover in the acutely morphine treated rat. Life Sci. 10, 977-983.

Yarbrough, G.G., Buxbaum, D.M. and Sanders-Bush, E. (1973) Biogenic amines and narcotic effects. II. Serotonin turnover in the rat after acute and chronic morphine administration. J. Pharmacol. Exp. Ther. 185, 328-335.

Zivkovic, B., Guidotti, A. and Costa, E. (1973) Increase of tryptophan hydroxylase activity elicited by reserpine. Brain Res. 57, 522-526.

E.E. Müller and R.M. MacLeod (eds) Neuroendocrine Perspectives Vol. 1
© Elsevier Biomedical Press, 1982

Chapter 3

Regulating mechanisms for oxytocin and prolactin secretion during lactation

Clark E. Grosvenor and Flavio Mena

INTRODUCTION

The various phases of the reproductive cycle of mammals, including lactation, become possible through the development of a variety of neuroendocrine mechanisms (Mena 1978). Specific external stimuli act upon the neuroendocrine substrates to regulate the responses of the various target organs, ovulation, milk secretion, etc. During lactation, the most important stimuli that the mother receives are those which activate specific receptors located in and around the nipple during suckling, and exteroceptive stimuli which emanate from the offspring and which are perceived by her special organ senses. These stimuli are responsible for the majority of the endocrine, metabolic and behavioral adjustments that develop in the lactating animal and which enable her to care for her offspring.

In the present review we present recent experimental data that relate to the afferent control and regulation of secretion of oxytocin and prolactin and to the regulatory influence exerted by the sympathetic nervous system upon milk ejection.

OXYTOCIN AND MILK EJECTION IN THE RAT

General

Suckling or exteroceptive stimuli associated with suckling activate a neuroendocrine reflex which results in the release of oxytocin from the neurohypophysis. Mechanoreceptors in the teat and in the skin overlying the mammary glands, as well as within the mammary parenchyma (Findlay 1966; Alekseev 1976, 1977), transform suckling stimuli into nerve impulses which, in turn, release oxytocin. These receptors are of both the rapid and fast-adapting type. Myoepithelial cells, which form a meshwork on the surface of the mammary alveoli and which also are found longitudinally aligned along the mammary ducts, are the elements within the gland which contract in response to oxytocin (Richardson 1949; Linzell 1955). Upon contraction, these cells compress the alveoli, thereby raising intraalveolar pressure, and also shorten and widen the ducts. A specific, high affinity receptor for oxytocin has been demonstrated in rat mammary tissue (Soloff and Swartz 1973). Abundant smooth muscle elements located in the mammary arterioles and larger ducts function to regulate the flow of blood to the gland, and milk from the gland, respectively. The tone of these elements is regulated principally by the sympathetic nervous system (Findlay and Grosvenor 1969). Both α- and β-adrenergic receptors have been found within the mammary gland (Vorherr 1971).

Afferent control of oxytocin release

It would appear that two systems of fibers, the spinothalamic tracts and the dorsal longitudinal fasciculus, are involved in the afferent flow of impulses from the mammary glands to the hypothalamic–hypophysial system involved in oxytocin release (see Grosvenor and Mena 1974).

Evidence obtained in several species with electrical stimulation and lesion techniques suggests that the functioning of the neurohypophysis also may be influenced by several extrahypothalamic regions. Thus, stimulation of the anterior cingulate gyrus, septum, hippocampus, and amygdala elicits oxytocin discharge (see Denamur 1965; Beyer and Mena 1969 for review), while bilateral lesions in the amygdala have been reported to block lactation in the rat by interference with milk ejection (Stutinsky and Terminn 1965). The importance of these structures for oxytocin release during lactation is, however, not clear, and apparently they are not essential for normal milk ejection. Removal of the entire telencephalon, including cerebral cortex, hippocampi, amygdala, and other parts, did not affect the release of oxytocin induced by electrical stimulation of the milk ejection pathway in the midbrain. This raises the possibility that within the forebrain the pathway is entirely diencephalic. Nevertheless, it is possible that the limbic forebrain participates in the conditioned release of oxytocin described by some workers (see Tindal 1978).

The fiber tracts in the pathway for oxytocin release may contain dopaminergic (Seybold et al. 1978; Clarke et al. 1979; Moos and Richard 1979a), adrenergic (Clarke and Lincoln 1976; Moos and Richard 1979b), and cholinergic (Clarke et al. 1978) components.

In certain species, (e.g. cow, pig, rabbit) milk ejection occurs soon after suckling or milking is initiated. In the rat, however, milk ejection does not occur as a reflex response after the onset of suckling, but rather after a latency of 10–15 min in the conscious animal (Deis 1968). Milk ejection does not occur until after more than 60 min in rats under deep anesthesia (Lincoln et al. 1973; Lincoln and Wakerley 1975); this is followed by a pattern in which milk is ejected at regular intervals of 3–5 min and in correlation with increased spike activity of neurohypophysial neurons. It was also reported that neither milk ejection nor neuronal activation occurred when less than six pups were suckling (Lincoln et al. 1973; Lincoln and Wakerley 1975), though this may be due to a lowered sensitivity of the milk ejection reflex in the anesthetized rat; suckling by two pups results in milk ejection in the conscious rat (Mena and Grosvenor 1968). Lincoln et al. (1973) proposed that the central mechanisms which normally inhibit oxytocin secretion (Cross 1955) can be counteracted by afferent stimulation from the mammary gland and thus account both for the delay and for the intermittent character of milk ejection (Lincoln et al. 1973). Tindal and Blake (1980) noted that discrete cuts in the forebrain of the anesthetized lactating rabbit caused spontaneous milk ejection responses every 1–5 min. They proposed that severance of the septo-hippocampal pathway frees the hippocampus from inhibition and allows oxytocin release to occur.

Observations by Voloschin and Tramezzani (1979) suggest that synchronization of the cerebral cortex precedes the discharge of oxytocin during suckling. They noted that the milk ejection reflex in the rat only occurred when the mother fell asleep, and not when she was awake or during paradoxical sleep. It is known that neurohypophysial neurosecretory neurons change their activity in relation to sleep and awake patterns in the monkey (Hayward and Jennings 1973).

Release of oxytocin in response to electrical stimulation of mammary nerve

We examined the relationship between oxytocin release and mammary contraction by using electrical stimulation of mammary nerve in the urethane anesthetized rat to release oxytocin. Previously, it had been shown by Richard (1970) that potentials could be recorded in the pituitary stalk in the ewe after electrical stimulation of the inguinal nerves or dilatation of the vagina. In a few instances, intramammary pressure (IMP) responses, apparently due to oxytocin, were obtained following nerve stimulation. In our study (Mena et al. 1978), we determined that parameters of electrical stimulation of 1-ms pulses, 10–20/s, at 5–30 volts applied for 5–10 s would elicit measurable and reproducible releases of oxytocin, as evidenced by rises in IMP within a contralateral mammary gland (Fig. 3.1). All responses were characterized by a single rise and fall in pressure, had a latency of 8–15 s, and could be mimicked by a single intravenous injection of 50–400 μU oxytocin.

Hypophysectomy or spinal cord transection above the level of the stimulated nerve blocked the IMP responses induced by mammary nerve stimulation (Fig. 3.1). The possibility that vasopressin, released by nerve stimulation, could have influenced the IMP responses was excluded since only a small amount of vasopressin was released (10–100 μU), and this amount had no effect upon IMP when injected into the circulation. It would appear, therefore, that IMP responses obtained by afferent mammary nerve stimulation are due mainly to oxytocin released from the neurohypophysis.

The IMP responses obtained with mammary nerve stimulation increased in amplitude by increasing either the frequency or the voltage of the electrical stimulus. Mechanoreceptors, which have been found in the teat and in the skin overlying the rat and rabbit mammary glands (see Introduction), may discharge over a similar range of frequencies in response to suckling. If so, this may be the mechanism whereby different amounts of oxytocin are released. The amount released in response to suckling of a single gland, however, would be small, judging from the amounts estimated to be discharged by stimulation of a single mammary nerve. Spatial summation, occuring when more than one gland is suckled, and temporal summation, taking place when the frequency changes at which a single gland is suckled, then could account for the release of quantitatively larger amounts of oxytocin. Further research will be necessary to clarify this point.

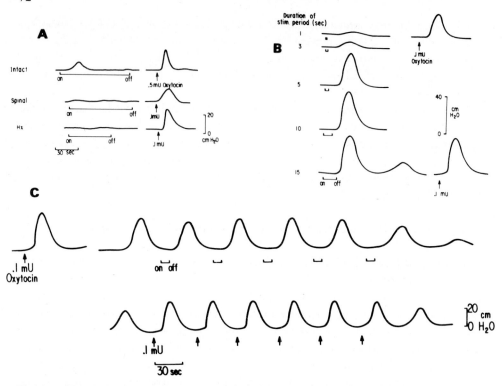

Fig. 3.1. Effect of electrical stimulation (5–30 V, 1-ms pulses, 10 per s) of an afferent mammary nerve upon intramammary pressure (IMP) in anesthetized lactating rats. (A) Failure of nerve stimulation to provoke a rise in IMP in spinal sectioned (spinal) (T_9–T_{10} level) and in hypophysectomized (Hx) rats. (B) Effect of varying the length of the period of mammary nerve stimulation upon IMP responses. (C) IMP responses evoked by repetitive stimulation (10 s on, 40 s off) and by oxytocin injections (0.1 mU, i.v.) applied at 40-s intervals (Mena et al. 1978).

In the rabbit, the low threshold, fast-adapting pressure receptors in the teat of the mammary gland fire rhythmically during a suckling episode (Findlay 1966); and, in the circulation of women and large domestic animals, small quantities of oxytocin appear transiently during suckling or milking (Tindal 1974). Analysis of suckling behavior in anesthetized rats revealed: (1) that the pups suck in bursts (each burst composed of an average of 2.7 sucks); (2) that each burst is applied at an average interval of 13.7 s; and (3) that asynchronous and non-synchronous suckling was characteristic of members of a litter of 10 pups, so that at any given time before milk ejection, only an average of one pup displayed actual suckling (Wakerley and Drewett 1975).

In our studies, IMP responses of similar amplitude were elicited repeatedly by short (5–10 s) periods of stimulation with 40-s intervals to permit return of the preceding pressure wave to baseline. A similar pattern was obtained when exogenous oxytocin was given at the same intervals (Fig. 3.1). On the other hand, when the interval was reduced to 20 s, the amplitude of the pressure responses either from mammary nerve stimulation or from exogenous oxytocin varied and often were greatly reduced. Thus, our data indicate that oxytocin may be released repeatedly provided that periodic short, rather than sustained, periods of stimulation are applied. They also suggest that during normal suckling in rats, the effective stimuli from the pups for oxytocin release may be applied for similar short periods to receptors within the mammary gland. In addition, it was found that when pups sucked occluded nipples of anesthetized rats, each burst of suckling apparently was stimulated by mammary contraction since the milk could not escape from the gland (Drewett et al. 1974). This suggests that small amounts of oxytocin sufficient to produce a slight contraction of the mammary myoepithelium and elevate IMP slightly, but too small perhaps to result in a noticeable ejection of milk to the exterior, could stimulate further suckling by the pups.

Role of the sympathetic nervous system in milk ejection

In rats and other species, it has been shown that a reduction in the rate of milk removal due either to increased ductal resistance and/or to mammary vasoconstriction is associated with increased activity, whereas either surgical or pharmacological sympathectomy results in a faster rate of milk flow to the exterior (Findlay and Grosvenor 1969; Cowie and Tindal 1971; Grosvenor and Mena 1974). In the anesthetized lactating rat, the IMP response induced by oxytocin rose faster and reached a higher amplitude following either injection of antiadrenergic drugs, spinal section above the gland whose pressure was being recorded, or after section of the dorsal roots or peripheral nerve supplying the gland (Grosvenor et al. 1972). Furthermore, ductal resistance as detected by the time taken for intraductal filling of the gland was reduced following sympatholytic drug treatment or local anesthesia (Grosvenor and Findlay 1968). These results suggested that the central nervous system, as well as the sympathetic system, could influence ductal and perhaps vascular smooth muscle tone in the rat. Moreover, based upon the effect of dorsal root sectioning, it was proposed that afferent mammary nerve fibers might have a facilitatory influence, via a spinal reflex arc, in the maintenance of smooth muscle tone of the mammary gland (Grosvenor et al. 1972).

Activation of the sympathetic system during suckling

We propose that an interplay normally exists between neurogenic sympathetic influences and oxytocin to determine the force and extent of milk ejection. In analyzing this interrelationship, we sought to determine the mechanisms involved in activation and control of sympathetic effects upon the contractile response of the rat mammary gland to oxytocin. In goats and cows, it has been shown that the motor inhibitory system of the mammary gland could be aroused in a reflex manner by activation of mammary receptors (Grachev 1949; Cochrane 1949). In addition, plasma catecholamine levels have been shown to increase following electrical stimulation of the teat in goats (Kuanyshbekova 1976) and during machine milking in sheep (Barowicz 1979).

In our studies, we applied manual compression for 10–15 s to two thoracic mammary glands in the anesthetized rat. This stimulation, which was designed to mimic the kneading action of the pups during a suckling, resulted in an immediate and significant reduction in amplitude of the IMP responses to oxytocin in cannulated abdominal mammary glands (Fig. 3.2). Following the period of reduced responsiveness to oxytocin, the IMP responses

74

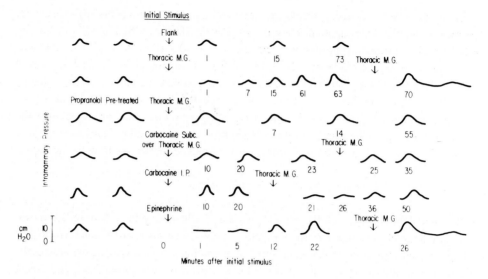

Fig. 3.2. Representative intramammary pressure responses of abdominal mammary glands in anesthetized lactating rats to oxytocin injections after the following procedures: 1st tracing, control compression of the flank; 2nd tracing, manual compression of thoracic mammary glands (10–15 s, denoted by Thoracic MG); 3rd tracing, Thoracic MG after propranolol pretreatment; 4th and 5th tracings, Thoracic MG after s.c. and i.p. injections of carbocaine, respectively; 6th tracing, epinephrine injection alone (0.5 µg, i.v.). Compression was applied or reapplied in all conditions but those represented in the 1st and 3rd tracings. Numbers below tracings indicate minutes elapsed after initial stimulus or injection (Grosvenor and Mena 1979).

gradually recovered; then a phase of increased contractile responsiveness occurred, during which the amplitude of the IMP responses to oxytocin progressively increased to a maximum, which was considerably above that seen prior to manual compression. A similar pattern of depression, recovery, and increased responsiveness of the IMP response to a given dose of oxytocin could be obtained by a single injection of epinephrine. The effect of manual compression upon IMP did not occur, however, if the rat was pretreated with propranolol or if the glands to be compressed were first locally anesthetized with carbocaine, or when manual compression was applied during the phase of increased responsiveness (Grosvenor and Mena 1979) (see Fig. 3.2). These results show that the sympathetic motor control of the mammary gland can be reflexively activated in an acute, i.e., phasic, manner by mechanical stimulation of the mammary gland area.

Further analysis of this mechanism was made by employing electrical stimulation of the mammary nerve. As indicated before (see Fig. 3.1), brief (5–10 s) periods of mammary nerve stimulation induced the release of 50–400 µU of oxytocin, and, a few seconds later, the IMP rose. However, when the mammary nerve was electrically stimulated for 120–140 s using the same parameters, the amplitude of IMP responses to a given dose of oxytocin became depressed by almost 50% after 60–120 s of such stimulation (Mena et al. 1979). The IMP recovered to the previous level 3–10 min after cessation of the stimulus (Fig. 3.3); the depressant effect of nerve stimulation then could be repeated. Bilateral

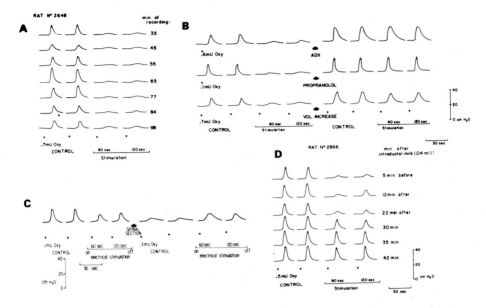

Fig. 3.3. The effect of electrical stimulation (5–30 V, 1-ms pulses, 10 per s) of a mammary nerve upon IMP responses to oxytocin (Oxy) injected 60 and 120 s after onset of stimulation in lactating rats. Solid dots indicate oxytocin injections. (A) Time control illustrating the ability of electrical stimulation of a mammary nerve to repeatedly depress the IMP response to injected oxytocin. (B) Responses obtained before and after bilateral adrenal ligature (ADX), propranolol injection, or increasing the volume of milk (Vol. increase) into an abdominal gland whose pressure is being recorded. (C) Responses obtained before and after spinal cord transection (T_9–T_{10}); note that the amplitude of IMP responses to oxytocin increase during nerve stimulation after the spinal section. (D) Effect of rapidly introducing 0.04 ml of milk intraductally into a thoracic gland on the IMP response to oxytocin of an abdominal gland after mammary nerve stimulation (Mena et al. 1979).

adrenal ligature, intravenous injection of 0.3 mg propranolol, or section of the spinal cord above the level of entry of the mammary nerve each completely blocked the depressant effect of nerve stimulation (see Fig. 3.3). In fact, the slope and amplitude of the IMP response increased above that found prior to mammary nerve stimulation following each of these procedures suggesting that the sympathetic tone within the ducts and arterioles of the mammary gland is maintained not only through direct innervation, but also through catecholamine-adrenal secretion. Moreover, the phasic, i.e. acute, sympathetic activation resulting from nerve stimulation appears to be mediated preferentially through epinephrine secretion, since ventral root section of the gland that was being recorded did not affect the depressant effect of nerve stimulation to any great extent.

Our data (Grosvenor and Mena 1979; Mena et al. 1979) therefore suggest that the sympathetic-adrenal system is activated during suckling and at the same time that oxytocin is being released. The small amounts of milk which are obtained during the first 10–15 min of suckling (Fig. 3.4) may be the result of a dominance of the sympathetic system. As the activity of the sympathetic system subsides, oxytocin becomes relatively more effective,

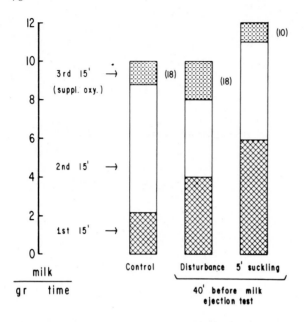

Fig. 3.4. Effect of disturbance (picking up rat) and 5 min of suckling upon average amount of milk obtained by 6 pups in three consecutive 15-min periods of suckling. Supplemental oxytocin (150 mU subcutaneously) given prior to the third period. (Grosvenor and Mena, unpublished results).

and much larger amounts of milk then can be obtained by the pups (Fig. 3.4). The delay in milk ejection noted earlier by Deis (1968) was partially prevented and milk ejection accomplished more quickly when suckling took place during the stage of depressed sympathetic activity (Fig. 3.4). In these experiments, the sympathetic system was activated 40 min before suckling either by disturbing the mother by picking her up or by providing a brief 5 min suckling. The 40 min period allowed the sympathetic system to pass through the inhibition and recovery stages and into the depression stage of activity as documented by our IMP studies. Recently, it was reported that milk ejection was facilitated in anesthetized rats during β-adrenergic depression (Tribollet and Dreifuss 1977). We noted also that the number of rats responding to nerve stimulation with a rise in IMP increased following adrenergic blockade (Mena et al. 1978). Clarke and Lincoln (1976) and Moos and Richard (1979b) showed that epinephrine or isoproterenol inhibited milk ejection in rats, an effect which was prevented with propranolol. These data further suggest that the relative activity of the sympathetic system influences the rate and extent of milk ejection.

Antagonistic mechanisms to sympathetic activity during milk ejection

We wished to analyze whether the stage of increased responsiveness to oxytocin was due to passive subsidence of sympathetic activity, perhaps related to gradual adrenergic receptor insensitivity (Lefkowitz et al. 1976), or whether antagonistic mechanisms exist within the mammary gland which operate to regulate sympathetic inhibitory influences (Mena et al. 1979). In the first experiment, a rapid increase in the volume of milk within the abdominal mammary gland whose pressure was being monitored immediately and effectively blocked the depressant effect of electrical stimulation upon the IMP response to exogenous oxytocin (Fig. 3.3). The mechanism of this effect probably is related to the sudden increase in alveolar diameter and, hence, in myoepithelial tension as the milk is introduced (DeNuccio and Grosvenor 1971). The subsequent greater elastic recoil of the myoepithelium following oxytocin stimulation probably was sufficient to override the increase in sympathetic tone induced by sympathetic activation following mammary nerve stimulation. In the second experiment, a small amount (0.04–0.06 ml) of milk was introduced intraductally into a thoracic gland while the pressure in an abdominal gland was being maintained. A gradual, rather than a rapid, disappearance of the depressant action of electrical stimulation ensued, starting a few minutes after the introduction of the milk into the thoracic gland, and attaining a complete blockade of the depressant effect 40–50 min later (Fig. 3.3). This result suggests that a reflex mechanism exists which when activated antagonizes the sympathetic system. Slowly adapting mammary gland mechanoreceptors may have been activated when the small volume was introduced into the thoracic gland, and thus initiated the reflex. In spinal cord transected rats whose central inhibitory control of ductal tone had been removed (Mena et al. 1979), leaving only segmental tone, stimulation of the mammary nerve provoked an increase, rather than a decrease, in slope and amplitude of IMP responses to oxytocin. Presumably, the sympathetic system was inhibited as a result of activation of afferent fibers from those mechanoreceptors.

It would therefore appear from the data in our studies (Grosvenor and Mena 1979; Mena et al. 1979) that impulses from mammary mechanoreceptors can regulate both tonic and phasic sympathetic activity upon the mammary gland. Moreover, since central mechanisms inhibiting oxytocin release may be adrenergic (Fuxe and Hökfelt 1967; Cross and Dyball 1974), it is possible that mechanoreceptor activity may also modulate central mechanisms and thus facilitate oxytocin release. Recently, Lincoln and Wakerley (1975) noted that introduction of 0.05 ml of saline into a thoracic gland provoked a rapid facilitation in the pattern of accelerated spike activity of neurohypophysial neurons induced by suckling of a small litter. As already mentioned, Tribollet and Dreifuss (1977) reported a similar effect following β-adrenergic depression in anesthetized rats. In view of the present data, it would appear that a fast, followed by a slow, long lasting depression of sympathetic tone results from mechanoreceptor activation, which leads to increased oxytocin secretion and to increased oxytocin effectiveness as a consequence of reduced ductal resistance. A combination of these effects would result in a faster rate of milk flow to the exterior.

PROLACTIN SECRETION

General

The secretion of prolactin by pituitary mammotrophs involves a series of interdependent, complex events including biosynthesis, packaging, maturation and transport of the hormone in granular form, and its release by exocytosis. Until recently, the pituitary has been considered as a passive target organ driven principally by blood-borne hypothalamic factors. However, it is becoming clear that the level of functioning of the mammotrophs may change drastically according to their physiological state. It is also becoming apparent that hypothalamic factors act at specific points in the secretory process and that any given effect upon release, biosynthesis, etc. might alter subsequent events in the sequence of secretion (Neill 1980). An understanding of the cellular events involved in prolactin secretion should allow better understanding of the sites and the mechanisms of action of hypothalamic factors. In this section, we will review recent data concerning afferent control of prolactin secretion and concerning factors within the mammotrophs which provide clues about pituitary-hypothalamic interactions regulating prolactin secretion during lactation.

Afferent control of prolactin secretion during lactation

In contrast to internal regulation of prolactin by ovarian steroids in the nonlactating female, secretion of the hormone during lactation is almost entirely under the control of afferent impulses generated in the periphery during suckling or from associated exteroceptive signals emanating from the litter (Grosvenor and Mena 1971; Grosvenor and Mena 1974; Neill 1974; Terkel et al. 1978; Mena et al. 1980; Neill 1980). As a reflection of the type of regulation, prolactin is not secreted tonically during lactation, but phasically in response to stimulation. Very low circulating titers of the hormone are to be found in the absence of suckling stimulation.

The release of prolactin from the anterior pituitary of the lactator occurs as a result of a neuroendocrine reflex activated by the neurogenic stimulus of suckling (Grosvenor and

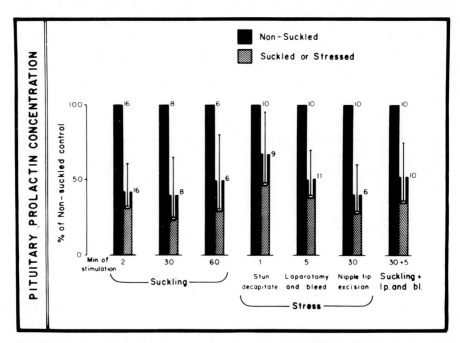

Fig. 3.5. Effect of duration and quality of stimulus upon fall in pituitary prolactin concentration in the postpartum day 14 rat. Values are means ±95% confidence limits; numbers alongside bars refer to numbers of rats (Grosvenor and Mena 1971).

Mena 1971; Grosvenor and Mena 1974). This reflex can be conditioned by olfactory (Grosvenor and Mena 1971; Grosvenor and Mena 1974) and auditory (Terkel et al. 1978) signals from the pups so that by mid-lactation the release of prolactin can occur in response to these exteroceptive stimuli (ECS) and in the absence of suckling (Grosvenor and Mena 1971; Grosvenor and Mena 1974).

The influence of suckling upon prolactin secretion consists of an initial rapid (1–2 min) and extensive (15–60 µg) depletion of the hormone within the anterior pituitary (Fig. 3.5). The effect of suckling and/or stress depletion, however, is not summating; that is, 2 min is as effective as 60 min of suckling, and suckling plus stress is no more effective than either stimulus by itself. Following depletion, anterior pituitary prolactin stores slowly reaccumulate, i.e. replete, to presuckled levels within the pituitary. The extent of depletion is directly related both to the intensity of suckling, i.e. number of pups, and to the length of the previous nonsuckling interval, but directly influenced by the intensity of suckling (Grosvenor and Mena 1971). In contrast, maximum concentrations of prolactin are reached in the plasma within 10–20 min of suckling. The pattern obtained with suckling could be mimicked by a steady, but not by a rapid, infusion of exogenous prolactin (Fig. 3.6). The secretion rate of prolactin during each min of suckling was estimated in rats in mid-lactation to be 400–600 ng min^{-1} (Grosvenor and Whitworth 1974).

Analysis of the afferent, reflex activation of prolactin secretion was made recently in

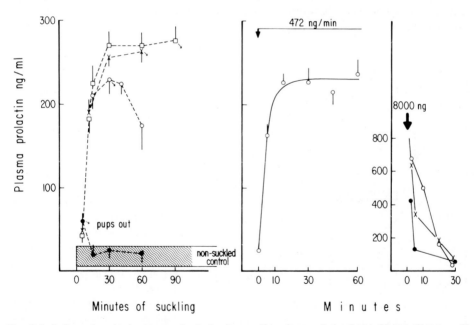

Fig. 3.6. Left panel, prolactin concentration in the plasma of lactating rats during 5 (○), 30 (●), 60 (×), or 90 (□) min of suckling following 8 h of nonsuckling on day 14 postpartum. Shaded area represents range prior to suckling. Arrows indicate the termination of suckling. Middle panel, prolactin concentration during constant 60 min intravenous infusion of rat prolactin (472 ng min^{-1}). Right panel, prolactin concentration after a single rapid intravenous injection of prolactin (8000 ng). Data in left and middle panels are expressed as means ±SEM for 5–8 rats; each symbol in the right panel represents a single rat (Grosvenor and Whitworth 1974).

urethane-anesthetized lactating rats. When suckling was applied, both intermittent milk ejection and prolactin release occurred (Burnet and Wakerley 1976). However, a latency of about 1 h preceded the release of each hormone, suggesting that anesthesia somehow slowed the effect of suckling. On the other hand, short (5–10 s) periods of adequate mammary nerve stimulation released small amounts of oxytocin without delay or refractoriness (Mena et al. 1978). Acute depletion, followed by prolactin repletion within the pituitary and release of prolactin into the circulation in amounts comparable to that in conscious rats following suckling, also resulted without delay from mammary nerve stimulation (Mena et al. 1980) (Fig. 3.7). Thus, it appears that oxytocin and prolactin may be released simultaneously in response to peripheral stimulation in the lactating rat. A similar conclusion was anticipated on the basis of overlapping afferent pathways (Tindal and Knaggs 1969) and also after simultaneous measurement of oxytocin and prolactin in the cow (Forsling et al. 1974).

It has been observed that the release of prolactin induced by peripheral stimulation in different species continues well beyond the period of actual stimulation. Thus, in the anesthetized rat, the plasma prolactin levels are maintained for up to 60 min after the end of suckling (Burnet and Wakerley 1976) or mammary nerve stimulation (Mena et al. 1980). In the conscious rat, the effect was observed only when suckling was maintained for 30, but not for 5, min which suggests that a threshold amount of stimulation from the pups was required (Grosvenor and Whitworth 1974) (Fig. 3.6). Recently, we exposed lactating rats to their pups for 10, 30, or 60 min to provoke the release of prolactin in the plasma. As seen

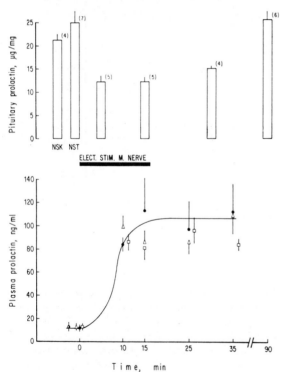

Fig. 3.7. The effect of 15 min of electrical stimulation (5–30 V, 1-ms pulses, 10 per s; 5 s on, 10 s off) of a mammary nerve upon pituitary and plasma prolactin concentrations in rats previously nonsuckled for 6–8 h. Upper panel, pituitary prolactin concentration in sham-stimulated (NST) and nonsuckled (NSK, all unlabelled points) rats. Numbers in parentheses refer to number of rats. Lower panel, plasma prolactin concentration in intact ($\bullet$, control; $n = 4$), adrenalectomized ($\triangle$, ADX performed 2 h before stimulation; $n = 4$), propranolol-treated ($\square$, 0.3 mg injected 20 min prior to stimulation; $n = 4$), and sham-operated (2 h before beginning of experiment) nonstimulated rats ($\bigcirc$; $n = 3$). Data are expressed as means $\pm$ SEM (Mena et al. 1980).

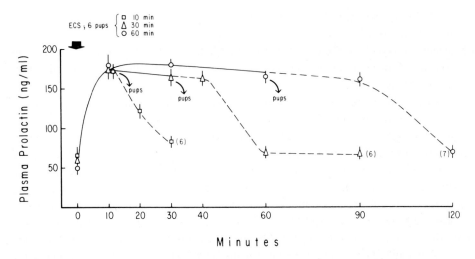

Fig. 3.8. Relationship between length of stimulation by exteroceptive stimulation (ECS) by 6 pups and extent of prolactin release after cessation of the stimulus. Values are means ±SEM; numbers in parentheses refer to numbers of rats (Grosvenor and Mena, unpublished results).

in Fig. 3.8, the plasma concentration of prolactin fell swiftly after 10 min of exposure, was maintained for at least 10 min before falling in those exposed for 30 min, and was maintained for at least 30 min before declining in those stimulated exteroceptively for 60 min. Thus, the length of time for which the release of prolactin continues following cessation of the stimulus is directly related to the length of the period of stimulation.

In contrast to that in the rat, this phenomenon was observed following a short suckling or milking stimulus in rabbits (McNeilly and Friesen 1978) and goats (Hart 1975). The possibilities of interpretation include: after-discharge of teat receptors in the goat following milking (Tindal 1978); reduction of prolactin metabolic clearance rate as a result of prolonged suckling (Burnet and Wakerley 1976); peripheral metabolic changes influencing immunodetectability (Nicoll 1975; Van Der Gugten 1976); activation by peripheral stimulation of central facilitatory mechanisms capable of remaining active and stimulating prolactin release once peripheral stimulation has subsided (Burnet and Wakerley 1976); and transfer and sequestering of plasma prolactin into the milk (McMurtry and Malven 1974; Grosvenor and Whitworth 1976) and subsequent return of the hormone to the circulation. Either one or several of these possibilities may contribute to the above phenomenon.

Autofeedback regulation of prolactin secretion in the lactating rat

Prolactin is thought to exert a negative feedback action on its own release. Evidence for this autoregulatory effect has been demonstrated in investigations where several parameters of prolactin secretion have been measured following different modes of prolactin administration to rats or mice. The effects of these treatments have been expressed at various levels, including enhanced hypothalamic prolactin inhibiting factor (PIF)-dopamine activity (Clemens and Meites 1968; Hökfelt and Fuxe 1972), depressed synthesis and reserve of adenohypophysial prolactin (Clemens and Meites 1968; MacLeod 1970), and, in lactating rats, lowered serum prolactin concentrations and milk rates (Clemens et al. 1969; Voogt and Meites 1973).

In general, these observations have been derived from studies in which prolactin was administered to rats by multiple systemic injections of 1 or more mg of prolactin, ectopic pituitary homografts, inoculation with prolactin-secreting tumors, or by median eminence implants of prolactin. While these procedures have unequivocally reduced the discharge of pituitary prolactin, their effects on systemic prolactin concentrations suggest that these treatments may not closely approximate normal patterns of prolactin release. A single 1 mg injection of prolactin elevates serum prolactin for several hours, with peak concentrations reaching 1200 ng ml^{-1} (Advis et al. 1977), and serum prolactin levels of hosts bearing prolactin-secreting tumors can approach 40 μg ml^{-1} (Lamberts and MacLeod 1979; Perkins et al. 1979). Although hormone diffusion and uptake rates are not known, median eminence implants of prolactin would seem likely to produce locally high concentrations of prolactin within the hypothalamus. Sustained high concentrations of circulating prolactin are not typically encountered in the male, the estrus cycling female, or even the lactating rat, where prolactin has been shown to quickly decline to basal levels during periods of nonsuckling (Neill 1974). Each of the above mentioned techniques would, therefore, not only raise systemic blood prolactin concentrations to levels well above normal, but may also expose prolactin autoregulatory pathways to unusually high and/or sustained levels of prolactin. For this reason, the role that prolactin feedback might actually play in the acute or chronic regulation of prolactin secretion has not been well defined. We therefore investigated this role. We found (Whitworth et al. 1981) that a single sc injection of 3 mg prolactin given 4 h beforehand was adequate to inhibit significantly the rise in plasma prolactin in response to subsequent suckling, as well as to ether, in lactating rats (Table 3.1). A comparable (56%) deficit in the suckling-induced rise in plasma prolactin was evident when mothers were injected with prolactin as long as 16 h prior to suckling. Injection of prolactin at 20 and 16 h

Table 3.1

THE PLASMA PROLACTIN RESPONSE TO SUCKLING OR ETHER STIMULATION 4 h AFTER sc INJECTION OF 3 mg oPRL

Treatment	Plasma prolactin (ng ml^{-1})		
	Pre-stimulation	30 min suckling	5 min ether
3 mg oPRL	21 ± 1(6)	105 ± 25(6)*	33 ± 3(5)*
Saline	24 ± 4(6)	273 ± 26(6)	77 ± 3(5)

Rats were nonsuckled 4 h before treatment. The values are means ±SEM; the number of rats is indicated in parentheses.
* Significantly less than saline treated control ($P<0.05$).

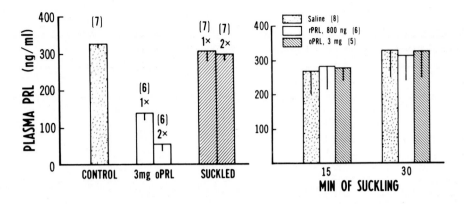

Fig. 3.9. (Left) The suckling induced rise in plasma PRL of lactating rats following injection of 3 mg oPRL or a 15 min nursing episode given 16 h (1×) or 16 and 20 h (2×) earlier. Plasma samples were obtained from trunk blood collected after 30 min of nursing. Mean plasma PRL values of non-suckled groups ranged from 20 to 27 ng ml⁻¹. The bars indicate the means and the vertical lines the SEM; the numbers in parentheses refer to the number of rats (Whitworth et al. 1981).

Fig. 3.10. (Right) The effect of oPRL or rPRL given 30 min before suckling upon the subsequent suckling induced rise in plasma PRL. The rats were nonsuckled 4 h before treatment. oPRL was given as a 3 mg subcutaneous injection, while rPRL was given as 5 intravenous injections, 800 ng each, at 1 min intervals. Each bar represents the mean, and vertical lines are the SEM. The number of rats is indicated in parentheses (Whitworth et al. 1981).

before nursing decreased the suckling-induced rise in prolactin to 17% of that of noninjected controls (Fig. 3.9), suggesting a dose–response relationship between injected prolactin and the extent to which the suckling-induced release of prolactin was subsequently inhibited. There was no inhibition, however, when 3 mg of prolactin were injected sc 30 min before suckling (see Fig. 3.10), despite the fact that other evidence (Advis et al. 1977) indicates that substantial concentrations of prolactin would have been present in the peripheral circulation during the course of this experiment. These observations are consistent with the previous report of Advis et al. (1977), who found that injection of 1 mg of prolactin did not inhibit the stress-induced rise in serum prolactin after administration. Lactating rats also fail to show blockage of the combined nursing- and stress-evoked depletion in pituitary prolactin when a total of 12 mg of prolactin are given sc over a 1 h period before exposure to these stimuli (Grosvenor et al. 1965). The latency between administration of prolactin and the onset of prolactin release inhibition would suggest that prolactin negative feedback mechanisms are not activated simultaneously with rising systemic titers of plasma prolactin. This conclusion may also be applicable to prolactin released in situ, since prolactin released endogenously by suckling stimulation continues unabated at least 30 and up to 90 min under a variety of conditions (Grosvenor and Whitworth 1974; Grosvenor et al. 1979). Furthermore, the stimulatory effect of prolactin on hypothalamic dopamine activity is not observed until 4 h after prolactin is administered

Table 3.2

CHANGES IN PLASMA PROLACTIN CONCENTRATION IN RESPONSE TO SUCKLING 4 h FOL-
LOWING 5 INTRAVENOUS INJECTIONS OF 400 OR 800 ng PROLACTIN

Dose/injection (ng)	Min of suckling		
	0	15	30
Saline (7)	26 ± 2	306 ± 20	383 ± 74
400 oPRL (5)	26 ± 5	296 ± 38	432 ± 70
400 rPRL (6)	32 ± 2	255 ± 62	396 ± 41
800 rPRL (6)	22 ± 2	298 ± 80	389 ± 95

The rats were nonsuckled for 4 h and injections were given at 1 min intervals. The values are means ±SEM of
plasma prolactin, ng ml^{-1}; the number of rats is referred to in parentheses.

or released (Hökfelt and Fuxe 1972; Perkins et al. 1979), a latency similar to that required
to inhibit prolactin release in the present study with high doses of prolactin. In view of the
above, it seems unlikely that prolactin autoregulation would provide acute negative feedback control, for example, to suppress prolactin release during a concurrent suckling
episode.

In further support of this view, we found that injection of 800 ng prolactin per min for
5 min, 30 min prior to suckling did not significantly inhibit the subsequent induced rise in
plasma prolactin (Fig. 3.10). There was also no indication of inhibited prolactin secretion
when 400 or 800 ng min^{-1} for 5 min prolactin were given if 4 h before suckling, even
though injection of these amounts raised plasma prolactin to levels comparable to those
following suckling (Table 3.2). Using a similar experimental technique, it has been
reported that a five- to eight-fold elevation in serum prolactin also does not prevent the
milking-induced release of prolactin in cows (Tucker et al. 1973).

Finally, we examined the effects of prolactin released endogenously by suckling on the
subsequent suckling-induced release of prolactin. When prolactin is released by this
stimulus, it would presumably reach autoregulatory sites, by retrograde circulation or
otherwise, under at least physiologic conditions, if not maximal concentrations. The
prolactin released in situ by one or two suckling episodes (15 min each) did not inhibit the
suckling-induced rise in plasma prolactin when tested 16 h later, yet when the animals were
injected with 3 mg prolactin instead of being suckled, the suckling-induced rise in prolactin
was clearly attenuated (Fig. 3.9). The rise in the lactating rat's plasma prolactin concentration in response to suckling generally exceeds the rise reported for nonlactating rats in
response to other naturally occurring prolactin-releasing stimuli, e.g. proestrus, copula-
tion, and pregnancy (Neill 1974). Assuming that the prolactin discharged in situ by
suckling is reaching prolactin autoregulatory sites at proportionate rates, the amount of
prolactin required to activate negative feedback mechanisms would therefore appear to be
quite high since prolactin released by suckling was not inhibitory.

Independence of prolactin depletion and release during suckling:
the multiphase pattern of prolactin secretion

Nicoll (1972) and Swearingen (1971) incubated pituitary tissue from lactating and estrogen–treated rats, respectively, and measured tissue and medium content of prolactin by disc electrophoresis and densitometry (E-D) at pH 7.0. They showed that temporal and quantitative discrepancies existed between depletion and release of the hormone and concluded that prolactin depletion within the pituitary could occur without concomitant release (Nicoll 1972) and that prolactin was released from a nondetectable (by E-D) pool (Swearingen 1971). We have obtained results in the lactating rat which support Nicoll's concept that during secretion, prolactin undergoes changes in form which may shift from one to another, without a great change in anterior pituitary hormone content.

As stated previously, there is a clear discrepancy between the amount of prolactin depleted from the pituitary after the onset of suckling and the amount of the hormone appearing in the circulation at the time. This is shown in Fig. 3.11, in which prolactin is maximally depleted (15–60 µg) within 1–2 min of suckling, yet little (1–2 µg) has appeared in the circulation within this time.

In our experiments with mammary nerve stimulation in rats, low plasma prolactin levels coincided with depleted anterior pituitary prolactin levels after 5 min of stimulation, and the high plasma prolactin seen after 90 and 180 min coincided with repleted levels of anterior pituitary prolactin (Mena et al. 1980) (Fig. 3.7). These results indicate that depletion, release, and repletion of the hormone are independent processes. In a recent study, the quantitative relationship between depleted and released prolactin was analyzed in rats suckled continuously for 90 min following 2, 4, or 8 h of nonsuckling. Since the amount of prolactin depleted by suckling is directly related to the length of the previous nonsuckling interval (see Grosvenor et al. 1979a for references) and since the depleted hormone does not leave the gland, but becomes undetected by current assay methods, the assumption was made that the undetected hormone would be released slowly and in small amounts in the circulation with continuous suckling. We found that 17, 32, and 48 µg of prolactin were released into the plasma in the 2, 4, and 8 h nonsuckled groups, respectively (Grosvenor et al. 1979a), values which were similar to amounts depleted from the pituitary during the first

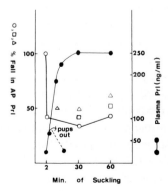

Fig. 3.11. Relationship between kinetics of depletion (○--○) of prolactin within the pituitary (AP) with that of release (●—●) of the hormone into the circulation.

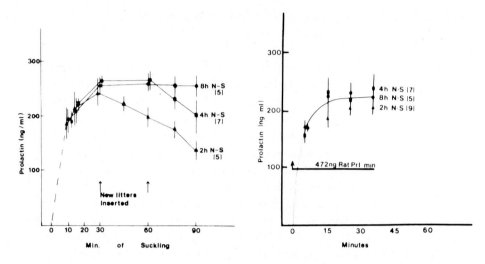

Fig. 3.12. Influence of increasing the length of the nonsuckling interval (N-S) from 2 (▲) to 4 (■) to 8 (●) h upon the plasma prolactin concentration induced by: left panel, suckling; right panel, continuous infusion of rat prolactin (472 ng min^{-1}). Values (minus plasma prolactin concentration at time 0) are expressed as means ± SEM. Numbers in parentheses refer to number of rats (Grosvernor et al. 1979a).

few min of suckling following similar nonsuckling periods (Amenomori et al. 1970; Subramanian and Reece 1975; Nicoll et al. 1976). Secretion rates (554, 530, and 537 ng min^{-1} for the three groups) as well as clearance rates of prolactin were similar for each group (Fig. 3.12). However, the time during which the rate of prolactin secretion remained constant varied directly with the length of the nonsuckling interval. A steady secretion was maintained for the entire 90 min suckling period in the 8 h group, for 60 min in the 4 h group, and for only 30 min in the 2 h group (Grosvenor et al. 1979a) (Fig. 3.12). These results indicated that a quantitative relationship existed between depleted and released prolactin provided their different secretory dynamics were taken into consideration. However, since depleted prolactin is not released directly into the circulation, it was reasoned that a transformation of depleted to releasable prolactin must occur before the hormone is released (Grosvenor et al. 1979a).

The relative significance of the depletion-transformation phase as a limiting event on the availability of prolactin for release was determined using ether as a stimulus that induces release, but not depletion, of prolactin. The results showed that a small, transient increase in prolactin occurred in the plasma when ether was applied after 5–6 h of nonsuckling (Fig. 3.13). This contrasted with a large, sustained release of prolactin similar to that induced by suckling when ether was administered to rats previously depleted of prolactin by 10 min of suckling. This resulted even if ether was applied 2 h after depletion (Grosvenor et al. 1979b). Similar results were obtained employing the ECS emanating from two rat pups or from laboratory personnel (Grosvenor et al. 1981). Neither stimulus provoked depletion or release of prolactin into the circulation when applied to nondepleted rats, but when applied after depletion had been effected by 10 min of suckling, large sustained elevations in

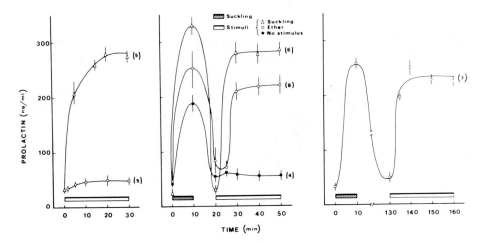

Fig. 3.13. Plasma prolactin concentration in lactating rats during: left panel, suckling (△) or ether (○) stimulation; middle panel, an initial 10-min period of suckling followed by 30 min of suckling (△), ether exposure (○), or no stimulus (●); right panel, ether exposure 130 min after an initial 10-min suckling period. Values are expressed as means ±SEM. Numbers in parentheses indicate number of rats (Grosvenor et al. 1979b).

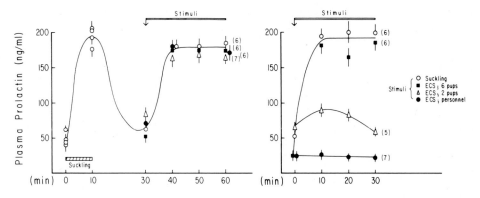

Fig. 3.14. Effect of exteroceptive stimulation (ECS) upon release of prolactin in conscious rats (right); same stimuli applied after a 10 min period of suckling (left) (Grosvenor et al. 1981).

plasma prolactin concentration occurred (Fig. 3.14). These data further support the concept that releasable prolactin derives from depleted prolactin and indicate that, once formed, releasable prolactin remains available for discharge into the circulation for a relatively long period of time. In addition, the observation that ECS from two pups will release prolactin, whereas ECS from six pups are required for depletion, suggests that the depletion-transformation phase may have a higher activation threshold than does the release phase.

Factors involved in depletion-transformation and release of prolactin

Recently, pituitary tissue from either nonsuckled or suckled (for 15 min after 8 h of non suckling) rats was incubated for 4 h in medium 199 containing 21.6 mM bicarbonate concentration. Both tissue and medium prolactin were measured by E-D at pH 7.0. Pituitary tissue from suckled rats exhibited an initial repletion and then a depletion of prolactin during the first 90 min of incubation, whereas that from nonsuckled rats first depleted, then repleted, and then depleted prolactin again during the same period. From 90 to 240 min, no further change of prolactin content occurred in either type of pituitary; in contrast, prolactin was released into the medium by each type at a similar constant rate (Mena et al. 1979) (Fig. 3.15). At the end of incubation, less prolactin was secreted than was depleted by pituitaries of suckled rats. These results show that prolactin within the lactating rat pituitary undergoes changes in detectability when devoid of regulatory controls.

Solubility of prolactin

Detectability of pituitary prolactin by E-D at pH 7.0 may be questioned on the grounds that not all the hormone present in the gland is extracted. Microsomal prolactin, for example, cannot be extracted unless sodium dodecyl sulfate (SDS) or other drastic methods are employed (Samli et al. 1972; Zanini et al. 1974a and b). Since E-D at pH 7 appears to

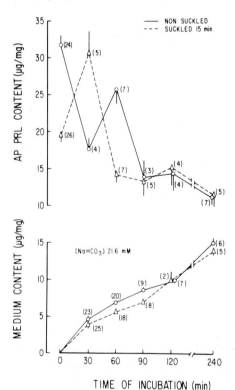

Fig. 3.15. Changes in AP PRL content (upper panel) and release (lower panel) during a 4 h incubation of hemipituitaries from lactating (pp. days 7–14) rats either untreated or suckled for 15 min after 8 h of non-suckling. Incubation was made at 37°C, in individual flasks, in medium 199 (21.6 mM bicarbonate concentration, pH 7.4) under 95% O_2, 5% CO_2; 125 rev. min⁻¹. Tissue and medium PRL were measured by E-D (pH 7). Numbers in parentheses refer to number of rats. Data are expressed as means ±SEM. (Mena et al. 1979).

Table 3.3

EFFECT OF SUCKLING AND SUBSEQUENT IN VITRO INCUBATION UPON ADENOHYPOPHYSIAL PROLACTIN CONTENT AND RELEASE ($\mu g\ mg^{-1}$)

Treatment	No. of rats	Anterior pituitary prolactin[B]		30 min incubation[A]		
				Anterior pituitary prolactin[B]		Medium prolactin
		pH 7	pH 10	pH 7	pH 10	
8 h Non-suckled[C]	5	48.3 ± 2.9	54.2 ± 1.8	27.7 ± 2.5	45.5 ± 4.2	6.3 ± 0.8
Suckled 15 min	5	31.9 ± 1.1	44.8 ± 2.0	31.2 ± 2.9	47.3 ± 2.0	6.2 ± 0.4

[A] Incubation was made in individual flasks at 37°C in medium 199 (21.6 mM bicarbonate concentration, pH 7.4) under 95 % O_2, 5 % CO_2; 125 rev. min^{-1}.

[B] Anterior pituitary prolactin content was measured by E-D (Nicoll et al. 1969). Extraction was made by homogenizing tissue in upper gel (pH 7) or in bicarbonate (pH 10).

[C] Rats employed were between day 7–14 postpartum. Each had 8–10 pup litters.

detect only that prolactin which has attained a certain degree of maturity, perhaps as granular prolactin, it is possible that the repletion of prolactin observed in vitro (see Fig. 3.15) may be accounted for in part by additional prolactin appearing in granule form (see Zanini et al. 1974b). On the other hand, in the experiments both in vivo and in vitro in which prolactin depletion was not accounted for in terms of released prolactin (Nicoll and Swearingen 1970; Swearingen 1971; Grosvenor et al. 1979b), one has to consider that the hormone has shifted within the pituitary from a detectable to a non detectable form (Nicoll 1972). Accordingly, the high degree of solubilization obtained by SDS alkaline extraction (see below) would render these methods inadequate to study transient changes of the hormone during secretion.

We recently observed that prolactin depleted by a 15 min period of suckling or that occurring after 30 min of incubation in pituitary glands of nonsuckled rats could be detected only when the pituitary tissue was extracted at pH 7.0 and not when extracted at pH 10 using bicarbonate buffer (Table 3.3). The amount of prolactin depleted from pituitaries of nonsuckled rats upon incubation was about 20 μg mg^{-1}, as detected at pH 7, whereas at pH 10, about 10 μg mg^{-1} were depleted. Since released prolactin accounted for only 6.3 μg mg^{-1}, it is clear that a large proportion, about 14 μg mg^{-1}, changed into a nondetectable form upon incubation. In the case of the suckled anterior pituitaries, the released prolactin (6.2 μg mg^{-1}) plus that detected in the pituitary at either pH did not equal the initial, preincubation content (Table 3.3), suggesting that some prolactin release may have occurred from a nondetectable pool. Also, new hormone, i.e. microsomal prolactin or that from de novo synthesis, may have been incorporated into granules and thus extracted at pH 10.

90

In vitro studies have revealed that most of the prolactin within the pituitary (~80% of total prolactin) is in granular form, that such prolactin is not soluble, but is a stable solid-state structure, and that solubilization of membraneless granules occurs only at a pH above pH 6, (Giannattasio et al. 1975). These results indicate that for prolactin to be released, solubilization of the hormone must take place during exocytosis, perhaps as a result of the alkaline environment of the extracellular space (Giannattasio et al. 1975). In support of this possibility, Lamberts and MacLeod (1979) reported that an increase in prolactin secretion occurred in vitro when anterior pituitary explants were incubated in medium containing high bicarbonate concentration. We have confirmed these results using lactating rat pituitaries incubated in low (4.16 mM) or high (21.6 mM) bicarbonate concentration; a direct dose-related effect of the ion upon both depletion and release of the hormone was noted (Mena et al. unpublished). These in vitro results, indicate that changes in solubility of the prolactin molecule are involved in the change from the depletion-transformation to the release phase, the former being prolactin which is relatively insoluble and the latter prolactin which has been solubilized, perhaps due to the high pH of the extracellular fluids.

Further analysis of the solubility factor was made recently by Zanini et al. (1980) using double-label techniques. They found that new granular prolactin is much less stable, i.e., more soluble, than older granular prolactin, thus demonstrating that the stability of the hormone is increased during maturation. The greater insolubility may have been the result of interactions between macromolecular carbohydrates and prolactin. Thus, sulfated glycosaminoglecans and glycoproteins were biochemically characterized in membraneless prolactin granules and in association with the hormone. The interactions between sugar macromolecules and prolactin may originate at the time of packaging of the hormone in the Golgi complex (see Zanini et al. 1980).

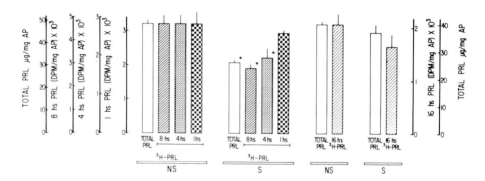

Fig. 3.16. Effect of 15 min suckling following 8 or 16 h of nonsuckling on pp days 7–14 upon either total unlabelled AP PRL (µg mg⁻¹) or PRL labelled with [³H]Leu either 1, 4, 8, or 16 h before suckling (DPM mg⁻¹). [³H]Leu (3 µCi g⁻¹ b.w.) was injected i.v. under light ether anesthesia. Each group was composed of 4–6 rats. Values are expressed as means ±SEM. * = significantly lower (P<0.05 or less) than their respective nonsuckled group. (Mena et al. unpublished results).

Age of prolactin

In recent experiments prolactin was labelled in vivo with [³H]leucine (3 μCi g⁻¹, body weight) at different times before suckling. We determined (Mena et al. unpublished) that in vivo depletion-transformation induced by suckling and subsequent in vitro release of the hormone varied according to the 'age' of the hormone within the pituitary. Thus, as shown in Fig. 3.16, [³H]prolactin labelled either 4 or 8 h before suckling was depleted in parallel to total unlabelled prolactin following a 15 min suckling period; however, there was no depletion of that [³H]prolactin labelled either 1 h or 16 h before suckling. These results show that only *some* of the prolactin present in the pituitary is transformed for subsequent release by the stimulus of suckling. Data obtained previously in vitro indicated that newly synthesized prolactin is preferentially released over old hormone (Swearingen 1971; Walker and Farquhar 1980). We had expected, therefore, that prolactin labelled 1 h before suckling would be depleted by suckling to a similar or greater extent than that labelled 4–8 h before suckling. This, however, did not occur. It appears likely instead that 1–4 h must elapse before prolactin can be depleted and subsequently transformed; hormone younger than 1 h in terms of its biosynthesis may require further maturation. We anticipated that prolactin labelled 16 h before suckling would not be depleted since previous work has shown that prolactin could not be depleted if 16–24 h had elapsed since the previous depletion (Grosvenor et al. 1967).

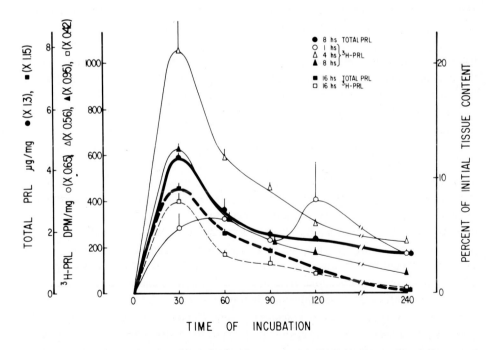

Fig. 3.17. Effect of 4 h incubation of hemipituitaries from rats in Fig. 3.16. Conditions of incubation were as described in legend of Fig. 3.15. Values are expressed as means ±SEM. Each group was composed of 4-hemipituitaries (Mena et al. unpublished).

The release of prolactin into the medium in vitro also was influenced by the age of the prolactin in general agreement with the above in vivo results (Fig. 3.17). Thus, prolactin labelled 4 h before incubation was secreted in relatively greater proportion than total prolactin. That labelled 8 h previously was secreted in about the same proportion as total prolactin during the first 90–120 min of incubation, whereas a much smaller amount of that prolactin labelled 16 h before incubation was secreted. Interestingly, the prolactin labelled 1 h before incubation also was secreted at a low rate, although, in contrast to the declining rate of release of all the other prolactins, its secretion rate was maintained at a constant level (Fig. 3.17). At the end of incubation, 33 % of 4 h prolactin remained unsecreted within the tissue, whereas 65 % of 8 h prolactin and 83 % of 16 h prolactin were retained within the gland. Finally, perhaps due to the fact that it was secreted at a constant rate, 61 % of 1 h prolactin was retained within the gland.

The results of the present in vivo and in vitro studies show some similarities, Thus, those prolactins that were not depleted by suckling, i.e., those labelled 1 and 16 h previously, were secreted in vitro in a comparatively low proportion; 8 h prolactin was intermediate. The prolactin labelled 4 h before suckling which, together with 8 h prolactin, was depleted by suckling showed the highest secretion in vitro. We suggest, therefore, that the mammotrophs possess intrinsic regulatory mechanisms for both 'protection' of the new hormone from premature release and 'retention' of the old hormone, presumably for disposal. The apparent contradiction of the in vitro results of other investigators (MacLeod 1976; Walker and Farquhar 1980) with this conclusion may be attributed to the particular experimental conditions. Isolated anterior pituitary cells obtained from estrogen-treated animals and/or isotopic labelling of only that hormone synthesized in vitro may yield results which, though valuable, are difficult to extrapolate to some physiological situations. It is possible, judging from our data, that newly synthesized prolactin may not be released preferentially over all other older prolactins, and that during secretion, transformations of prolactin may occur which, if not taken into consideration, may result in inaccurate estimates of hormonal turnover.

Recent morphological studies of mammotrophs of lactating rats in our laboratory have yielded results which appear to correlate with physiological and biochemical data on the dynamics of prolactin secretion. As expected from previous studies of Farquhar's laboratory (Farquhar et al. 1978) we noted that [3H]prolactin labelled 8 h previously was observed in large granules (Fig. 3.18A), suggesting that depletion-transformation and release occurred principally at the expense of mature hormone. The use of horseradish peroxidase (HRP) as a tracer added in vivo indicates that granule extrusion occurs in response to suckling. Although such extrusion is extensive (see Fig. 3.18B), it is a very slow process, allowing time for the extracellular fluid to interact with the granule content (Vila-Porcile and Olivier 1980), and presumably contributing to granule solubilization. The diffusion tracer progressively penetrates the granules to attain a complete impregnation (Fig. 3.18C). Interestingly, at the end of a 2-h suckling period, positive horseradish peroxidase granules were found (Fig. 3.18D), similar to those observed previously in vitro (Pelletier 1973). This suggests either retention of stained granules and/or recycling of membrane material through endocytosis and subsequent incorporation into prolactin granules (Pelletier 1973).

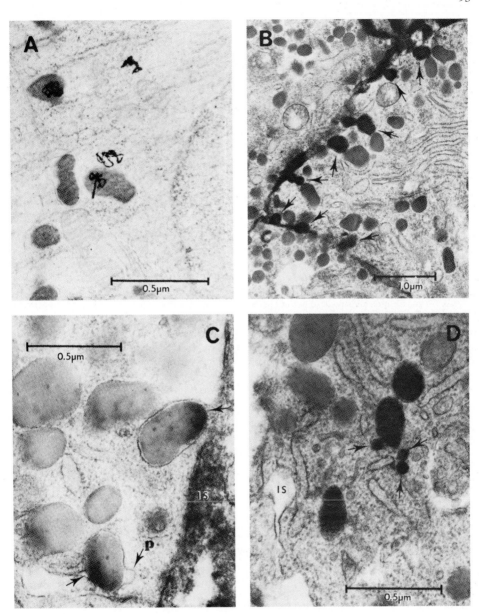

Fig. 3.18. (A) Electron micrograph (EM) of part of a prolactin cell from a lactating rat nonsuckled for 8 h and then suckled for 15 min. [^{3}H]Leucine was injected i.p. ($3\ \mu$Ci g^{-1} b.w.) at the time of removing the pups. Two mature secretory granules appear labelled. (B) EM of part of a prolactin cell from a lactating rat nonsuckled for 8 h and then suckled for 15 min. Horseradish peroxidase (HPR) (Sigma type II) was injected i.v. (15 mg 100 g^{-1} b.w.) 30 min before, i.e. 15 min before suckling commenced. Note that the granules which open towards the intercellular space have taken the HRP (arrows). (C) Higher magnification of a prolactin cell from a rat treated as in Fig. 3.18B. HPR seems to have penetrated two secretory granules (arrows) from the intercellular space (IS). A pinocytotic vesicle has been formed in one of them (P). (D) EM of part of a prolactin cell from an HRP-injected rat fixed two hours after onset of suckling. At this time there is no HRP in the intercellular space (IS) but several positive granules are found in the cytoplasm. Some small HRP positive vesicles of unknown origin (Golgi, endocytocis, ?) are also seen (arrows) (Unpublished data from H. Merchant, D. Aguayo and F. Mena).

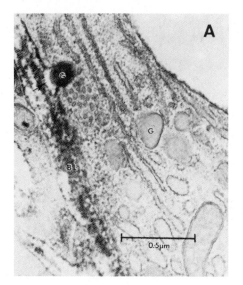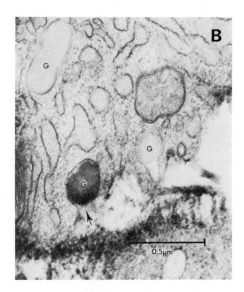

Fig. 3.19. (A) Electron micrograph of part of a prolactin cell (rat nonsuckled for 8 h then suckled 15 min) treated with Concanavalin A and developed with HRP in 40 μm aldehyde-fixed sections. The basal lamina (BL) and an open secretory granule (G-arrow) are positive. Close secretory granules (G) are negative. (B) Exocytosis of a wheat-germ–agglutinin–HRP positive prolactin secretory granule (G-arrow) from a lactating rat (nonsuckled 8 h and then suckled 15 min). 40 μm sections were exposed to HRP-conjugated lectin after aldehyde fixation. Closed secretory granules (G) are negative, even those very near the plasmalemma. (Merchant, Aguayo and Mena, unpublished).

The possibility that, during exocytosis, glycoconjugated macromolecules from the extracellular space may enter into the exocytotic pouch and interact with the prolactin granule is suggested by the finding that only granules undergoing exocytosis, and not those within the cell, gave positive reaction to lectins like concanavalin A and wheat-germ-agglutinin, well known for their specificity for the above compounds (Sharon and Lis 1972), (see Fig. 3.19A and B). These results (Merchant et al. unpublished) suggest that depletion-transformation and release of prolactin by the lactating rat pituitary may occur in the mature, large granules. These perhaps interact with glycoconjugates originating either from the membrane itself and/or from the intercellular space, following which proteases and/or alkaline extracellular fluids may solubilize the granules permitting the hormone to be released.

Lysosomal destruction of prolactin

Granule breakup may occur both in the extracellular space and in the lysosomal compartment, the latter being an important intracellular regulatory mechanism responsible for digesting excess hormone (Smith and Farquhar 1966). Lysosomal degradation of prolactin, i.e. crinophagy (see Farquhar 1977), was demonstrated in mammotrophs 24–36 h after removing the pups from the mother. Recently, the possibility has been explored in several laboratories, including ours, that crinophagy may actively participate in the short-term

Table 3.4

EFFECT OF 15 min OF SUCKLING, HALOPERIDOL OR CHLOROQUINE ADMINISTRATION, APPLIED MIDWAY DURING A 16 h NON-SUCKLING PERIOD, UPON SUCKLING-INDUCED DEPLETION OF ANTERIOR PITUITARY PROLACTIN AND UPON SUBSEQUENT 4 h RELEASE OF PROLACTIN

Treatment	No. of rats[A]	Effect of 15 min-suckling Anterior pituitary prolactin (μg mg^{-1})[B]	Effect of 4 h incubation Medium prolactin (μg mg^{-1})[C]
8 h nonsuckled	6	48.7 ± 1.5	20.7 ± 1.6
Suckled 15 min	5	31.5 ± 1.2	18.7 ± 0.8
16 h nonsuckled	4	39.8 ± 1.0	10.4 ± 0.2
Suckled 15 min	6	37.0 ± 2.5	8.1 ± 0.6
16 h nonsuckled	3	40.3 ± 1.9	16.4 ± 1.2[D]
Suckled 15 min (Both groups suckled 15 min after first 8 h NS)	3	29.4 ± 0.9	14.1 ± 0.6[D]
16 h nonsuckled	5	46.2 ± 3.7	17.3 ± 0.9
Suckled 15 min (Haloperidol (100 μg kg^{-1} b.w.) injected i.p. both groups after first 8 h NS)	5	25.9 ± 2.2	16.3 ± 0.7
16 h nonsuckled	5	56.0 ± 1.7[E]	21.3 ± 1.8
Suckled 15 min (Chloroquine (10 mg kg^{-1} b.w.) injected i.p. into both groups after first 8 h NS)	5	33.7 ± 0.4	20.6 ± 1.1

[A] Rats employed were 7–14 days postpartum. Each had 8–10 pup litters. Groups nonsuckled for 16 h had their pups with foster mothers for the first 8 h of separation.

[B] Anterior pituitary prolactin content was measured by E-D (pH 7).

[C] 4 h incubation was made at 37°C in medium 199 (21.6 mM bicarbonate concentration, pH 7.4) under 95 % O_2, 5 % CO_2; 125 rev. min^{-1}.

[D] Significantly higher ($p<0.05$ or less) than 16 h nonsuckled control group.

[E] Significantly higher ($p<0.05$ or less) than other groups.

regulation of prolactin. As already described, depletion-transformation induced by suckling no longer occurs (Grosvenor et al. 1967; Fig. 3.16, present study), and in vitro secretion is greatly reduced from pituitaries of rats nonsuckled for 16 h (Fig. 3.17). However, a short 15–30 min suckling applied midway during the 16 h nonsuckling interval, restored the functioning of the prolactin depletion mechanism to suckling (Grosvenor et al. 1967). Recently, we found that a single injection of chloroquine, a well-known lysosomal inactivator, to rats midway during a 16 h non-suckling period resulted in a high prolactin content and in prolactin depletion-transformation when suckling was applied at the end of the 16 h period (Table 3.4). In addition, a release of prolactin, similar to that following 8 h of non-suckling, occurred in vitro from pituitaries of rats not suckled for 16 h but treated with chloroquine midway during the 16 h period (Table 3.4). These results (Mena et al. unpublished) confirm concepts derived from previous morphological studies (Smith and Farquhar 1966) and also indicate that lysosomal activation may operate in the short-term regulation of prolactin secretion.

The mechanisms which trigger lysosomal action upon prolactin granules are not known. However, since both suckling and haloperidol as well as chloroquine applied midway during the 16 h nonsuckling period, were effective in restoring both depletion-transformation and, at least partially, in vitro release of prolactin (see Table 3.4), it is possible that removal of the suckling stimulus and the maintenance of dopaminergic tone upon the pituitary are factors which favor crinophagy. It is probable that suckling-induced depletion-transformation is effected through transient depression of dopamine secretion (see Neill 1980). On the other hand, another factor which might also favor prolactin crinophagy may be related with the stability and age of the hormone since, as already discussed, these appear to be directly related (Zanini et al. 1980). The older and more insoluble the prolactin becomes, the more easily it is retained and therefore susceptible to lysosomal digestion. The absence of suckling also would be associated with a lack of PRF and/or TRH and this may contribute as well to retention of the hormone within the pituitary. In the reverse situations, i.e. that of actively secreting mammotrophs, a triggering of endocytotic-related lysosomal activation by TRH has been suggested (Tixier-Vidal and Gourdji 1980), on the basis of in vitro work. A clear increase in acid phosphatase activity around secretory granules was associated with both increased endocytosis and blockage of prolactin release in normal prolactin cells incubated with Concanavalin A and an increased number of lysosomes were visualized following exposure to TRH (Tixier-Vidal and Gourdji 1980). These results suggest the possibility that during TRH-induced prolactin release a concomitant retention and subsequent degradation of prolactin by lysosomes may take place.

Pituitary–hypothalamic interactions regulating multiphasic secretion of prolactin

In vivo data

The nature of the hypothalamic control of prolactin secretion is complex and is still far from being fully elucidated. In the lactating rat, evidence has been obtained implicating the hypothalamus in the control of prolactin depletion, release, and repletion. Part of this control is inhibitory, mediated by a hypothalamic factor (PIF) and/or by dopamine (see Grosvenor et al. 1980, for references). Recently, changes in dopamine levels in the hypothalamus, hypophysial stalk blood, or in the adenohypophysis have been reported following suckling or peripheral stimulation (Mena et al. 1976; Gibbs and Neill 1978; Chiocchio et al. 1979; deGreef and Neill 1979; Plotsky et al. 1979; also see Neill 1980). In addition, strong experimental evidence supports the existence of factors, including TRH (Nicoll et al. 1970; Valverde et al. 1972; Boyd et al. 1976; Koch et al. 1977; Vale et al. 1977),which stimulate the release of prolactin. Serotonin has been linked to the control mechanism for prolactin release (Kordon et al. 1973; Mena et al. 1976). Serotonin also stimulated the release of TRH from rat hypothalamus in vitro (Chen and Ramírez 1979) and of a PRF, presumably from the hypothalamus, in vivo (Clemens et al. 1978; Garthwaite and Hagen 1979). TRH will induce action potentials in prolactin-secreting rat pituitary cells when placed directly into the cell membrane (Dufy et al. 1979), suggesting TRH may be the terminal link in a serotonin–PRF–TRH system initiating release of the hormone. Finally, data indicate that circulating prolactin may feed back upon the hypothalamus and indirectly regulate its own rate of repletion by the pituitary (Grosvenor et al. 1970). The repletion of prolactin following its depletion may be accounted for by de novo synthesis, though a retransformation to depletable prolactin may be involved (Nicoll 1972).

In recent experiments using lactating rats, depletion-transformation and subsequent release of prolactin into the bloodstream were blocked when either stalk-median eminence (SME) extracts or the dopamine agonist, bromocriptine, was injected before suckling, whereas normal release of prolactin into the circulation occurred during suckling when they were given after an initial 10 min suckling (Figs 3.20 and 3.21) (Grosvenor et al. 1980). These data indicate that in the lactating rat, the dopamine–PIF hypothalamic control is exerted only upon the depletion-transformation, and not upon the release, phase of prolactin secretion.

In other experiments, either TRH or an extract of rat hypothalamus largely free of TRH was injected into lactating rats either after 4–5 h of nonsuckling or after anterior pituitary prolactin depletion had been first effected by prior short-term (10 min) suckling. Depletion-transformation did not occur, and only a small, transient release occurred when the TRH-free extract of SME or 1250 ng of TRH were injected after the period of nonsuckling

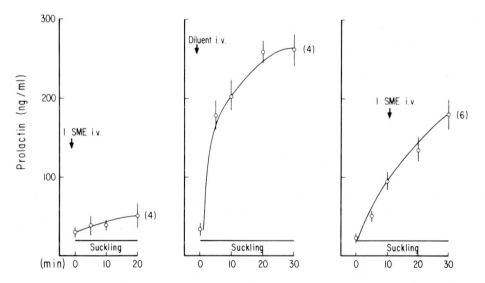

Fig. 3.20. Effect of stalk median eminence (SME) extract upon the suckling-induced release of prolactin in conscious rats. Left and right panels, SME extract injected i.v. before and 10 min after the suckling stimulus has begun, respectively. Note that the effect of suckling is blocked only under the former condition. Middle panel, controls injected i.v. with diluent before suckling. Values are expressed as means ±SEM. Numbers in parentheses refer to number of rats (Grosvenor et al. 1980).

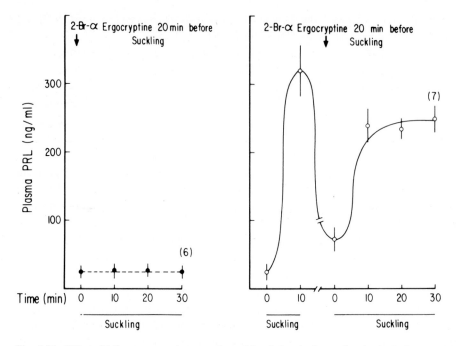

Fig. 3.21. Effect of 2-Br-α-ergocryptine upon the suckling-induced release of prolactin. Left panel, injection i.v. 20 min before a 30-min suckling period. Right panel, injection i.v. after an initial 10-min suckling period, 20 min before a 30-min suckling period. Values are expressed as means ±SEM. Numbers in parentheses refer to number of rats (Grosvenor et al. 1980).

(Fig. 3.22). However, when either the extract or 2, 10, 50, or 250 ng of TRH were injected after depletion-transformation of prolactin had taken place, a large and sustained release of prolactin was obtained similar to that induced by a second suckling (Fig. 3.22) (Grosvenor and Mena 1980). Neither 1.25 μg of TRH nor cerebral cortical extract previously incubated in rat serum released prolactin into the circulation when injected after depletion had taken place. Likewise, oxytocin, dopamine, and LH-RH were ineffective (Fig. 3.23). Thus, TRH and a TRH-free hypothalamic extract have a stimulatory action on the releasable phase of prolactin secretion in the lactating rat which is comparable to that of suckling; neither of these two compounds, however, has any effect on the depletion-transformation phase. These results recently have been corroborated by Plotsky and Neill (1981). They found that TRH failed to alter plasma prolactin levels in lactating rats treated with α-methyl p-tyrosine and infused continuously with dopamine. However, when the dopamine was stopped for 5 min and then resumed at the original level, injections of TRH resulted in a three-fold increase in plasma PRL levels lasting 20–30 min.

In conclusion, there appears to be a selective hypothalamic control upon the compartmentalized phases of anterior pituitary prolactin depletion and release, in vivo; a PIF-dopaminergic inhibition being exerted upon depletion and a TRH-PRF stimulatory control upon release.

In vitro data

Dopamine and its agonist bromocriptine depress both prolactin release and synthesis in vitro whereas lisuride, another agonist, inhibits only prolactin release (MacLeod et al. 1980). In our laboratory we tested the effect of dopamine upon prolactin depletion, repletion and release in incubated pituitaries from suckled and nonsuckled rats. Under the influence of dopamine in high concentration (5×10^{-5} M), neither prolactin depletion nor repletion occurred, and release of the hormone into the medium was greatly inhibited in both types of anterior pituitary glands (Fig. 3.24) suggesting, in support of in vivo findings (Grosvenor et al. 1980), that dopamine blocks release secondarily to blockade of depletion. A large amount of dopamine was required to depress depletion, repletion and release; lower amounts produced only partial inhibition (data not shown). By contrast, 2 SME equivalents caused the same degree of inhibition as that of 5×10^{-5} M dopamine (data not shown). Although these results (Mena et al. unpublished) support the view that inhibition of prolactin is not exclusively under dopaminergic control (see Kordon and Enjalbert 1980), it is also possible that within the framework of a multiphasic secretory process, dopamine and other proposed PIFs may contribute to inhibition of prolactin by acting upon separate intermediate steps. Thus, inhibition of prolactin synthesis and release by dopamine may be related to the recent finding that the amine is internalized by the lactotrophs, presumably through endocytosis, and becomes associated with prolactin granules (Nansel et al. 1979). Therefore, if a dopamine–prolactin complex is formed, it might be maintained, at least in the lactating rat pituitary, until the time dopamine secretion becomes transiently suppressed by suckling (see Neill 1980), i.e., at the time of depletion-transformation. However, as already discussed, the dopaminergic system inhibits depletion and not release of prolactin in lactating rats. Since releasable prolactin derives from transformed prolactin, it is possible that other mechanisms, those relating to age, solubility and susceptibility to lysosomes, and non-dopaminergic PIFs may contribute to prevention of prolactin release. Recently, we observed that dopamine (at 5×10^{-5} M) effectively inhibited prolactin depletion, repletion

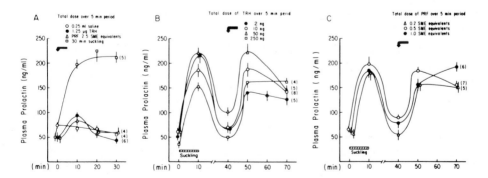

Fig. 3.22. Effect of TRH and a hypothalamic PRF which contains little if any TRH upon the release of PRL into the circulation of lactating rats. Injections were made either before the depletion of PRL (A) or after depletion has been effected by prior suckling (B and C). Values are means ±SEM; the numbers of rats are in parentheses (Grosvenor and Mena 1980).

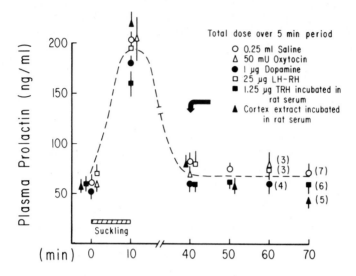

Fig. 3.23. Lack of effect of TRH upon PRL release in the depleted lactating rat after TRH has been incubated in fresh rat serum at 37°C for 1 h. Data also illustrate that stimulation of PRL release by TRH and hypothalamic PRF shown in Fig. 3.22 are not nonspecific responses. Values are the means ±SEM; the numbers of rats are in parentheses (Grosvenor and Mena 1980).

and release in pituitaries from chloroquine-injected rats and to the same extent as in anterior pituitaries from normal animals (unpublished). These results suggest independent mechanisms of action of dopamine and lysosomes upon prolactin secretion.

Recent in vitro studies, using clonal cell lines, have shown that TRH exerts complex, multiple effects upon mammotrophs. There is an initial short term effect upon prolactin release (150–350% of the control) and a secondary longer term stimulation of prolactin synthesis (130–500% of the control) which involves an increase of mRNA coding for prolactin in GH_3 cells (see reviews by Vale et al. 1977; Gourdji 1980; Tixier-Vidal and Gourdji 1980). Concomitant with the prolactin response, short and long-term effects have been observed upon GH release and synthesis (Tashjian et al. 1971). Also TRH-involved morphological changes, alterations in membrane properties and growth modifications of pituitary cells in culture have been reported. At the present time the mechanisms by which TRH exerts these multiple effects are unclear although it is possible that the action of TRH is effected at several levels, including the nucleus (see Gourdji 1980).

We found that TRH (7.5–37.5 ng) stimulated the pituitaries of lactating rats to secrete prolactin in vitro (Mena et al. unpublished). The pituitaries from suckled rats were stimulated to secrete an amount of prolactin that corresponded quantitively to that depleted by suckling (Fig. 3.25). Further analysis of the TRH effect was made upon both [3H]prolactin labelled 8 h beforehand and de novo synthesized [3H]prolactin. The data revealed that the release of both old and new prolactin was stimulated by the tripeptide. Newly synthesized [3H]prolactin could be detected in the tissue after only 5 min of incubation with [3H]Leu (50–500 µCi ml[-1]), thus confirming previous work (Zanini et al. 1974). Release of prolactin

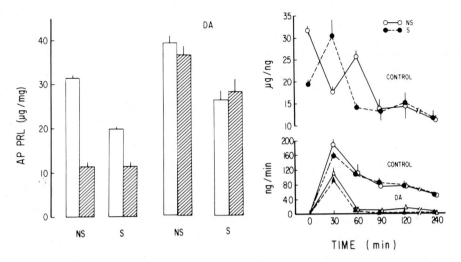

Fig. 3.24. Effect of 4 h incubation of hemipituitaries from nonsuckled (8 h) or suckled (15 min) rats in the presence or absence of dopamine (5×10^{-5} M) to which ascorbic acid (13.3 μg ml^{-1}) was added. Conditions of incubation were as described in Fig. 3.15. Bars in left panel refer to AP PRL concentration in hemipituitaries, before (open) and after (hatched bars) incubation with DA. Right panel shows PRL release in vitro in the presence of DA. Note that no change in AP PRL content occurred under DA. Values are expressed as means ±SEM. (Mena et al. unpublished).

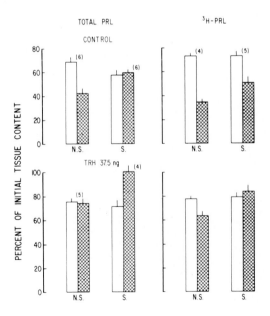

Fig. 3.25. Tissue loss (open) and medium gain (cross hatched bars) of total PRL and of [³H]PRL (expressed as percent of initial tissue content) from APs of either nonsuckled (8 h) or suckled (15 min) rats. [³H]Leucine (3 μCi g^{-1} b.w.) was injected i.v. 8 h before suckling. Hemipituitaries were incubated for 4 h as described in Fig. 3.15, with or without TRH (37.5 ng) added to the medium. Values are expressed as means ±SEM. Each group was composed of 4–6 hemipituitaries (Mena et al. unpublished).

into the medium did not occur in non-TRH-treated pituitaries, until after 90 min of incubation whereas, by contrast, [³H]prolactin was secreted 30 min earlier, i.e. after 60 min of incubation, in pituitaries incubated with TRH (Fig. 3.26). Since in vitro secretion of prolactin is composed by prolactin of different maturities (ages), including that from de novo synthesis, our results indicate that TRH is capable of stimulating the release of all of them, but in a varied manner. Moreover, since de novo synthesized prolactin was released faster under the influence of TRH, it is possible that TRH-induced release in vitro is exerted through an acceleration of transport of the hormone.

SEQUENCING OF MULTIPHASIC CONTROL OF PROLACTIN SECRETION

Evidence suggests that depletion occurs quickly following the onset of suckling (Grosvenor et al. 1967; Subramanian and Reece 1975) or electrical stimulation of mammary nerve (Mena et al. 1980). However, suckling, stress or electrical stimulation of mammary nerve applied continuously for periods of more than 60 min does not provoke depletion of more prolactin than does 1–2 min of stimulation (Figs 3.5, 3.7) (Grosvenor and Mena 1971; Subramanian and Reece 1975; Mena et al. 1980).

We demonstrated with bioassay techniques that if the suckling-induced depletion was blocked with SME extracts 2–4 h had to lapse before a second depletion could take place (Grosvenor and Mena 1971). We recently noted, using RIA, that the suckling induced rise in plasma prolactin concentration was prevented if depletion of prolactin was prevented

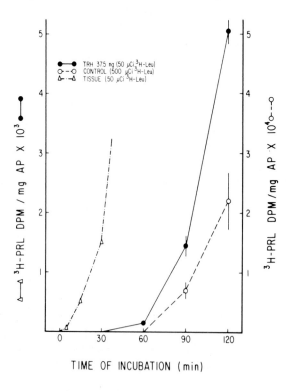

Fig. 3.26. PRL radioactivity (DPM mg⁻¹ tissue) in tissue and medium after 5–30 min (tissue) or at different times (medium) following incubation of ¹/₂ AP explants from lactating rats in medium containing 50-500 μCi of [³H]leucine with or without TRH (37.5 ng). Values are expressed as means ±SEM. Each group was composed of 4–6 hemipituitaries (Mena et al. unpublished).

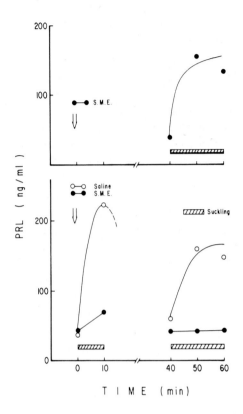

Fig. 3.27. Illustration of refractoriness in prolactin secretory mechanism. Bottom panel: Prolactin can be released once depletion has occurred with initial 10 min suckling. Blockade of suckling-induced depletion with acidic extracts of rat stalk median eminence (SME) though results in failure of subsequent suckling to deplete and, subsequently, to release prolactin. Top panel shows that SME extract does not carry over 40 min to block prolactin. Five rats in each group (Grosvenor and Mena unpublished).

during an earlier suckling with SME extracts (Fig. 3.27). In neither study did the extract itself carry over to prevent prolactin depletion at the second suckling. These data therefore suggest that the failure of suckling to effect a second depletion until 2–4 h has elapsed is not due to an insufficient amount of 'depletable' hormone but rather the neural stimulus in some manner has rendered the depletion mechanism inoperative for a period of time, i.e. it has become refractory to further neurogenic stimulation. During the 2–4 h refractory period the previously depleted, and subsequently transformed into releasable prolactin, is discharged into the circulation (see Grosvenor et al. 1979b). The period of refractoriness also permits the depleted stores of prolactin to replete to pre-depleted levels (see Mena et al. 1980). In sum, the refractory period insures that prolactin stores are not exhausted in the face of continuous or short-interval neurogenic stimulation through regulating the sequencing of the depletion-transformation and release phases of prolactin secretion.

The mechanism by which depletion of prolactin is prevented during the refractory period is largely unknown at the present time. Prolactin depletion by neurogenic stimulation in the lactating rat more than likely involves suppression of a PIF–dopaminergic inhibitory mechanism within the hypothalamus (Grosvenor et al. 1980) accompanied by a rapid uncoupling of dopamine from its receptor within the pituitary (MacLeod and Leymeyer 1974; Calabro and MacLeod 1978; Caron et al. 1978; Cronin et al. 1978; Nansel et al. 1979). Plotsky et al. (1981) (see also Neill 1980) recently noted that the dopamine levels in

104

the median eminence fell quickly after the onset of a prolactin-depleting stimulus (electrical stimulation of mammary nerve), then after about 5 min dopamine levels returned to prestimulus levels though the stimulus continued to be applied. Chiocchio et al. (1979) showed that the concentration of dopamine in the anterior pituitary fell within 5 min after the onset of suckling. These important observations not only add considerable support to the concept that the initial depletion phase of prolactin secretion results from a transient suppression of the PIF–dopaminergic system and subsequent rapid reduction of pituitary dopamine levels, but also suggests that the neural mechanism responsible for suppressing dopamine release from the hypothalamus does not respond to neurogenic stimulation for a period of time after the initial suppression.

The refractory period may thus be due in part to the inability of a neurogenic stimulus to suppress tonic dopamine secretion from the hypothalamus. However, changes in binding of dopamine and/or other PIFs to receptors within the pituitary also may be implicated. Evidence in support of this postulate stems from experiments using haloperidol, a drug known to prevent the physiological expression of dopamine at the pituitary level. Injecting haloperidol (0.2 mg) i.v. into lactating rats on day 14 of lactation after 4–5 h of nonsuckling resulted in a rapid prolactin depletion and in a rise in plasma concentration of the hormone within 10–15 min to levels 3–5 times those seen in suckled rats (Fig. 3.28). Other lactating rats first were injected i.v. with either saline, dopamine (500 ng min^{-1}×5 min) or SME extracts (containing the equivalent of 1 rat SME), then suckled by their 6 pups for 10 min.

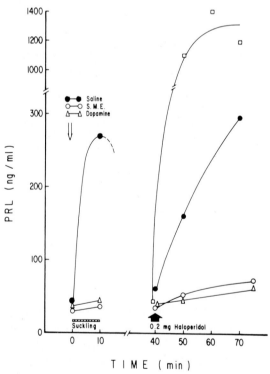

Fig. 3.28. Failure of haloperidol to deplete and release prolactin when suckling-induced depletion is blocked previously with either acidic extracts of rat stalk median eminence or dopamine. The open squares represent rats with no prior suckling; 5–8 rats per group (Grosvenor and Mena unpublished).

The subsequent blockade of depletion prevented the release of prolactin into the circulation. When these rats subsequently (30 min later) were injected i.v. with 0.2 mg of haloperidol, little or no elevation in plasma prolactin above basal levels occurred (Fig. 3.28). Saline-injected rats, whose depletion of prolactin was not blocked had a much reduced plasma elevation of prolactin in response to the drug. Thus, haloperidol appears to be less effective in uncoupling dopamine from the pituitary dopamine receptor in lactating rats rendered refractory by the previous suckling.

If the dopamine receptor is involved in the failure of haloperidol under these conditions to deplete and subsequently to release prolactin then one would have to assume that with reoccupation of the dopamine receptor there is a change in binding affinity which thereby renders it more difficult for dopamine to become uncoupled by the drug. Alternatively, dopamine might be involved only in the initial depletion of prolactin and not in development of the refractory period. Another prolactin-inhibiting substance, released from the hypothalamus during neurogenic stimulation, might occupy a receptor in the pituitary which functions to inhibit prolactin depletion and which is not sensitive to uncoupling by haloperidol. Such a substance may be present in crude acidic extracts of rat hypothalamus which exert powerful inhibitory effects upon prolactin depletion and subsequent release in vivo (Grosvenor et al. 1979) and in vitro (Mena et al. unpublished) since the prolactin blocking activity could not be easily accounted for on the basis of the dopamine contained in the extracts.

REFERENCES

Advis, J.P., Hall, T.R., Hodson, C.A., Mueller, G.P. and Meites, J. (1977) Temporal relationship and role of dopamine in 'short-loop' feedback of prolactin. Proc. Soc. Exp. Biol. Med. 155, 567-570.

Alekseev, N.P., Velling, V.A. and Grachev, I.I. (1976) Functional characteristics of rapidly adapting mechano-receptors in the teat of the mammary gland of the rat. Fiziol. Zh. Mosk. 62, 375-381.

Alekseev, N.P., Alieva, S.A., Grachev, I.I., Darinskaya, V.S., Kamezhukova, E.F. and Epshtein, N.Z. (1977) Properties of mechanoreceptor units of the mammary gland parenchyma. Fiziol. Zh. SSSR imeni I. H. Sechenova 63, 673-680.

Amenomori, Y., Chen, C.L. and Meites, J. (1970) Serum prolactin levels in rats during the different reproductive states. Endocrinology 86, 506-510.

Barowicz, T. (1979) Changes of blood catecholamine levels in the sheep during machine milking. J. Dairy Res. 46, 555-557.

Beyer, C. and Mena, F. (1969) Neural substrate of oxytocin and prolactin secretion during lactation. In: Progress in Endocrinology (Gual, C. ed.), pp. 952-958. Internat. Congr. Ser. No. 184, Excerpta Medica, Amsterdam.

Boyd III, A.E., Spencer, E., Jackson, I.M.D. and Reichlin, S. (1976) Prolactin-releasing factor (PRF) in porcine hypothalamic extract distinct from TRH. Endocrinology 99, 861-871.

Burnet, F.R. and Wakerly, J.B. (1976) Plasma concentrations of prolactin and thyrotropin during suckling in urethane-anaesthetized rats. J. Endocrinol. 70, 429-437.

Calabro, M.A. and MacLeod, R.M. (1978) [^{3}H]Dopamine binding to bovine anterior pituitary membranes. Neuroendocrinology 25, 32-46.

Caron, M.G., Beaulieu, M., Raymond, V., Gagne, B., Drouin, J., Lefkowitz, R.J., Labrie, F. (1978) Identification of dopaminergic receptors in anterior pituitary: correlation with the dopaminergic control of prolactin release. J. Biol. Chem. 253, 2224-2253.

Chen, N.F. and Ramirez, V.D. (1979) Serotonin stimulates TRH release from rat hypothalami in perifusion. Program of the 61st Annual Meeting of the Endocrine Society. Anaheim, CA. p. 178.

Chiocchio, S.R., Cannata, M.A., Cordero-Funes, J.R., Tramezzani, J.H. (1979) Involvement of adenohypo-physial dopamine in the regulation of prolactin release during suckling. Endocrinology 105, 544-547.

Clarke, G. and Lincoln, D.W. (1976) Central and peripheral inhibition of the milk-ejection reflex: studies with α-adrenoceptor antagonists. Br. J. Pharmacol. 58(3), 464P-465P.

Clarke, G., Fall, C.H.D., Lincoln, D.W. and Merrick, L.P. (1978) Effects of cholinoceptor antagonists on the suckling-induced and experimentally evoked release of oxytocin. Br. J. Pharmacol. 63, 519-527.

Clarke, G., Lincoln, D.W. and Merrick, L.P. (1979) Dopaminergic control of oxytocin release in lactating rats. J. Endocrinol. 83, 409-420.

Clemens, J.A. and Meites, J. (1968) Inhibition by hypothalamic prolactin implants of prolactin secretion, mammary growth and luteal function. Endocrinology 82, 878-881.

Clemens, J.A., Sar, M. and Meites, J. (1969) Inhibition of lactation and luteal function in postpartum rats by hypothalamic implantation of prolactin. Endocrinology 84, 868-872.

Clemens, J.A., Roush, M.E., Fuller, R.W. (1978) Evidence that serotonin neurons stimulate secretion of prolactin releasing factor. Life Sci. 22, 2209-2214.

Cochrane, E.R. (1949) Observations on a reflex controlling milk flow in the individual mammary gland of the cow. Br. Vet. J. 105, 320.

Cowie, A.T. and Tindal, J.S. (1971) The physiology of lactation. Monographs of The Physiological Society. Arnold, London.

Cronin, M.J., Roberts J. and Weiner, R.I. (1978) Dopamine receptor binding to the anterior pituitary in the rat. Endocrinology 103, 302-309.

Cross, B.A. (1955) Neuroendocrine mechanisms in emotional inhibition of milk ejection. J. Endocrinol. 12, 29-37.

Cross, B.A. and Dyball, R.E.J. (1974) Central pathways for neurohypophyseal hormone release. In: Handbook of Physiology (Knobil, E. and Sawyer, W.H. eds) Vol. 4, Sect. 7, pp. 269-285. American Physiological Society, Washington.

deGreef, W.J. and Neill, J.D. (1979) Dopamine levels in hypophysial stalk plasma of the rat during surges of prolactin secretion induced by cervical stimulation. Endocrinology 105, 1093-1099.

deGreef, W.J., Plotsky, P.M. and Neill, J.D. (1981) Dopamine levels in hypophysial stalk plasma and prolactin levels in peripheral plasma of the lactating rat: Effects of a simulated suckling stimulus. Neuroendocrinology 32, 229-233.

Deis, R.P. (1968) The effect of an exteroceptive stimulus on milk ejection in lactating rats. J. Physiol. 197, 37-46.

Denamur, R. (1965) The hypothalamo-neurohypophysial system and the milk-ejection reflex. Dairy Sci. Abstr. 27, 193-224.

DeNuccio, D.J. and Grosvenor, C.E. (1971) Effect of volume and distribution of milk on the oxytocin-induced contraction of the lactating rat mammary gland in vivo. J. Endocrinol. 51, 437-446.

Drewett, R.F., Statham, C. and Wakerly, J.B. (1974) A quantitative analysis of the feeding behavior of suckling rats. Anim. Behav. 22, 907-913.

Dufy, B., Vincent, J-D., Fleury, H., DuPasquier, P., Gourdji, F. and Tixier-Vidal, A. (1979) Membrane effects of thyrotropin-releasing hormone and estrogen shown by intracellular recording from pituitary cells. Science 204, 509-511.

Farquhar, M.G. (1977) Secretion and crinophagy in prolactin cells. In: Comparative Endocrinology of Prolactin (Dellman, H.D., Johnson, J.A. and Klachko, D.M. eds) pp. 37-94, Plenum Press, New York.

Farquhar, M.G., Reid, J.J. and Daniell, L.W. (1978) Intracellular transport and packaging of prolactin: a quantitative electron microscope autoradiographic study of mammotrophs dissociated from rat pituitaries. Endocrinology 102, 296-311.

Findlay, A.L.R. (1966) Sensory discharges from lactating mammary glands. Nature (London) 211, 1183-1184.

Findlay, A.R.L. and Grosvenor, C.E. (1969) The role of mammary gland innervation in the control of the motor apparatus of the mammary gland: A review. Dairy Sci. Abstr. 3, 109-116.

Forsling, M.L., Reinhardt, V. and Himmler, V. (1974) Neurohypophysial hormones and prolactin release. J. Endocrinol. 63, 579-580.

Fuxe, K. and Hökfelt, T. (1967) The influence of central catecholamine neurons on the hormone secretion from anterior and posterior pituitary. In: Neurosecretion (Stutinsky, F. ed.) pp. 165-177, Springer-Verlag, Heidelberg.

Garthwaite, T.L. and Hagen, T.C. (1979) Evidence that serotonin stimulates a prolactin-releasing factor in the rat. Neuroendocrinology 29, 215-220.

Giannattasio, G., Zanini, A. and Meldolesi, J. (1975) Molecular organization of rat prolactin granules. I. In vitro stability of intact and 'membrane-less' granules. J. Cell Biol. 64, 246-251.

Gibbs, D.M. and Neill, J.D. (1978) Dopamine levels in hypophysial stalk blood in the rat are sufficient to inhibit prolactin secretion in vivo. Endocrinology 102, 1895-1900.

Gourdji, D. (1980) Characterization of thyroliberin (TRH) binding sites and coupling with prolactin and growth hormone secretion in rat pituitary cell lines. In: Synthesis and Release of Adenohypophyseal Hormones. (Jutisz, M. and McKerns, K.W. eds), pp. 463-493, Plenum Press, New York.

Grachev, I.I. (1949) O refleksakh s molochnoi zhelezy (Reflexes from the mammary gland). Ih. Obsheh. Biol. 10, 401-420.

Grosvenor, C.E. and Findlay, A.L.R. (1968) Effect of denervation on fluid flow into rat mammary gland. Am. J. Physiol. 214, 820-824.

Grosvenor, C.E. and Mena, F. (1970) Alterations in the oxytocin induced intramammary pressure response after mechanical stimulation of the mammary gland of the anesthetized lactating rat. Endocrinology 104, 443-447.

Grosvenor, C.E. and Mena F. (1971) Effect of suckling upon the secretion and release of prolactin from the pituitary gland of the lactating rat. J. Anim. Sci. 32, suppl. 1, pp. 115-136.

Grosvenor, C.E. and Mena, F. (1974) Neural and hormonal control of milk secretion and milk ejection in lactation. A comprehensive treatise. (Larson, B.L. and Smith, V.R. eds), Vol. 1, pp. 227-276, Academic Press, New York.

Grosvenor, C.E. and Whitworth, N. (1974) Evidence for a steady rate of secretion of prolactin following suckling in the rat. J. Dairy Sci. 57, 900-904.

Grosvenor, C.E. and Whitworth, N.S. (1976) Incorporation of rat prolactin into rat milk in vivo and in vitro. J. Endocrinol. 70, 1-9.

Grosvenor, C.E., McCann, S.M. and Nallar, R. (1965) Inhibition of nursing-induced and stress-induced fall in pituitary prolactin concentration in lactating rats by injection of acid extracts of bovine hypothalamus. Endocrinology 76, 883-889.

Grosvenor, C.E., Mena, F. and Schaefgen, D.A. (1967) Effects of nonsuckling interval and duration of suckling on the suckling-induced fall in pituitary prolactin concentration in the rat. Endocrinology 81, 449-453.

Grosvenor, C.E., Mena, F., Maiweg, H., Dhariwal, A.P.S. and McCann, S.M. (1970) Effect of hypothalamic extracts and exogenous prolactin on reaccumulation of prolactin in the pituitary of the lactating rat after suckling. J. Endocrinol. 47, 339-346.

Grosvenor, C.E., DeNuccio, D.J., King, S.F., Maiweg, H. and Mena, F. (1972) Central and peripheral neural influences on the oxytocin-induced pressure response of the mammary gland of the anaesthetized lactating rat. J. Endocrinol. 55, 299-309.

Grosvenor, C.E., Mena, F. and Whitworth, N.S. (1979a) The secretion rate of prolactin in the rat during suckling and its metabolic clearance rate after increasing intervals of nonsuckling. Endocrinology 104, 372-376.

Grosvenor, C.E., Mena, F. and Whitworth, N.S. (1979b) Ether releases large amounts of prolactin from rat pituitaries previously depleted by short-term suckling. Endocrinology 105, 884-887.

Grosvenor, C.E., Mena, F. and Whitworth, N.S. (1980) Evidence that the dopaminergic-PIF mechanism regulates the depletion-transformation phase and not the release phase of prolactin secretion during suckling in the rat. Endocrinology 106, 481-485.

Grosvenor, C.E., Whitworth, N.S. and Mena, F. (1981) Evidence that the depletion and release phases of prolactin secretion in the lactating rat have different thresholds in response to exteroceptive stimulation from rat pups. Endocrinology 108, 820-824.

Hart, J.C. (1975) Concentrations of prolactin in serial blood samples from goats before, during, and after milking throughout lactation. J. Endocrinol. 64, 305-312.

Hayward, N. and Jennings, D.P. (1973) Influence of sleep-waking and nociceptor-induced behavior on the activity of supraoptic neurons in the hypothalamus of the monkey. Brain Res. 57, 461-466.

Hökfelt, T. and Fuxe, K. (1972) Effects of prolactin and ergot alkaloids on the tubero-infundibular dopamine

(DA) neurons. Neuroendocrinology 9, 100-122.

Koch, Y., Goldhaber, G., Fireman, I., Zor, U., Shani, J. and Tal, E. (1977) Suppression of prolactin and thyrotropin secretion in the rat by antiserum to thyrotropin-releasing hormone. Endocrinology 100, 1476-1478.

Kordon, C. and Enjalbert, A. (1980) Prolactin inhibiting and stimulating factors. In: Central and Peripheral Regulation of Prolactin Function (MacLeod, R.M. and Scapagnini, U. eds), pp. 69-78, Raven Press, New York.

Kordon, C., Blake, C.A., Terkel, J. and Sawyer, C.H. (1973/4) Participation of serotonin-containing neurons in the suckling-induced rise in plasma prolactin levels in lactating rats. Neuroendocrinology 13, 213-223.

Kuanyshbekova, G.A. (1976) Reflex discharge of catecholamines during milk ejection inhibition in goats. Izv. Akad. Nauk. SSR (Biol.) 14, 62-65, 90-91.

Lamberts, S.W.J. and MacLeod, R.M. (1979a) The inability of bromocriptine to inhibit prolactin secretion by transplantable rat pituitary tumors: observations on the mechanism and dynamics of the autofeedback regulation of prolactin secretion. Endocrinology 104, 65-70.

Lamberts, S.W.J. and MacLeod, R.M. (1979b) Stimulation of prolactin release by the bicarbonate ion. Proc. Soc. Exp. Biol. Med. 101, 495-497.

Lefkowitz, R.J., Murkherjee, C., Limbird, L.E., Caron, H.G., Williams, L.T., Alexander, R.W., Mickey, J.V., Tate, R. (1976) Regulation of adenyl cyclase-coupled beta adrenergic receptors. Recent Prog. Horm. Res. 32, 597-632.

Lincoln, D.W. and Wakerly, J.B. (1975) Factors governing the periodic activation of supraoptic and paraventricular neurosecretory cells during suckling in the rat. J. Physiol. Lond. 250, 443-461.

Lincoln, D.W., Hill, A. and Wakerly, J.B. (1973) The milk-ejection reflex of the rat: An intermittent function not abolished by surgical levels of anaesthesia. J. Endocrinol. 57, 459-476.

Linzell, J.L. (1955) Some observations on the contractile tissues of the mammary glands. J. Physiol. 130, 257-267.

MacLeod, R.M. (1970) Inhibition of the in vitro synthesis of pituitary prolactin and growth hormone by mouse pituitary isografts. Proc. Soc. Exp. Biol. Med. 133, 339-341.

MacLeod, R.M. (1976) Regulation of prolactin secretion. In: Frontiers in Neuroendocrinology (Martini, L. and Ganong, W.F. eds), Vol. 4, pp. 169-194. Raven Press, New York.

MacLeod, R.M. and Lehmeyer, J.E. (1974) Studies on the mechanisms of the dopamine-mediated inhibition of prolactin secretion. Endocrinology 94, 1077-1085.

MacLeod, R.M., Nagy, I., Login, I.S., Kimura, H., Valdenegro, C.A. and Thorner, M.O. (1980) The roles of dopamine, cAMP and calcium on prolactin secretion. In: Central and Peripheral Regulation of Prolactin Function (MacLeod, R.M. and Scapagnini, V.eds), pp. 27-42, Raven Press, New York.

McMurtry, J.P. and Malven, P.V. (1974) Experimental alterations of protein levels in goat milk and blood plasma. Endocrinology 95, 559-564.

McNeilly, A.S. and Friesen, H.G. (1978) Prolactin during pregnancy and lactation in the rabbit. Endocrinology 102, 1548-1554.

Mena, F. and Grosvenor, C.E. (1968) Effect of number of pups upon suckling induced fall in pituitary concentrations and milk yield in the rat. Endocrinology 82, 623-626.

Mena, F., Enjalbert, A., Carbonell, L., Priam, M. and Kordon, C. (1976) Effect of suckling on plasma prolactin and hypothalamic monoamine levels in the rat. Endocrinology 99, 445-451.

Mena, F., Pacheco, P., Aguayo, D., Clapp, C. and Grosvenor, C.E. (1978) A rise in intramammary pressure follows electrical stimulation of mammary nerve in anesthetized rats. Endocrinology 103, 1929-1956.

Mena, F., Pacheco, P., Aguayo, D., Martinez-Escalera, G. and Grosvenor, C.E. (1979) Reflex regulation of autonomic influences upon the oxytocin-induced contractile response of the mammary gland in the anesthetized rat. Endocrinology 104, 751-756.

Mena, F., Pacheco, P. and Grosvenor, C.E. (1980) Effect of electrical stimulation of mammary nerve upon pituitary and plasma prolactin concentrations in anesthetized lactating rats. Endocrinology 106, 458-462.

Mena, F., Pacheco, P., Whitworth, N.S. and Grosvenor, C.E. (1980) Recent data concerning the secretion and function of oxytocin and prolactin during lactation in the rat and rabbit. In: Frontiers in Hormone Research (Valverde-Rodriquez C. and Arechiga, H. eds), Vol. 6, pp. 217-250, Karger, Basel.

Moos, F. and Richard, P. (1979a) Effect of dopaminergic antagonist and agonist on oxytocin release induced by various stimuli. Neuroendocrinology 28, 138-144.

Moos, F. and Richard, P. (1979b) The inhibitory role of β-noradrenergic receptors in oxytocin release during suckling. Brain Res. 169, 595-599.

Nansel, D.D., Gudelsky, G.A. and Porter, J.C. (1979) Subcellular localization of dopamine in the anterior pituitary gland of the rat: Apparent association of dopamine with prolactin secretory granules. Endocrinology 105, 1073-1077.

Neill, J.D. (1974) Prolactin: its secretion and control. In: Handbook of Physiology (Knobil, E. and Sawyer, W.H. eds), Vol. 4, Sect. 7, pp. 469-488. American Physiological Society, Washington D.C.

Neill, J.D. (1980) Neuroendocrine Regulation of Prolactin Secretion. In: Frontiers in Neuroendocrinology (Martini, L. and Ganong, W.F. eds), Vol. 6, pp. 129-155. Raven Press, New York.

Nicoll, C.S. (1972) Some observations and speculation on the mechanism of 'depletion', 'repletion', and release of adenohypophyseal hormones. Gen. Comp. Endocrinol. (Suppl.) 3, 86-96.

Nicoll, C.S. (1975) Radioimmunoassay and radioreceptor assays for prolactin and growth hormones: a critical appraisal. Am. Zool. 15, 881-903.

Nicoll, C.S. and Swearingen, K. (1970) Preliminary observations on prolactin and growth hormone turnover in rat adenohypophyses in vivo. In: The Hypothalamus (Martini, L., Motta, M. and Fraschini, F. eds) pp. 449-462, Academic Press, New York.

Nicoll, C.S., Fiorindo, R.P., McKennee, C.F. and Parsons, J.A. (1970) Assay of hypothalamic factors which regulate prolactin secretion. In: Hypophysiotropic Hormones of the Hypothalamus: Assay and Chemistry (Meites, J. ed.), pp. 115-150. Williams and Wilkins, Baltimore.

Nicoll, C.S., Mena, F., Nichols, C.W., Jr., Green, S.H., Thai, M. and Russell, S.M. (1976) Analysis of suckling-induced changes in adenohypophyseal prolactin concentration in the lactating rat by three assay methods. Acta Endocrinol. (Copenhagen) 83, 512-521.

Pelletier, G. (1973) Secretion and uptake of peroxidase by rat adenohypophyseal cells. J. Ultrastruct. Res. 43, 445-459.

Perkins, N.A., Westfall, T.C., Paul, C.V., MacLeod, R.M. and Rogol, A.D. (1979) Effect of prolactin on dopamine synthesis in medial basal hypothalumus: evidence for a short loop feedback. Brain Res. 160, 431-444.

Plotsky, P.M., deGreef, W.J., Neill, J.D. (1979) The role of dopamine in suckling-induced prolactin secretion. 61st Annual Meeting of the Endocrine Society. Anaheim, CA. p. 185.

Richard, P. (1970) An electrophysiological study in the ewe of the tracts which transmit impulses from the mammary glands to the pituitary stalk. J. Endocrinol. 47, 37-44.

Richardson, R.C. (1949) Contractile tissues in the mammary gland with special reference to myoepithelium in the goat. Proc. R. Soc. Lond. Ser. B. 136, 30-45.

Samli, M.H., Lai, M.F. and Barnett, C.A. (1972) Protein synthesis in the rat anterior pituitary: II. Solubility studies on total protein, growth hormone and prolactin labelled in an in vitro incubation. Endocrinology 91, 227-232.

Seybold, V.S., Miller, J.W. and Lewis, P.R. (1978) Investigation of a dopaminergic mechanism for regulating oxytocin release. J. Pharmacol. Exp. Ther. 207(2), 605-610.

Sharon, N. and Lid, H. (1972) Lectins: Cell agglutinating and sugar-specific proteins. Science 177, 949-959.

Smith, R.E. and Farquhar, M.G. (1966) Lysosome function in the regulation of the secretory process in cells of the anterior pituitary gland. J. Cell Biol. 31, 319-347.

Soloff, M.S. and Swartz, T.L. (1973) Characterization of a proposed oxytocin receptor in rat mammary gland. J. Biol. Chem. 248, 6471-6478.

Stutinsky, F. and Terminn, Y. (1965) Effets des lesions du complexe amygdalien sur le reflexe d'ejection de lait chez la ratte. J. Physiol. (Paris) 57, 279-284.

Subramanian, M.G. and Reece, R.P. (1975) Anterior pituitary and plasma prolactin in rats after 2 to 90 minutes of suckling. Proc. Soc. Exp. Biol. N.Y. 149, 754-756.

Swearingen, K. (1971) The heterogenous turnover of adenohypophysial prolactin. Endocrinology 89, 1380-1388.

Tashjian, A.H., Jr., Barowsky, N.J. and Jensen, D.K. (1971) Thyrotropin releasing hormone: Direct evidence for stimulation of prolactin production by pituitary cells in culture. Biochem. Biophys. Res. Commun. 81,

798-806.

Terkel, J., Damassa, D.A. and Sawyer, C.H. (1979) Ultrasonic vocalizations of infant rats stimulate prolactin release in lactating females. Horm. Behav. 12, 95-102.

Tindal, J.S. (1974) Stimuli that cause the release of oxytocin. In: Handbook of Physiology (Knobil, R. and Sawyer, W.H. eds), Vol. 4, Sect. 7, pp. 257-269. American Physiological Society, Washington, D.C.

Tindal, J.S. (1978) Neuroendocrine control of lactation in lactation: A Comprehensive Treatise (Larson, B.L. and Smith, V.R. eds), Vol. 1, pp. 239-256, Academic Press, New York.

Tindal, J.S. and Blake, C.A. (1980) A neural basis for central inhibition of milk-ejection in the rabbit. J. Endocrinol. 86, 525-531.

Tindal, J.S. and Knaggs, G.S. (1969) An ascending pathway for release of prolactin in the brain of the rabbit. J. Endocrinol. 45, 111-120.

Tixier-Vidal, A. and Gourdji, D. (1980) Endocytosis in cultured prolactin cells. In: Central and Peripheral Regulation of Prolactin Function (MacLeod, R.M. and Scapagnini, V. eds), pp. 125-140, Raven Press, New York.

Tribollet, E. and Dreifuss, J.J. (1977) Effect of propranolol on reflex milk-ejection and on paraventricular neurones. Experentia 33, 786.

Tucker, H.A., Convey, E.M. and Koprowski, J.A. (1973) Milking-induced release of endogenous prolactin in cows infused with exogenous prolactin. Proc. Soc. Exp. Biol. Med. N.Y. 142, 72-75.

Vale, W., Rivier, C. and Brown, M. (1977) Regulatory peptides of the hypothalamus. Annu. Rev. Physiol. 39, 473-527.

Valverde, C., Chieffo, V. and Reichlin, S. (1972) Prolactin releasing factor in porcine and rat hypothalamic tissue. Endocrinology 91, 982-993.

Vila-Porcile, E. and Oliver, L. (1980) Exocytosis and related membrane events. In: Synthesis and Release of Adenohypophyseal Hormones. (Jutisz, M. and McKerns, K.W. eds), pp. 67-104, Plenum Press, New York.

Voloschin, L.M. and Tramezzani, J.H. (1979) Milk ejection reflex linked to slow wave sleep in nursing rats. Endocrinology 105, 1202-1207.

Voogt, J.L. and Meites, J. (1973) Suppression of proestrous and suckling-induced increase in serum prolactin by hypothalamic implant of prolactin. Proc. Soc. Exp. Biol. Med. N.Y. 142, 1056-1058.

Vorherr, H. (1971) Catecholamine antagonism to oxytocin-induced milk ejection. Acta Endocrinol. (Copenhagen) Suppl. 154, 5-38.

Walker, A.M. and Farquhar, M.G. (1980) Preferential release of newly synthesized prolactin granules is the result of functional heterogeneity among mammotrophs. Endocrinology 107, 1095-1104.

Wakerly, J.B. and Drewett, R.F. (1975) Pattern of suckling in the infant rat during spontaneous milk-ejection. Physiol. Behav. 15, 277-281.

Whitworth, N.S., Grosvenor, C.E. and Mena, F. (1981) Autofeedback regulation of prolactin secretion: effect of prolactin (PRL) prior to suckling on the subsequent nursing-induced release of PRL in the lactating rat. Endocrinology, 108, 1279-1284.

Zanini, A., Giannattasio, G. and Meldolesi, J. (1974a) Separation of rat pituitary growth hormone and prolactin by SDS polyacrylamide gel electrophoresis. Endocrinology 94, 594-598.

Zanini, A., Giannattasio, G. and Meldolesi, J. (1974b) Studies on in vitro synthesis and secretion of growth hormone and prolactin. II. Evidence against the existence of precursor molecules. Endocrinology 94, 104-111.

Zanini, A., Giannattasio, G. and Meldolesi, J. (1980) Intracellular events in prolactin secretion. In: Synthesis and Release of Adenohypophyseal Hormones (Jutisz, M. and McKerns, K.W. eds), pp. 105-123, Plenum Press, New York.

E.E. Müller and R.M. MacLeod (eds) Neuroendocrine Perspectives Vol. 1
© Elsevier Biomedical Press, 1982

Chapter 4

In vitro systems for the study of secretion and synthesis of hypothalamic peptides

Richard Robbins and Seymour Reichlin

INTRODUCTION

Cellular mechanisms which regulate hypothalamic hormone secretion are difficult to study in whole animals. As a consequence, many investigators have begun in recent years to use isolated preparations in order to elucidate the physiologic, pharmacologic, and biochemical characteristics of the tuberoinfundibular system.

Sufficient information has now accumulated to permit a critical review of the data on regulation of endogenous neuropeptides derived from in vitro hypothalamic models, and to outline promising lines for future work. Although of great importance for the understanding of hypothalamic physiology, we will not consider regulation of biogenic amines (for recent reviews see Moore and Bloom 1978, 1979; Krulich 1979; Chapter 2).

IN VITRO SYSTEMS

The first studies on the isolated hypothalamus to be reported were those of Hild (1954), who employed a plasma-coated 'flying' coverslip method to maintain explants of paraventricular and supraoptic nuclei in Gey's solution supplemented by embryo extracts. In the outgrowth zone, he noted axonal processes in which axoplasmic transport of cell particles was visualized, as well as outpouchings reminiscent of Herring bodies in the neurohypophysis. Cultures were successfully maintained for up to 8 weeks.

The feasibility of such an in vitro approach had been suggested half a century earlier by the pioneering work of Ross Harrison (1906), who validated the independent neuron unit theory of Cajal and His by demonstrating that neurons at the edge of frog spinal cord explants had the capacity to extend axons and processes. Subsequent success in maintaining neural tissue in vitro depended on the development of optimum media, the design of various types of culturing chambers and the use of cellular or non-cellular substrates (for review see Thomas 1956; Murray 1965; May 1966; Lumsden 1968). More recent developments in work with in vitro systems exploring molecular neurobiology have been extensively reviewed by Herschman (1973), Mandel (1976), and Tixier-Vidal and DeVitry (1979).

Reports of experiments that employed hypothalamic models began to appear, concomitant with and shortly after isolation and characterization of the hypothalamic hormones: vasopressin (VP), thyrotropin releasing hormone (TRH), somatostatin, and gonadotropin releasing hormone (GnRH). Many groups applied the knowledge derived from in vitro studies of other brain areas to the hypothalamus (Masurovsky et al. 1971; Sobkowicz et al. 1974).

Although diverse approaches have been made over the past 20 years to maintain the hypothalamus in vitro, these techniques can be divided into a few general categories: tissue culture (explants, organ culture, slices, fragments) in which the histotypic organization is maintained; cell culture, in which cells, usually of fetal origin, are mechanically or enzymatically dispersed and grown dissociated in monolayers or reaggregated into organotypic structures (tumor lines and transformed primary cells cultures will be considered with this group); and lastly, synaptosomal and other subcellular preparations. In general, the type of preparation dictates the time frame of the experiments, synaptosomes being used within minutes to hours, tissue cultures within hours to days, and cell cultures from days to weeks after establishment.

Tissue culture

In addition to being relatively easy to set up, the use of small hypothalamic explants or fragments maintained for hours to days takes advantage of the intrinsic neuron-to-neuron network, while affording precise control of the physical and chemical environment in a model system which, when properly maintained, retains a high degree of cellular integrity. Furthermore, the normal intimate relationship among neurons, supporting glia, and other non-neuronal cells is preserved. This kind of preparation, quickly removed from normal animals or from those with induced hormonal or metabolic derangements (e.g. Berelowitz et al. 1980a), probably reflects most closely of all in vitro systems the prior physiologic state, if only for short intervals. When derived from an embryonic source, tissue culture provides a valuable tool for examining neuronal differentiation or ontogenesis of individual cell components such as enzymes, neuropeptides, and neurotransmitters.

The size of the explant is a major consideration in the successful use of this method; the extensive experience of Lumsden (1968) indicates that 1 mm^3 is the maximum volume of brain tissue which will maintain cellular integrity for days in vitro. This has been histologically verified in hypothalamic organ cultures, which are considerably larger than 1 mm^3 (Sachs et al. 1971; Silverman et al. 1973; McKelvy et al. 1975). The study of Sachs (1971) in particular demonstrated that extensive neuronal and non-neuronal damage occurred rapidly throughout the explant of hypothalamic-neurohypophysial blocks, but magnocellular neurons located near the edge of the explant maintained morphologic and biosynthetic characteristics for up to 12 days in vitro. This is presumably due to a gradient of diffusion of nutrients into and of toxic metabolites out from the center as compared with the periphery of the explant.

In addition to the heterogeneity brought about by variability of cell survival related to distance of individual cells from the edge of the explant, some of the neurons in any explant will be severed fragments undergoing various degrees of degeneration and chromatolysis. In explant cultures of the median eminence, which include virtually no neuronal perikarya, most of the total weight of the explant consists of severed nerve endings which are involuting, not from lack of nutrients, but because of their loss of anatomical, electrophysiological, and trophic connections with the cell soma. Therefore, the possibility must be considered that much of the peptide released by these explants may be leakage from dying fragments (Kelly et al. 1979), despite the fact that peptide content is stable (Iversen et al. 1978) and oxygen consumption linear over time (Berelowitz et al. 1978).

Precise definition of nutrient media is essential because one of the main advantages of in vitro work is that the environment can be controlled. Most short-term, tissue culture experiments employ a bathing solution which is an isosmotic buffer, such as Krebs–Ringer bicarbonate solution, containing glucose and physiologic concentrations of Na^+, Cl^-, K^+ and CO_2. On the other hand, a number of studies have attempted to maintain explants for more than 24 h and these have required the additional presence of serum for optimal survival (Sachs et al. 1971; Sladek and Joynt 1979a; Richardson et al. 1980). This ill-defined but necessary constituent contains a number of hormones, neurotransmitters and growth factors, as well as peptide- and protein-degrading enzymes essential to long-term preservation of in vitro preparations. These problems with tissue culture may be obviated by the use of media supplemented with serum-free growth factor in which neural tissue can be maintained for prolonged periods (Bottenstein and Sato 1979a; Honnegar et al. 1979; Messer et al. 1980). This approach has been pioneered by Sato and colleagues (Rizzino and Sato 1978).

Primary cell cultures

The term primary indicates that the cells in these cultures are derived directly from the organism and not from any other in vitro preparation. It also implies that the cells are non-neoplastic, and in general, for neurons, nondividing.

This type of preparation, first described by Moscona (1952), using trypsin dispersal in a medium devoid of Ca^{2+} and Mg^{2+}, provides a dimension beyond that of tissue culture. The characteristics and capacities of individual cells, apart from the complex in vivo interconnections, can now be examined. This technique was first applied to the nervous system by Pomerat (1952), and to the hypothalamus by Wilkinson (1974) and Benda (1975). The advantages of this system have been reflected in the rapid accumulation of literature using this model (for reviews see Mandel et al. 1976; Tixier-Vidal and De Vitry 1979; Dreifuss and Gahwiler 1979).

Dispersal of hypothalamic tissue can provide a suspension of viable cells which can be divided as aliquots into replicate cultures for more reproducible experimental design. When grown as monolayers, the exchange of nutrients, secreted products and catabolites with the media is rapid. In addition to these theoretical advantages to cell survival, as compared with the use of explants, monolayer culture allows one to monitor morphologic integrity while cells are still surviving in vitro.

When embryonic cells are the source, dispersed cell cultures also provide a means of examining the morphogenesis of individual neurons, and synaptogenesis. Autoradiographic or immunohistochemical approaches can also define regions of the cell body or its processes in which metabolic functions or transport of molecules are occurring (Amaldi and Rusca 1970; Tixier-Vidal and DeVitry 1979; Delfs et al. 1980; Denizeau et al. 1981).

The long life of dispersed cell preparations is important because the influence of extrahypothalamic structures on biochemical or physiologic characteristics of the cells declines with time. Dispersed cell cultures can also be used for the isolation of sub-populations of cells with special characteristics. Attempts to achieve this end have been successfully attained by modification of the media (Mains and Patterson 1973; Honeggar et al. 1979), by sucrose gradient separation (Varon and Raiborn 1969; Lloyd et al. 1979), and by affinity chromatography (Dvorak et al. 1978; Au and Varon 1979). Unfortunately, quantitative recoveries have been low, precluding proper biochemical analysis. As a consequence, studies of 'sorted' neurons have centered on developmental requirements.

An important potential drawback to interpretation of results from primary cell cultures is that the cells, having lost their customary inputs from other hypothalamic structures, may show responses that do not resemble those of normal cells in situ. Attempts must be made, therefore, with each model, to determine how closely it resembles the in vivo situation and how these characteristics change with time in vitro. Even in cultures with no obvious changes of phenotypic expression, it must be emphasized that any particular biological event reflects only the capacity of the cells and does not indicate that that function is expressed in vivo. The use of neurotoxic enzymes in dispersal solutions, such as trypsin (Hemminki, 1971; Althaus 1977) may inadvertently select out neuronal or non-neuronal subsets to survive in the cultures. Beyond immediate cytotoxic insults, the possibility must be considered that certain subsets of hypothalamic cells, such as neurosecretory cells, have greater plasticity and may survive better in any given medium.

An additional limitation to the applicability of dispersed cell cultures is that embryonic or neonatal tissue must be used. This eliminates characteristics programmed into fully differentiated hypothalamic cells by humoral or structural extrahypothalamic inputs.

Growth factors in serum may be involved in differentiation and may provide continuing trophic influences. For this reason, as well as for the others cited above, serum-free, chemically defined media with growth supplements should be designed and tested for each individual hypothalamic model.

Cell lines

Continuous neuronal tumor cell lines were developed by Augusti-Tocco and Sato (1969) because they provided a homogenous cell population which retained a number of biochemical characteristics ordinarily ascribed to neurons. The mouse neuroblastoma line (C 1300) was shown to contain enzymes necessary for the formation of dopamine (Prasad et al. 1973), norepinephrine (Anagoste et al. 1972) and acetylcholine (Amano et al. 1972).

Other tumor lines have been shown to produce the hypothalamic releasing factors, TRH (Grimm-Jorgensen et al. 1976) and somatostatin (DeVitry et al. 1979). The advantage of using spontaneous or transformed cell lines is that the neurochemist can select out a clone which retains the ability to produce a particular molecule or family of molecules; by growing large quantities of that line, sufficient material can be produced for biochemical analysis. The major drawback to this approach is the limited applicability to studies of normal physiological regulation. It has also been demonstrated that certain biochemical characteristics may only be present in certain phases of growth (Grimm-Jorgensen et al. 1976).

Synaptosomes

Synaptosomes are cellular fragments, generally obtained by homogenization and differential sucrose sedimentation, which contain mainly synaptic elements (including pre- and postsynaptic membranes). However, many of the structures present are not synaptosomes (Morgan 1976; Warberg et al. 1977). Nevertheless, many investigators have found that this sub-cellular compartment contains in particulate form the bulk of the neurotransmitters (DeRobertis et al. 1963) and many neuropeptides (Ramirez et al. 1975; Epelbaum et al. 1977; Lee et al. 1978).

The main theoretical advantages are that results from experiments with these sub-cellular particles represent molecular events which occur at nerve endings and by implication exclude a nuclear or perikaryal level of control. Synaptosomes are relatively easy to work with, provide minimal barriers to diffusion, and allow good experimental design because of the ability to generate exact replicates.

The major and possibly overwhelming drawbacks are the marked heterogeneity of the preparation and uncertainty of what fraction of released product represents leakage from damaged membranes (see Kelly et al. 1979 for review). The report of Tytell et al. (1980) for example, documents a substantial proportion of GnRH release from these preparations as being non-specific and calcium independent.

IN VITRO STUDIES OF INDIVIDUAL NEUROPEPTIDES

In the foregoing sections we have considered the general aspects of various types of in vitro preparations for the study of hypothalamic peptide secretion. This section will summarize what is known about the control of secretion and synthesis of individual neuropeptides.

Although studies of neuropeptide release from isolated hypothalamic preparations are often technically straightforward, studies of de novo biosynthesis can be very difficult. Apart from the numerous preliminary studies necessary to characterize the conditions for maximum precursor incorporation, rigorous isolation methods are also required to eliminate contaminating counts (see Table 4.1). In addition to many technical problems, the theoretical considerations of the relatively small percentage of overall synthesis in a small number of cells in the hypothalamus are formidable. For an elegant analysis of this problem, with respect to synthesis of hypothalamic peptides, see McKelvy et al. (1979).

A newer approach for unravelling the regulation of biosynthesis of small peptides, using recombinant DNA techniques, has also recently been reviewed by Habener (1981) and is

Table 4.1

REQUIREMENTS FOR DEMONSTRATING THE PURITY OF BIOSYNTHETICALLY LABELLED NEUROPEPTIDES (McKelvy et al. 1979)

1. The neuropeptide is isolated by a sequential purification which may require the use of carrier synthetic peptide
2. Purification is carried out until constant specific activity (cpm per unit of biological or radioimmunological activity, or mass of peptide by amino acid analysis) is achieved. Assessment of purity is a *quantitative* matter: the qualitative demonstration of the co-migration of putative labelled biosynthetic product with synthetic peptide in several solvent systems is an inadequate criterion.
3. Further proof of radiochemical purity is obtained by appropriate derivatization of the putatively pure biosynthetic product. Assessment of the rate of derivatization of the biosynthetic product relative to that of pure synthetic peptide should be carried out as well as assessment of the chromatographic behavior of the derivative.
4. Rapid purification methodologies, emphasizing High Performance Liquid Chromatography should be favored to avoid the problem of peptide instability during the course of purification.

now being applied to the study of hypophysiotropic peptides (Joseph-Bravo et al. 1980).

Since a number of peptides and proteins ordinarily associated with other organ systems (e.g. gastrointestinal tract and pancreas) are localized in the hypothalamus, the in vitro approach becomes essential in establishing them as authentic hypothalamic factors. In general, the following criteria for proof of the hypothalamic origin of a peptide should be met.

1. Determination of its presence in the tissue by a well characterized radioimmunoassay system, including documentation of dilution curves parallel to those of a synthetic standard.
2. Localization in hypothalamic cells by immunohistochemical techniques; presumably for putative neuromodulators this localization should include distribution in nerve processes and terminals.
3. Demonstration of biological activity in conventional assays or of binding to specific receptor sites in the brain area to which immunohistochemically positive nerve terminals have been localized.
4. Incorporation of labelled amino acid precursors into the molecule (or its precursors) by hypothalamic tissue.
5. Documentation of the presence of mRNA in the tissue encoding precursors of the molecule.

Vasopressin

Synthesis

The first studies on biosynthesis of hypothalamic hormones were those of Sachs and co-workers (1971), who demonstrated that organ cultures of anterior hypothalamic-neurohypophysial blocks incorporated radiolabelled amino acid precursors into vasopressin (VP) for up to 12 days in vitro, despite extensive cellular degeneration. These workers suggest that VP might be synthesized as a prohormone because they identified a larger form of VP by means of neurophysin affinity columns. They also drew attention to the need for rigorous purification techniques of newly labelled peptides in such preparations. Using similar hypothalamic-neurohypophysial organ cultures, Pearson (1977) later demonstrated that during the first few days in vitro virtually no 'cytoplasmic' RNA was present, and that this type of RNA appeared after day 5, in vitro, when the culture began to synthesize VP. Studies by DeVitry et al. (1974) on a VP and neurophysin producing SV40-transformed hypothalamic cell line demonstrated at least three types of neurophysins. They restricted their biochemical studies to newly synthesized material in the 10 000 dalton range, and although they demonstrated newly synthesized materials co-eluting with neurophysin (I–III) and vasopressin, larger forms were excluded by the first gel filtration step.

The most complete studies of vasopressin synthesis were not carried out in vitro, but are the results of in vivo labelling of rat hypothalamic tissue by intrahypothalamic injection of labelled hormone precursors. These have shown that vasopressin and oxytocin, and their respective associated neurophysins, are each synthesized as part of precursors, each about 20 000 molecular weight. As summarized by Gainer (1981) and Russell et al. (1980), the vasopressin prohormone ('propressophysin') appears to be a glycoprotein, whereas the oxytocin prohormone is not glycosylated. It has been further shown by cell-free translation experiments that pre-proneurophysin forms exist (Guidice and Chaiken 1979; Gainer 1981) and can be membrane processed (Gainer 1981).

That the microtubular axonal system is involved in delivering newly synthesized VP from the perikaryon to the nerve terminal has been demonstrated by Pearson (1977) using stalk transection and colchicine.

Secretion

The classical studies by Douglas (1964) on the demonstration of stimulation-secretion coupling in VP release were not only the first complete studies on direct VP release from the isolated neurohypophysis, but they also established a standard for investigating release mechanisms which is still applicable to all neurotransmitters and neuropeptides today.

Consistent with its role as an osmoregulator, isolated hypothalamic tissue has been shown to release VP in response to osmotic stimuli (Ishikawa et al. 1980). The VP response to osmotic stimuli can be blocked by both indomethacin (Ishikawa et al. 1981) and the nicotinic receptor antagonist hexamethonium (Sladek and Joynt 1979b). Angiotensin II also stimulates VP release, an effect blocked by indomethacin but not by hexamethonium (Ishikawa et al 1981). Cyclic AMP and theophylline both increase the amount of VP released during depolarization (Mathison and Lederis 1980). Prostaglandins (PGE_2 and $PGF_{2\alpha}$) have been shown to enhance VP release from neural explants (Gagnon et al. 1973; Ishikawa et al. 1981) and picomolar concentrations of dopamine (DA) and acetylcholine (Ach) were also found to stimulate the release of VP from anterior hypothalamic organ cultures (Bridges et al. 1976).

Somatostatin

Synthesis

In vitro systems are being used to study the mechanisms of somatostatin biosynthesis in hypothalamic cells. The first report was that of Ensinck et al. (1978), who incubated [³H]phenylalanine with hypothalamic slices. They found that anterior hypothalamic tissue synthesized more immunoadsorbable somatostatin than did posterior hypothalamic slices, a result consistent with immunohistochemical reports that the highest number of somatostatin perikarya are located in the anterior periventricular nucleus. Chromatography of pulse-labelled slices revealed counts in three molecular species, one approximately 160 000 daltons, one in the 1600–3500 dalton range, and one peak co-eluting with somatostatin-14. They demonstrated that it took up to 4 h for new counts to be incorporated into the somatostatin-14 area, whereas counts were incorporated sooner into the two larger peaks. Their findings are consistent with a precursor–product relationship in the somatostatin biosynthetic pathway.

We have carried out similar studies using dissociated fetal rat cerebro-cortical cells and demonstrated two forms of immunoreactive somatostatin (IRS) with mobility different from that of somatostatin-14 on high performance liquid chromatography (HPLC). In a pulse-chase experiment, at least one of these forms was shown to be a precursor to somatostatin-14. Further analysis of the types of IRS in these cell cultures revealed three distinct types of IRS, one with an apparent molecular weight of 11 500, one co-eluting with synthetic somatostatin 25/28 (both kindly provided by Dr R. Guillemin, Salk Institute) and one co-eluting with somastostatin-14. These in vitro labelling experiments conform well with information accumulating about the biosynthesis of somatostatin from a number of approaches. Gel filtration studies to size extracts of hypothalamus and cerebral cortex (Lauber et al. 1979; Rorstad et al. 1979; Zingg and Patel 1980) have identified several larger IRS forms which may be precursors, or somatostatin bound to a binding protein (Ogawa et al. 1977). mRNAs encoding larger somatostatin precursors have been found in angler fish islets (Goodman et al. 1980; Shields 1980) and in rodent hypothalamus (Joseph-Bravo et al. 1980). Recombinant DNA techniques have been used to construct cDNAs which encode preprosomatostatins (in the M_r 14 000–16 000 range) (Goodman et al. 1980; Hobart et al. 1980). Conventional protein isolation and sequencing techniques also provide evidence for biologically active somatostatin prohormones (Oyama et al. 1980; Meyers et al. 1980; Bohlen et al. 1980). Results from the foregoing studies form a basis from which in vitro methods can explore potential post-transcriptional and post-translational regulatory sites in somatostatin biosynthesis.

Secretion

The most consistent effects on somatostatin secretion have been those elicited from in vitro hypothalamic preparations by membrane depolarization brought about by high extracellular potassium (Iversen et al. 1978; Berelowitz et al. 1978; Terry et al. 1980; Richardson et al. 1980), by the sodium ionophore veratridine (Maeda and Frohman 1980; Gamse et al. 1980), or by electrical stimuli (Patel et al. 1978). In all of these studies, (see Table 4.2) the depolarization-induced somatostatin secretion can be prevented by withdrawing calcium ions or by blocking their flow with agents such as cobalt or verapamil. It is presumed, therefore, that somatostatin release under these conditions is mediated by inward calcium flux through voltage-dependent channels. Studies in our own laboratory

Table 4.2

SUBSTANCES WHICH AFFECT SOMATOSTATIN RELEASE FROM IN VITRO HYPOTHALAMIC PRE-
PARATIONS

Study	Stimulatory	Inhibitory	No effect
Iversen et al. 1978	K^+		
	Neurotensin		
Berelowitz et al. 1978	K^+		
Negro-Vilar et al. 1978	DA		
	NE		
Sheppard et al. 1978	Growth hormone		TSH
Sheppard et al. 1979	Substance P		Met-enkephalin
	Neurotensin		Leu-enkephalin
Epelbaum et al. 1979	K^+	VIP	GABA
Turkelson et al. 1979	GABA		
Bennett et al. 1979	K^+	NE	
	Veratridine	5-HT	
		DA	
Richardson et al. 1979		5-HT	
		Ach	
Richardson et al. 1980	K^+	Ach	Atropine
		Neostigmine	
Berelowitz et al. 1980a	DA	Hypothyroidism	TRH
	T_3		TSH
Terry et al. 1980	K^+		Ach, DA, GABA
			Morphine, NE, PGE_2,
			Neostigmine, Glu, Gly
Gamse et al. 1980	K^+	Tetrodotoxin	
	Veratridine	Cobalt	
	Bicuculline	GABA	
Maeda and Frohman 1980	K^+, DA, L-dopa		cAMP, NE
	Bromocriptine,		5-HT, Ach
	Neurotensin		Substance P
	Veratridine		
Berelowitz et al. 1980b	Growth hormone		
Ojeda et al. 1980	Indomethacin		PGE_2, $PGF_{2\alpha}$
	DA		NE

using dispersed hypothalamic and cerebral cortical cells have likewise demonstrated
enhanced IRS release after exposure to elevated potassium concentrations, and to veratridine in a calcium-dependent manner (Robbins et al. 1981). In addition, we have shown
that sodium-induced depolarization can be blocked by both sodium channel blockade with
tetrodotoxin (see also Gamse et al. 1980) and the calcium channel blocker, verapamil.

Studies utilizing classical neurotransmitters on the other hand, have produced contradictory results. Ach has been reported to inhibit IRS release from hypothalamic frag-

ments (Richardson et al. 1980), or to have no effect in similar preparations (Terry et al. 1980; Maeda and Frohman. 1980), and in our own studies, in dispersed cell cultures to stimulate IRS release (Robbins et al. 1981). Enhanced IRS release after Ach has also been noted in hypophysial portal vein collections (Chihara et al. 1979). The response to Ach in our studies was predominantly muscarinic, a result also noted by Richardson et al. (1980). Aside from technical problems, these apparently contradictory results may be due to the possibility that in organized tissue explants, Ach may be stimulating IRS release and also neurons inhibitory to somatostatinergic cells. For instance, Ach stimulates gamma amino-butyric acid (GABA) via enhanced glutamic acid decarboxylase activity (Sze 1979), a known inhibitor of IRS release (see below). Since normal intercellular connections may not be operating in dispersed cells, these responses may be absent.

Dopamine in micromolar concentrations has been reported to be stimulatory to IRS release from hypothalamic explants (Wakabayashi et al. 1977; Negro-Vilar et al. 1978; Bennett et al. 1979; Maeda and Frohman 1980; Berelowitz et al. 1980a), an effect which can be blocked by prostaglandin PGE_2 (Ojeda et al. 1980). Terry et al. (1980), however, found no effect of DA on IRS release from perfused hypothalamic fragments. Preliminary results of studies of dispersed hypothalamic cells in our laboratory also demonstrate IRS release by similar, but not by lower, concentrations of DA.

Except for a weak stimulatory response in one report (Negro-Vilar et al. 1978), NE has been found to have no direct effect on IRS release (Terry et al. 1980; Maeda and Frohman 1980; Ojeda et al. 1980). Our studies on cerebral cortical cell cultures likewise show no change in IRS release in response to NE.

Gamma-aminobutyric acid was reported to inhibit somatostatin release from dispersed hypothalamic cells by Gamse et al. (1980), a finding we have been able to confirm. We have shown that picrotoxin, a blocker of GABA action, produces striking stimulation of IRS release from cortical cells.

The influence of hormones thought to be involved in the feedback control of growth hormone (GH) and TSH control (both regulated by somatostatin) have also been studied. IRS release from hypothalamic blocks was reportedly increased by prior exposure to triiodothyronine (Sheppard et al. 1978; Berelowitz et al. 1980a) or to GH (Berelowitz et al. 1980b). These findings support the hypothesis that both thyroid hormones and GH are autoregulatory in part at the hypothalamic level by increasing somatostatin secretion.

A miscellaneous group of factors has also been studied with respect to their abilities to modify somatostatin release in vitro. These were chosen for examination because they are known to modify GH secretion in vivo. Neurotensin, substance P, morphine and the enkephalins have all been reported to stimulate GH release through effects on the hypo-thalamus (see Imura et al. 1981 and Chapter 1). However, neurotensin (Iversen et al. 1978; Sheppard et al. 1979; Maeda and Frohman 1980), and substance P (Sheppard et al. 1979) apparently increase IRS release, whereas Met- or Leu-enkephalin (Sheppard et al. 1979) or morphine (Terry et al. 1980) have no effect on basal IRS release. If the in vitro studies can be taken as indicators of function in vivo they indicate that these GH regulatory peptides are not acting through changes in somatostatin release, but rather through modifications of the secretion of GH releasing factors(s).

Thyrotropin releasing hormone

Synthesis

As initially reported by Reichlin and collaborators (Mitnick and Reichlin 1971; Reichlin and Mitnick 1973; Reichlin 1976) fragments of rat hypothalamic tissue were found to incorporate labelled amino acid precursors into peptides that had the same chromatographic behavior as authentic thyrotropin releasing hormone. Many other peptides were found in the same system. Grimm and Reichlin (1973) also found that mouse hypothalamic fragments incubated in labelled histidine incorporated this amino acid into a substance with the mobility of TRH on thin-layer chromatography, and that the product, labelled with [^{14}C]histidine, chromatographed to constant specific activity with [^{3}H]TRH.

Subsequently, McKelvy (McKelvy 1974; McKelvy 1977) and McKelvy and Grimm-Jorgensen (Grimm-Jorgensen and McKelvy 1974; McKelvy and Grimm-Jorgensen, 1975; McKelvy et al. 1975) criticized the earlier work from this laboratory on rat TRH biosynthesis on the basis that the proof of identity of the labelled product had not been rigorous enough and that only a small fraction of the radioactivity moving with TRH on electrophoresis or thin-layer chromatography was authentic TRH. The problems in identification of a labelled product were emphasized in recent publications by Mc Kelvy and collaborators (Table 4.2). Their studies were carried out using much more sophisticated chemical separation methods than were the first studies done in our laboratory. In vitro incorporation of precursors into a compound that migrates with TRH, at least in some chromatographic systems, was reported by Guillemin (1971) and by Knigge and collaborators (1974) (see Reichlin 1976, for review), but the same reservations about isolation of product undoubtedly apply to these reports as well. Using guinea pig hypothalamic cultures, Mc Kelvy et al. (1975) showed that [^{3}H]proline was incorporated into a compound that moved with TRH in at least nine separate chromatographic steps and formed an *n*-trifluoroacetyl *n*-butyl-ester derivative that had chromatographic properties identical with those of TRH. Using the whole newt brain, Grimm-Jorgensen and McKelvy (1974) conducted a similar study using extensive chromatographic procedures including derivatization and proved the identity of the compound. From these experiments and those of Grimm-Jorgensen and Reichlin, it seems reasonable to conclude that isolated hypothalamic tissue is capable of forming new TRH, but that the most rigorous separation methods are needed to establish the identity of the compound in view of the large number of new peptides that are formed by such systems. In incubations of rat brain fragments we reported that puromycin (an inhibitor of translation) did not block the incorporation of amino acids into a peptide separable as TRH by thin-layer chromatography and electrophoresis (Mitnick and Reichlin 1971, Reichlin et al. 1972). Since the identity of the compound isolated as TRH is now in doubt because of the more recent findings alluded to, the significance of this result can now be questioned. On the other hand, Grimm-Jorgensen and McKelvy (1974) found that newt brain TRH formation was blocked neither by incubation with puromycin nor by diphtheria antitoxin, a potent ribosomal poison, also indicating a nonribosomal form of biosynthesis. Kubek et al. (1977) reported that rat hypothalamic fragments incubated in vitro with [^{3}H]proline incorporated the amino acid into a product separated by affinity chromatography on anti-TRH columns. Although this may well be TRH, the occurrence of some non-TRH compounds that react with anti-TRH antisera make it essential to carry out more extensive separation methods than simple affinity chromatography. In this system, incorporation of counts into 'TRH' was not blocked by cycloheximide, indicating a nonribosomal form of biosynthesis.

The actual nature of TRH biosynthesis has not been elucidated by study of whole hypothalamic incubates. A number of workers have studied TRH biosynthesis in subcellular fractions. In our initial studies (Mitnick and Reichlin 1971), incorporation of labelled amino acids into material with 'TRH'-like properties was demonstrated, but the separation techniques used were inadequate to assure specificity. More recent studies from this laboratory (summarized in Reichlin 1976), using a variety of subcellular preparations and more specific methods for separation, have failed to demonstrate de novo TRH biosynthesis. Similarly, other workers have failed to demonstrate TRH biosynthesis by incubation of hypothalamic extracts with precursors of TRH. Restudy of this question by McKelvy and associates (1975), utilizing large amounts of homogenate prepared from mammalian hypothalamus, and bacitracin to inhibit TRH breakdown, led to the demonstration that [^{3}H]proline was incorporated into a TRH-like material, rigorously separated from the reaction mixture. In this system, the addition of inhibitors of protein synthesis, or of ribonuclease A (which would destroy mRNA-directed peptide synthesis) decreased the synthesis of 'TRH', a finding interpreted to mean that this peptide is synthesized as part of a larger precursor molecule analogous to other peptides such as neurophysin (McKelvy et al. 1979). These studies have not yet been reported in extenso.

That TRH may be formed from a precursor molecule is further suggested by recent studies of Rupnow et al. (1979), who showed that frog brain extracts, treated with proteolytic enzymes, followed by procedures that convert glutamic acid residues to pyroglutamic acid and that amidate carboxyterminal amino acids, generated a compound with the properties of TRH as determined by immunoassay, chromatography and binding properties. This work means that there is a protein sequence corresponding to Glu–His–Pro in brain extract, but does not prove that this is the normal route by which TRH is synthesized. There are, in fact, several proteins naturally occurring in mammalian tissue that include this sequence.

It must be concluded that at this time, and despite a decade of work in a number of laboratories, studies of TRH synthesis, utilizing either in vitro incubation techniques or subcellular fractionation methods have not fully clarified the mechanisms of TRH biosynthesis.

Secretion

Several authors have studied in vitro TRH release from various kinds of hypothalamic incubation preparations (Table 4.3). The first of these studies (Grimm and Reichlin 1973), utilized mouse hypothalamic incubates which had been pulse labelled with [^{14}C]histidine, a precursor of TRH. The discharge of radioactivity associated with chromatographically separated 'TRH' was shown to be stimulated by exposure to NE and to DA. The effect of DA was blocked if disulfiram, an agent that blocks conversion of DA to NE, was added to

Table 4.3

SUBSTANCES WHICH INFLUENCE THE RELEASE OF TRH FROM IN VITRO HYPOTHALAMIC PREPARATIONS

Study	Stimulatory	Inhibitory	No effect
Grimm and Reichlin 1973	NE	5HT	Ach
	DA		Carbamylcholine
Warberg et al. 1977	K^+		PGE_2
Hirooka and Hollander 1978	NE	Somatostatin	
Joseph-Bravo et al, 1979	K^+	DA	NE, 5HT, GABA
	H_2 agonists	DA antagonists	Ach
Maeda and Frohman 1980	K^+		Neurotensin, NE
	Veratridine		5HT, Ach
	DA		
	cAMP		

the media. The technique used to isolate the TRH has subsequently been criticized by McKelvy and Grimm-Jorgensen because of its lack of specificity; the limitations of this technique have been further considered by Reichlin et al. (1978). DA-stimulated release of TRH-like material has also been reported from hypothalamic synaptosomes (Schaeffer et al. 1977).

Hirooka and Hollander (1978) reported recently that immunoreactive TRH is released from hypothalamic fragments by NE, but Joseph-Bravo et al. (1979) and Maeda and Frohman (1980) failed to confirm this finding, utilizing rather similar methods. Reports of the effects of neurotransmitters on TRH release in vitro show many discrepancies. Joseph-Bravo et al. (1979) studied a series of neurotransmitters, including 5HT, GABA, Ach, DA, DA agonists, and histamine. Histamine exerted a stimulatory effect, a response mediated by H_2 receptors, and DA was inhibitory. On the other hand, Maeda and Frohman (1980) reported that DA, bromocriptine, and L-dopa were stimulatory to TRH release. In common with the findings of Joseph-Bravo et al. (1979), NE, 5HT, and Ach were without effect, as were neurotensin or substance P. In contrast to the work of Hirooka and Hollander (1978), who reported that somatostatin inhibited TRH release, Maeda and Frohman (1980) found no effect.

It is apparent from this brief review that a consensus on the effects of neurotransmitters on TRH secretion in vitro has not been reached. The influence of neurotransmitters on TRH secretion inferred from studies of TSH secretion in whole animals utilizing neuropharmacological agents is also difficult to elucidate because both somatostatin and TRH are involved in TSH regulation, as is DA through direct effects on the pituitary (Ford et al. 1981). These questions are considered in detail by Müller and colleagues (1977) and by Reichlin et al. (1978).

Gonadotropin releasing hormone

Synthesis

The first demonstration that radioactive precursors of gonadotropin releasing hormone were incorporated by hypothalamic-fragment incubates into peptides with the chromatographic properties of GnRH was that of Johannsson et al. (1972), a finding confirmed by Sachs (1974), by Moguilevsky et al. (1974), by Hall and Steinberger (1976), and by Reichlin (1976). Incorporation appeared to be greater in hypothalamic fragments removed from long term castrated animals (Reichlin 1976), although the studies were not subject to statistical analysis. The addition of testosterone to hypothalami from castrated rats was reported to reduce incorporation of precursor into GnRH (Moguilevsky 1975), but Hall and Steinberger (1977) have failed to find any effects of short term castration on subsequent in vitro incorporation of precursor amino acids into GnRH.

None of the above cited studies utilizing short term incubation methods indicate the mode of synthesis of GnRH. The relatively large size of this molecule, ten amino acid residues, suggests that synthesis is most likely by classical peptide synthetic pathways. Several

Table 4.4

GONADOTROPIN RELEASING HORMONE RELEASE FROM IN VITRO HYPOTHALAMIC PREPARATIONS

Study	Stimulatory	Inhibitory	No effect
Schneider and McCann 1969	DA		NE 5HT
Bennett and Edwardson 1975	DA		K^+
Rotsztejn et al. 1976	K^+ DA		DA (OVX rats)
Kao and Weisz 1977	Melatonin		NE, DA, 5HT, Ach
Rotsztejn et al. 1977	DA		NE
Warberg et al. 1977	K^+		PGE_2
Bigdeli and Snyder, 1978	K^+ Ouabain Melatonin PGE_2		
Negro-Vilar et al. 1979	DA NE		Epinephrine
Ojeda et al. 1979	DA NE PGE_2	Indomethacin	$PGF_{2\alpha}$
Hartter and Ramirez 1980	K^+ Dinitrophenol Colchicine (100 μM)	Cyanide Iodoacetic acid Colchicine (1 and 10 μM)	Ouabain
Tytell 1980		Estradiol	

authors have, in fact, observed GnRH immunoreactivity in hypothalamic extracts to occur in a 'large' as well as a small form; the latter corresponding to decapeptide GnRH (Fawcett et al. 1975; Millar et al. 1977). Moreover, generation of bioactive GnRH from incubated hypothalami suggest the possibility that a precursor form has broken down to GnRH (Seyler et al. 1973).

Further support for the view that GnRH is synthesized as part of a larger molecule is the observation by McKelvy (1979) that a cell-free particulate preparation of hypothalamus from the rat incorporates labelled tyrosine into chromatographically separated GnRH and this incorporation is prevented by incubation with puromycin and cycloheximide (protein synthesis inhibitors), or by ribonuclease A, a blocker of ribosomal synthesis.

Finally, several recent reports of GnRH production by dissociated primary fetal rat hypothalamic cells suggest that such preparations may be useful for study of GnRH biosynthesis (Daikoku et al. 1978; Feldman et al. 1980; Denizeau et al. 1981).

Secretion

Schneider and McCann (1969) performed the earliest studies on in vitro GnRH release by co-incubating stalk median eminence and pituitary with or without various neurotransmitters and monitoring LH release as a measure of GnRH secretion (Table 4.4). They found a significant enhancement of LH release when DA was added to the incubation. Although the α-blocker, phentolamine, could block the DA-induced response, NE and α-receptor agonist applied directly had no effect. Subsequent studies in a synaptosomal preparation (Bennett and Edwardson 1975b) and in hypothalamic explant incubations (Rotsztejn et al. 1976; 1977; Negro-Vilar et al. 1979; Ojeda et al. 1980) have confirmed the stimulatory effect of DA on GnRH release. Kao and Weisz (1977) have reported, however, that short pulses of DA onto superfused rat hypothalami do not stimulate GnRH. The hypothalami of ovariectomized rats likewise seem refractory to DA (Rotsztejn et al. 1976).

The initial demonstration by Schneider and McCann (1969) that NE does not mimic the effect of DA, thereby excluding conversion of DA to NE as the mode of action, was confirmed by Rotsztejn (1977). Two reports from McCann's laboratory, however, suggest that not only are DA and NE direct secretagogues, but that their effects may be mediated by prostaglandin E_2 (Negro-Vilar et al. 1979: Ojeda et al. 1980). The stimulatory effect of prostaglandin E_2 has been confirmed in hypothalamic fragment incubations (Gallardo and Ramirez 1977; Bigdeli and Snyder 1978) and in hypophysial portal blood collection studies (Eskay et al. 1975), but not in synaptosomes (Warberg et al. 1977). Melatonin has also been found to directly stimulate GnRH release (Kao and Weisz 1977; Bigdeli and Snyder 1978). The following compounds have been reported to have no effect on GnRH release: ouabain, (Hartter and Ramirez 1980), serotonin (Schneider and McCann 1969; Kao and Weisz 1977), epinephrine (Negro-Vilar et al. 1979), $PGF_2\alpha$ (Ojeda et al. 1980), and Ach (Kao and Weisz 1977). The only direct inhibitors of LH-RH release described to date, other than calcium flux blockers, are cyanide, iodoacetic acid, colchicine (Hartter and Ramirez, 1980), and indomethacin (Ojeda et al. 1980).

The effect of gonadal steroids on GnRH release was examined by Rotsztejn et al. (1976). These workers noted that basal GnRH release was higher in hypothalamic explants from castrate rats, but that the putative GnRH secretagogue, DA, was ineffective unless the rats had been pretreated with estradiol. These observations were extended by Tytell et al. (1980), who noted that hypothalamic synaptosomal preparations from ovariectomized rats released more GnRH than those from similar rats who had received estradiol benzoate up to 48 h prior to sacrifice.

These studies, taken together, support a direct action of gonadal steroids at the level of the hypothalamus, influencing both the rate of synthesis and release of GnRH. The possibility that estrogens might modify DA-induced GnRH release (Rotsztejn et al. 1976), may be related to the competition between the estrogen metabolites, catecholestrogens, and catecholamines for the enzyme catechol-*o*-methyl transferase at nerve terminals (Foreman and Porter 1980). Recent preliminary reports have also implicated cyclic AMP (Burrows and Barnea 1980), Met-enkephalin (Drouva et al. 1980) and vasoactive intestinal peptide (VIP) (Samson et al. 1980) as regulators of GnRH secretion.

Corticotropin releasing factor

Synthesis

Because corticotropin releasing factor (CRF(s)) has only been chemically defined recently (Vale et al. 1981), specific studies of amino acid precursor incorporation by hypothalamic tissue have not been done. Studies employing bioassay, however, have demonstrated that adrenalectomy results in elevated bioassayable CRF release without changing hypothalamic CRF content, suggesting that glucocorticoid deficiency causes increased CRF synthesis (Jones et al. 1976b). Jones and Hillhouse (1977) have investigated the mechanism of CRF synthesis further and concluded that non-ribosomal synthesis of CRF was excluded because cycloheximide prevented 5HT-induced CRF release. In their in vitro system, a 5-min stimulation by Ach caused release of an amount of CRF corresponding to the total stored CRF, but within that time there was no change in tissue content. They conclude, therefore, that a prohormone (presumably biologically inactive) is cleaved under the influence of Ach stimulation to maintain a steady intracellular level of CRF.

Secretion

The characteristics of CRF release have been extensively studied by Jones and colleagues. Utilizing a well characterized in vitro hypothalamic explant system, they have demonstrated that CRF release can be modulated only in the whole explant and not in smaller explants (including ventromedial, dorsomedial, periventricular, and arcuate nuclei, as well as the median eminence) (Jones et al 1976b). In contrast, hypothalamic synaptosomal preparations have been shown to release CRF in response to potassium and DA (Edwardson and Bennett 1974; Bennett and Edwardson 1975).

Ach (Bradburg, 1974; Hillhouse et al. 1975) was found to be an effective secretagogue, acting predominantly through nicotinic receptors (Jones et al. 1976b). The action of Ach was blocked by NE (via an α receptor mechanism) and melatonin. 5HT was also found to be stimulatory, but the fact that its action could be antagonized by atropine and hexamethonium indicates that its mode of action may be via activation of cholinergic neurons (Jones et al. 1976a).

Although the extensive studies of Jones et al. (1976a) failed to find any direct inhibitors of basal CRF release, NE, melatonin and GABA were able to block the stimulatory effects of Ach and 5HT. Corticosterone was also a potent blocker of cholinergically induced release (Jones and Hillhouse 1977). The latter effect is consistent with the recent demonstration that bioassayable CRF release by hypothalamic tissues from adrenalectomized rats is increased, and that release is reduced by dexamethasone (Vermes et al. 1977). Analysis of the feedback of corticosteroids on CRF release has been made by Jones et al. (1977).

The most recent studies of CRF regulation by Fehm et al. (1980) failed to confirm the studies of Jones and co-workers, in that they found NE to be stimulatory and Ach and 5HT to be without effect on CRF release. In addition, they concluded that the NE effect was at the nerve terminal, because experiments with median eminence slices reproduced the results with whole hypothalamic explants.

The effects of two neuropeptides on CRF release were investigated by Jones and Hillhouse (1977). They determined that neither VP (a putative direct stimulator of ACTH release) nor angiotensin II had any role in the regulation of CRF release.

Taken together, these experiments can be interpreted as demonstrating steroid feedback directly at the hypothalamic level, as well as noradrenergic and GABA-ergic inhibitory influences on cell bodies, but not on nerve terminals, in response to a putative cholinergic final excitatory pathway. These results are in good agreement with in vivo animal and human studies, as recently reviewed by Krieger (1977) and Ganong (1980).

Other peptides in the hypothalamus

A large number of peptides and protein molecules in the hypothalamus are now being studied in vitro. These include substance P (Iversen et al. 1976; Fishbach et al. 1981), VIP (Giachetti et al. 1977), bombesin (Moody et al. 1980), GH (Pacold et al. 1978), ACTH (Krieger and Liotta. 1979; Robbins et al. 1979; Liotta et al. 1979), an ACTH precursor (Liotta et al. 1980), and β-endorphin (Osborne et al. 1979; Fukata et al. 1980).

SUMMARY

In this review, we have attempted to describe the various model systems which have been employed to examine regulation of peptide secretion by the isolated hypothalamus. Although each has its advantages and limitations, no single system used to date affords optimal, simultaneous analysis of synthesis, processing, secretion and physiological relevance. The information gained with respect to each individual peptide has served to establish it as a true hypothalamic secretion and to provide insight into the levels of neuroendocrine feedback regulation. Although results from these in vitro preparations define intrinsic biochemical and physiologic mechanisms, complementary in vivo studies are necessary to define the level of their phenotypic expression.

128

ACKNOWLEDGEMENTS

Richards Robbins is a Trainee, USPHS. Work from the authors' laboratory alluded to in this paper was supported by USHS Grants No. AM 16684 and T32 AM 07039.

REFERENCES

Althaus, H.H., Huttner, W.B. and Neuhoff, V. (1977) Neurochemical and morphological studies of bulk isolated rat brain cells. Hoppe-Seyler's Physiol. Chem. 358, 1155-1159.

Amaldi, P. and Rusca, G. (1970) Autoradiographic study of RNA in nerve fibers of embryonic sensory ganglia culture in vitro under NGF stimulation. J. Neurochem. 17, 767-771.

Amano, T., Richelson, E. and Nirenberg, M. (1972) Neurotransmitter synthesis by neuroblastoma clones. Proc. Natl. Acad. Sci. USA 69, 258-263.

Anagoste, B., Freedman, L.S., Goldstein, M., Broome, J. and Fuxe, K. (1972) Dopamine-β-hydroxylase activity in mouse neuroblastoma tumors and in cell cultures. Proc. Natl. Acad. Sci. USA 69, 1883-1886.

Au, A.J. and Varon, S. (1979) Neural cell sequestration on immunoaffinity columns. Exp. Cell. Res. 120, 269-272.

Augusti-Tocco, G. and Sato, G. (1969) Establishment of functional clonal lines of neurons from mouse neuroblastoma. Proc. Natl. Acad. Sci. USA 64, 311-315.

Benda, P., DeVitry, F., Picart, R. and Tixier-Vidal, A. (1975) Dissociated cell cultures from fetal mouse hypothalamus: Patterns of organization and ultrastructural features. Exp. Brain Res. 23, 29-47.

Bennett, G.W. and Edwardson, J.A. (1975) Release of corticotrophin releasing factor and other hypophysiotrophic substances from isolated nerve endings. J. Endocrinol. 65, 33-44.

Bennett, G.W., Edwardson, J.A., Holland, D., Jeffcoate, S.L. and White, N. (1975) Release of immunoreactive LHRH and TRH from hypothalamic synaptosomes. Nature (London) 257, 323-325.

Bennett, G.W., Edwardson, J.A., Marcano De Cotte, D., Berelowitz, M., Pimstone, B. and Kronheim, S. (1979) Release of somatostatin from rat brain synaptosomes. J. Neurochem. 32, 1127-1131.

Berelowitz, M., Kronheim, S., Pimstone, B. and Sheppard, M. (1978) Potassium stimulated calcium dependent release of immunoreactive somatostatin from incubated rat hypothalamus. J. Neurochem. 31, 1537-1539.

Berelowitz, M., Kiyoshi, M., Harris, S. and Frohman, L.A. (1980a) The effect of alterations in the pituitary-thyroid axis on hypothalamic content and in vitro release of somatostatin-like immunoreactivity. Endocrinology 107, 24-29.

Berelowitz, M., Harris, S.L. and Frohman, L.A. (1980b) Modification of somatostatin homeostasis by growth hormone: Effect of GH excess and deficiency on hypothalamic SRIF content and release and tissue SRIF distribution. 62nd Annual Meeting of the Endocrine Society p. 261.

Bigdeli, H. and Snyder, P.J. (1978) Gonadotropin-releasing hormone release from rat hypothalamus: Dependence on membrane depolarization and calcium influx. Endocrinology 103, 281-286.

Bohlen, P., Brazeau, P., Benoit, R., Ling, N., Esch, F. and Guillemin, R. (1980) Isolation and amino acid composition of two somatostatin-like peptides from ovine hypothalamus: Somatostatin-28 and somatostatin-25. Biochem. Biophys. Res. Comm. 96, 725-734.

Bottenstein, J.E. and Sato, G.H. (1979) Growth of a rat neuroblastoma cell line in serum-free supplemented medium. Proc. Natl. Acad. Sci. USA 76, 514-517.

Bradbury, M.W.B., Burden, J., Hillhouse, E.W. and Jones, M.T. (1974) Stimulation electrically and by acetylcholine of the rat hypothalamus in vitro. J. Physiol. (London) 239, 269-283.

Bridges, T.E., Hillhouse, E.W. and Jones, M.T. (1976) The effect of dopamine on neurohypophysial hormone release in vivo and from the rat neural lobe and hypothalamus in vitro. J. Physiol. (London) 260, 647-666.

Burrows, G.H. and Barnea, A. (1980) Effect of divalent cations and ATP on the release of LHRH from isolated secretory granules. 62nd Annual Meeting of the Endocrine Society, p. 109.

Chihara, K., Arimura, A. and Schally, A.V. (1979) Effect of intraventricular injections of dopamine, norepinephrine, acetylcholine, and 5-hydroxy-tryptamine on immunoreactive somatostatin release into rat hypophysial portal blood. Endocrinology 104, 1656-1662.

Daikoku, S., Kawano, H., Matsumura, H. and Saito, S. (1978) In vivo and in vitro studies on the appearance of LHRH neurons in the hypothalamus of perinatal rats. Cell. Tissue Res. 194, 433-445.

Delfs, J., Robbins, R., Connolly, J.L., Dichter, M. and Reichlin, S. (1980) Somatostatin production by rat cerebral neurons in dissociated cell cultures. Nature (London) 283, 676-677.

Denizeau, F., Dube, D., Antakly, T., Lemay, A., Parent, A., Pelletier, G. and Labrie, F. (1981) Attempts to demonstrate peptide localization and secretion in primary cell cultures of fetal rat hypothalamus. Neuroendocrinology 32, 96-102.

DeRobertis, E., DeLores, A., Salganicoff, L. DeIraldi, A. and Zieher, L.M. (1963) Isolation of synaptic vesicles and structural organization of the acetylcholine system within brain nerve endings. J. Neurochem. 10, 225-235.

DeVitry, F., Camier, M., Czernichow, P., Benda, P. and Tixier-Vidal, A. (1974) Establishment of a clone of mouse hypothalamic neurosecretory cells synthesizing neurophysin and vasopressin. Proc. Natl. Acad. Sci. USA 71, 3575-3579.

DeVitry, F., Dubois, M. and Tixier-Vidal, A. (1979) Immunological detection of somatostatin in a primitive hypothalamic mouse cell line, precursor of a neurophysin cell lineage. J. Physiol. (Paris) 75, 11-13.

Douglas, W.W. (1974) Mechanism of release of neurohypophysial hormones: Stimulus secretion coupling. In: Handbook of Physiology (Greep, R.O. and Astwood, E.B. eds), Vol. 4, Sect. 7, pp. 191-224 Am. Physiol. Soc., Washington, D.C.

Dreifuss, J.J. and Gahwiler, B.H. (1979) Hypothalamic neurons in culture I: A short review of the literature. J. Physiol. (Paris) 75, 15-21.

Drouva, S.V., Epelbaum, J., Tapia-Arancibia, L., LaPlante, E. and Kordon, C. (1980) Met-enkephalin inhibition of K^+-induced LHRH and SRIF release from rat mediobasal hypothalamic slices. Eur. J. Pharmacol 61, 411-412.

Dvorak, D.J., Gipps, E. and Kidson, C. (1978) Isolation of specific neurons by affinity methods. Nature (London) 271, 564-566.

Edwardson, J.A. and Bennett, G.W. (1974) Modulation of corticotropin-releasing factor release from hypothalamic synaptosomes. Nature 251, 425-427.

Ensinck, J.W., Laschansky, E.C., Kanter, R.A., Fujimoto, W.Y., Koerker, D.J. and Goodner, C.J. (1978) Somatostatin biosynthesis and release in the hypothalamus and pancreas of the rat. Metabolism 27, 1207-1210.

Epelbaum, J., Brazeau, P., Tsang, D., Brawer, J. and Martin, J. (1977) Subcellular distribution of radioimmunoassayable somatostatin in rat brain. Brain Res. 126, 309-323.

Eskay, R.L., Warberg, J., Mical, R. and Porter, J.C. (1975) Prostaglandin E_2-induced release of LHRH into hypophysial portal blood. Endocrinology 97, 816-820.

Fawcett, C.P., Beezley, A.E. and Wheaton, J.E. (1975) Chromatographic evidence for the existence of another species of LRF. Endocrinology 96, 1311-1314.

Fehm, H.L., Voigt, K.H., Lang, R.E. and Pfeiffer, E.F. (1980) Effects of neurotransmitters on the release of corticotrophin releasing hormone (CRH) by rat hypothalamic tissue in vitro. Exp. Brain Res. 39, 229-234.

Feldman, S.C., Johnson, A.B., Bornstein, M.B. and Campbell, G.T. (1979) Luteinizing hormone releasing-hormone neurons in cultures of fetal rat hypothalamus. Neuroendocrinology 28, 131-137.

Fischbach, G.D., Dunlap, K., Mudge, A. and Leeman, S. (1981) Peptide and amine transmitter effect on embryonic chick sensory neurons in vitro. In: Neurosecretion and Brain Peptides. (Martin, J. B., Reichlin, S. and Bick, K.L. eds), pp. 175-198. Raven Press, New York.

Foord, S.M., Peters, J., Scanlon, M.F., Rees Smith, B. and Hall, R. (1980) Dopaminergic control of TSH secretion in isolated rat pituitary cells. FEBS Lett. 121, 257-259.

Foreman, M.M. and Porter, J.C. (1980) Effects of catechol estrogens and catecholamines on hypothalamic and corpus striatal tyrosine hydroxylase activity. J. Neurochem. 34, 1175-1183.

Fukata, J., Nakai, Y. and Imura, H. (1980) Release of immunoreactive β-endorphin from rat hypothalamic fragments in vitro. Brain Res. 201, 492-496.

Gagnon, D.J., Cousineau, D. and Boucher, P.J. (1973) Release of vasopressin by angiotensin II and prostaglandin E_2 from the rat neurohypophysis in vitro. Life Sci. 12, 487-489.

Gainer, H. (1981) The biology of neurosecretory neurons. In: Neurosecretion and Brain Peptides (Martin, J. B., Reichlin, S. and Bick, K.L. eds), pp. 5-20, Raven Press, New York.

Gallardo, E. and Ramirez, V.D. (1977) A method for superfusion of rat hypothalami: Secretion of luteinizing hormone releasing hormone. Proc. Soc. Exp. Biol. Med. 155, 79-82.

Gamse, R., Vaccaro, D.E., Gamse, G., DiPace, M., Fox, T.O. and Leeman, S.E. Release of immunoreactive somatostatin from hypothalamic cells in culture: Inhibition by gamma amino butyric acid. Proc. Natl. Acad. Sci. USA 77, 5552-5556.

Ganong, W.F. (1980) Neurotransmitters and pituitary function: Regulation of ACTH secretion. Fed. Proc. 39, 2923-2930.

Giachetti, A., Said, S., Reynolds, R. and Koniges, F.C. (1977) Vasoactive intestinal polypeptide in brain: Localization in and release from isolated nerve terminals. Proc. Natl. Acad. Sci. USA 74, 3424-3428.

Giudice, L.C. and Chaiken, I.M. (1979) Immunological and chemical identification of a neurophysin containing protein coded by mRNA from bovine hypothalamus. Proc. Natl. Acad. Sci. USA 76, 3800-3804.

Goodman, R.H., Jacobs, J.W., Chin, W.W., Lund, P.K., Dee, P.C. and Habener, J.F. (1980) Nucleotide sequence of a cloned structural gene coding for a precursor of pancreatic somatostatin. Proc. Natl. Acad. Sci. USA 77, 5869-5873.

Grimm, Y. and Reichlin, S. (1973) Thyrotropin-releasing hormone (TRH): Neurotransmitter regulation of secretion by mouse hypothalamic tissue in vitro. Endocrinology 93, 626-631.

Grimm-Jorgensen, Y. and McKelvy, J.F. (1974) Biosynthesis of thyrotropin releasing factor by newt brain in vitro. Isolation and characterization of thyrotropin releasing factor. J. Neurochem. 23, 471-478.

Grim-Jorgensen, Y. and McKelvy, J.F. (1976) TRF biosynthesis in vitro. Effect of inhibitors of protein synthesis. Brain Res. Bull. 1, 171-175.

Guillemin, R. (1971) Biosynthesis of the hypothalamic tripeptide-amide TRF. Abstr. Soc. Neurosci., p. 70.

Habener, J.F. (1981) Principles of peptide hormone biosynthesis. In: Neurosecretion and Brain Peptides (Martin, J.B., Reichlin, S. and Bick, K.L. eds), pp. 21-34, Raven Press, New York.

Hall, R.W. and Steinberger, E. (1976) Synthesis of LHRH by rat hypothalamic tissue in vitro: Use of a specific antibody to LHRH for immunoprecipitation. Neuroendocrinology 21, 111-119.

Hall, R.W. and Steinberger, E. (1977) Synthesis of LHRH by rat hypothalamic tissue in vitro: Effect of short-term orchiectomy and estradiol benzoate therapy. Neuroendocrinology, 24, 325-332.

Harrison, R. (1906) Observations on the living developing nerve fiber. Proc. Soc. Exp. Biol. Med. 4, 140-143.

Hartter, D.E. and Ramirez, V.D. (1980) The effects of ions, metabolic inhibitors and colchicine on luteinizing hormone-releasing hormone release from superfused rat hypothalami. Endocrinology 107, 375-382.

Hemminki, K., Huttonen, M.D. and Jarnefett, J. (1970) Some properties of brain cell suspensions prepared by a mechanical enzymatic method. Brain Res. 23, 23-24.

Herschman, H.R. (1973) Culture of neural tissue and cells. In: Research Methods in Neurochemistry (Marks, N. and Rodnight, R. eds.), Vol. II, pp. 101-160, Plenum Press, New York.

Hild, W. (1954) Das morphologische, kinetische und endokrinologische verhalten von hypothalamischem und neurohypophysarem gewebe in vitro. Zellforsch. 40, 257-312.

Hillhouse, E.W., Burden, J. and Jones, M.T. (1975) Effect of various putative neurotransmitters on the release of CRH from the hypothalamus of the rat in vitro. Neuroendocrinology 17, 1-11.

Hirroka, Y., Hollander, C.S., Suzuki, S., Ferdinand, P. and Juan, S.I. (1978) Somatostatin inhibits release of thyrotropin releasing factor from organ cultures of rat hypothalamus. Proc. Natl. Acad. Sci. USA 75, 4509-4514.

Hobart, P., Crawford, R., Shen, L., Pictet, R. and Ritter, W.J. (1980) Cloning and sequence analysis of cDNAs encoding two distinct somatostatin precursors found in the endocrine pancreas of anglerfish. Nature (London) 288, 137-141.

Honegger, P., Lenoir, D. and Favrod, P. (1979) Growth and differentiation of aggregating fetal brain cells in a serum-free defined medium. Nature (London) 282, 305-308.

Imura, H., Kato, Y., Katakami, H. and Matsushita, N. (1981) Effect of CNS peptides on hypothalamic regulation of pituitary secretion. In: Neurosecretion and Brain Peptides (Martin, J.B., Reichlin, S. and Bick, K.L. eds), pp. 557-570. Raven Press, New York.

Ishikawa, S., Saito, T. and Yoshida, S. (1980) The effect of osmotic pressure and angiotensin II on arginine vasopressin release from guinea pig hypothalamo–neurohypophyseal complex in organ culture. Endocrinology 106, 1571-1578.

Ishikawa, S., Saito, T. and Yoshida, S. (1981) The effect of prostaglandins on the release of arginine vasopressin from the guinea pig hypothalamo-neurohypophyseal complex in organ culture. Endocrinology 108, 193-198.

Iversen, L.L., Jessell, T. and Kanazawa, I. (1976) Release and metabolism of substance P in rat hypothalamus. Nature 264, 81-84.

Iversen, L.L., Iversen, S.D., Bloom, F., Douglas, C. Brown, M. and Vale, W. (1978) Calcium dependent release of somatostatin and neurotensin from rat brain in vitro. Nature 273, 161-163.

Jackson, I.M.D. and Reichlin, S. (1979) Distribution and biosynthesis of TRH in the nervous system. In: Central Nervous System Effects of Hypothalamic Hormones and Other Peptides (Collu, R., Barbeau, A., Rochefort, J.-G. and Ducharme, J.R. eds), pp. 3-54, Raven Press, New York.

Johansson, N.G., Hooper, F., Sievertsson, Currie, B.C. and Folkers, K. (1972) Biosynthesis in vitro of luteinizing hormone releasing hormone by hypothalamic tissue. Biochem. Biophys. Res. Commun. 49, 656-660.

Jones, M.T. (1978) Control of corticotropin (ACTH) secretion. In: The Endocrine Hypothalamus, (Jeffcoate, S.L. and Hutchinson, J.S.M. eds), pp. 386-418, Academic Press, New York.

Jones, M.T. and Hillhouse, E.W. (1977) Neurotransmitter regulation of corticotropin releasing factor in vitro. Ann. N.Y. Acad. Sci. 297, 536-558.

Jones, M.T., Hillhouse, E.W. and Burden, J. (1976a) Effect of various putative neurotransmitters on the secretion of corticotrophin-releasing hormone from the rat hypothalamus in vitro – a model of the neurotransmitter involved. J. Endocrinol. 69, 1-10.

Jones, M.T., Hillhouse, E.W. and Burden, J.L. (1976b) Secretion of corticotrophin releasing factor in vitro. In: Frontiers of Neuroendocrinology, (Ganong, W.F. and Martini, L. eds), pp. 195-226, Raven Press, New York.

Jones, M.T., Hillhouse, E.W. and Burden, J.L. (1977) Structure-activity relationships of corticosteroid feedback at the hypothalamic level. J. Endocrinol. 74, 415-424.

Joseph-Bravo, P. Charli, J.L., Palacios, J.M. and Kordon, C. (1979) Effect of neurotransmitters on the in vitro release of immunoreactive thyrotropin-releasing hormone from rat mediobasal hypothalamus. Endocrinology 104, 801-806.

Joseph-Bravo, P., Charli, J.L., Sherman, T., Boyer, H., Bolivar, F. and McKelvy, J.F. (1980) Identification of a putative hypothalamic mRNA coding for somatostatin and of its product in cell-free translation. Biochem. Biophys. Res. Comm. 94, 1004-1012.

Kao, L.W.L. and Weisz, J. (1977) Release of GnRH from isolated, perifused medial-basal hypothalamus by melatonin. Endocrinology 100, 1723-1727.

Kelly, R.B., Deutsch, J.W., Carlson, S.S. and Wagner, J.A. (1979) Biochemistry of neurotransmitter release. Annu. Rev. Neurosci. 2, 399-446.

Knigge, K.M., Joseph, S.A., Schock, D., Silverman, A.J., Ching, M.C.H., Scott, D.E., Zeman, D. and Krobisch-Dudley, G. (1974) Role of the ventricular system in neuroendocrine process: Synthesis and distribution of TRF in the hypothalamus and third ventricle. Can. J. Neurol. Sci. 1, 74-85.

Krieger, D.T. (1977) Serotonin regulation of ACTH secretion. Ann. N.Y. Acad. Sci. 297, 527-533.

Krieger, D.T. and Liotta, A.S. (1979) Pituitary hormones in brain: Where, how and why? Science 205, 366-372.

Krulich, L. (1979) Central neurotransmitters and the secretion of prolactin, GH, LH and TSH. Annu. Rev. Physiol. 41, 603-615.

Kubek, M., Lorincz, M., Emanuele, N., Shambaugh, G.E. and Wilbur, J. (1977) Thyrotropin releasing hormone: Biosynthesis by extrahypothalamic and hypothalamic tissues in vitro. Abstracts, 59th Annual Meeting Endocrine Society, p. 125.

Lauber, M., Camier, M. and Cohen, P. (1979) Immunological and biochemical characterization of distinct high molecular weight forms of neurophysin and somatostatin in mouse hypothalamic extracts. FEBS Lett. 97, 343-347.

Lee, S., Havlicek, V., Panerai, A. and Friesen, H.G. (1978) High K^+-induced release of somatostatin from the cortical preparation of rat brain. Experientia 35, 351-352.

Liotta, A.S., Gildersleeve, D., Brownstein, M.J. and Krieger, D.T. (1979) Biosynthesis in vitro of immuno-reactive 53,000 dalton corticotropin β-endorphin-like material by bovine hypothalamus. Proc. Natl. Acad. Sci. USA 76, 1448-1452.

Liotta, A.S., Loudes, C., McKelvy, J.F. and Krieger, D.T. (1980) Biosynthesis of precursor corticotropin/en-dorpin, corticotropin-, α-melanotropin-, β-lipotropin-, and β-endorphin-like material by cultured neonatal rat hypothalamic neurons. Proc. Natl. Acad. Sci. USA 77, 1880-1884.

Lloyd, R.V., Gilles, P.A. and Karavolas, H.J. (1979) Uptake and metabolism of female sex steroids by isolated small neurons and other cell fractions from the rat medial basal hypothalamus. Steroids 19, 97-113.

Lumsden, C.L. (1968) Nervous tissue in culture. In: Structure and Function of Nervous Tissue (Bourne, G.H. ed.), p. 67-140, Academic Press, New York.

Maeda, K. and Frohman, L.A. (1980) Release of somatostatin and thyrotropin–releasing hormone from rat hypothalamic fragments in vitro. Endocrinology 106, 1837-1842.

Mains, R.E. and Patterson, P.H. (1973) Primary cultures of dissociated sympathetic neurons. J. Cell. Biol. 59, 329-366.

Mandel, P., Ciesielski-Treska, J. and Sensenbrenner, M. (1976) Neurons in vitro. In: Molecular and Functional Neurobiology (Gispen, W.H. ed.), pp. 112-160, Elsevier, Amsterdam.

Masurovsky, E.B., Benitez, H.H. and Murray, M.R. (1971) Synaptic development in long-term organized cultures of murine hypothalamus. J. Comp. Neurol. 143, 263-278.

Mathison, R. and Lederis, K. (1980) A mechanism for adenosine 3',5'-monophosphate regulation of vasopressin secretion. Endocrinology 106, 842-848.

May, R.M. (1966) Culture et greffe des cellules nerveuses chez les vertebres superieures. In: Monographs de Physiologie Causale, Vol. VI, pp. 1-207, Ganthier, Paris.

Messer, A., Maskin, P. and Mazurkiewicz, J. (1980) Effects of using a chemically defined medium for primary rat monolayer cerebellar cultures: Morphology, GABA uptake, and kainic acid sensitivity. Brain Res. 184, 243-247.

Meyers, C.A., Murphy, W.A., Redding, T.W., Coy, D.H. and Schally, A.V. (1980) Synthesis and biological actions of prosomatostatin. Proc. Natl. Acad. Sci. USA 77, 6171-6174.

McKelvy, J.F. (1974) Biochemical neuroendocrinology. I. Biosynthesis of TRH by organ cultures of mammalian hypothalamus. Brain Res. 65, 489-502.

McKelvy, J.F. (1977) Biosynthesis of hypothalamic peptides. Adv. Exp. Med. Biol. 87, 77-98.

McKelvy, J.F. and Grimm-Jorgensen, Y. (1975) Studies on the biosynthesis of thyrotropin releasing hormone in vitro. In: Hypothalamic Hormones (Motta, M., Crosignani, P. and Martini, L. eds), pp. 13-25, Academic Press, London.

McKelvy, J.F., Sheridan, M., Joseph, S., Phelps, C.H. and Perrie, S. (1975) Biosynthesis of thyrotropin-releasing hormone in organ cultures of the guinea pig median eminence. Endocrinology 97, 908-918.

McKelvy, J.F., Lin, C.F., Chan, L., Joseph-Bravo, P., Charli, J.L., Pacheco, M., Paulo, M., Neale, J. and Barker, J. (1979) Biosynthesis of brain peptides. In: Brain Peptides: A new endocrinology (Gotto Jr, A.M., Peck, E.J. and Boyd III, A.E. (eds), pp. 183-196, Elsevier, Amsterdam.

Millar, R.P., Aehnelt, C., and Rossier, G. (1977) Higher molecular weight immunoreactive species of luteinizing hormone releasing hormone: possible precursors of the hormone. Biochem. Biophys. Res. Commun 74, 720-731.

Mitnick, M., and Reichlin, S. (1971) Biosynthesis of TRH by rat hypothalamic tissue in vitro. Science 172, 1241-1243.

Moguilevsky, J.A., Enero, M.A., and Szwarcfarb, B. (1974) Luteinizing hormone releasing hormone biosynthesis by rat hypothalamus in vitro. Influence of castration. Proc. Soc. Exp. Biol. Med. 147, 434-437.

Moguilevsky, J.A., Scacchi, P., Debeljuk, L. and Faigon, M.R. (1975) Effect of castration upon hypothalamic luteinizing hormone releasing factor (LH-RF). Neuroendocrinology 17, 189-192.

Moody, T.W., Thoa, N.B., O'Donohue, T.Z., Pert, C.B. (1980) Bombesin-like peptides in the rat brain: Localization in synaptosomes and release from hypothalamic slices. Life Sci. 26, 1707-1712.

Moore, R.Y. and Bloom, F.E. (1978) Central catecholamine neuron systems: Anatomy and physiology of the dopamine systems. Annu. Rev. Neurosci. 129-170.

Moore, R.Y. and Bloom, F.E. (1979) Central catecholamine neuron systems: Anatomy and physiology of the norepinephrine and epinephrine systems. Annu. Rev. Neurosci. 113-168.

Morgan, I.G. (1976) Synaptosomes and cell separation. Neuroscience 1, 159-165.

Moscona, A.A. (1952) Cell suspensions from organ rudiments of chick embryos. Exp. Cell. Res. 3, 535-558.

Müller, E.E., Nisticò, G. and Scapagnini, U. (1977) Neurotransmitters and Anterior Pituitary Function, Academic Press, New York.

Murray, M. (1965) Nervous tissue in vitro. In: Cells and Tissues in Culture, (Willmer, E.N. ed), Vol. II, pp. 373-455, Academic Press, New York.

Negro-Vilar, A., Ojeda, S.R., Arimura, A. and McCann, S.M. (1978) Dopamine and norepinephrine stimulate somatostatin release by median eminence fragments in vitro. Life Sci. 23, 1493-1495.

Negro-Vilar, A., Ojeda, S.R., McCann, S.M. (1979) Catecholaminergic modulation of luteinizing hormone-releasing hormone release by median eminence terminals in vitro. Endocrinology 104, 1749-1752.

Ogawa, N., Thompson, T., Friesen, H., Martin, J.B. and Brazeau, P. (1977) Properties of soluble somatostatin binding protein. Biochem. J. 165, 269-277.

Ojeda, S.R., Negro-Vilar, A., Arimura, A. and Mc Cann, S.M. (1980) On the hypothalamic mechanism by which prostaglandin E_2 stimulates growth hormone release. Neuroendocrinology 31, 1-7.

Osborne, H., Przewlocki, R., Hollt, V. and Herz, A. (1979) Release of β-endorphin from rat hypothalamus in vitro. Eur. J. Pharmacol 55, 425-428.

Oyama, H., Hirsch, H.J., Gabbay, K.H. and Permutt, A. (1980) Isolation and characterization of immunoreactive somatostatin from fish pancreatic islets. J. Clin. Invest. 65, 993-1002.

Pacold, S.T., Kirsteins, L., Jojvat, S. and Lawrence, A.M. (1978) Biologically active pituitary hormones in the rat brain amygdaloid nucleus. Science 199, 804-806.

Patel, Y.C., Zingg, H.H. and Dreifuss, J.J. (1978) Somatostatin secretion from the rat neurohypophysis and stalk median eminence in vitro: Calcium-dependent release by high potassium and electrical stimulation. Metabolism 27, 1243-1246.

Pearson, D. (1977) Neurosecretion in cultured systems. In: Cell, Tissue and Organ Culture in Neurobiology (Fedoroff, S. and Hertz, L. eds), pp. 573-587, Academic Press, London.

Pomerat, C.M. (1952) Dynamic neurogliology. Tex. Rep. Biol. Med. 10, 885-913.

Prasad, K.N., Mandel, B., Waymire, J.C., Lees, G.J., Vernadakis, A. and Weiner, N. (1973) Basal level of neurotransmitter synthesizing enzymes and effect of cyclic AMP agents on the morphological differentiation of isolated neuroblastoma clones. Nature (London) 241, 117-119.

Ramirez, V.D., Epelbaum, J., Gantrou, J.P., Pattou, E., Zamora, A. and Kordon, C. (1975) Distribution of LHRH in subcellular fractions of the basomedial hypothalamus. Mol. Cell. Endocrinol. 3, 339-351.

Reichlin, S. (1976) Biosynthesis and degradation of hypothalamic hypophysiotrophic factors. In: Subcellular Mechanisms in Reproductive Neuroendocrinology (Naftolin, F. ed), pp. 109-127, Elsevier, Amsterdam.

Reichlin, S., Martin, J.B., Mitnick, M., Boshans, R., Grimm-Jorgensen, Y., Bollinger, J., Gordon, J. and Malacara, J. (1972) The hypothalamus in pituitary-thyroid regulation. Recent Prog. Horm. Res. 28, 229-277.

Reichlin, S., Martin, J.B. and Jackson, I.M.D. (1978) Regulation of thyroid stimulating hormone secretion. In: The Endocrine Hypothalamus (Jeffcoate, S. and Hutchinson, J.S.M. eds), pp. 230-237, Academic Press, London.

Reichlin, S. and Mitnick, M.A. (1973) Biosynthesis of thyrotropin releasing hormone and its control by hormones, central monoamines and external environment. In: Hypothalamic Hypophysiotropic Hormones, (Gual, C. and Rosemberg, E. eds), pp. 122-135. Excerpta Medica, Amsterdam.

Richardson, S.B., Hollander, C.S., D'Eletto, R., Greenleaf, P.W. and Thaw, C. (1980) Acetylcholine inhibits the release of somatostatin from rat hypothalamus in vitro. Endocrinology 107, 122-129.

Rizzino, A. and Sato, G. (1978) Growth of embryonal carcinoma cells in serum free medium. Proc. Natl. Acad. Sci. USA 75, 1844-1848.

Robbins, R.J., Kapcala, L.P., Goodman, R.H. and Reichlin, S. (1979) Synthesis of ACTH by rat neuronal cell cultures. 9th Annual Meeting of the Society for Neuroscience, p. 456.

Robbins, R.J. and Reichlin, S. (1980) Synthesis of somatostatin prohormones in cerebral cortical cell cultures. 10th Annual Meeting of the Society for Neuroscience, p. 30.

Robbins, R.J., Sutton, R.E., King, L.W. and Reichlin, S. (1981) Stimulation of somatostatin release from cerebral cortical cells by acetylcholine and by calcium and sodium ionophores. 63rd Annual Meeting of the Endocrine Society, p. 104.

Rorstad, O.P., Epelbaum, J., Brazeau, P., and Martin, J.B. (1979) Chromatographic and biological properties of immunoreactive somatostatin in hypothalamic and extrahypothalamic brain regions of the rat. Endocrinology 105, 1083-1092.

Rotsztejn, W.H., Charli, J.L., Patton, E., Epelbaum, J. and Kordon, C. (1976) In vitro release of LH-RH from rat mediobasal hypothalamus: Effect of potassium, calcium and dopamine. Endocrinology 99, 1663-1666.

Rotsztejn, W.H., Charli, J.L., Patton, E. and Kordon, C. (1977) Stimulation by dopamine of LH-RH release from the mediobasal hypothalamus in male rats. Endocrinology 101, 1475-1483.

Rotsztejn, W.H., Drouva, S.V., Patton, E. and Kordon, C. (1978) Met-enkephalin inhibits in vitro dopamine-induced LHRH release from mediobasal hypothalamus of male rats. Nature 274, 281-285.

Rupnow, J.H., Hinkle, P.K. and Dixon, J.E. (1979) A macromolecule which gives rise to thryrotropin releasing hormone. Biochem. Biophys. Res. Comm. 89, 721-728.

Russell, J.T., Brownstein, M.J. and Gainer, H. (1980) Biosynthesis of vasopressin, oxytocin and neurophysins: Isolation and characterization of two common precursors (propressophysin and prooxyphysin). Endocrinology 107, 1880-1891.

Sachs, H., Goodman, R., Osinchak, J. and McKelvy, J. (1971) Supraoptic neurosecretory neurons of the guinea pig in organ culture. Biosynthesis of vasopressin and neurophysin. Proc. Natl. Acad. Sci. USA 68, 2782-2786.

Sachs, H., Pearson, D., Schanberg, A., Shin, S., Bryce, G., Malamed, S. and Mowles, T. (1974) Studies on the hypothalamo-neurohypophysial complex in organ culture. In: Recent Studies of Hypothalamic Function (Lederis, K. and Copper, K.E. eds), pp. 50-66, Karger, Basel.

Samson, W.K., Koenig, J., Reeves, J. and McCann, S.M. (1980) Vasoactive intestinal peptide stimulates LHRH release from hypothalamic synaptosomes. 62nd Annual Meeting of the Endocrine Society, p. 261.

Schaeffer, J.M., Axelrod, J. and Brownstein, M.J. (1977) Regional differences in dopamine-mediated release of TRH-like material from synaptosomes. Brain Res. 138, 571-575.

Schneider, H.P.G. and McCann, S.M. (1969) Possible role of dopamine as a transmitter to promote discharge of LH-releasing factor. Endocrinology 85, 121-136.

Seyler, L.E., Mitnick, M.A., Gordon, J. and Reichlin, S. (1973) Hypothalamic LRF biosynthesis in vitro and plasma LRF in orchidectomized hypophysectomized estrogen treated rats. 55th Annual Meeting of the Endocrine Society, p. 144.

Sheppard, M.C., Kronheim, S. and Pimstone, B.L. (1978) Stimulation by growth hormone of somatostatin release from the rat hypothalamus in vitro. Clin. Endocrinol. 9, 583-590.

Sheppard, M.C., Kronheim, S. and Pimstone, B.L. (1979) Effect of substance P, neurotensin and the enkephalins on somatostatin release from the rat hypothalamus in vitro. J. Neurochem. 32, 647-651.

Shields, D. (1980) In vitro biosynthesis of fish islet preprosomatostatin: Evidence of processing and segregation of a high molecular weight precursor. Proc. Natl. Acad. Sci. USA 77, 4074-4078.

Silverman, A.J., Knigge, K.M., Ribas, J.L. and Sheridan, M.N. (1973) Transport capacity of median eminence: III. Amino acid and thyroxine transport of organ-cultured median eminence. Neuroendocrinology 11, 107-118.

Sladek, C.D. and Joynt, J.R. (1979a) Angiotensin stimulation of vasopressin release from the rat hypothalamo-neurohypophysial system in organ culture. Endocrinology 104, 148-153.

Sladek, C.D. and Joynt, J.R. (1979b) Characterization of cholinergic control of vasopressin release by the organ-cultured rat hypothalamo-neurohypophysial system. Endocrinology 104, 659-663.

Sobkowicz, H.M., Bleir, R. and Monzain, R. (1974) Cell survival and architectonic differentiation of the hypothalamic mammillary region of the newborn mouse in culture. J. Comp. Neurol. 155, 355-376.

Sze, P.Y. (1979) L-glutamate decarboxylase. In: GABA-Biochemistry and CNS Function (Mandel, P. and De Feudis, F.V. eds), pp. 59-78, Plenum Press, New York.

Terry, L.C., Rorstad, O.P. and Martin, J.B. (1980) The release of biologically and immunologically reactive somatostatin from perifused hypothalamic fragments. Endocrinology 107, 794-800.

Thomas, G.A. (1956) Tissue culture in the study of the nervous system. Guy's Hosp. Rep. 105, 14-26.

Tixier-Vidal, A. and DeVitry, F. (1979) Hypothalamic neurons in cell culture. Internat. Rev. Cytology 58, 291-331.

Tytell, M., Clark, J.H. and Peck, E.J. (1980) Effects of estrogen and progesterone on LHRH release from a hypothalamic synaptosomal fraction of ovariectomized rats. Neurochem. Res. 5, 493-504.

Vale, W., Spiess, J., Rivier, C. and Rivier, J. (1981) Characterization of a 41-residue ovine hypothalamic peptide that stimulates secretion of corticotropin and β-endorphin. Science 213, 1394-1397.

Varon, S. and Raiborn, C.W. (1969) Dissociation, fractionation and culture of embryonic brain cells. Brain Res. 12, 180-199.

Vermes, I., Mulder, G.H. and Smelik, P.G. (1977) A superfusion system technique for the study of the sites of action of glucocorticoids in the rat hypothalamus-pituitary-adrenal system in vitro. Endocronology 100, 1153-1159.

Wakabayashi, T., Miyazawawa, H., Kanda, M., Miki, N., Demura, R., Demura, H. and Shizume, K. (1977) Stimulation of immunoreactive somatostatin release from hypothalamic synaptosomes by high K^+ and dopamine. Endocrinol. Jpn 24, 601-606.

Warberg, J., Eskay, R.L., Barnea, A., Reynolds, R. and Porter, J.C. (1977) Release of luteinizing hormone releasing hormone and thyrotropin releasing hormone from a synaptosome-enriched fraction of hypothalamic homogenates. Endocrinology 100, 814-825.

Wilkinson, M., Gibson, C.J., Breesler, B.H. and Inman, D.R. (1974) Hypothalamic neurons in dissociated cell culture. Brain Res. 82, 129-138.

Zingg, H.H. and Patel, Y.C. (1980) Processing of somatostatin precursors: Evidence of enzymatic cleavage by hypothalamic extract. Biochem. Biophys. Res. Comm. 93, 1274-1279.

E.E Müller and R.M. MacLeod (eds) Neuroendocrine Perspectives Vol. 1
© Elsevier Biomedical Press, 1982

Chapter 5

Control of biosynthesis and secretion of ACTH, endorphins and related peptides

Hiroo Imura, Yoshikatsu Nakai, Kazuwa Nakao, Shogo Oki, Issei Tanaka

INTRODUCTION

Adrenocorticotropin (ACTH) is a peptide that has been isolated from the pituitary gland of several species and its nature has been extensively studied. The pituitary is also known to contain such hormones as β-lipotropin (β-LPH), β-melanotropin (β-MSH) and α-melanotropin (α-MSH), which share several amino acids with ACTH. The recent discovery of peptides with opiate-like activity from the pituitary gland or the hypothalamus by Li and Chung (1976) and Guillemin et al. (1976) has drawn attention to β-LPH, because these opioid peptides, called endorphins, consist of the C-terminal portion of the β-LPH molecule. It is now known that all these peptides are derived from the common precursor molecule, proACTH-β-LPH (Nakanishi et al. 1979). The precursor contains another melanotropin-like substance, γ-melanotropin (γ-MSH). This was first predicted from the nucleotide sequence of complementary DNA (cDNA) coding for the precursor molecule (Nakanishi et al. 1979) and later confirmed by radioimmunoassay (Tanaka et al. 1980; Shibasaki et al. 1980).

It is well-known that secretion of ACTH from the anterior pituitary gland is controlled by the central nervous system and by the negative feedback mechanism of adrenal steroids. Accumulating evidence has suggested that putative neurotransmitters in the brain play an important role in the regulation of ACTH secretion, although corticotropin-releasing factor (CRF) responsible for the regulation of ACTH secretion as a final mediator has not yet been identified. Regulation of secretion of other peptides derived from the ACTH-β-LPH precursor has been studied in recent years. This chapter deals with the regulation of biosynthesis and secretion of ACTH, endorphins and related peptides, focusing mainly on regulation in man.

BIOSYNTHESIS

Structure of the common precursor for ACTH and β-LPH

ACTH is a 39-amino acid peptide with a molecular weight of approximately 4500 (4.5k). The presence of a large molecular form of immunoreactive ACTH was first reported by Yalow and Berson (1971) using gel chromatography, and the precursor role of this large molecular form in the biosynthesis of ACTH has been demonstrated in our laboratory by observing the incorporation of a labelled amino acid into the big ACTH molecule (Hirata et al. 1975a). Later studies on the cell-free biosynthesis of the precursor molecule directed by messenger RNA (mRNA) obtained from pituitary tissue, and the kinetics of ACTH biosynthesis in pituitary tumor cells using a labelled amino acid, have demonstrated that big ACTH is the precursor in the biosynthesis of ACTH, although there also exist high molecular weight intermediate forms (Nakanishi et al. 1976; Mains and Eipper 1976). Moreover, using the same techniques, these authors and others have demonstrated that the precursor molecule contains not only ACTH but also endorphins in its moiety (Nakanishi et al. 1977a; Mains et al. 1977; Roberts and Herbert 1977).

The structure of the bovine precursor molecule has been identified by Nakanishi et al. (1979) based on the nucleotide sequence of complementary DNA produced against mRNA coding for the precursor molecule. This sequence is considered to be preproACTH-β-LPH, having a signal peptide at the N-terminus. The N-terminus of proACTH-β-LPH could not be determined from the nucleotide sequence. However, Keutman et al. (1979) have determined a partial sequence of the N-terminal portion of proACTH-β-LPH and decided the N-terminal amino acid to be Trp. In addition, Håkanson et al. (1980) purified a peptide with Trp at the N-terminus from porcine pituitary glands. Thus, the 26 amino acids at the N-terminus are considered to be a signal peptide. Fig. 5.1 shows schematically the structure of bovine preproACTH-β-LPH. Although the complete amino acid sequence of proACTH-β-LPH of other species has not been determined yet, partial sequences reported

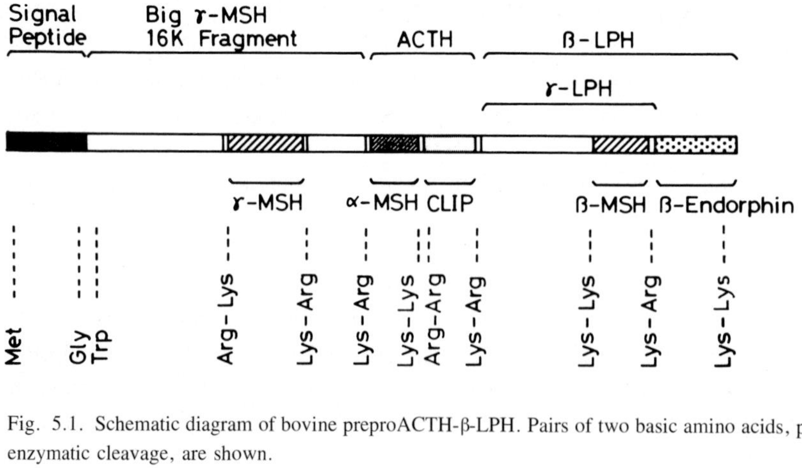

Fig. 5.1. Schematic diagram of bovine preproACTH-β-LPH. Pairs of two basic amino acids, possible sites of enzymatic cleavage, are shown.

Table 5.1

ACTH-LI, β-EP-LI AND γ-MSH-LI IN BOVINE AND HUMAN PITUITARIES

	No.	ACTH-LI (ng/100 µg prot.)	β-EP-LI (ng/100 µg prot.)	γ-MSH-LI (ng/100 µg prot.)
Bovine pituitary				
Ant. lobe	3	712 ± 139.1	463 ± 86.0	93 ± 24.4
Neuroint. lobe	3	204 ± 12.1	1041 ± 287.9	560 ± 86.4
Human pituitary	3	1241 ± 228.9	631 ± 228.9	126 ± 6.1

The pituitary tissue was homogenized in 0.2 N HCl and centrifuged. The supernatant was neutralized with 0.1 N NaOH immediately before assay. γ-MSH-LI was expressed as ng of $γ_3$-MSH per 100 µg protein. Values in the table are means ±SEM.

suggest that bovine, porcine, human, rat and mouse proACTH-β-LPHs have very similar sequences (Keutman et al. 1979; Håkanson et al. 1980; Nakanishi et al. 1979; Gossard et al. 1980; Benjannet et al. 1980; Drouin and Goodman 1980). At the C-terminus of preproACTH-β-LPH, there exists β-LPH, of which the C-terminal portion is β-endorphin. Next to β-LPH is a sequence of Lys–Arg, a possible cleavage site by proteolytic enzymes, and then there is ACTH. At the N-terminus of ACTH there exists again Lys–Arg and then there is the sequence of a previously unknown peptide. This cryptic portion contains four Cys residues and at least one carbohydrate moiety. Murine but not human prohormone has another sugar moiety in the ACTH portion. In the cryptic N-terminal portion, there exists another melanotropin-like sequence, Met–X–His–Phe–Arg–Trp, and this portion is named γ-MSH. There are three pairs of two basic amino acids in this cryptic N-terminal portion, suggesting that two to four peptides can be derived from this portion. The existence of more than two forms of proACTH-β-LPH is suggested (Gossard et al. 1980; Drouin and Goodman 1980).

Nature of immunoreactive ACTH, β-endorphin and γ-MSH

Since the size of native γ-MSH was unknown, Ling et al. (1979) synthesized three possible peptides of different lengths, $γ_1$, $γ_2$ and $γ_3$-MSH*. We have produced antiserum against $γ_3$-MSH and set up a radioimmunoassay for γ-MSH. Table 5.1 shows concentrations of immunoreactive ACTH, β-endorphin and γ-MSH in the anterior and neurointermediate lobes of bovine pituitary and the anterior lobe of human pituitary. Besides

* $γ_1$-MSH(Tyr–Val–Met–Gly–His–Phe–Arg–Trp–Asp–Arg–Phe–NH₂),
$γ_2$-MSH(Tyr–Val–Met–Gly–His–Phe–Arg–Trp–Asp–Arg–Phe–Gly–OH),
and $γ_3$-MSH(Tyr–Val–Met–Gly–His–Phe–Arg–Trp–Asp–Arg–Phe–Gly–Arg–Arg–Asn–Gly–Ser–Ser–Ser–Ser–Gly–Val–Gly–Gly–Ala–Ala–Gln–OH)

ACTH-like immunoreactivity (ACTH-LI)** and β-endorphin-like immunoreactivity (β-EP-LI), all pituitary extracts contained γ-MSH-like immunoreactivity (γ-MSH-LI). To further clarify molecular forms of ACTH-LI, β-EP-LI and γ-MSH-LI, gel exclusion chromatography of pituitary extracts were performed on a Bio-Gel P-60 column. γ-MSH-LI, ACTH-LI and β-EP-LI of each fraction were assayed by radioimmunoassays. As shown in Fig. 5.2, bovine anterior pituitary extract gave a single peak of γ-MSH-LI (big γ-MSH) eluted near the elution position of β-LPH and two peaks of ACTH-LI, big and little ACTH. β-EP-LI was composed of two peaks, β-LPH and β-endorphin, the former of which was predominant. The gel chromatographic pattern of human anterior pituitary was similar to that of bovine anterior pituitary, although β-LPH is more predominant, as shown in Fig. 5.3. On the other hand, gel chromatography of bovine neurointermediate lobe revealed two peaks of γ-MSH-LI, big and little γ-MSHs, the latter emerging near the position of β-endorphin (Fig. 5.4). Differing from the pattern of the anterior lobe, β-endorphin predominated in β-EP-LI. These results suggest different processing of proACTH-β-LPH between the anterior and neurointermediate lobes. Concanavalin A affinity chromatography revealed

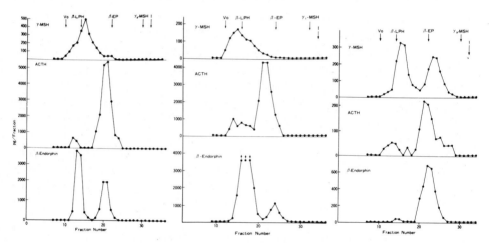

Fig. 5.2. (left) Gel chromatographic pattern of γ-MSH-LI, ACTH-LI and β-EP-LI of bovine anterior pituitary. Gel chromatography of HCl extract of the pituitary was performed on a column of Bio-Gel P-60 (0.7×52 cm) and each fraction was assayed for immunoreactive γ-MSH, ACTH and β-endorphin. Elution positions of markers are shown by arrows in the upper frame.

Fig. 5.3. (centre) Gel chromatographic pattern of γ-MSH-LI, ACTH-LI and β-EP-LI of human pituitary. See legend for Fig. 5.2.

Fig. 5.4. (right) Gel chromatographic pattern of γ-MSH-LI, ACTH-LI, and β-EP-LI of bovine neurointermediate lobe. See legend for Fig. 5.2.

** ACTH-LI represents the sum of authentic 39-amino-acid ACTH, precursor and intermediate forms measured by radioimmunoassay for ACTH. Likewise, β-EP-LI consists of β-endorphin, β-LPH and precursor form measured by radioimmunoassay for β-endorphin. γ-MSH-LI is composed of big and little γ-MSH, measured by radioimmunoassay for γ₃- MSH.

that both big and little γ-MSHs were bound to the lectin column, suggesting their glycoprotein nature. The big γ-MSH was similar in size and immunoreactivity to the 16 k fragment purified from AtT-20 cells by Eipper and Mains (1978b) and, therefore, considered to be the complete N-terminal sequence of proACTH-β-LPH. On the other hand, little γ-MSH can be assumed to be a glycosylated form of γ₃-MSH, since γ_3-MSH contains the amino acid sequence Asn–X–Ser, a glycosylation site in glycoproteins.

Zakarian and Smyth (1979) reported that rat pituitary endorphins are heterogenous in nature, consisting of β-endorphin (61-91 β-LPH), δ-endorphin (61-87 β-LPH), N-acetylated β-endorphin and N-acetylated δ-endorphin. We studied β-EP-LI in human pituitary by isoelectric focusing and observed four peaks, two of which were identified as β-endorphin and δ-endorphin (unpublished observation). These results indicate that pituitary endorphins are heterogenous in nature.

Summary of the biosynthetic pathway of ACTH, endorphins and related peptides

The translation product of mRNA coding for the bovine precursor molecule, preproACTH-β-LPH, consists of 265 amino acids, with the molecular weight of 29 300. The structure of human preproACTH-β-LPH has not yet been elucidated, although it is very similar to the bovine one because of the similarity of the N-terminal portion (Benjannet et al. 1980). The N-terminal 26 amino acids of preproACTH-β-LPH are cleaved when the newly synthesized peptide penetrates the membrane of endoplasmic reticulum. The remaining portion is glycosylated probably in the region of γ₃-MSH in human and bovine proACTH-β-LPH, although the ACTH region is also glycosylated in some of the mouse precursors. The C-terminal portion, β-LPH, is first cleaved from the proACTH-β-LPH, then the intermediate form is converted to ACTH and big γ-MSH (16 k fragment). β-LPH is

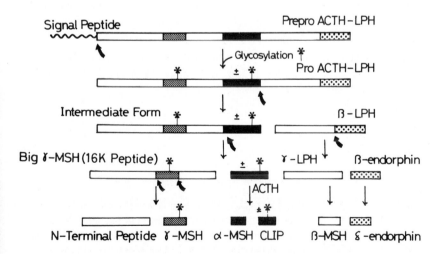

Fig. 5.5 Biosynthetic pathway of ACTH, β-LPH, β-endorphin and γ-MSH. Arrows show possible sites of enzymatic cleavage.

142

further cleaved into γ-LPH and β-endorphin, although this processing is very limited in the anterior lobe and almost complete in the intermediate lobe. ACTH is further split into α-MSH and a corticotropin-like intermediate lobe peptide (CLIP) in the intermediate lobe but not in the anterior lobe. β-MSH may also be produced in the intermediate lobe from γ-LPH, although this has not been demonstrated by pulse-chase experiments. Big γ-MSH is further cleaved into little γ-MSH and possibly the N-terminal peptide in the intermediate lobe. The main final products in the anterior pituitary are ACTH, β-LPH, big γ-MSH, and a small amount of β-endorphin, whereas they were α-MSH, CLIP, β-endorphin, big and little γ-MSHs and possibly β-MSH, with lesser amounts of ACTH, in the intermediate lobe (Fig. 5.5). Since mRNA and its translation product are identical in the anterior and intermediate lobes (Taii et al. 1979), the difference in final products between the anterior and inter-mediate lobes is considered to be caused by different post-translational processing. This has been demonstrated by pulse-chase experiments using rat pars intermedia (Crine et al. 1978; Mains and Eipper 1979).

REGULATION OF BIOSYNTHESIS

Biosynthesis of ACTH, endorphins and related peptides in the pituitary seems to be regulated by at least two factors; stimulatory and inhibitory. What stimulates biosynthesis of these peptides has not yet been clarified. CRF is a possible stimulating agent, but it is still unclear whether or not it acts directly on the biosynthesis of ACTH.

On the other hand, it has been known for many years that glucocorticoids lower pituitary ACTH content in vivo, or intracellular ACTH concentration in cultured pituitary cells in vitro (Fortier 1959; Watanabe et al. 1973a). The latter observation suggests the direct inhibitory effect of glucocorticoids on the biosynthesis of ACTH. These studies were performed before the discovery that β-LPH or β-endorphin is derived from the same precursor protein as ACTH. More recently, glucocorticoids added to the culture medium of AtT-20 cells have been shown to decrease intracellular endorphin and 16 k fragment levels (Sabol 1978; Roberts et al. 1979; Simantov 1979).

In order to elucidate the mechanism of action of glucocorticoids, we measured translata-ble ACTH mRNA activity in rat pituitaries following adrenalectomy and glucocorticoid

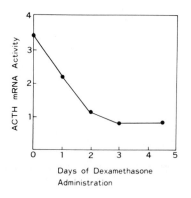

Fig. 5.6. Changes in the level of ACTH mRNA activity in the anterior pituitary of adrenalectomized rats following the admini-stration of dexamethasone. Rats 10 days after adrenalectomy re-ceived dexamethasone in the drinking water (10 μg ml⁻¹). Reprodu-ced from Proc. Natl. Acad. Sci. USA 74, 3285 (1977) with permis-sion.

Table 5.2

EFFECT OF VARIOUS STEROIDS ON THE AMOUNT OF mRNA CODING FOR proACTH-β-LPH AND DISPLACEMENT OF [³H]TRIAMCINOLONE BOUND TO CYTOPLASMIC STEROID RECEPTORS IN AtT-20 CELLS

Steroid hormones	mRNA for proACTH-β-LPH*	% of [³H]triamcinolone bound to receptors**
None	100%	100%
Dexamethasone	30	33
Corticosterone	46	53
Cortisol	74	86
Testosterone	90	86
Estradiol-17β	93	87

Cells were exposed to steroid hormones at a concentration of 0.1 μg ml⁻¹ for 4 days.

* Nakamura et al. 1978.

** Watanabe et al. 1973b.

treatment (Nakanishi et al. 1977b). The pituitary ACTH mRNA activity increased progressively during the first 4 days after adrenalectomy and a high level was maintained thereafter. Following oral administration of dexamethasone, pituitary ACTH mRNA activity in adrenalectomized rats decreased within a day and reached the minimal value 3 days after the initiation of the treatment (Fig. 5.6). A dose-response relationship was observed between the amount of dexamethasone and the decrease of mRNA activity. To clarify whether glucocorticoids act directly on the pituitary or via the hypothalamus, we then studied the effect of various glucocorticoids on AtT-20 cells in vitro (Nakamura et al. 1978). The translatable ACTH mRNA activity in the pituitary tumor cells decreased dose-dependently after the addition of dexamethasone, although 30–40% remained unsuppressed. Table 5.2 compares the effect of various steroids. Dexamethasone was the most effective in suppressing ACTH mRNA activity, followed by corticosterone and cortisol. The relative potency of steroids correlated with the affinity in binding cytoplasmic steroid hormone receptors that was reported by Watanabe et al. (1973b). These results indicate that glucocorticoids act directly on the pituitary corticotrophs to decrease mRNA activity through glucocorticoid receptors.

Roberts et al. (1979) studied the effect of glucocorticoids on the translatable ACTH mRNA actitvity and biosynthesis of ACTH and β-endorphin in AtT-20 cells. They found no change in post-translational processing of proACTH-β-LPH studied by the incorporation of a labelled amino acid. They also observed that the change of mRNA activity was parallel with ACTH content, following the addition of dexamethasone, and that the change of mRNA activity occurred on both cytoplasmic and ribosomal RNA fractions. All these results obtained by us and Roberts et al. suggest that glucocorticoids inhibit the biosynthesis of ACTH and β-endorphin by reducing the amount of mRNA acting at the transcriptional level. At the moment, there is no evidence suggesting that glucocorticoids alter the translation of mRNA by shifting mRNA from an actively translating form to an inactive form. This type of translational regulation was observed by Civelli et al. (1976) and Yap et al. (1978) in the biosynthesis of other proteins. The RNA–DNA hybridization study using a cDNA probe to proACTH-β-LPH will clarify the presence or absence of translational regulation in the biosynthesis of ACTH and related peptides.

It is of interest to point out that glucocorticoids cannot lower translatable ACTH mRNA activity to less than 20% of control values (Nakanishi et al. 1977b; Nakamura et al. 1978; Roberts et al. 1979). There seem to be several possible explanations for this phenomenon, one such is that two or more genes for proACTH-β-LPH are being expressed and that glucocorticoids are able to regulate only one gene. The existence of two genes has been suggested by Haralson et al. (1979), Gossard et al. (1980) and Drouin and Goodman (1980). Another question remaining to be solved is how glucocorticoids influence transcriptional activity of the gene for proACTH-β-LPH. The steroid–receptor complex bound to the acceptor site of DNA may directly suppress the expression of the ACTH gene. Alternatively, a more complicated process, including the biosynthesis of an inhibitory protein, may be involved in the regulation of gene expression by the steroid–receptor complex.

PHYSIOLOGICAL MECHANISMS REGULATING SECRETION

Plasma levels

Plasma ACTH levels oscillate throughout the day, but in most instances they are below 100 pg ml^{-1}. There is little disagreement in plasma ACTH levels measured by different radioimmunoassay systems. Immunoreactive β-MSH in human plasma is now considered to be larger molecules, LPHs, after the artifactual nature of human β-MSH was discovered (Scott and Lowry 1974). Since plasma LPH consists of β-LPH (1–91) and γ-LPH (1–58), plasma LPH levels vary when measured by different radioimmunoassay systems. Most of the antisera against β-MSH (37–58 β-LPH) react well with γ-LPH, but less well with β-LPH (Gilkes et al. 1975). On the other hand, most currently available β-LPH antisera cross-react with γ-LPH, so that values obtained by these antisera represent the sum of β- and γ-LPH. Anti-β-endorphin antisera usually cross-react well with β-LPH, thus giving the sum of β-LPH and β-endorphin when used for radioimmunoassay. In spite of such complexity in the nature of antisera, values obtained by anti-β-LPH or anti-β-MSH antisera are in relatively good agreement when the latter are corrected for cross-reactivity to β-LPH (Abe et al. 1969; Hirata et al. 1975b; Bachelot et al. 1977; Gilkes et al. 1977; Jeffcoate et al. 1978; Wiedeman et al. 1978; Tanaka et al. 1978a; Krieger et al. 1979). Plasma β-LPH levels in the morning are 25–200 pg ml^{-1} in most instances.

There is little information on plasma levels of γ-LPH. Earlier studies of Gilkes et al. (1975) suggested no significant amount of γ-LPH in circulating plasma. On the other hand, Tanaka et al. (1978b) demonstrated the presence of a significant amount of γ-LPH in two normal human plasmas by gel filtration. Bertagna et al. (1980) reported plasma γ-LPH levels of < 12.5–21 fmol ml^{-1}, while Yamaguchi et al. (1980) reported levels of 4.4 ± 0.5 fmol ml^{-1}. These γ-LPH levels are higher than β-endorphin levels, although both hormones are considered to be produced in equimolar amounts by the proteolysis of β-LPH. β-LPH and possibly γ-LPH also exist in plasma in animals, but little is known about their levels.

The plasma level of β-endorphin is a matter of dispute. At first, Suda et al. (1978) reported that β-endorphin was virtually absent in human plasma. On the other hand, we observed the existence of β-endorphin distinct from β-LPH on gel filtration in normal subjects and obtained morning basal β-endorphin levels of 5.8 ± 1.1 pg ml^{-1} (Nakao et al. 1978). Utilizing similar methods, Höllt et al. (1979) and Wardlaw and Frantz (1979) reported values of 11.8–21.6 pg ml^{-1} and 21 ± 7.3 pg ml^{-1}, respectively. Somewhat higher values were reported when direct radioimmunoassay utilizing specific antisera was employed (Wiedeman et al. 1979; Wilkes et al. 1980). These discrepancies can be explained in part by the difference in reactivity of heterogenous β-endorphin moieties (β-, δ-endorphins and their acetylated forms) with different antisera. Plasma levels of β-endorphin are higher in animals, approximately 400 pg ml^{-1} in rats (Höllt et al. 1978), probably because of its secretion from the intermediate lobe.

Big γ-MSH also exists in human plasma. Fig. 5.7 shows the gel chromatographic pattern of plasma obtained from a patient with Addison's disease. There exists a single peak of big γ-MSH in plasma, as in the pituitary, and the β-endorphin peak distinct from β-LPH is also observed. However, plasma γ-MSH levels in normal subjects could not be measured because of the limited sensitivity of our assay system. Bertagna et al. (1980) also reported the existence of a 16 k fragment in human plasma.

Negative feedback mechanism

It is well-known that ACTH secretion from the pituitary gland is controlled by plasma levels of corticosteroids, thus maintaining homeostasis of the pituitary–adrenal system. There is evidence both in man and animals that there are two types of feedback me-

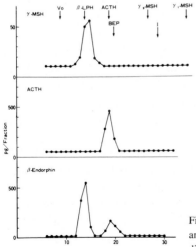

Fig. 5.7. Gel chromatographic pattern of γ-MSH-LI, ACTH-LI and β-EP-LI of plasma obtained from a patient with Addison's disease. See legend for Fig. 5.2.

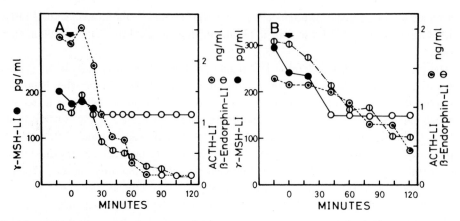

Fig. 5.8. Effect of intravenous injection of 100 mg of cortisol on plasma levels of γ-MSH-LI, β-EP-LI and ACTH-LI in patients with Addison's disease (A) and Nelson's syndrome (B). The limit of detection for each immunoreactivity is indicated by open circles. Reproduced from J. Clin. Endocrinol. Metab. 51, 1206, 1980, with permission.

chanisms, fast and delayed (Dallman and Yates 1969; Jones et al. 1972). The fast mechanism exerts its effect immediately after steroid administration, whereas the delayed feedback appears some hours later. In humans, it is known that intravenous administration of cortisol causes a prompt cessation of ACTH secretion, occurring within 2 min (Rees et al. 1973). Plasma β-LPH measured directly or as β-MSH disappears parallel with ACTH with slower disappearance half-time (Tanaka et al. 1978a; Krieger et al. 1979). We observed that the injection of cortisol lowered plasma levels of ACTH-LI, β-EP-LI, γ-MSH-LI in patients with Addison's disease and Nelson's syndrome, as shown in Fig. 5.8 (Nakao et al. 1980). All these results indicate that secretion of all hormones derived from proACTH-β-LPH is promptly inhibited by the rise of plasma cortisol level in man.

Metyrapone is a substance that blocks 11β-hydroxylation involved in the final step of cortisol biosynthesis. The resultant fall in plasma cortisol in turn stimulates secretion of ACTH via the negative feedback mechanism. We have demonstrated that plasma β-LPH and β-endorphin measured separately by gel chromatography increase parallel with ACTH in response to metyrapone as shown in Table 5.3 (Nakao et al. 1978). Other investigators also reported the increase of β-LPH, γ-LPH, β-endorphin or immunoreactive β-MSH following the administration of metyrapone (Hirata et al. 1975b; Krieger 1978; Jeffcoate et al. 1978). Although the response of γ-MSH-LI or the 16 k fragment to metyrapone has not yet been studied, all other peptides derived from proACTH-β-LPH increase in response to the decrease of plasma cortisol levels.

The negative feedback control of ACTH secretion has been extensively studied in experimental animals (for review, see Kendall 1971; Jones 1978). Bilateral adrenalectomy raises plasma ACTH (Matsuyama et al. 1971; Dallman et al. 1972), whereas the administration of glucocorticoids suppresses it to undetectable levels (Ruhmann-Wennhold and Nelson 1977). Although the intermediate lobe of rat pituitary secretes ACTH in vitro, in vivo secretion into blood, if it exists at all, is in very small amounts. In fact, plasma ACTH levels become very low after glucocorticoid treatment even though in vitro release of

Table 5.3

PLASMA ACTH, β-LPH AND β-ENDORPHIN LEVELS IN NORMAL SUBJECTS BEFORE AND AFTER
METYRAPONE ADMINISTRATION

	No.	Before metyrapone	After metyrapone
ACTH (pg ml^{-1})	5	73 ± 4	269 ± 41
β-LPH (pg ml^{-1})	5	111.2 ± 17.4	1356.1 ± 252.0
β-endorphin (pg ml^{-1})	5	5.8 ± 1.1	48.9 ± 3.8

Plasma β-LPH and β-endorphin were measured after gel exclusion chromatography by radioimmunoassay for
β-endorphin. Values are means ± SEM.

ACTH from the intermediate lobe is not affected by glucocorticoids (Fischer and Moriarty
1977).

The effect of glucocorticoids on the secretion of β-endorphin, α- and β-MSH in animals
has also been studied. Höllt et al. (1978) reported that either metyrapone administration or
adrenalectomy raised plasma β-EP-LI in rats. On the other hand, the administration of
glucocorticoids lowers plasma ACTH-LI and β-EP-LI concomitantly (Guillemin et al.
1977). These changes of plasma hormones may be ascribed to the changes of hormone
release from the anterior pituitary, as will be discussed later.

The precise site and mode of feedback action of glucocorticoids are still not completely
elucidated. By reviewing the literature, Kendall (1971) postulated the direct action of
glucocorticoids on the pituitary. This was further supported by the effect of glucocorticoids
on AtT-20 cells in vitro, and the control of biosynthesis at the transcriptional level has been
demonstrated, as mentioned above. However, Sayers and Portanova (1974) have shown
that corticosterone reduces CRF-induced ACTH release from the pituitary cells within
15 min, suggesting that fast feedback occurs at the pituitary levels. Moreover, the hypothalamic CRF content was observed to increase after adrenalectomy and to decrease after
corticosterone treatment (Buckingham 1979). In addition, corticosterone inhibits in vitro
CRF release from, but not its synthesis in, the hypothalamus (Buckingham and Hodges
1977). These results suggest that the negative feedback mechanism is a complex phenomenon and that glucocorticoids act on the hypothalamus or even higher centers to modulate
ACTH release, besides the direct inhibitory action on the pituitary.

Stress

A variety of systemic, neural and psychological stresses stimulate ACTH secretion. In
man, insulin-induced hypoglycemia is a systemic stress most commonly used to test the
response of the hypothalamo-pituitary system. The administration of pyrogen is another
type of systemic stress which stimulates ACTH secretion. We observed that insulin-induced hypoglycemia raised not only plasma ACTH but also β-LPH and β-endorphin in a
parallel fashion in normal subjects and patients with Graves' disease (Nakao et al. 1979).
Similar concomitant increases of plasma ACTH and β-LPH (or measured as β-MSH) in
response to insulin-induced hypoglycemia have previously been observed by ourselves and
others (Hirata et al. 1975b; Gilkes et al. 1975; Krieger et al. 1979). Moreover, we observed

148

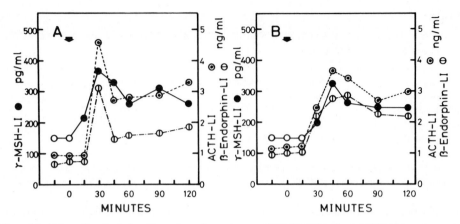

Fig. 5.9. Effect of insulin-induced hypoglycemia on plasma γ-MSH-LI, β-EP-LI and ACTH-LI in patients with Addison's disease (A) and Nelson's syndrome (B). The limit of detection for each immunoreactivity is indicated by open circles. Reproduced from J. Clin. Endocrinol. Metab. 51, 1206, 1980, with permission.

that plasma γ-MSH-LI, another peptide derived from proACTH-β-LPH, increased parallel with ACTH-LI and β-EP-LI in patients with Addison's disease, as shown in Fig. 5.9 (Nakao et al. 1980). It can be concluded, therefore, that all peptides derived from the common precursor concomitantly increase in response to systemic stresses.

Neural stresses are also known to stimulate ACTH secretion in man. At least some types of surgical stress are considered to be a neural stress, which augments plasma ACTH through neural pathway. Vaginal or caesarian delivery is also known to be associated with an increase of plasma ACTH, which is blocked by lumbar anesthesia (Berson and Yalow 1968; Nakai 1976). Plasma β-endorphin and β-LPH were also reported to increase during labour and parturition in parallel with plasma ACTH (Csontos et al. 1979). Although the response of plasma γ-MSH-LI to neural stresses has not been studied yet, it is likely that all peptides derived from proACTH-β-LPH are elevated in parallel by neural stresses.

In animals, extensive studies have been done to elucidate the response of plasma ACTH and related peptides to a variety of stresses. Concomitant increases of plasma ACTH and β-EP-LI induced by electrical foot shock or bone fracture have been reported (Guillemin et al. 1977; Höllt et al. 1978). The increase occurred within a few minutes following the application of neural stresses.

The exact mechanism by which a variety of stresses stimulate secretion of ACTH and related peptides has not been fully understood yet. Certain humoral substances may reach the pituitary ACTH-producing cells, bypassing the central nervous system. However, most stresses, even so-called systemic stresses like hypoglycemia and pyrogen, are considered to act through the neural mechanisms. Lesions of the medial basal hypothalamus abolish the ACTH secretion induced by various stimuli (McCann 1953). Certain stresses activate the neural pathways that reach the hypothalamus from the midbrain and the pons, originating from the spinal cord. They enter the hypothalamus mainly from the antero-lateral (Palkovits 1977). Hemorrhage or other stress stimulates ACTH secretion through the visceral reflex, originating from baroreceptors and volume receptors (Gann et al. 1977).

Circadian rhythm

The existence of a circadian periodicity of ACTH and cortisol secretion is well establis-hed in man. The highest levels occur between 0400 and 0800 in subjects on a normal sleep–wake schedule. Studies with frequent blood samplings have revealed that an ul-tradian periodicity is superimposed on this circadian periodicity, with 5–10 secretory episodes over the 24-h period (Hellman et al. 1970; Krieger et al. 1971). No apparent regularity is observed in the interepisode intervals. Similar episodicity and circadian periodicity are also observed in plasma β-LPH (Krieger et al. 1979).

The circadian periodicity is retained in patients with Addison's disease, although plasma levels are elevated and the circadian change is exaggerated. Therefore, we studied the circadian changes of plasma ACTH-LI, β-EP-LI and γ-MSH-LI in patients with Addison's disease. As shown in Fig. 5.10, all these hormones clearly showed the circadian periodi-city. Although there are no data on the episodicity of plasma β-endorphin and γ-MSH-LI, it is likely that these hormones are secreted in an episodic fashion as ACTH and β-LPH.

The circadian periodicity of plasma ACTH and corticosteroids is also observed in infra-human mammalian species. In rats, the peak value occurs before or immediately after the onset of darkness. It is widely believed that periodicity of CRF secretion from the hypothalamus is involved in the ACTH circadian rhythm. In fact, hypothalamic CRF content shows circadian periodicity in rats (David-Nelson and Brodish 1969; Hiroshige et al. 1969). Therefore, a periodic firing of CRF neurons may cause episodic secretion of ACTH, that is, the ultradian rhythm. The center of the circadian rhythm is considered to affect this episodic secretion of ACTH. The major neural area responsible for the circadian periodicity seems to be the suprachiasmatic nucleus, since the destruction of this nucleus resulted in the loss of circadian periodicity of adrenal corticosterone in rats (Moore and Eichler 1972). This nucleus receives projections from the retina via a retino-hypothalamic tract, and from the midbrain. Both light–dark and sleep–wake cycles are known to be implicated as regulators of circadian periodicity of ACTH secretion. In addition, time of

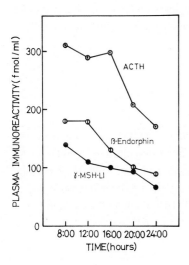

Fig. 5.10. Circadian changes of plasma γ-MSH-LI, β-EP-LI and ACTH-LI in a patient with Addison's disease.

food presentation is known to affect the circadian periodicity of adrenal steroids in rats (Krieger 1974). Interestingly, the effect of food restriction on the circadian periodicity was not affected by the destruction of the suprachiasmatic nucleus, suggesting a different neural pathway to CRF neurons (Krieger et al. 1977a).

Summary

Secretion of ACTH from the pituitary gland is regulated by three physiological regulators; a negative feedback mechanism, stress and circadian periodicity. There are complicated interrelationships between these regulators (for review see Jones 1978). For example, the suppressive effect of corticoids on ACTH secretion varies according to the time of day, being maximal when administered 4–8 h before the circadian peak (Grant et al. 1965). There is also circadian variation in the magnitude of corticotropic response to stress in man (Clayton et al. 1963).

As mentioned above, not only ACTH but also other peptides such as β-LPH, β-endorphin and γ-MSH-LI, all of which are derived from proACTH-β-LPH, respond to the physiological regulators. It is difficult to compare plasma levels of these peptides on a molar basis, because (1) plasma hormones have heterogenous molecular forms with different cross-reactivity with antisera and (2) each of these peptides has a different half-life in blood. Nevertheless, a parallel change of plasma peptides under various conditions in man and animals suggests that they are secreted in equimolar amounts from the pituitary gland. Only a few papers reported the dissociation in plasma levels of these peptides. Kalin et al. (1980) reported that a small dose of dexamethasone decreased plasma cortisol levels but did not alter circulating β-EP-LI in man and monkeys. The possibility that ACTH and β-endorphin are secreted discordantly from the pituitary cells can not be ruled out completely, since recent immunohistochemical studies revealed that ACTH-LI and β-EP-LI are not necessarily present in the same cells simultaneously (Mendelsohn et al. 1979; Osamura et al. 1980). However, nonspecific interference of radioimmunoassay for β-EP-LI by plasma factors must be excluded. It appears, therefore, that at least under most circumstances ACTH and other peptides derived from the common precursor are secreted concomitantly.

HYPOTHALAMIC CONTROL OF SECRETION

Corticotropin-releasing factor

It is generally accepted that the hypothalamus regulates ACTH secretion from the pituitary gland via the release of corticotropin-releasing factor into pituitary portal vessels. Although CRF is the hypothalamic-releasing factor that was first studied, the exact chemical nature has not yet been elucidated*. CRF-like activity has been demonstrated in the central nervous system both within and outside the hypothalamus (Yasuda and Greer 1976; Krieger et al. 1977b). There have also been reports of CRF-like activity present in

* See p. 58, Note added in proof.

tissue other than the central nervous system, that is, tissue CRF (Brodish 1977). However, the nature of CRFs has not yet been elucidated, because of the instability during the process of purification. Pearlmutter et al. (1975) reported that gel chromatography yielded two separable zones with no CRF activity when assayed separately but showed high CRF activity when administered together. Since then, existence of a potentiator or multi-factor system has been repeatedly reported (Jones et al. 1977; Vale and Rivier 1977; Schally et al. 1979). In a recent report, Sayers et al. (1980) isolated two CRFs and a potentiator from the hypothalamus.

Early suggestions that vasopressin might be the CRF have been refuted by several observations. Although vasopressin invariably releases ACTH from the anterior pituitary, the dose–response curve and the maximal secretory rate are different from those of partially purified CRF (Vale and Rivier 1977). In addition, rats which do not synthesize vasopressin have essentially normal ACTH secretory patterns (Arimura et al. 1967) and have CRF in the hypothalamus in an amount not significantly different from that in control rats (Pearlmutter et al. 1980). However, the role of vasopressin in regulating ACTH release is still a subject of controversy. Gillies and Lowry (1979) postulated that vasopressin is the major component of CRF whose potency is modulated by synergistic factors present in the hypothalamus. Immunohistochemical studies have revealed that vasopressin neurons terminate around the portal capillaries of the median eminence where large amounts of the hormone can be secreted (for review see Zimmerman et al. 1977). These observations suggest the role of vasopressin in regulating anterior pituitary function. Further studies should clarify the interaction between vasopressin and CRF.

Release of ACTH and related peptides in vitro

The mechanism of release of ACTH and related peptides from the pituitary has been studied by in vitro systems using anterior pituitary cells. Cultures of normal or tumorous

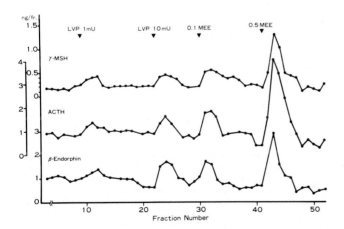

Fig. 5.11. Effect of rat MEE and vasopressin on release of γ-MSH-LI, β-EP-LI and ACTH-LI from perfused, dispersed, pituitary adenoma cells obtained from a patient with Cushing's disease. See text for details.

mouse pituitary cells and dispersed rat anterior pituitary cells have been most extensively used. Recently, human ACTH-producing adenoma cells obtained at surgery for Cushing's disease have become available.

Studies on human ACTH-producing pituitary adenoma cells

We obtained isolated human pituitary ACTH-producing adenoma cells by mechanical agitation of pituitary tumor tissue in trypsin solution. The cells were placed on a Sephadex column and perfused with buffer solution containing various substances (Oki et al. 1981a). As shown in Fig. 5.11, rat median eminence extract (MEE) containing CRF dose-dependently increased the release of ACTH-LI, β-EP-LI and γ-MSH-LI from tumor cells. Gel chromatographic studies revealed that ACTH-LI consisted mainly of little ACTH with a minor peak of big ACTH, that β-EP-LI had two components of β-LPH and β-endorphin, and that γ-MSH-LI consisted of big γ-MSH. Lysine vasopressin also enhanced release of these peptides, although it was less potent than MEE and the dose–response relationship was not clear cut. Although not shown in the figure, we observed in one case that thyrotropin-releasing hormone (TRH) and luteinizing hormone-releasing hormone (LH-RH) enhanced the release of ACTH and related peptides. In all experiments, secretory patterns of ACTH-LI, β-EP-LI and γ-MSH-LI were in general parallel.

Gillies et al. (1980) also studied the effect of rat MEE and arginine vasopressin on release of ACTH, LPH and β-endorphin from human adenoma cells. They also observed parallel releases of these hormones and different dose–response relationship between MEE and vasopressin. Mashiter et al. (1980) used primary cell cultures of human pituitary adenoma cells and observed that rat MEE and arginine vasopressin caused a parallel increase of ACTH and LPH release from tumor cells. They further reported that hydrocortisone did not suppress basal but only the stimulated release of ACTH and LPH, whereas serotonin had no significant effect.

All these results indicate that (1) MEE (CRF) and vasopressin stimulate release of ACTH and related peptides from human pituitary tumor cells; (2) peptides derived from the common precursor are released in a parallel fashion; (3) glucocorticoids inhibit release of ACTH and related peptides induced by MEE. Although the mechanism of hormone release from adenoma cells may not be the same as that from intact cells, these results essentially agree with those obtained with intact animal pituitary cells. It can be concluded, therefore, that CRF is an important factor which stimulates ACTH release in man. The parallel release of all peptides derived from the common precursor is in accordance with the observation in normal subjects in vivo, as mentioned in the preceding section and in Nelson's syndrome as reported by us (Oki et al. 1980).

Another observation that deserves discussion is the release from adenoma cells of ACTH and related peptides by TRH or LH-RH. The result is compatible with the paradoxical response of plasma ACTH to TRH or LH-RH in Nelson's syndrome or Cushing's disease (Krieger et al. 1977c; Matsukura et al. 1977). These results can be explained by the abnormalities in receptor mechanisms in tumor cells, since we observed that adenylate cyclase was activated by LH-RH in a tumor obtained from a patient with Cushing's disease who showed a paradoxical response of plasma ACTH to LH-RH (Matsukura et al. 1977).

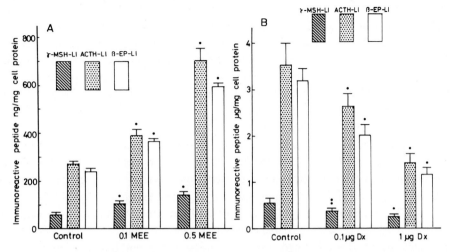

Fig. 5.12. Effect of rat MEE (A) and glucocorticoids (B) on the release of γ-MSH-LI, β-EP-LI and ACTH-LI from AtT-20 cells into the medium. Rat MEE (National Pituitary Agency) dissolved in serum-free medium was added to AtT-20 cells and incubated for 2 h. Dexamethasone (Dx) dissolved in the conventional medium was incubated with AtT-20 cells for 48 h. The hormone contents in the medium were assayed by radioimmunoassay. •P < 0.05; ••P < 0.01

Another abnormality in the receptor mechanism in tumor cells is the response to bromo-criptine, a dopaminergic agonist. Bromocriptine is known to lower plasma ACTH in some patients with Cushing's disease and Nelson's syndrome (Lamberts and Birkenhäger 1976a and 1976b). Evidence suggesting the direct action of bromocriptine on tumor cells has recently been provided by Lamberts et al. (1980).

Studies on murine ACTH-producing pituitary adenoma cells

Mouse ACTH-producing pituitary adenoma cells in culture (AtT-20) have been most extensively used for the study of the mechanism of hormone release. The tumor cells produce and secrete ACTH, 31 k precursor, β-LPH, β-endorphin and γ-MSH-LI (Mains et al. 1977; Allen et al. 1978; Oki et al 1981b). Fig. 5.12 illustrates release of ACTH-LI, β-EP-LI and γ-MSH-LI into the medium of AtT-20 cell cultures. Rat MEE containing CRF dose-dependently enhanced the release of all hormones derived from proACTH-β-LPH, whereas glucocorticoids suppressed them. Release of ACTH-LI, β-EP-LI and γ-MSH-LI was coupled in the stimulated and suppressed states.

The stimulatory effect of crude or purified CRF on release of ACTH and β-endorphin from AtT-20 cells has been observed consistently (Allen et al. 1978; Oki et al. 1981b). Vasopressin is also active in stimulating the release of ACTH and β-endorphin (Allen et al. 1978). The suppressive effect of glucocorticoids has been repeatedly demonstrated (Watanabe et al. 1973b; Allen et al. 1978). These results are in accordance with those obtained in human pituitary adenoma cells as mentioned above and those in intact rat pituitary, as will be discussed below.

However, tumor cells have some characteristics that are different from those of intact cells. TRH is known to stimulate ACTH release from mouse pituitary tumor cells, being a potential model for the study of the paradoxical response to TRH in Cushing's disease (Gershengorn et al. 1980). Lamberts et al. (1980) observed that bromocriptine and cyproheptadine inhibited release of ACTH from dispersed rat pituitary tumor cells, 7315a. This system may also be a possible model for the study of the anomalous response of plasma ACTH to various stimuli in patients with Cushing's syndrome.

Studies on rat anterior pituitary cells

Rat anterior pituitary slices and more recently, dispersed pituitary cells and their primary cultures, have been extensively used for the study of ACTH release. As in AtT-20 cells, rat MEE containing CRF or partially purified CRF dose-relatedly increases the release of ACTH and related peptides from anterior pituitary cells (Portanova and Sayers 1973; Allen et al. 1978; Vale et al. 1978; Raymond et al. 1979). In addition, vasopressin is also capable of enhancing ACTH release from isolated pituitary cells, although its dose–response curve and relative potency as compared with CRF varied in different reports (Portanova and Sayers 1973; Vale and Rivier 1977; Vale et al. 1978; Kendall et al. 1979; Voigt et al. 1980). Norepinephrine is another secretagogue for ACTH release in vitro, although the dose–response relationship is different from that of CRF (Vale et al. 1978; Voigt et al. 1980). In many experiments, the maximum secretion rates of ACTH and β-EP-LI induced by vasopressin or norepinephrine were lower than those induced by CRF, suggesting different mechanisms of hormone release.

As non-specific secretagogues, cyclic nucleotide derivatives such as dibutyryl cyclic AMP and phosphodiesterase inhibitors such as theophylline are also known to stimulate release of ACTH and related peptides in vitro (Eipper and Mains 1978a; Vale et al. 1978; Raymond et al. 1979). This suggests that cyclic AMP mediates the action of CRF.

Glucocorticoids are well-known inhibitory agents in regulating the release of ACTH and related peptides (Sayers and Portanova 1974; Vale et al. 1978; Allen et al. 1978; Raymond et al. 1979). In such in vitro experiments, two phases of glucocorticoid inhibition were observed; one of rapid onset and the other of long duration (Sayers and Portanova 1974). This suggests that at least two sets of negative feedback mechanisms discussed in the preceding section are operating at the level of the pituitary. The latter phase may be ascribed to the inhibition of biosynthesis of proACTH-β-LPH, as discussed above.

In these in vitro experiments, basal, stimulated and inhibited releases of ACTH, β-LPH, β-endorphin, α-MSH and γ-LPH (measured as β-MSH-like immunoreactivity) were all parallel (Vale et al. 1978; Allen et al. 1978; Raymond et al. 1979), supporting the concept that all these peptides are derived from the common precursor.

Studies on rat neurointermediate pituitary in vitro

As mentioned previously, the neurointermediate lobe of rat and bovine pituitary contains ACTH, α-MSH, corticotropin-like intermediate lobe peptide, β-LPH, γ-LPH and β-endorphin, all of which are derived from proACTH-β-LPH, as in the anterior pituitary. However, the secretory mechanism in the neurointermediate lobe is quite different from that in the anterior lobe. Some in vivo studies indicate that the neurointermediate lobe does

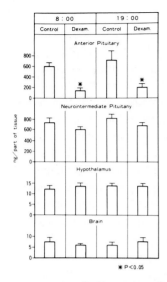

Fig. 5.13. Effect of oral administration of dexamethasone (1 µg ml⁻¹ in drinking water) for 2 weeks on the content of β-EP-LI in the anterior and neurointermediate lobes of the pituitary, hypothalamus and other parts of the brain.

not secrete ACTH one or several days after the removal of the anterior lobe, even after stress (Mialhe-Voloss 1958; Fisher and de Salva 1959; Greer et al. 1975). These results are in accordance with the observation that plasma ACTH levels in rats in stimulated or inhibited states can be explained by altered release from the anterior pituitary.

However, in vitro studies show that the neurointermediate lobe releases ACTH and related peptides. In a pulse-chase experiment using a tracer amino acid, Mains and Eipper (1979) were able to observe the release of ACTH, α-MSH, β-LPH, β-endorphin and the 16 k fragment (big γ-MSH) from isolated neurointermediate cells. The parallel release of peptides derived from proACTH-β-LPH was observed in other studies (Voigt et al. 1980; Sueoka et al. 1981). However, the neurointermediate lobe predominantly releases α-MSH, CLIP and β-endorphin, whereas the anterior lobe predominantly releases ACTH and β-LPH.

The mechanism of hormone release from the neurointermediate lobe is not fully understood. Crude MEE stimulated hormone release in some studies (Kraicer et al. 1978; Briaud et al. 1978; Sueoka et al. 1981) but not in others (Voigt et al. 1980; Prezewłocki et al. 1978). Since vasopressin had no effect on ACTH release from the neurointermediate lobe, the effect of crude MEE should be ascribed to component(s) other than vasopressin. The effect of glucocorticoids on the content and release of ACTH and related peptides is still contradictory. In most of the studies reported neither adrenalectomy nor long-term glucocorticoid treatment was shown to affect the ACTH, α-MSH and β-endorphin contents (Moriarty and Moriarty 1975; Kraicer et al. 1977; Rossier et al. 1979; Lépine and Dupont 1980). Fig. 5.13 shows our experiment in which neither adrenalectomy nor the administration of dexamethasone affected the ACTH and β-endorphin contents of rat neurointermediate lobes, although they affected the hormone contents of the anterior lobe (Imura 1980). However, Sueoka et al. (1981) observed that the addition of dexamethasone to the culture medium of neurointermediate pituitary cells partially but significantly lowered basal releases of ACTH-LI and β-EP-LI, as well as their responses to MEE. Further studies, especially on the level of mRNA, should clarify the effect of glucocorticoids on the intermediate lobe.

It has been known that the intermediate lobe cells are innervated by both peptidergic and aminergic nerve fibers and, therefore, are considered to be regulated by neural inputs. In fact, neurogenic stress causes a marked change of the ACTH content in the intermediate lobe (Mialhe-Voloss 1955). Kraicer (1977) and Fisher and Moriarty (1977) reported that dopamine inhibited the release of ACTH from the neurointermediate lobe, whereas Briaud et al. (1979) found a stimulatory effect. In vivo studies rather favor the inhibitory action of dopamine, since a dopaminergic antagonist, haloperidol, raised plasma α-MSH in rats (Usategui et al. 1976). These results suggest the existence of a dopaminergic inhibitory system. Norepinephrine had no effect in Kraicer's experiment but showed a stimulatory effect in the study of Briaud et al. (1979). Serotonin had a stimulatory effect in the study of Kraicer (1977) but no effect in the experiment of Briaud et al. (1979). Thus, the effect of neurotransmitters other than dopamine is still controversial.

Summary

ACTH, β-endorphin and other peptides derived from proACTH-β-LPH are released in vitro in the basal, stimulated and inhibited states from the non-tumorous or tumorous anterior lobe of man, mouse and rat, and the non-tumorous intermediate lobe of rat. CRF and glucocorticoids are major regulators for the control of release from the anterior pituitary, although other factors such as vasopressin and norepinephrine may also be involved. In adenoma cells, other agents such as TRH or LH-RH may stimulate hormone release, at least in some cases.

The control of release of ACTH and related peptides from the neurointermediate lobe is different. Although results are still contradictory, neural inputs from the hypothalamus or the higher centers seem important.

NEUROTRANSMITTERS INVOLVED IN THE CONTROL OF SECRETION

As discussed in the preceding section, release of ACTH and related peptides is considered to be regulated mainly by CRF, an as yet unidentified hypothalamic hormone. Like other hypothalamic hormones, CRF is present widely in the brain, being highest in content at the median eminence (Krieger et al. 1977b). Studies on the subcellular localization of CRF revealed its presence in the synaptosomal fraction (Mulder et al. 1970). These results suggest that neural inputs into CRF neurons stimulate the release of CRF into the portal vessels, with possible mediation of neurotransmitters. A considerable body of evidence exists suggesting that neurotransmitters are involved in the regulation of ACTH secretion in man and animals.

Role of neurotransmitters in the regulation of secretion of ACTH and related peptides in man

The role of adrenergic mechanisms in the regulation of ACTH secretion is still controversial. In our previous studies, we observed that plasma ACTH response to insulin-induced hypoglycemia was augmented by propranolol, a beta-adrenergic blocking agent, and suppressed by phentolamine, an alpha-adrenergic blocking agent (Nakai et al. 1973). An alpha-stimulating agent, methoxamine, also raised plasma ACTH, though inconsistently (Nakai et al. 1973). Similarly, Rees et al. (1970) found that the elevation of plasma ACTH and corticosteroid induced by methylamphetamine was exaggerated by propranolol and attenuated by thymoxamine, an alpha-adrenergic blocking agent. These results suggest the presence of alpha-adrenergic stimulatory and beta-adrenergic inhibitory mechanisms regulating ACTH secretion in man. On the other hand, Nakagawa et al. (1971) failed to find any significant change in the corticosteroid response to insulin-induced hypoglycemia during the infusion of phentolamine. More recently, Lancranjan et al. (1979) observed that plasma ACTH and cortisol responses to insulin-induced hypoglycemia were blunted by an alpha-adrenergic agonist, guanfacine. This suggests the presence of an alpha-adrenergic inhibitory mechanism in man. These results are compatible with the finding of Wilcox et al. (1975) that the infusion of norepinephrine lowers plasma ACTH in man. It seems premature to draw any conclusion from these results.

The role of the dopaminergic mechanism in regulating ACTH secretion in man is still obscure. Intravenous or oral administration of L-dopa, a precursor of dopamine, had no significant effect on plasma ACTH and corticosteroids in man (Wilcox et al. 1975).

We observed that the oral administration of 5-hydroxytryptophan (5-HTP), the immediate precursor of serotonin, increased plasma ACTH and cortisol, in most of the normal subjects studied (Imura et al. 1973). In addition, intravenous infusion of cyproheptadine, a serotonin antagonist, blocked the circadian rise of plasma cortisol (Chihara et al. 1976). Cyproheptadine is also known to blunt the plasma cortisol response to insulin-induced hypoglycemia (Plonk et al. 1974). Another more specific serotonin antagonist, metergoline, has also been reported to reduce the increment in plasma corticosteroids produced by metyrapone (Cavagnini et al. 1975). Since these anti-serotoninergic agents did not alter plasma ACTH response to vasopressin (Cavagnini et al. 1976; George et al. 1976), the site of action of the drug is considered to be higher than the pituitary.

It is likely that β-LPH, β-endorphin and other peptides derived from proACTH-β-LPH change in parallel with ACTH under the various conditions mentioned above. However, to our knowledge, this has not been confirmed yet.

The intravenous injection of methionine-enkephalin (Met-enkephalin) or its potent analogue (D-Ala^2,MePhe^4,Met(o)-ol)-enkephalin, has been reported to decrease plasma ACTH and corticosteroid levels (Stubbs et al. 1978) or to blunt the plasma ACTH response to vasopressin (del Pozo et al. 1980). This action of the Met-enkephalin analogue was completely counteracted by the administration of naloxone, an opiate antagonist (Stubbs et al. 1978). This suggests that Met-enkephalin acts through opiate receptors to lower ACTH release. Although the site of action of Met-enkephalin is not clear, it may act at the level of the central nervous system or the pituitary (del Pozo et al. 1980). This action of Met-enkephalin may be of physiological significance, since the intravenous infusion of naloxone significantly raises plasma cortisol (Kato et al. 1979). It is possible, however, that other opioid peptides such as β-endorphin might be involved also in the regulation of ACTH secretion in man.

Role of neurotransmitters in the regulation of secretion of ACTH and related peptides in animals

In spite of a large number of studies regarding the role of neurotransmitters in regulating ACTH secretion in experimental animals, the results obtained are still contradictory. Since there are several reviews on this subject (Van Loon 1974; Jones 1978; Weiner and Ganong 1978; Ganong 1980), we need discuss it only briefly in this chapter.

Ganong and his associates (Ganong 1972; Weiner and Ganong 1978) performed extensive studies in dogs and have postulated that central catecholamines inhibit ACTH secretion. Catecholamines seem to exert their effect through alpha-adrenergic receptors, because the alpha-adrenergic agonist, clonidine, inhibits stress-induced ACTH secretion (Ganong et al. 1976). Jones et al. (1976a; 1976b) found that norepinephrine incubated with rat hypothalamic tissue in vitro blocked the release of CRF stimulated by serotonin and acetylcholine. However, not all reports have supported the concept of a noradrenergic-inhibitory system. For example, intraventricular administration of 6-hydroxydopamine in rats decreases hypothalamic norepinephrine levels, but does not affect basal corticosterone levels nor their response to stress (Kumeda et al. 1974).

The implantation of serotonin in the brain has been shown to result in the activation of the pituitary–adrenal system in cats (Krieger and Krieger 1970). Intraventricular injection of serotonin increased ACTH secretion in rats (Rose and Ganong 1976). Moreover, Jones et al. (1976b) observed that serotonin enhanced CRF release from the hypothalamus in vitro. On the other hand, Telegdy and Vermes (1976) and Vernikos-Danellis et al. (1977) have postulated that serotonin inhibits ACTH secretion in rats. More recently, Ganong (1980) failed to find any significant effect of serotonin on ACTH secretion in dogs.

Rudolph et al. (1979) reported that intraventricular injection of histamine produced a significant increase in plasma ACTH and corticosteroids in dogs. This effect was blocked by mepyramine, a H_1 receptor blocker, but not by metiamide, a H_2 receptor blocker. However, mepyramine failed to produce any effect on stress-induced ACTH secretion.

There is evidence that acetylcholine, when injected into the third ventricle, stimulates ACTH release (Krieger and Krieger 1970). In addition, acetylcholine enhanced CRF release from rat hypothalamus in vitro (Jones et al. 1976b), supporting the stimulatory action of acetylcholine on ACTH secretion.

Although amino acids do not affect the basal release of CRF in vitro, gamma-aminobutyric acid (GABA) reduces the stimulatory effect of acetylcholine and serotonin (Jones et al. 1976b). It appears, therefore, that GABA acts directly on the CRF neurons. These results are in accordance with the finding that the intraventricular injection of GABA inhibits ACTH secretion (Makara and Stark 1974).

A peptide which plays a potential stimulatory role in regulating ACTH secretion is angiotensin II (see Chapter 8). Systemic administration of this peptide has been reported to increase ACTH secretion (Ramsey et al. 1978). However, the results of the intraventricular injection of angiotensin II are conflicting (Ganong 1980) and further studies are required to clarify the role of this peptide.

Other peptides possibly involved in the regulation of ACTH secretion are opioid peptides and substance P. Different from human studies, as mentioned above, opioid peptides injected intraventricularly rather enhanced plasma corticosterone response to stress (Gibson et al. 1979). The reason for such a discrepancy is unknown. On the other hand, substance P appears to inhibit ACTH secretion by acting directly on the pituitary (Jones et al. 1978b), since it has no effect on CRF release in vitro. The effect of other neuropeptides on ACTH secretion must be studied in the future.

Summary

Secretion of ACTH from the pituitary gland is considered to be controlled by CRF released from the median eminence into the pituitary portal vessels. There seem to be complicated neural pathways connecting with CRF neurons, and there are probably stimulatory and inhibitory neurotransmitters that regulate CRF release. However, the results so far obtained are still contradictory and it is difficult to draw any conclusion at the moment. These neurotransmitters may affect also the release of β-endorphin and other related peptides derived from proACTH-β-LPH, although these studies are only now starting to be performed (Sapun et al. 1981).

ACKNOWLEDGEMENTS

We are greatly indebted to Drs. S. Numa, S. Nakanishi, T. Kita, S. Taii and M. Nakamura, Department of Medical Chemistry, Kyoto University Faculty of Medicine, for their collaboration on a part of the studies mentioned in this chapter. These studies were supported in part by research grants from the Ministry of Education, Science and Culture in Japan.

NOTE ADDED IN PROOF

While we were correcting the proofs of this chapter, Vale et al. (1981) reported the purification and primary structure of a peptide with 41 residues from ovine hypothalami that stimulates release of ACTH and β-endorphin from cultured anterior pituitary cells. They reported also that the synthetic peptide was active both in vitro and in vivo at an apparently physiological dose.

REFERENCES

Abe, K., Nicholson, W.E., Liddle, G.W., Orth, D.N. and Island, D.P. (1969) Normal and abnormal regulation of β-MSH in man. J. Clin. Invest. 48, 1580-1585.
Allen, R.G., Herbert, E., Hinman, M., Shibuya, H. and Pert, C. (1978) Coordinate control of corticotropin, β-lipotropin, and β-endorphin release in mouse pituitary cell cultures. Proc. Natl. Acad. Sci. USA 75, 4972-4976.
Arimura, A., Saito, T., Bowers, C.Y. and Schally, A.V. (1967) Pituitary-adrenal activation in rats with hereditary hypothalamic diabetes insipidus. Acta Endocrinol. (Copenhagen) 54, 155-165.
Bachelot, I., Wolfsen, A.R. and Odell, W.D. (1977) Pituitary and plasma lipotropins: demonstration of the artifactual nature of β-MSH. J. Clin. Endocrinol. Metab. 44, 939-946.

160

Benjannet, S., Seidah, N.G., Routhier, R. and Chrétien, M. (1980) A novel human pituitary peptide containing γ-MSH sequence. Nature 285, 415-416.

Berson, S.A. and Yalow, R.S. (1968) Radioimmunoassay of ACTH in plasma. J. Clin. Invest. 47, 2725-2751.

Bertagna, X., Girard, F., Seurin, D., Luton, J.-P., Bricaire, H., Mains, R.E. and Eipper, B.A. (1980) Evidence for a peptide similar to 16 k fragment in man. Its relationship to ACTH. J. Clin. Endocrinol. Metab. 51, 182-184.

Bertagna, X.Y., Stone, W.J., Nicholson, W.E., Mount, C.D. and Orth, D.N. (1981) Simultaneous assay of immunoreactive β-lipotropin, γ-lipotropin, and β-endorphin in plasma of normal human subjects, patients with ACTH/lipotropin hypersecretory syndromes, and patients undergoing chronic hemodialysis. J. Clin. Invest. 67, 124-135.

Briaud, B., Koch, B., Lutz-Bucher, B. and Mialhe, C. (1978) In vitro regulation of ACTH release from neurointermediate lobe of rat hypophysis. I. Effect of crude hypothalamic extracts. Neuroendocrinology 25, 47-63.

Briaud, B., Koch, B., Lutz-Bucher, B. and Mialhe, C. (1979) In vitro regulation of ACTH release from neurointermediate lobe of rat hypophysis. II. Effect of neurotransmitters. Neuroendocrinology 28, 377-385.

Brodish, A. (1977) Tissue corticotropin releasing factors. Fed. Proc. 36, 2088-2093.

Buckingham, J.C. and Hodges, J.R. (1977) Production of corticotropin releasing hormone by the isolated hypothalamus of the rat. J. Physiol. (London) 272, 469-479.

Buckingham, J.C. (1979) The influence of corticotropin and its hypothalamic releasing hormone. J. Physiol. (London) 286, 331-342.

Cavagnini, F., Panerai, A.E., Valentini, F., Bulgheroni, P., Peracchi, M. and Pinto, M. (1975) Inhibition of ACTH response to oral and intravenous metyrapone by antiserotoninergic treatment in man. J. Clin. Endocrinol. Metab. 41, 143-148.

Cavagnini, F., Raggi, U., Micossi, P., DiLandro, A. and Invitti, C. (1976) Effect of an antiserotoninergic drug, metergoline, on the ACTH and cortisol response to insulin hypoglycemia and lysine-vasopressin in man. J. Clin. Endocrinol. Metab. 43, 306-312.

Chihara, K., Kato, Y., Maeda, K., Matsukura, S. and Imura, H. (1976) Suppression by cyproheptadine of human growth hormone and cortisol secretion during sleep . J. Clin. Invest. 57, 1393-1402.

Civelli, O., Vincent, A., Buri, J.-F. and Scherrer, K. (1976) Evidence for a translational inhibitor linked to globin mRNA in untranslated free cytoplasmic messenger ribonucleoprotein complexes. FEBS Lett. 72, 71-76.

Clayton, G.W., Librik, L., Gardner, R.L. and Guillemin, R. (1963) Studies on the circadian rhythm of pituitary adrenocorticotropic release in man. J. Clin. Endocrinol. Metab. 23, 975-980.

Crine, P., Gianoulakis, C., Seidah, N.G., Gossard, F., Pezalla, P.D., Lis, M. and Chrétien, M. (1978) Biosynthesis of β-endorphin from β-lipotropin and a larger molecular weight precursor in rat pars intermedia. Proc. Natl. Acad. Sci. USA 75, 4719-4723.

Csontos, K., Rust, M., Höllt, V., Mahr, W., Kromer, W. and Teschemacher, H.J. (1979) Elevated plasma β-endorphin levels in pregnant women and their neonates. Life Sci. 25, 835-844.

Dallman, M.F. and Yates, F.E. (1969) Dynamic asymmetries in the corticosteroid feedback path and distribution-metabolism-binding elements of the adrenocortical system. Ann. N.Y. Acad. Sci. 156, 696-721.

Dallman, M.F., Jones, M.T., Vernikos-Danellis, J. and Ganong, W.F. (1972) Corticosteroid feedback control of ACTH secretion: rapid effects of bilateral adrenalectomy on plasma ACTH in the rat. Endocrinology 91, 961-968.

David-Nelson, M.A. and Brodish, A. (1969) Differences in corticosterone and dexamethasone binding to rat brain and pituitary. Endocrinology 96, 598-609.

del Pozo, E., Martin-Perez, J., Stadelmann, A., Girard, J. and Brownell, J. (1980) Inhibitory action of a met-enkephalin on ACTH release in man. J. Clin. Invest. 65, 1531-1534.

Drouin, J. and Goodman, H.M. (1980) Most of the coding region of rat ACTH β-LPH precursor gene lacks intervening sequences. Nature 288, 610-613.

Eipper, B.A. and Mains, R.E. (1978a) Existence of a common precursor to ACTH and endorphin in the anterior and intermediate lobes of the rat pituitary. J. Supramol. Struct. 8, 247-262.

Eipper, B.A. and Mains, R.E. (1978b) Analysis of the common precursor to corticotropin and endorphin. J. Biol. Chem. 253, 5732-5744.

Fisher, J.D. and de Salva, S.J. (1959) Plasma corticosterone and adrenal ascorbic acid levels in adeno- and neurohypophysectomized rats given epinephrine postoperatively. Am. J. Physiol. 197, 1263-1264.

Fisher, J.L. and Moriarty, C.M. (1977) Control of bioactive corticotropin release from the neuro-intermediate lobe of the rat pituitary in vitro. Endocrinology 100, 1047-1054.

Fortier, C. (1959) Pituitary ACTH and plasma free corticosteroids following bilateral adrenalectomy in the rat. Proc. Soc. Exp. Biol. Med. 100, 13-16.

Gann, D.S., Ward, D.G., Baertschi, A.J., Carlson, D.E. and Maran, J.W. (1977) Neural control of ACTH release in reponse to hemorrhage. Ann. N.Y. Acad. Sci. 297, 477-497.

Ganong, W.F. (1972) Evidence for a central noradrenergic system that inhibits ACTH secretion. In: Brain-Endocrine Interaction: Median Eminence: Structure and Function (Knigge, K.M., Scott, D.E. and Weindl, A. eds), pp. 254-266, Karger, Basel.

Ganong, W.F., Kramer, N., Salmon, J., Reid, I.A., Lovinger, R., Scapagnini, U., Boryczka, A.T. and Shackelford, R. (1976) Pharmacological evidence for inhibition of ACTH secretion by a central adrenergic system in the dog. Neuroscience 1, 167-174.

Ganong, W.F. (1980) Neurotransmitters and pituitary function: regulation of ACTH secretion. Fed. Proc. 39, 2923-2930.

George, W.F., Husain, M., Lock, J.P. and Katz, F.H. (1976) Failure of cyproheptadine to inhibit vasopressin-stimulated cortisol release in a patient with Cushing's disease. Hormone Res. 7, 308-312.

Gershengorn, M.C., Arevalo, C.D., Geras, E. and Rebecchi, M.J. (1980) Thyrotropin-releasing hormone stimulation of adrenocorticotropin production by mouse pituitary tumor cells in culture. J. Clin. Invest. 65, 1294-1300.

Gibson, A., Ginsburg, M., Hall, M. and Hart, S.L. (1979) The effect of intracerebroventricular administration of methionine-enkephalin on the stress-induced secretion of corticosterone in mice. Br. J. Pharmacol. 66, 164-166.

Gilkes, J.J.H., Bloomfield, G.A., Scott, A.P., Lowry, P.J., Ratcliffe, J.G., Landon, J. and Rees, L.H. (1975) Development and validation of a radioimmunoassay for peptides related to β-melanocyte-stimulating hormone in human plasma: the lipotropins. J. Clin. Endocrinol. Metab. 40, 450-457.

Gilkes, J.J.H., Rees, L.H. and Besser, G.M. (1977) Plasma immunoreactive corticotrophin and lipotrophin in Cushing's syndrome and Addison's disease. Brit. Med. J. 1, 996-998.

Gillies, G. and Lowry, P. (1979) Corticotrophin releasing factor may be modulated by vasopressin. Nature 278, 463-464.

Gillies, G., Ratter, S., Grossman, A., Gaillard, R., Lowry, P.J., Besser, G.M. and Rees, L.H. (1980) Secretion of ACTH, LPH and β-endorphin from human pituitary tumors in vitro. Clin. Endocrinol. 13, 197-205.

Gossard, F., Seidah, N.G., Crine, P., Reuthier, R. and Chrétien, M. (1980) Partial N-terminal amino acid sequence of pro-opio-melanocortin (ACTH/Beta-LPH precursor) from rat pars intermedia. Biochem. Biophys. Res. Commun. 92, 1042-1051.

Grant, S.D., Forsham, P.H. and DiRaimondo, V.C. (1965) Suppression of 17-hydroxy-corticosteroid in plasma and urine by single and divided doses of triamcinolone. N. Engl. J. Med. 273, 1115-1117.

Greer, M.A., Allen, C.F., Panton, P. and Allen, J.P. (1975) Evidence that the pars intermedia and the pars nervosa of the pituitary do not secrete functionally significant quantities of ACTH. Endocrinology 96, 718-724.

Guillemin, R., Ling, N. and Burgus, R. (1976) Endorphines, peptides, d'origine hypothalamique et neurohypophysaire à activité morphinomimetique. Isolement et structure moleculaire de l'alpha-endorphine. C.R. Acad. Sci. Paris, 282, 783-785.

Guillemin, R., Vargo, T., Rossier, V., Minick, S., Ling, N., Rivier, C., Vale, W. and Bloom, F. (1977) β-endorphin and adrenocorticotropin are secreted concomitantly by the pituitary gland. Science 197, 1367-1369.

Håkanson, R., Ekman, R., Sundler, F. and Nilsson, R. (1980) A novel fragment of the corticotropin-beta-lipotropin precursor. Nature 283, 789-792.

Haralson, M.A., Fairfield, S.J., Nicholson, W.E., Harrison, R.W. and Orth, D.N. (1979) Cell-free synthesis of mouse corticotropin. J. Biol. Chem. 254, 2172-2175.

Hellman, L.T., Nikada, F., Curti, J., Weitzman, E.D., Kream, J., Roffwarg, K., Ellman, S., Fukushima, D.K. and Gallagher, D.T. (1970) Cortisol is secreted episodically by normal man. J. Clin. Endocrinol. Metab. 30,

411-422.

Hirata, Y., Yamamoto, H., Matsukura, M. and Imura, H. (1975a) In vitro release and biosynthesis of tumor ACTH in ectopic ACTH producing tumors. J. Clin. Endocrinol. Metab. 41, 106-114.

Hirata, Y., Sakamoto, N., Matsukura, S. and Imura, H. (1975b) Plasma levels of β-MSH and ACTH during acute stresses and metyrapone administration in man. J. Clin. Endocrinol. Metab. 41, 1092-1097.

Hiroshige, T., Sakakura, M. and Itoh, S. (1969) Diurnal variation of corticotropin-releasing activity in the rat hypothalamus. Endocrinol. Jpn. 16, 465-467.

Höllt, V., Przewłocki, R. and Herz, A. (1978) Radioimmunoassay of β-endorphin basal and stimulated levels in extracted rat plasma. Naunyn-Schmiedeberg's Arch. Pharmacol. 303, 171-174.

Höllt, V., Müller, O.A. and Fahlbusch, R. β-endorphin in human plasma: basal and pathologically elevated levels. Life Sci. 25, 37-44.

Imura, H., Nakai, Y. and Yoshimi, T. (1973) Effect of 5-hydroxytryptophan (5-HTP) on growth hormone and ACTH release in man. J. Clin. Endocrinol. Metab. 36, 204-206.

Imura, H. (1980) ACTH, β-endorphin and related peptides. In: Endocrinology 1980 (Cumming, I.A., Funder, V.W. and Mendelson, F.A.O. eds), pp. 58-65, Australian Academy of Science, Canberra.

Jeffcoate, W.J., Rees, L.H., Lowry, P.J. and Besser, G.M. (1978) A specific radioimmunoassay for human β-lipotropin. J. Clin. Endocrinol. Metab. 47, 160-167.

Jones, M.T., Brush, F.R. and Neame, R.L.B. (1972) Characteristics of fast feedback control of corticotrophin release by corticosteroids. J. Endocrinol. 55, 489-497.

Jones, M.T., Hillhouse, E.W. and Burden, J. (1976a) Secretion of corticotropin-releasing hormone in vitro. In: Frontiers in Neuroendocrinology (Martini, L. and Ganong, W.F. eds), pp. 195-226, Raven Press, New York.

Jones, M.T., Hillhouse, E.W. and Burden, J. (1976b) Effect of various putative neurotransmitters on the secretion of corticotrophin-releasing hormone from the rat hypothalamus in vitro – a model of the neuro-transmitters involved. J. Endocrinol. 69, 1-10.

Jones, M.T., Gillham, B. and Hillhouse, E.W. (1977) The nature of corticotropin-releasing factor from rat hypothalamus in vitro. Fed. Proc. 36, 2104-2109.

Jones, M.T. (1978a) Control of corticotrophin (ACTH) secretion. In: The Endocrine Hypothalamus (Jeffcoate, S.L. and Hutchinson, J.S.M. eds), pp. 385-419, Academic Press, London.

Jones, M.T., Gillham, B., Holmes, M.C., Hodges, J.R. and Buckingham, J.C. (1978b) Influence of substance P on hypothalamo-pituitary-adrenocortical activity in the rat. J. Endocrinol. 76, 183-184.

Kalin, N.H., Risch, S.C., Cohen, R.M., Insel, T. and Murphy, D.L. (1980) Dexamethasone fails to suppress β-endorphin plasma concentrations in humans and rhesus monkeys. Science 209, 827-828.

Kato, Y., Katagami, H., Matsushita, N., Waseda, N., Imura, H. and Shimbo, S. (1979) Effect of naloxone and an enkephalin analog (FK33824) on secretion of pituitary hormones in man. Folia Endocrinol. Jpn 55, 404 (Abstract).

Kendall, J.W. (1971) Feedback control of adrenocorticotropic hormone secretion. In: Frontiers in Neuroendoc-rinology, 1971 (Martini, L. and Ganong, W.F. eds), pp. 177-207, Oxford University Press, New York.

Kendall, J.W., Gray, D.K., Gaudette, N.D. and Orwoll, E.S. (1979) ACTH: recent advances in biochemistry and physiology. In: Recent Advances in the Diagnosis and Treatment of Pituitary Tumors (Linfoot, J.A. ed.), pp. 83-92, Raven Press, New York.

Keutmann, H.T., Eipper, B.A. and Mains, R.E. (1979) Partial characterization of a glycoprotein comprising the NH2-terminal region of mouse tumor cell pro-adrenocorticotropic hormone/endorphin. J. Biol. Chem. 254, 9204-9208.

Kraicer, J. (1977) ACTH and MSH release from pars intermedia. In: Melanocyte Stimulating Hormone: Control. Chemistry and Effects (Tilders, F.J.H., Swaab, D.F. and Van Wimersma Greidanus, Tj.B. eds), pp. 200-207, Karger, Basel.

Kraicer, J., Briaud, G. and Lywood, D.W. (1977) Pars intermedia ACTH and MSH content: effect of adrenalectomy, gonadectomy and neurotropic (noise) stress. Neuroendocrinology 23, 352-367.

Kraicer, J., Elliot, N.L. and Zimmerman, A.E. (1978) In vitro release of ACTH from dispersed rat pars intermedia cells. III Multiple forms of ACTH biological activity. Neuroendocrinology 27, 86-96.

Krieger, H.P. and Krieger, D.T. (1970) Chemical stimulation of the brain: effect on adrenal corticoid release. Am. J. Physiol. 218, 1632-1641.

Krieger, D.T., Allen, W., Rizzo, F. and Krieger, H.P. (1971) Characterization of the normal temporal pattern of plasma corticosteroid levels. J. Clin. Endocrinol. Metab. 32, 266-284.

Krieger, D.T. (1974) Food and water restriction shifts corticosterone, temperature, activity and brain amine periodicity. Endocrinology 95, 1195-1201.

Krieger, D.T., Hanser, H. and Krey, L.C. (1977a) Suprachiasmatic nuclear lesions do not abolish food-shifted circadian adrenal and temperature rhythmicity. Science 197, 398-399.

Krieger, D.T., Liotta, A. and Brownstein, M.J. (1977b) Corticotropin releasing factor distribution in normal and Brattleboro rat brain, and effect of deafferentation, hypophysectomy and steroid treatment in normal animals. Endocrinology 100, 227-237.

Krieger, D.T. and Luria, M. (1977c) Plasma ACTH and cortisol responses to TRF, vasopressin or hypoglycemia in Cushing's disease and Nelson's syndrome. J. Clin. Endocrinol. Metab. 44, 361-368.

Krieger, D.T. (1978) Plasma lipotropin and endorphin in the human. In: Endorphins '78 (Gráf, L., Palkovits, M. and Rónai, A.Z. eds), pp. 275-290, Excerpta Medica, Amsterdam.

Krieger, D.T., Liotta, A., Suda, T., Goodgold, A. and Condon, E. (1979) Human plasma immunoreactive lipotropin and adrenocorticotropin in normal subjects and in patients with pituitary-adrenal disease. J. Clin. Endocrinol. Metab. 48, 566-571.

Kumeda, H., Uchimura, H., Kawabata, T., Maeda, Y., Okamoto, O., Kawa, A. and Kanehisa, T. (1974) Role of brain noradrenaline in the regulation of pituitary-adrenocortical functions. J. Endocrinol. 62, 161-162.

Lamberts, S.W.J. and Birkenhäger, J.C. (1976a) Effect of bromocriptine in pituitary-dependent Cushing's syndrome. J. Endocrinol. 70, 315-316.

Lamberts, S.W.J. and Birkenhäger, J.C. (1976b) Bromocriptine in Nelson's syndrome and Cushing's disease. Lancet 2, 811 (letter).

Lamberts, S.W.J., Klijn, J.G.M., De Quijada, M., Timmermans, H.A.T., Uitterlinden, P., De Jong, F.H. and Birkenhäger, J.C. (1980) The mechanism of the suppressive action of bromocriptine on adrenocorticotropin secretion in patients with Cushing's disease and Nelson's syndrome. J. Clin. Endocrinol. Metab. 51, 307-311.

Lancranjan, I., Ohnhaus, E. and Girard, J. (1979) The α-adrenoceptor control of adrenocorticotropin secretion in man. J. Clin. Endocrinol. Metab. 49, 227-230.

Lépine, J. and Dupont, A. (1980) Influence of dexamethasone, 17β-estradiol and haloperidol on the pituitary content of β-LPH, β-endorphin, ACTH and related peptides. 62nd Annu. Meet. Endocrine Society, p. 152.

Li, C.H. and Chung, D. (1976) Isolation and structure of an untriakontapeptide with opiate activity from camel pituitary glands. Proc. Natl. Acad. Sci. USA 73, 1145-1148.

Ling, N., Ying, S., Minick, S. and Guillemin, R. (1979) Synthesis and biological activity of four γ-melanotropin derived from the cryptic region of the adrenocorticotropin/β-lipotropin precursor. Life Sci. 25, 1773-1780.

Mains, R.E. and Eipper, B.A. (1976) Biosynthesis of adrenocorticotropic hormone in mouse pituitary tumor cells. J. Biol. Chem. 251, 4115-4120.

Mains, R.E., Eipper, B.A. and Ling, N. (1977) Common precursor to corticotropins and endorphins. Proc. Natl. Acad. Sci. USA 74, 3014-3018.

Mains, R.E. and Eipper, B.A. (1979) Synthesis and secretion of corticotropins, melanotropins, and endorphins by rat intermediate pituitary cells. J. Biol. Chem. 254, 7885-7894.

Makara, G.B. and Stark, E. (1974) Effects of gamma-aminobutyric acid (GABA) and GABA antagonist drugs on ACTH release. Neuroendocrinology 16, 178-190.

Mashiter, K., Adams, E.F., Gilles, H., Van Noorden, S. and Ratter, S. (1980) Adrenocorticotropin and lipotropin secretion by dispersed cell cultures of a human corticotropic adenoma: effect of hypothalamic extract, arginine vasopressin, hydrocortisone and serotonin. J. Clin. Endocrinol. Metab. 51, 566-572.

Matsukura, S., Kakita, T., Hirata, Y., Yoshimi, H., Fukase, M., Iwasaki, Y., Kato, Y. and Imura, H. (1977) Adenylate cyclase of GH and ACTH producing tumors of human: activation by non-specific hormones and other biological substances. J. Clin. Endocrinol. Metab. 44, 392-397.

Matsuyama, H., Mims, R.B., Ruhmann-Wennhold, A. and Nelson, D.H. (1971) Bioassay and radioimmunoassay of plasma ACTH in adrenalectomized rats. Endocrinology 88, 696-701.

McCann, S.M. (1953) Effect of hypothalamic lesions on adrenal cortical response to stress in rats. Am. J. Physiol. 175, 13-20.

Mendelsohn, G., D'Agostino, R., Eggleston, J.C. and Baylin, S.B. (1979) Distribution of β-endorphin immunoreactivity in normal human pituitary. J. Clin. Invest. 63, 1297-1301.

Mialhe-Voloss, C. (1955) Variations des teneurs en hormone corticotrope des lobes antérieur et postérieur de l'hypophyse du rat soumis a differents types d'agressions. C.R. Hebd. Séanc. Acad. Sci. 241, 105-107.

Mialhe-Voloss, C. (1958) Posthypophyse et activité corticotrope. Acta Endocrinol. 35 (suppl.), 1-96.

Moore, R.Y. and Eichler, V.B. (1972) Loss of a circadian adrenal corticosterone rhythm following suprachiasmatic lesions in the rat. Brain Res. 42, 201-206.

Moriarty, C.M. and Moriarty, G.C. (1975) Bioactive and immunoactive ACTH in the rat pituitary: influence of stress and adrenalectomy. Endocrinology 96, 1419-1425.

Mulder, A.H., Geuze, J.J. and De Wied, D. (1970) Studies on the subcellular localization of corticotropin releasing factor (CRF) and vasopressin in the median eminence of the rat. Endocrinology 87, 61-79.

Nakagawa, K., Horiuchi, Y. and Mashimo, K. (1971) Further studies on the relation between growth hormone and corticotropin secretion in insulin-induced hypoglycemia. J. Clin. Endocrinol. Metab. 32, 188-191.

Nakai, Y. (1976) Studies on the regulatory mechanism of ACTH secretion in man. Part 6. Control mechanism of ACTH secretion in fetus and pregnant women. Jpn Arch. Intern. Med. 23, 153-157.

Nakai, Y., Imura, H., Yoshimi, T. and Matsukura, S. (1973) Adrenergic control mechanism for ACTH secretion in man. Acta Endocrinol. (Copenhagen) 74, 263-270.

Nakamura, M., Nakanishi, S., Sueoka, S., Imura, H. and Numa, S. (1978) Effects of steroids hormones on the level of corticotropin messenger RNA activity in cultured mouse pituitary-tumor cells. Eur. J. Biochem. 86, 61-66.

Nakanishi, S., Taii, S., Hirata, Y., Matsukura, S., Imura, H. and Numa, S. (1976) A large product of cell-free translation of messenger RNA coding for corticotropin. Proc. Natl. Acad. Sci. USA 73, 4319-4323.

Nakanishi, S., Inoue, A., Taii, S. and Numa, S. (1977a) Cell-free translation product containing corticotropin and β-endorphin encoded by messenger RNA from anterior lobe and intermediate lobe of bovine pituitary. FEBS Lett. 84, 105-109.

Nakanishi, S., Kita, T., Taii, S., Imura, H. and Numa, S. (1977b) Glucocorticoid effect on the level of corticotropin messenger RNA activity in rat pituitary. Proc. Natl. Acad. Sci. USA 74, 3283-3286.

Nakanishi, S., Inoue, A., Kita, T., Nakamura, M., Chang, A.C.Y., Cohen, S.N. and Numa, S. (1979) Nucleotide sequence of cloned cDNA for bovine corticotropin-β-lipotropin precursor. Nature 278, 423-427.

Nakao, K., Nakai, Y., Oki, S., Horii, K. and Imura, H. (1978) Presence of immunoreactive β-endorphin in normal human plasma: a concomitant release of β-endorphin with adrenocorticotropin after metyrapone administration. J. Clin. Invest. 62, 1395-1398.

Nakao, K., Nakai, Y., Jingami, H., Oki, S., Fukata, J. and Imura, H. (1979) Substantial rise of plasma β-endorphin levels after insulin-induced hypoglycemia in human subjects. J. Clin. Endocrinol. Metab. 49, 838-841.

Nakao, K., Oki, S., Tanaka, I., Nakai, Y. and Imura, H. (1980) Concomitant secretion of γ-MSH with ACTH and β-endorphin in humans. J. Clin. Endocrinol. Metab. 51, 1205-1207.

Oki, S., Nakai, Y., Nakao, K. and Imura, H. (1980) Plasma β-endorphin responses to somatostatin, thyrotropin-releasing hormone, or vasopressin in Nelson's syndrome. J. Clin. Endocrinol. Metab. 50, 194-197.

Oki, S., Nakao, K., Tanaka, I., Horii, K., Nakai, Y., Shimbo, S., Watanabe, M., Nakane, T., Kuwayama, A., Kageyama, N. and Imura, H. (1981a) Concomitant secretion of adrenocorticotropin, β-endorphin, and γ-melanotropin from perfused pituitary tumor cells of Cushing's disease: effects of lysine vasopressin, rat median eminence extracts, thyrotropin-releasing hormone, and luteinizing hormone-releasing hormone, J. Clin. Endocrinol. Metab. 52, 42-49.

Oki, S., Nakao, K., Tanaka, I., Nakai, Y., Kinoshita, F. and Imura, H. (1981b) Characterization of γ-melanotropin-like immunoreactivity and its secretion in ACTH-producing mouse pituitary tumor cell line. To be published.

Osamura, Y., Watanabe, K., Nakai, Y. and Imura, H. (1980) Adrenocorticotropic hormone cells and immunoreactive β-endorphin cells in the human pituitary gland: normal and pathologic conditions studied by the peroxidase-labelled antibody method. Am. J. Pathol. 99, 105-124.

Palkovits, M. (1977) Neural pathways involved in ACTH regulation. Ann. N.Y. Acad. Sci. 297, 455-476.

Pearlmutter, A.F., Rapino, E. and Saffran, M. (1975) The ACTH-releasing hormone of the hypothalamus requires a co-factor. Endocrinology 97, 1336-1339.

Pearlmutter, A.F., Dokas, L.A. and Saffran, M. (1980) Purification of CRF in normal and Brattleboro rats by neurophysin-affinity chromatography. 62nd Annu. Meet. Endocrine Society 239.

Plonk, J.W., Bivens, C.H. and Feldman, J.M. (1974) Inhibition of hypoglycemia induced cortisol secretion by the serotonin antagonist cyproheptadine. J. Clin. Endocrinol. Metab. 38, 836-840.

Portanova, R. and Sayers, G. (1973) Isolated pituitary cells: CRF-like activity of neural hypophysial and related peptides. Proc. Soc. Exp. Biol. Med. 143, 661-666.

Przewłocki, R., Höllt, V. and Herz, A. (1978) Release of β-endorphin from rat pituitary in vitro. Eur. J. Pharmacol. 51, 179-183.

Ramsey, P.J., Keil, L., Sharpe, M.C., Shinsako, J. (1978) Angiotensin II infusion increases vasopressin, ACTH and 11-hydroxycorticosteroid secretion. Am. J. Physiol. 234, R66-R71.

Raymond, V., Lépine, J., Lissitzky, J.-C., Côté, J. and Labrie, F. (1979) Parallel release of ACTH, β-endorphin, α-MSH and β-MSH-like immunoreactivities in rat anterior pituitary cells in culture. Mol. Cell Endocrinol. 16, 113-122.

Rees, L.H., Holdaway, I.M., Besser, G.M., Kramer, R., Landon, J. and Chayen, J. (1973) Comparison of the redox assay for ACTH with previous assays. Nature 241, 84-85.

Rees, L.H., Butler, P.W.P., Gosling, C. and Besser, G.M. (1976) Adrenergic blockade and the corticosteroid and growth hormone responses to methylamphetamine. Nature 228, 565-566.

Roberts, J.L. and Herbert, E. (1977) Characterization of a common precursor to corticotropin and β-lipotropin: cell-free synthesis of the precursor and identification of corticotropin peptides in the molecule. Proc. Natl. Acad. Sci. USA 74, 4826-4830.

Roberts, J.L., Budarf, M.L., Baxter, J.D. and Herbert, E. (1979) Selective reduction of proadrenocorticotropin/endorphin proteins and messenger ribonucleic acid activity in mouse pituitary tumor cells by glucocorticoids. Biochemistry 18, 4907-4915.

Rose, J.C. and Ganong, W.F. (1976) Neurotransmitter regulation of pituitary secretion. In: Current Developments in Psychopharmacology (Essman, W.F. and Valzelli, L. eds), pp. 87-123, Holliswood, New York.

Rossier, J., French, E., Gros, C., Minick, S., Guillemin, R. and Bloom, F.E. (1979) Adrenalectomy, dexamethasone or stress alters opioid peptide levels in rat anterior pituitary but not intermediate lobe or brain. Life Sci. 25, 2105-2112.

Rudolph, C., Richards, G.E., Kaplan, S. and Ganong, W.F. (1979) Effect of intraventricular histamine on hormone secretion in dogs. Neuroendocrinology 29, 169-177.

Ruhmann-Wennhold, A. and Nelson, D.H. (1977) Plasma ACTH levels in stressed and nonstressed adrenalectomized rats. Ann. N.Y. Acad. Sci. 297, 498-506.

Sabol, S.L. (1978) Regulation of endorphin production by glucocorticoids in cultured pituitary tumor cells. Biochem. Biophys. Res. Commun. 82, 560-567.

Sapun, D.L., Farah, J.M. and Mueller, G.P. (1981) Evidence that a serotoninergic mechanism stimulates the secretion of pituitary β-endorphin-like immunoreactivity in the rat. Endocrinology 109, 421-426.

Sayers, G. and Portanova, R. (1974) Secretion of ACTH by isolated anterior pituitary cells: kinetics of stimulation by corticotropin-releasing factor and of inhibition by corticosterone. Endocrinology 94, 1723-1730.

Sayers, G., Hanzmann, E. and Bodansky, M. (1980) Hypothalamic peptides influencing secretion of ACTH by isolated adenohypophysial cells. FEBS Lett. 116, 236-238.

Schally, A.V., Chang, R.C.C., Huang, W.Y., Redding, T.W., Carter, W.H., Coy, D.H. and Saffran, M. (1979) Isolation, structure and biological activities of several hypothalamic peptides. 61st Annu. Meet. Endocrine Society, p. 78.

Scott, A.P. and Lowry, P.J. (1974) Adrenocorticotrophic and melanocyte-stimulating peptides in the human pituitary. Biochem. J. 139, 593-602.

Shibasaki, T., Ling, N. and Guillemin, R. (1980) Pituitary immunoreactive γ-melanotropins are glycosylated oligopeptides. Nature 285, 416-417.

Simantov, R. (1979) Glucocorticoids inhibit endorphin synthesis by pituitary cells. Nature 280, 684-685.

Stubbs, W.A., Delitala, G., Jones, A., Jeffcoate, W.J., Edwards, C.R.W., Ratter, S.J., Besser, G.M., Bloom, S.R. and Alberti, K.G.M.M. (1978) Hormonal and metabolic responses to an enkephalin analogue in normal man. Lancet 2, 1225-1227.

Suda, T., Liotta, A.S. and Krieger, D.T. (1978) β-endorphin is not detectable in plasma from normal human subjects. Science 202, 221-223.

Sueoka, S., Matsukura, S., Hirata, Y., Yoshimi, H., Yokota, M. and Fujita, T. (1981) Differential glucocorticoid suppression of the release of ACTH and β-endorphin from cultured rat anterior and neuro-intermediate pituitary cells. Submitted for publication.

Taii, S., Nakanishi, S. and Numa, S. (1979) Distribution of the messenger RNA coding for the common precursor of corticotropin and β-lipotropin within the bovine pituitary. Eur. J. Biochem. 93, 205-212.

Tanaka, I., Nakai, Y., Jingami, H., Fukata, J., Nakao, K., Oki, S., Nakanishi, S., Numa, S. and Imura, H. (1980) Existence of γ-melanotropin (γ-MSH)-like immunoreactivity in bovine and human pituitary glands. Biochem. Biophys. Res. Commun. 94, 211-217.

Tanaka, K., Nicholson, W.E. and Orth, D.N. (1978a) Diurnal rhythm and disappearance half-time of endogenous plasma immunoreactive β-MSH (LPH) and ACTH in man. J. Clin. Endocrinol. Metab. 46, 883-890.

Tanaka, K., Nicholson, W.E. and Orth, D.N. (1978b) The nature of the immunoreactive lipotropins in human plasma and tissue extracts. J. Clin. Invest. 62, 94-104.

Telegdy, G. and Vermes, I. (1976) Changes induced by stress in the activity of the serotoninergic system in limbic brain structures. In: Catecholamines and Stress (Usdin, E., Kvetňanský, R.K. and Kopin, I.J. eds), pp. 145-156, Pergamon Press, Oxford.

Usategui, R., Oliver, C., Vaudry, H., Lombardi, G., Rozenberg, I. and Mourre, A.M. (1976) Immunoreactive α-MSH and ACTH levels in rat plasma and pituitary. Endocrinology 98, 189-196.

Vale, W. and Rivier, C. (1977) Substances modulating the secretion of ACTH by cultured anterior pituitary cells. Fed. Proc. 36, 2094-2099.

Vale, W., Rivier, C., Yang, L., Minick, S. and Guillemin, R. (1978) Effects of purified hypothalamic corticotropin-releasing factor and other substances on the secretion of adrenocorticotropin and β-endorphin-like immunoactivities in vitro. Endocrinology 103, 1910-1915.

Vale, W., Spiess, J., Rivier, C. and Rivier, J. (1981). Characterization of a 41-residue ovine hypothalamic peptide that stimulates secretion of corticotrophin and β-endorphin. Science 213, 1394-1397.

Van Loon, G.R. (1974) The role of brain catecholamines in the regulation of ACTH secretion. Adv. Neurol. 5, 479-486.

Vernikos-Danellis, J., Kellar, K.J., Kent, D., Gonzales, C., Berger, P.A. and Barchas, J.D. (1977) Serotonin involvement in pituitary-adrenal function. Ann. N.Y. Acad. Sci. 297, 518-526.

Voight, K.H., Weber, E., Fehn, H.L. and Martin, R. (1980) The concomitant storage and simultaneous release of ACTH and β-endorphin. In: Brain and Pituitary Peptides (Wuttke, W., Weindl, A., Voight, K.H. and Dries, R.-R. eds), pp. 54-64, Karger, Basel.

Wardlaw, S.L. and Frantz, A.G. (1979) Measurement of β-endorphin in human plasma. J. Clin. Endocrinol. Metab. 48, 176-180.

Watanabe, H., Nicholson, W.E. and Orth, D.N. (1973a) Inhibition of adrenocorticotropic hormone production by glucocorticoids in mouse pituitary tumor cells. Endocrinology 93, 411-416.

Watanabe, H., Orth, D.N. and Taft, D.O. (1973b) Glucocorticoid receptors in pituitary tumor cells. I. Cytosol receptors. J. Biol. Chem. 248, 7625-7630.

Weiner, R.I. and Ganong, W.F. (1978) Role of brain monoamines and histamine in regulation of anterior pituitary secretion. Physiol. Rev. 58, 905-976.

Wiedeman, E., Saito, T. and Linfoot, J. (1978) Elevated plasma β-lipotropin in Cushing's disease due to pituitary adenoma. 60th Annu. Meet. Endocrine Society p. 227.

Wiedeman, E., Saito, T., Linfoot, J.A. and Li, C.H. (1979) Specific radioimmunoassay of human β-endorphin in unextracted plasma. J. Clin. Endocrinol. Metab. 49, 478-480.

Wilcox, C.S., Aminoff, M.J., Millar, J.G.B., Keenan, J. and Kremer, M. (1975) Circulating levels of corticotrophin and cortisol after infusions of L-DOPA, dopamine and noradrenaline in man. Clin. Endocrinol. 4, 191-198.

Wilkes, M.M., Stewart, R.D., Bruni, J.F., Quigley, M.E., Yen, S.S.C., Ling, N. and Chrétien, M. (1980) A specific homologous radioimmunoassay for human β-endorphin: direct measurement in biological fluids. J. Clin. Endocrinol. Metab. 50, 309-315.

Yamaguchi, H., Liotta, A.S. and Krieger, D.T. (1980) Simultaneous determination of human plasma immunoreactive β-lipotropin, γ-lipotropin, and β-endorphin using immune-affinity chromatography. J. Clin. Endocrinol. Metab. 51, 1002-1008.

Yap, S.H., Strair, R.K. and Shafritz, D.A. (1978) Effect of a short term fast on the distribution of cytoplasmic albumin messenger ribonucleic acid in rat liver. J. Biol. Chem. 253, 4944-4950.

Yasuda, N. and Greer, M.A. (1976) Distribution of corticotropin relasing factor(s) activity in neural and extraneural tissues of the rat. Endocrinology 99, 944-948.

Zakarian, S. and Smyth, P. (1979) Distribution of active and inactive forms of endorphins in rat pituitary and brain. Proc. Natl. Acad. Sci. USA 76, 5972-5976.

Zimmerman, E.A., Stillman, M.A., Recht, L.D., Antunes, J.L., Carmel, P.W. and Goldsmith, P.C. (1977) Vasopressin and corticotropin-releasing factor: an axonal pathway to portal capillaries in the zona externa of the median eminence containing vasopressin and its interaction with adrenal corticoids. Ann. N.Y. Acad. Sci. 297, 405-419.

E.E. Müller and R.M. MacLeod (eds) Neuroendocrine Perspectives Vol. 1

Chapter 6

The role and direct measurement of the dopamine receptor(s) in the anterior pituitary

Michael J. Cronin

INTRODUCTION

Historical consideration

Less than a century ago, Langley (1906) distinguished two characteristics of biological receptors based on his work with cholinergic agents. He concluded: (1) "It is convenient to have a term for the specifically excitable constituent, and I have called it the receptive substance. It receives the stimulus, and by transmitting it causes contraction." (2) "Since the formation of nicotine compounds causes contraction, and that of the curare compounds does not, it is obvious that the chemical rearrangements set up in the muscle molecule by the combination of one of its radicals are different in the two cases." (Langley 1906). Those two traits, the ability to initiate a biological response and the capacity to distinguish specific ligands, will be the focus of this chapter on the dopamine receptor of the anterior pituitary.

Before the study of catecholamine receptors became glamorous, as judged by the mass of experimental effort directed toward this area, there was a rather slow progression of key observations which prepared the field for the bonanza of the last twenty years. In 1906, Dale (1906) noted that ergot alkaloids block some catecholamine responses but not others. He suggested the possibility of multiple types of receptors in responsive cells. This concept was confirmed and extended by Ahlquist (1948) when he was able to partition catecholamine responses into alpha and beta types, based on findings with several catecholamines in a variety of tissues. Antagonists were discovered which could block the norepinephrine and epinephrine responses, and the relationship between catecholamine concentration and the magnitude of the biological response was quantified in some instances. It was not until the First Symposium on Catecholamines in 1958 that dopamine was suggested to have effects independent of norepinephrine and epinephrine. At this meeting, Carlson described the regional distribution of dopamine in nine species and showed that dopamine was not correlated with the norepinephrine content. In addition, Carlson suggested that a deficit of dopamine in the corpus striatum may contribute to Parkinsonism (Carlson, 1958). At this same meeting, Vogt cautioned: "Whether it (dopamine) is both a precursor of norepinephrine and an active agent in its own right is also uncertain" (Vogt 1959). Subsequent to this, a multitude of localization and functional studies endowed dopamine with the status of a neurotransmitter–neuromodulator in its own right, with a receptor species distinct from the alpha and beta adrenergic receptors. Dopamine receptors are characterized by their higher affinity for dopamine than for norepinephrine, epinephrine and isoproterenol, while alpha adrenergic receptors show higher affinities for norepinephrine and epinephrine with lower attraction to isoproterenol and dopamine. Beta adrenergic receptors bind isoproterenol with relatively higher affinity than the catecholamines norepinephrine, epinephrine and dopamine. Specific antagonists such as haloperidol (dopamine), phentolamine (alpha adrenergic) and propranolol (beta adrenergic) aid in this delineation.

Scope of the review

This chapter will be limited to a discussion of the responses of the prolactin secreting mammotroph (also called lactotroph) which are initiated by dopamine agonist activity in the anterior pituitary, and the characterization of the dopamine receptor with radioligand binding and immunocytochemical techniques. The mammotroph is selectively discussed because of the overwhelming volume of data which support dopamine's role in this cell type and the paucity of studies on dopamine's effect on other anterior pituitary cell types. This survey is meant to highlight several levels (e.g. hormone release, cell growth) upon which dopamine has some inhibitory influence in the mammotroph. It is not an exhaustive treatise on all known effects.

Furthermore, it is recognized that there may be other physiological prolactin inhibitory hormones, such as gamma amino butyric acid (Enjalbert et al. 1979a) and a metabolite of thyrotropin releasing hormone (Enjalbert et a. 1979b), that contribute to the final response of the mammotroph.

The majority of this presentation will then discuss the radioligand and immunoligand binding techniques that have been utilized to characterize the anterior pituitary dopamine receptor in the recent past. Comparisons of the dopamine receptor of the anterior pituitary with dopamine receptors present in other organs will not be rigorous because of the strong probability that there are multiple subtypes of dopamine receptors present in these other areas (e.g. corpus striatum). Until these receptor entities can be individually dissected out to study, it would be unwise to relate the summed effect of pre- and postsynaptic dopamine receptors in the striatum to the effects observed in the anterior pituitary, an organ devoid of presynaptic dopamine receptors.

DOPAMINE AND THE PROLACTIN-SECRETING MAMMOTROPH

Historical consideration

It was recognized some time ago (Nikitovitch-Winer and Everett 1958; Meites et al. 1961) that the mammalian hypothalamus exerts a predominantly inhibitory influence over the mammotroph by releasing a prolactin inhibitory factor or factors from the median eminence into the hypophyseal portal vessels (Pasteels 1961; Talwalker et al. 1963). This is unique in that all other known anterior pituitary hormones are under a dominant stimulatory influence by the basal hypothalamus. The first legitimate candidate for prolactin inhibitory hormone was dopamine, when it was determined that dopamine could reduce prolactin secretion from the anterior pituitary in vitro in a dose dependent and pharmacologically reversible manner (MacLeod and Lehmeyer 1970, 1974; Quijada et al. 1973). Furthermore, the catecholamine content of the hypothalamus is more than adequate to cause these effects (Shaar and Clemens 1974).

Tuberoinfundibular dopamine neurons

Dopamine containing neurons of the arcuate nucleus and adjacent periventricular zone project a dense terminal array to the external layer of the median eminence (Fuxe 1964; Björklund and Nobin 1973), in close apposition to the fenestrated primary hypophyseal portal capillaries (Hökfelt 1967). The hypothesis that these neurons' primary function is to release dopamine into the portal blood is supported by the observation that there is a poor reuptake capacity in these neurons when compared to the high affinity reuptake system in the mesolimbic and nigrostriatal dopamine terminals (Annunziato 1979). Therefore, extracellular dopamine would be more likely to gain access to the portal blood than be taken up and reutilized or inactivated. This is a design consistent with the concept that dopamine is predominantly a neurohormone in this system, not a neurotransmitter. Direct measurements prove that dopamine concentrations are substantially higher in hypophyseal-stalk blood than in the systemic circulation (Ben-Jonathan et al. 1977; Plotsky et al. 1978) and that changes in hypophyseal-stalk dopamine content are inversely correlated with prolactin secretion (Ben-Jonathan et al. 1977; DeGreef and Neill 1979). Feedback regulation by prolactin on the activity in the tuberoinfundibular neurons has also been described. Both acute (Perkins and Westfall 1978) and chronic (Hökfelt and Fuxe 1972; Gudelsky et al. 1976; Annunziato and Moore 1977; Perkins et al. 1979) increases in extracellular prolactin enhance dopamine turnover in and release from hypothalamic fragments. This response would provide a greater inhibitory tonus to the mammotroph so as to lower extracellular prolactin concentration, a classic short feedback loop (see also Chapter 2).

Effects of dopamine on the mammotroph

This section will cite several examples of how mammotrophs respond to dopaminergic agents, or the lack of dopamine stimulation, in order to highlight the strong linkage that exists between dopamine and the mammotroph. The biochemistry of the dopamine receptor is discussed in a later section.

Appropriate concentrations of dopamine can markedly inhibit prolactin release within 3–6 min, as shown in enzymatically dispersed rat anterior pituitary glands. Upon release of the dopamine challenge, prolactin secretion is rapidly restored to high basal rates (Yeo et al. 1979; Thorner et al. 1980a). This is a dose-dependent phenomenon (Yeo et al. 1979; Caron et al. 1978) which is readily reversible with pre- or cotreatment with dopamine antagonists (MacLeod 1976; Caron et al. 1978; Denef and Follebouckt 1978; Rick et al. 1979). In addition to the acute effects on prolactin release, dopamine and dopamine agonists have recently been shown to decrease prolactin synthesis (MacLeod et al. 1980b; Maurer 1980b; Cheung et al. 1981) and increase prolactin degradation (Dannies and Rudnick 1980; Maurer 1980a). It is of interest regarding prolactin degradation that dopamine may stimulate the activity of lysosomal enzyme activity in mammotrophs (Nansel et al. 1980).

A morphological correlate of the inhibited release with acute dopamine treatment is the accumulation of prolactin granules. Interestingly, dopamine itself is associated with prolactin granules and not with other anterior pituitary hormone secretory granules. Pretreatment of anterior pituitary glands with the dopamine precursor L-dopa enhances but pretreatment with the dopamine agonist bromocriptine blocks dopamine content in prolactin secretory granules, indicating the mediation of a dopamine receptor (Gudelsky et al. 1979; Nansel et al. 1979). This situation is not unique in that dopamine is also associated with secretory granules in the islet of Langerhans (Ericson et al. 1977), and dopamine content in these granules can be increased with L-dopa treatment (Zern et al. 1979). What this association represents in the anterior pituitary is unknown. It may contribute to the sequestration of granules and thus to the inhibition of prolactin release.

Beyond the acute effects on prolactin release and synthesis, dopamine agents can also apparently affect cell division, most likely in mammotrophs. With chronic treatment, the dopamine agonist bromocriptine inhibits DNA synthesis (Davies et al. 1974) and cell proliferation in the anterior pituitary (Stepien et al. 1978). On the other hand, the dopamine antagonists sulpiride and pimozide enhance DNA synthesis (Kalberman et al. 1979) and mitotic index (Stepien et al. 1978) respectively in the anterior pituitary. A lesion of the medial basal hypothalamus, which eliminates the tuberoinfundibular dopamine neurons, also causes a significant increase in the density of immunostained mammotrophs (Cronin et al. 1980c). Although the morphometric studies are tedious, these initial results offer encouragement to those who seek to determine the circumstances which will induce endocrine cell division in a mature mammalian anterior pituitary.

As in other dopamine systems, chronic pharmacological (Annunziato and Moore 1977) or physical (Cheung and Weiner 1976; Cheung and Weiner 1978; Cheung et al. 1981) lesions of the tuberoinfundibular dopamine neurons render the mammotroph supersensitive to the inhibitory action of dopamine and dopamine agonists. It remains unclear whether chronic treatment with dopamine antagonists can also induce this state in the anterior pituitary (Lal et al. 1977; Ravitz and Moore 1977; Meltzer et al. 1978) as it does in the striatum (Müller and Seeman 1978).

Finally, attempts have been made to correlate electrical activity of pituitary cells with dopamine inhibition of prolactin secretion. Unfortunately, no one to date has verified that the recording electrode was in a normal mammalian mammotroph. Taraskevich and Douglas (1978) found that dopamine slowed or stopped spontaneous action potentials in pituitary cells of the alewife fish. These cells were presumed to be prolactin-secreting due to their anatomical location. Dufy and associates (1979) recorded action potentials from neoplastic cells of the GH_3B6 clone which secretes prolactin and growth hormone.

Dopamine slowed or stopped spontaneous action potentials in some cells, while treatment with the dopamine antagonist haloperidol either blocked dopamine's effect or induced some silent cells to fire. However, none of these effects were shown to be reversible or repeatable in the same cell. It is also bothersome that all of the above studies used nonphysiological concentrations of either sodium or calcium with only calcium, chloride, potassium and sodium in the bathing buffer. A third group recorded from about 1,000 unidentified cells in the anterior pituitary of an anesthetized rat and found no spontaneous action potentials (York et al. 1973). We also have attempted to record spontaneous action potentials from the anterior pituitary of an anesthetized rat with no success (I. Login, P. Guyenet and M. Cronin, unpublished observations). Thus, the suggestion that prolactin secretion from the mammalian anterior pituitary is coupled to an action potential and that the rate of occurrence of these depolarizations can be physiologically modulated by dopamine agents remains to be demonstrated.

MEASUREMENT OF DOPAMINE RECEPTORS

Radioligand binding studies

Criteria

We started with an indirect knowledge of certain characteristics of the dopamine receptors based on the ability of various dopamine agents to modulate prolactin release. The desire was to identify the dopamine receptor directly by measurement of dopamine ligand binding. It was assumed that the dopamine receptor was present in trace quantities, as had already been shown with other catecholaminergic receptors, especially if the dopamine receptor population existed on only one of six or more cell types of the anterior pituitary. Therefore, radiolabelled ligands were the obvious choice as an initial probe.

The decision to measure dopamine receptor binding and consider it as biologically relevant in the anterior pituitary requires that one be able to correlate kinetic and equilibrium binding events with a biological response, such as the release of prolactin. It is unfortunate in this system that the second messenger(s) is not known, because the stoichiometry between the binding and a proximal process is likely to be tighter than the distal consequence of prolactin synthesis or release. This is one compelling reason why it is imperative to determine second messenger(s) so that this new tool of radioligand receptor labelling can be applied to rigorous studies of the initial transduction process. Key questions which could then be addressed include: What is the ratio of dopamine receptor to second messenger molecules and the affinity of this interaction in normal mammotrophs? Do these values change under hormonal stimulation or pathological conditions?

The initial criteria to be satisfied in order to identify a dopamine receptor population in the anterior pituitary included the following: (1) The binding sites should exist in limited numbers (i.e. saturable binding sites) and the rates of association and dissociation of binding should parallel the biological response in the mammotroph (i.e. appropriate kinetics). (2) The order of affinity of a large number of interactive agents should equal the

Table 6.1A

ASSAY CONDITIONS FOR DOPAMINE RECEPTOR BINDING IN THE ANTERIOR PITUITARY

	[³H]Dihydroergocriptine	[³H]Dihydroergocriptine
Buffer composition		
Buffer	15 mM TRIS	25 mM TRIS
pH	7.4	7.4
MAO Inhibitor	13 μM nialamide	—
EDTA	5 mM	—
Guanine nucleotides		—
Ascorbate	1.1 mM	—
NaCl	—	—
CaCl$_2$	—	—
MgCl$_2$	—	2 mM
KCl	—	—
Other	—	—
Subcellular fractionation	multiple	multiple
Assay conditions		
Time (min)	60	60
Temperature (°C)	22–24	25
Volume (ml)	0.6	0.5
Protein (mg/tube)	0.2–0.8	0.7–2.0
Blank (% specific binding)	apomorphine, 60–70	d-butaclamol, 60–70
Isolation conditions		
Wash buffer	same as above	same as above
Volume (ml), temperature (°C)	20, iced	18, iced
Speed (s)	15–20	10
Filter type	GF/C	GF/C
Reference	Cronin et al. 1978	Caron et al. 1978

ASSAY CONDITIONS FOR DOPAMINE RECEPTOR BINDING IN THE ANTERIOR PITUITARY

	[3H]Spiperone					
Buffer composition						
Buffer	50 mM TRIS	15 mM TRIS	25 mM TRIS	50 mM TRIS	26 mM NaHCO₃, 1.2 mM KH₂PO₄	5 mM TRIS
pH	7.1	7.3	7.4	7.1	7.4	7.4
MAO inhibitor	10 μM pargyline	13 μM nialamide	2 μM pargyline	—	—	1 μM pargyline
EDTA	+/−	+/−	—	—	—	—
Guanine nucleotides						
Ascorbate	5.7 mM	5.7 mM	5.7 mM	5.7 mM	5.7 mM	5.7 mM
NaCl	120 mM	120 mM		120 mM	124 mM	2,10,60,120 mM
CaCl₂	1 mM	2 mM	2 mM	2 mM	0.8 mM	
MgCl₂	1 mM	1 mM				100 mM
KCl	5 mM	5 mM		5 mM	5 mM	100 mM
Other	—	—	—	—	1.3 mM MgSO₄	± 100 mM Na₂CO₃ ± 100 mM KCO₃
Subcellular fractionation	simple	multiple	simple	simple	simple	multiple
Assay conditions						
Time (min)	10–15	90	60	10	15	12
Temperature (°C)	37	22–24	25	37	37	37
Volume (ml)	2	0.6	0.5	0.4	1	1.1
Protein (mg/tube)	?	0.2–1.0	0.4–0.7	0.5	1	?
Blank (% specific binding)	d-butaclamol, 70–90	d-butaclamol, 70–90	spiperone, ?	d-butaclamol, ?	d-butaclamol, 80	d-butaclamol, ?
Separation conditions						
Wash buffer	50 mM TRIS	same as above	same as above	50 mM TRIS	same as above	same as above
Volume (ml), temperature (°C)	15, iced	20, iced	18, cold	7, cold	15, iced	10, cold
Speed (s)	'rapidly'	15	10	'rapidly'	'rapid'	?
Filter type	GF/B	GF/C	GF/C	GF/B	GF/B	GF/C
Reference	Creese et al. 1977; Sibley and Creese 1979	Cronin and Weiner 1979; Beach et al. 1979	DiPaolo et al. 1979	Meltzer et al. 1979	Schaeffer and Hsueh 1979	Stefanini et al. 1980a, b

biological order of potency of these agents, and the physiological substance (i.e., dopamine) must interact with the sites. The binding sites should be stereoselective, which implies greater pharmacological activity in one optical isomer than the other. (3) With present knowledge, the binding sites should be associated with plasma membranes of the mammotroph (i.e. cell specificity). (4) Other measurements, such as protein linearity, pH, temperature sensitivity and ion dependence, should be determined before the assay becomes routine.

Most of these criteria have been satisfied in the initial series of experiments in several independent laboratories, as will be described below. Recently published books on the measurement of receptors offer more details on both the criteria and the methodology of such studies (Smythies and Bradley 1978; Williams and Lefkowitz 1978; Yamamura et al. 1978; O'Brien 1979).

Methodology

1. *Cell preparation.* It is imperative to dissect the neurointermediate lobe from the anterior pituitary if one expects to define binding that is exclusive to the anterior pituitary. All students of the dopamine receptor in the anterior pituitary have been mindful of the fact that tuberoinfundibular dopamine neurons also terminate in the pars nervosa (Björklund and Nobin 1973; Ben-Jonathan et al. 1977) and that dopamine has many potential physiological actions in the neurointermediate lobe including inhibition of melanocyte stimulating hormone secretion (Tilders and Smelik 1978). We first reported dopaminergic binding in the neurointermediate lobe (Cronin et al. 1978; Cronin and Weiner 1979), but Creese and associates (Creese et al. 1977b) measured no dopamine receptors here. Recently, Stefanini and colleagues (1980b) reported on dopamine receptors in the rat neurointermediate lobe, and Sibley and Creese (1980a) have shown dopamine receptors in the steer intermediate lobe.

As listed in Table 6.1 A and B, all studies of the dopamine receptor to date have been on subcellular preparations of the anterior pituitary. The simple homogenates involve breaking of the cells and pelleting the particulate with a high speed centrifugation. This pellet is then rehomogenized and the concentration or character of the binding sites is determined. The multiple fractionations range from a slow speed centrifugation in sucrose buffer that removes nuclei, unbroken cells and debris, to a refined preparation of the plasmalemma. By isolating plasmalemma and other cell constituents, Caron and associates (1978) elegantly demonstrated that the binding of the dopamine agonist [^{3}]dihydroergocriptine is primarily associated with plasmalemma; the dopamine receptor is located on the surface membrane of the cell (Fig. 6.1). Furthermore, no binding is coincident with the secretory granules. Recall that dopamine gains access to the prolactin secretory granule through the mediation of a dopamine receptor in the anterior pituitary (Gudelsky et al. 1979; Nansel et al. 1979). If the dopamine receptor shuttles the ligand to the granule and remains complexed there, one may have expected some binding to be present in the granule fraction.

These various fractionation methods of obtaining dopamine receptors make it nearly impossible to compare binding site numbers between laboratories. Table 6.2 documents

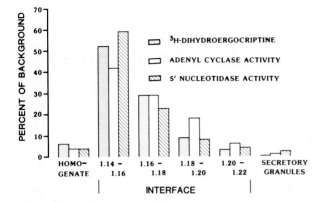

Fig. 6.1. Dopamine receptor localization and marker enzyme activity of subcellular fractions of the bovine anterior pituitary. The greatest dopamine receptor activity is correlated with the plasmalemma fractions, while there is no activity associated with the secretory granules. The enzyme marker data are taken from Poirier and coworkers (1974), while the binding data are those of Caron and associates (1978).

this dilemma. Now that the initial surge of studies has been accomplished, some standardization should be accepted so that these comparisons can be made more easily.

It is apparent that the homogenization and washing procedures remove endogenous dopamine from the receptors because the addition of dopamine to some of the initial homogenate does not decrease the binding in the final particulate preparation. This may not be the case with drug studies with high affinity competitors at the dopamine receptor (e.g. spiperone). Under these circumstances, it is imperative to show that the withdrawal period or the washing procedure is adequate to remove all ligand, especially before measuring receptor density.

Changes in binding with ultracold storage (i.e. −40 to −80°C) of the anterior pituitary homogenates is negligible over a two (Caron et al. 1978) and three (Cronin, unpublished observation) month period. However, critical studies have not been performed to determine whether there is any modification of the dopamine receptor activity when fresh homogenates are compared to frozen homogenates. The tissue is maintained on ice throughout the homogenization process to keep degradative enzyme activity to a minimum, and it may be advisable to add some inhibitors of lysosome function (e.g., chloroquine, NH_4Cl) to the initial preparation.

Dopamine receptor studies on pituitary cells maintained in primary or longer term culture have been initiated. Because this approach may become attractive, one should realize: (1) No serum-medium combination can totally replace the components found in extracellular fluid in vivo; nor can a plastic substrate replace basement membrane or special attachment to other cells. Consequently, measurements on cells cultured on plastic are probably never entirely representative of the in vivo condition. (2) Serum proteins bind ligands such as bromocriptine (M.O. Thorner, unpublished observation) and spiperone (J. Ramsdell and R.I. Weiner, unpublished observation) so that final free concentrations of ligand available to a receptor may be grossly different than total extracellular ligand concentration. This is especially crucial in dose response experiments which include serum or protein, such as

Table 6.2

DOPAMINERGIC LIGAND BINDING TO THE ANTERIOR PITUITARY

Species	[³H]Ligand	K_d (nM)	Site number	Rate constants		Temperature	Reference
				Association	Dissociation		
Human	Domperidone	0.2 ± 0.04	690 ± 82 fm/mg? protein	—	—	30°C	Bression et al. 1980
	Domperidone	4.0 ± 0.4	2069 ± 245 fm/mg? protein	—	—	30°C	Bression et al. 1980
	Spiperone	2.2 ± 0.7	141 ± 22 fm/mg assay protein	—	—	22–24°C	Cronin et al. 1980d
Rat	Dihydro-ergocriptine	3.7	260 fm/mg insoluble protein	—	—	22–24°C	Cronin et al. 1978
	Dopamine	50 ± 6	408 ± 130 fm/mg insoluble protein	—	—	22–24°C	Cronin et al. 1978
	Spiperone	0.63	81 fm/mg? protein	—	—	37°C	Meltzer et al. 1979
	Spiperone	0.2	215 fm/mg? protein	—	—	37°C	Schaeffer and Hsueh 1979
	Spiperone	0.2	3.8 pm/gm tissue	—	—	37°C	Stefanini et al. 1980a
Sheep	Dihydro-ergocriptine	4.7 ± 2.2	150 ± 20 fm/mg insoluble protein	—	—	22–24°C	Cronin et al. 1978
	Dihydro-ergocriptine	5.2 ± 1.1	373 ± 40 fm/mg fractionated protein	—	—	22–24°C	Cronin et al. 1978
	Dopamine	80 ± 18	267 ± 147 fm/mg insoluble protein	—	—	22–24°C	Cronin et al. 1978
	Spiperone	0.85 ± 0.09	343 ± 10 fm/mg fractionated protein	—	—	22–24°C	Cronin and Weiner 1979
Bovine	Dihydro-ergocriptine	2.2 ± 0.6	600 fm/mg plasmalemma protein	7.2×10^6/M per min	0.004 per min	25°C	Caron et al. 1978
	Dopamine	0.4	336 fm/mg? protein	—	—	30°C	Calabro and MacLeod 1978
	Dopamine	47	2,340 fm/mg? protein	—	—	30°C	Calabro and MacLeod 1978
	Spiperone	0.1 – 0.2	7 pmol/gm wet weight	0.8×10^9/M per min	0.1 per min	37°C	Creese et al. 1977
	Spiperone	0.38 ± 0.15	210 ± 30 fm/mg assay protein	2.2×10^7/M per min	0.02 per min	22–24°C	Cronin and Weiner 1979
Porcine	Spiperone	0.1	124 fm/mg assay protein	—	—	22–24°C	Cronin, unpublished observations

bovine serum albumin. (3) Hormones that are known to affect dopamine receptor activity, such as estradiol, vary in concentration between batches of sera. Every effort should be made to control this or to use a chemically defined serum substitute (Sato and Ross 1979). (4) Trypsinization of cells, a common method of dispersing endocrine cells and harvesting plated cells, may affect surface receptors acutely (Moriarty et al. 1978; El-Refai and Exton 1980; Hoeffler and Ben-Jonathan 1980) or permanently, especially in clones that have been maintained for years.

Experiments on whole cells from the normal anterior pituitary are in progress in order to find out whether broken cell binding of dopamine ligands is completely representative of the interactions which occur in living cells and to determine the number of dopamine receptors per cell. Insel and Stoolman (1978) discovered that breaking cells reduces total beta-adrenergic binding per cell and hormone sensitive adenylate cyclase activity by greater than 70%, as well as increasing the affinity of agonists for the receptors. More relevant is the observation that a large change in pharmacological specificity occurs when striatal dopamine receptors are compared in a slice and homogenate preparation (Saiani et al. 1979). When using whole cells of the anterior pituitary, one must control uptake of the ligand by the use of specific inhibitors or by performing the binding at 0°C. Another possibility is to lightly fix the cells as has been done for prolactin receptors (Salih et al. 1979), although this itself may modify certain dynamic parameters which participate in living cell binding.

2. *Species, time of sacrifice and hormonal status.* As in many other biological systems, species differences may exist in dopamine receptors of the anterior pituitary. In particulate preparations, differences in agonist and antagonist activity at dopamine receptors are observed between calf, rat and human corpus striatum. For example, sulpiride and meto-clopramide (dopamine antagonists) are 3–10 times more potent in rat and human than in calf homogenates (Creese et al. 1979c), although these differences may be attributable to the immaturity of the calf striatum. In our initial studies of the porcine anterior pituitary, dopamine itself is a much more potent agonist in displacing antagonist binding in the pig than in the steer. Detailed analyses are required to determine whether this phenomenon is based on artifact (e.g., washing out endogenous guanine nucleotide, species difference in particulate sedimenting properties) or is truly a species difference in the nature of the receptor complex.

In addition to species variation, there may be a diurnal rhythm in dopamine receptor activity in the anterior pituitary as there is for alpha- and beta-adrenergic receptors in the brain (Wirz-Justice et al. 1980). This possibility should be strictly controlled in studies that are designed to specify whether receptor numbers change after a perturbation. The light–dark schedule and hour of sacrifice should be consistent between groups and should be reported. The only publication listed in Table 6.1A and B which states when the animals were sacrificed indicates that the anterior pituitary glands were obtained in the 'morning' (DiPaolo et al. 1979), as was the case in our studies of sheep (Cronin et al. 1978) and steer (Cronin and Weiner 1979b) anterior pituitary. It is well known that there is a diurnal pattern of prolactin release from the anterior pituitary, and it is within the realm of possibility that this is partially mediated by dopamine receptor modifications.

It is also probably wise to design binding experiments that wish to show receptor number changes with the hormonal status of the animal under control. A general example: The sex and age of the animals as well as the stage of the reproductive cycle in the case of females should be reported. Whole anterior pituitary measurements of dopamine receptor density, which show no change in ovariectomized versus estradiol treated ovariectomized rats (DiPaolo et al. 1979; Cronin et al. 1980a), may be dramatically different if the data are expressed per mammotroph rather than per whole anterior pituitary or protein. Our work shows that there is a highly significant decrease in mammotroph density in an ovariectomized rat when compared to random cycling female rats (Cronin et al. 1980c).

3. *Radioactive dopaminergic ligands.* Logically, [³H]dopamine itself was first employed in an attempt to directly measure this catecholamine receptor (Seeman et al. 1974; Burt et al. 1975; Brown et al. 1976; Calabro and MacLeod 1976; Cronin et al. 1978). This ligand has been generally abandoned in dopamine receptor systems because of (in part): (1) the generally low affinity measured which made filter separation of bound from free at equilibrium hazardous (Table 6.2); (2) active uptake processes known to exist in dopamine terminal fields; (3) the specter of covalent bonding of the catecholamine to the membrane, as has been shown to occur (Saner and Thoenen 1971; Rotman et al. 1976). An excellent example of this phenomenon is the initial attempts to measure the beta-adrenergic receptor with [³H]catecholamines. This body of work is critically analyzed in two papers (Haber and Wrenn 1976; Lefkowitz et al. 1976). In brief, no stereoselectivity of agonists or antagonists was found in the early studies. The numbers of sites measured in some studies are orders of magnitude greater than calculated values or experience with other receptor systems would dictate. Abuse of the membranes with prolonged incubations at 100°C often increased the amount of [³H]catecholamine that was bound. It must be added as a qualification that

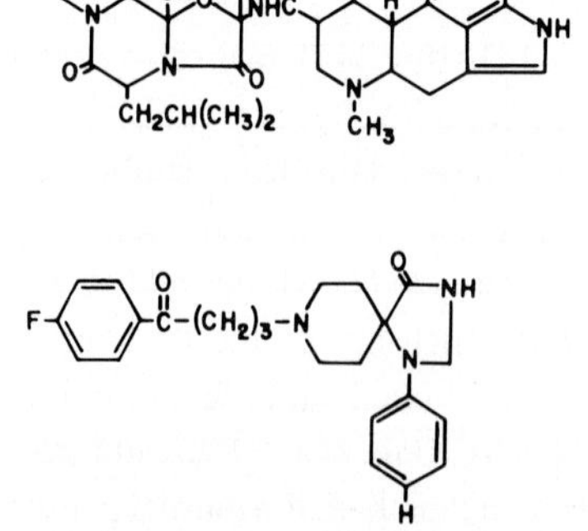

Fig. 6.2. The molecular structures of the three commonly used ³H-labelled ligands for dopamine receptor labelling in the anterior pituitary.

although receptologists have recently avoided the use of [³H]dopamine to label dopamine receptors (see discussion in Creese, 1980), it appears that catecholamine receptors can be measured with some [³H]catecholamine ligands under certain conditions (U'Prichard and Snyder 1978; Titeler et al. 1979a).

As listed in Tables 6.1 and 6.2, ³H-labelled ligands dihydroergocriptine and spiperone (also named spiroperidol) have been extensively utilized to characterize the dopamine receptor in the anterior pituitary. Their structures as well as that of dopamine are shown in Fig. 6.2. Dihydroergocriptine, an ergot alkaloid, functions strictly as a dopamine agonist in the anterior pituitary, inhibiting prolactin release in a dose-dependent manner between 0.1 and 1 nM (Caron et al. 1978). Dihydroergocriptine also labels the alpha-adrenergic receptor in uterine smooth muscle, parotid acinar cells, platelets and brain. In the anterior pituitary, dihydroergocriptine binds predominantly if not exclusively to dopamine receptors (Caron et al. 1978; Cronin et al. 1978; Fig. 6.3). The tritiated molecule not only is stable after freeze–thawing, storage and the conditions of the binding incubation, but also maintains biological potency equal to that of nonradioactive dihydroergocriptine (Caron et al. 1978). Spiperone, a butyrophenone (Fig. 6.2), is the most potent dopamine antagonist known in the anterior pituitary (Denef and Follebouckt 1978). [³H]Spiperone is the ligand of choice by most investigators because of its high affinity and specificity for the dopamine receptor of the anterior pituitary (Tables 6.2, 6.3). This ligand may label serotonin receptors as well (Creese and Snyder 1978a; Leysen et al. 1979), but this is not an issue in the anterior pituitary because of the relatively poor ability of serotonin to displace [³H]spiperone binding (Creese et al. 1977b; Cronin and Weiner 1979; Stefanini et al. 1980b).

Other [³H]labelled ligands which have been applied to the anterior pituitary or may be useful in labelling the dopamine receptors are mentioned here. The original attempts at dopamine receptor binding in the anterior pituitary was with one concentration of [³H]haloperidol (dopamine antagonist) and [³H]dopamine (Brown et al. 1976). To my knowledge, [³H]haloperidol has only been used once since then (Friend et al. 1978), probably because

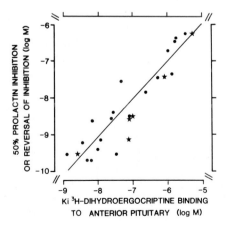

Fig. 6.3. The potency of various agents to compete for [³H]dihydroergocriptine binding to the bovine (closed circles; Caron et al. 1978) and sheep (open circles; Cronin et al. 1978) anterior pituitary is compared with these agents' ability to either inhibit prolactin release or reverse inhibited prolactin release from rat anterior pituitaries in vitro (Caron et al. 1978). The correlation coefficient is 0.93.

Table 6.3

APPARENT INHIBITORY CONSTANTS (nM) OF SELECTED COMPETITORS FOR [³H]SPIPERONE BINDING TO ANTERIOR PITUITARY

	Steer	Steer	Pig	Rat	Rat	Dog
Agonists						
bromocriptine	3	19	6	—	—	—
dl-6,7 ADTN	—	—	23	385	—	890
d-6,7 ADTN	—	—	7	—	—	—
l-6,7 ADTN	—	—	180	—	—	—
apomorphine	300	220	660	247/820	—	420
dl-5,6 ADTN	—	—	308	—	—	—
dopamine	9 000	1 300	—	3 100/5 600	1 800	—
l-epinephrine	81 000	22 000	—	50 000	100 000	—
l-norepinephrine	260 000	18 000	—	50 000	100 000	—
serotonin	68 000	40 000	—	40 000	21 000	40 000
Antagonists						
spiperone	0.4	0.8	—	—	0.2	—
d-butaclamol	1	2	—	1/1	3.2	1
fluphenazine	3	—	—	8	—	—
haloperidol	4	12	—	13/12	—	10
chlorpromazine	22	16	—	—	1,6	—
l-sulpiride	—	220	21	204/460	—	230
metoclopramide	—	—	110	—	—	—
l-butaclamol	12 000	17 000	—	13 000/15 000	—	13 000
d-sulpiride	—	40 000	570	36 000/35 000	—	27 000
References	Creese et al. 1979b	Cronin and Weiner 1979	Cronin, unpubl.	Stefanini et al. 1980a, b	Schaeffer and Hsueh 1979	Stefanini 1980a

of the availability of [³H]spiperone, a more potent dopamine antagonist than haloperidol. The dopamine antagonist [³H]domperidone apparently binds with high affinity to human pituitary homogenates (Bression et al. 1980), but the benefit of this ligand over [³H]spiperone is not apparent. The only dopamine agonist that has come into use in the anterior pituitary other than [³H]dopamine and [³H]dihydroergocriptine is N-n-propyl-N-phenyl-ethyl-beta-(3-hydroxyphenyl) ethylamine hydrochloride ([³H]RU24213). However, it is bothersome that: (1) apomorphine (dopamine agonist) is as potent as clonidine (alpha adrenergic agonist) and phentolamine (alpha adrenergic antagonist) in competing for [³H]RU24213 binding to the anterior pituitary; (2) dihydroergocriptine does not compete for the binding; (3) dopamine's ability to compete for [³H]RU24213 was either not tested or not reported (Di Paolo et al. 1979). Consequently, this ligand remains to be validated as a dopaminergic ligand in the anterior pituitary. Other ligands which have not been applied or not applied successfully to the anterior pituitary, but are useful in other tissues, include the agonists N-[³H]propylapomorphine (Creese et al. 1979a; Titeler and Seeman 1979b) and (±)-2-amino-6,7[³H]dihydroxy-1,2,3,4-tetrahydronapthalene or ADTN (Creese and Snyder 1978b). A possible explanation of the failure to find appropriate binding of [³H]ADTN to the anterior pituitary (M.J. Cronin and R.I. Weiner, unpublished observation) is that ascorbate may have destroyed these sites (Kayaalp and Neff, 1980), as discussed below. Radiolabelled bromocriptine binding studies would be well received due to the vast literature on bromocriptine's biological properties (Goldstein et al. 1980), but the ability to tritiate the molecule to a high specific activity is limiting at the moment.

4. *Ions and other ingredients of the assay:* As Table 6.1A highlights, there is no consensus on the appropriate ingredients or conditions for the dopamine receptor assay in homogenates of the anterior pituitary. It was not apparent when the first studies were accomplished, but these variables may seriously affect many binding parameters. For example, incubation of porcine anterior pituitary homogenates in a Tris (15 mM), ascorbate (0.1 %), EDTA (0.1 mM), pH 7.4 solution rather than our standard buffer with salts (Table 6.1A, B) and EDTA (0.1 mM) roughly doubles the percent of [³H]spiperone binding which is not displaceable with 2 μM d-butaclamol. The affinity of the receptors for dopamine decreases nonsignificantly in the unsalted buffer from 310 ± 100 nM ($n = 8$) to 180 nM ($n = 2$) (M.J. Cronin, unpublished observation). In the striatum, [³H]spiperone binding is augmented by monovalent and divalent cations as well as chelating agents. Mono- and divalent cations also appear to enhance agonist affinity while having no effect on antagonist affinity for the dopamine receptor (Usdin et al. 1980). Added to these probable effects in the anterior pituitary, sodium is required for the interaction of benzamides (e.g. sulpiride and metoclopramide, dopamine antagonists) with the dopamine receptors of the anterior pituitary, while sodium has no apparent effect on neuroleptic (e.g., butaclamol, chlorpromazine, dopamine antagonists) binding to the anterior pituitary (Stefanini et al. 1980a).

Ascorbic acid has been included as an antioxidant in solutions for binding studies (Table 6.1A, B), especially when monoamines were tested for activity. It has been appreciated lately, first with opiate receptors and then with dopamine receptors, that ascorbate can destroy binding sites. In the case of the opiate receptors, irreversible damage to stereoselective binding sites is rapid (i.e., up to 50 % loss in 1 min) as well as oxygen and pH dependent (Dunlap et al. 1979). The concentrations of ascorbate (i.e., mM range) that are reported in the dopamine receptor studies (Table 6.1A and B) cause a 70–90% reduction in opiate receptor binding. This is cause for great concern. A 0.1 mM concentration of EDTA protects the opiate receptor from the ascorbate effects, and this is now a standard constituent of our ion-buffer solution. In the case of the dopamine receptors of the striatum, similar concentrations of ascorbate irreversibly damage the specific binding of the agonists ADTN and apomorphine but have no effect on the antagonists spiperone and haloperidol. Furthermore, other reducing agents, which may have substituted for ascorbate, cause the same decrease in binding (Kayaalp and Neff 1980). Thus, although some investigators may have been fortunate by using the antagonist [^{3}H]spiperone in the anterior pituitary with ascorbate and without EDTA, we recommend that this interaction be critically tested before conclusions are made about a ligand's interaction in the anterior pituitary.

Binding properties of the dopamine receptors in the anterior pituitary

1. *Kinetics.* The measured rate constants of association and dissociation of [^{3}H]dihydroergocriptine and [^{3}H]spiperone in the anterior pituitary are listed in Table 6.2. Some of the studies did not calculate these values because of tissue volume limitations (i.e., human and rat anterior pituitary) or the speed of the events (i.e., [^{3}H]dopamine binding). The association of spiperone is very fast, to a great extent limited by the speed of diffusion, while dissociation caused by the addition of excess *d*-butaclamol is a protracted event. The association of both ^{3}H-labelled ligands is also temperature sensitive (Cronin et al. 1978; Cronin and Weiner 1979b).

In an ideal situation, the rate of dopamine binding to the receptor in the anterior pituitary would coincide with the rate of prolactin inhibition. These measurements have not been made because of the speed at which prolactin is inhibited by dopamine (Thorner et al. 1980a) and the inherent methodological problems with [^{3}H]dopamine binding (see above). This study may be best performed with an ergot alkaloid at less than 37°C because of the relatively slow on-rate of binding at 30°C (Caron et al. 1978) and onset of prolactin inhibition (Yeo et al. 1979). On the other hand, as with other catecholamine receptor systems, the more utilitarian ligands for careful kinetic experiments are antagonists because of their high affinity binding. In association reactions, one is condemned to correlate antagonist binding with disinhibition of prolactin release in the presence of agonist inhibitor. The dissociation of antagonists seems to be more amenable to quantitation because of the slow rates of dissociation measured. This could be correlated with the rate of appearance of dopamine inhibited prolactin release. It is worth noting that the kinetics of binding of experimental ligands are usually not applicable to the kinetics of the naturally occurring agonists, since the physiological effect is rapid in occurrence and cessation, by design. The existence of other mechanisms for inactivation in an intact system (e.g., reuptake, catabolism) and the absence of many of these properties in homogenates or the inability of these mechanisms to act on synthetic ligands is also a confounding factor.

2. *Equilibrium studies.* (2i). *Saturation isotherms.* Saturation isotherms of a variety of ligands and in various species have been generated to estimate dissociation constants (K_d) and numbers of binding sites in the anterior pituitary and tumors (Tables 6.2, 6.4; Fig. 6.4).

Table 6.4

DOPAMINERGIC LIGAND BINDING TO ALTERED PROLACTIN SECRETING CELLS

Cell type	[3H]-labelled ligand	K_d (nm)	Binding sites	Temperature	Reference
Human prolactinomas	Domperidone	0.29/4.19	513/1134 fm/mg protein	30°C	Bression et al. 1980
	Spiperone	3.1	707 fm/mg assay protein	22–24°C	Cronin et al. 1980d
Rat GH$_3$ clone	Spiperone	570	7×10^6 sites/cell (broken)	37°C	Cronin et al. 1980e
	Spiperone	830	4×10^7 sites/cell (intact)	23°C	Cronin et al. 1980e
Rat 7315a tumor	Spiperone	0.1	66 fm/mg assay protein	22–24°C	Cronin, Valdenegro, Perkins and MacLeod, unpublished observations
Rat MtTW15 tumor	Spiperone	0.2	143 fm/mg assay protein	22–24°C	Cronin, Valdenegro and MacLeod, unpublished observations

186

The usual method of defining saturable binding has been with an excess of nonradioactive competitor, but mathematical estimations of saturable binding can also be made (Fig. 6.4). There are fewer total dopamine receptors in the anterior pituitary than in the corpus striatum (Creese et al. 1977b; Cronin et al. 1980b), but the affinities of the sites for many agents appear to be comparable, suggesting that a similar species of receptor exists in both tissues (Creese et al. 1977b).

The majority of authors interpret their saturation data in terms of one class of dopamine receptor in the anterior pituitary based on the apparent linearity of Scatchard plots. However, some investigators suggest the existence of more than one class of dopamine receptor based on a nonlinear Scatchard plot when low concentrations of [3H]-labelled ligand are used (Calabro and MacLeod 1978; Cronin and Weiner 1979a; DiPaolo et al. 1979; Bression et al. 1980). This observation has also been made in the corpus striatum (Briley and Langer 1978; Pedigo et al. 1978; Cronin and Weiner 1979a), where it is postulated that the two putative sites represent pre- and post-synaptic receptors. This interpretation cannot be made in the anterior pituitary, since there are no presynaptic dopamine terminals here. At this juncture, no one has resolved whether the phenomenon of a nonlinear Scatchard plot in the anterior pituitary is due to two populations of binding sites, negative cooperativity in one class of binding sites, or an artifact. This will be important to resolve in the near future. If there are two receptors in the anterior pituitary, both will have to be accurately monitored after a perturbation to be able to conclude that there is an effect on either or both of the receptor types. It is technically difficult to do this at present because of limitations of resolution and the specific activity of the ligands. In addition, a nonlinear Scatchard plot is not consistently observed.

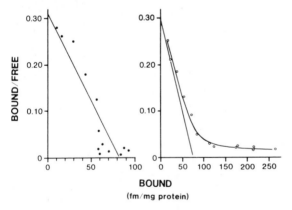

Fig. 6.4. A saturation isotherm of [3H]spiperone binding to the porcine anterior pituitary has been generated in two ways. On the left, the specific binding points on the Scatchard plot were derived with a 1000-fold K_d excess of d-butaclamol as is commonly done (see Table 6.1). On the right, the specific or saturable binding was estimated by fitting the total binding data (i.e. open circles with fitted curved line) by a nonlinear least squares program (Cronin et al. unpublished observation). The derived fit is the straight line in the right graph which numerically matches the same experiment depicted in the left plot. In this and other experiments, both the site numbers and K_d values defined by both methods are identical, and the fit is best to one class of binding sites. An advantage of the least squares fitted design is that it requires half the tissue that the drug-displacement design requires for the same number of points.

Finally, based on the ability of one concentration of nonradioactive agonist to reduce the [³H]spiperone site number without changing [³H]spiperone's K_d in an anterior pituitary homogenate, Sibley and Creese (1980b) conclude that the "... correct interpretation of this data then is that agonists *competitively* displace [³H]spiperone from two binding sites, one which has a high and one which has a low agonist affinity (p. 132)." One cannot make this exclusive judgement based on the data shown. An equally tenable hypothesis to explain these data is that an agonist site allosterically modulates the binding of [³H]spiperone to another site which has relatively low affinity for agonist.

(2ii). *Competiton studies.* The potency with which a large array of agents competes for ³H-labelled agonist or ³H-labelled antagonist binding to the anterior pituitary has been exploited to characterize these sites. To satisfy the criteria of pharmacological and biological specificity, the rank order of potency of these agents should coincide with the order expected of a dopamine interaction, as well as parallel the ability of agonists to inhibit and antagonists to reverse inhibited prolactin release in vitro.

In the most elegant work to date, Caron and associates (1978) report a strong correlation between an agent's potency for the [³H]dihydroergocriptine binding sites and the agent's ability to modulate prolactin release. This relationship is depicted graphically in Fig. 6.3. The two studies of [³H]dihydroergocriptine binding to anterior pituitary homogenates strongly suggest that this ergot binds to a stereoselective dopamine receptor (Caron et al. 1978; Cronin et al. 1978).

The characteristics of [³H]spiperone binding to the anterior pituitary have been more intensely studied. Table 6.3 lists the apparent inhibitory constants (K_i) for selected agonists and antagonists. The order of agonist potency (e.g., bromocriptine > apomorphine > dopamine > epinephrine ≥ norepinephrine) is appropriate for a dopaminergic interaction and is consistent with the order of potency of these agents to inhibit prolactin release in vitro. In addition, there is a strong intrinsic selectivity revealed with the alpha rotamer of ADTN (Table 6.3). The relative potency with which several species of ADTN compete for [³H]spiperone binding to the anterior pituitary (Table 6.3) parallels their potency to inhibit prolactin secretion (Thorner, unpublished observations; Rick et al. 1979 for 5,6- and 6,7-ADTN). Regarding antagonist competition for [³H]spiperone binding, the order of potency at the [³H]spiperone labelled sites (e.g., spiperone > d-butaclamol > haloperidol > chlorpromazine > 1-sulpiride > 1-butaclamol) is identical to the order of disinhibition of prolactin release by these agents (Denef and Follebouckt 1978).

Other agents which can affect prolactin secretion in vivo have little or no effect on binding to the dopamine receptor. These include the following (extracted from Caron et al. 1978; Cronin et al. 1978; Cronin and Weiner 1979b; Schaeffer and Hsueh 1979; Cronin et al. 1980a): catecholamine precursors and metabolites, carbidopa, reserpine, thyrotropin-releasing hormone, substance P, neurotensin, somatostatin, gamma aminobutyric acid, morphine, beta-endorphin, endorphin analogs, melanocyte stimulating hormone, triiodo-thyronine, estrone, 17β-estradiol, estriol, methoxyestrone and 2-hydroxyestrone. The catecholestrogen 2-hydroxyestradiol competes for [³H]spiperone binding with an apparent K_i of about 10 μM (Schaeffer and Hsueh, 1979).

(2iii). *Guanine nucleotides.* A plasmalemma guanine nucleotide binding protein (Ross et al. 1978; Howlett et al. 1979) appears to influence agonist receptor binding properties in many diverse systems, both adenylate cyclase linked (e.g. beta-adrenergic, glucagon) and unlinked (e.g. alpha-adrenergic, opiate, angiotensin II). In general, the addition of guanosine triphosphate to subcellular preparations decreases agonist affinity, while there is no effect on antagonist affinity for ^{3}H-labelled agonist or labelled antagonist receptors.

The dopamine receptors of the anterior pituitary are also sensitive to this guanine nucleotide phenomenon (Beach et al. 1979; Caron 1979; Sibley and Creese 1979). Guanosine triphosphate and diphosphate as well as the non-hydrolysable analog 5′-guanylimide-diphosphate (i.e. Gpp(NH)p) increase the apparent K_i for dopamine and apomorphine 2–7 fold (Beach et al. 1979) or 40–80 fold (Caron 1979), while there is no effect with guanosine monophosphate, guanosine or adenosine triphosphate (Beach et al. 1979). Antagonist affinity is not affected by guanosine triphosphate (Beach et al. 1979; Caron 1979; Sibley and Creese 1979), nor is the affinity of bromocriptine (Beach et al. 1979; Sibley and Creese 1979) or dihydroergocriptine (Beach, Cronin and Weiner, unpublished observation), a curious finding. This property suggests that ergots may: (1) bind to the dopamine receptor at the site that dopamine binds, because bromocriptine competes for [^{3}H]dopamine binding in the anterior pituitary (Calabro and MacLeod 1978), as well as bind to another site on the receptor which mimics or prevents the action of guanine nucleotides; (2) bind to the dopamine receptor as well as to the regulatory protein, thus mimicking or preventing the action of guanine nucleotides. This is a fascinating property which hopefully can be exploited in dissecting the initial mechanisms of transduction.

The function of the guanine nucleotide shift at the level of the receptor may be to increase the off-rate of the agonist (U'Prichard and Snyder 1979), so that a change in extracellular ligand concentration can be rapidly sensed. In fact, the high agonist affinities observed in broken cells may be artifactually increased by washing out endogenous guanine nucleotides. For example, the beta-adrenergic agonist affinity in intact cells is similar to the guanine nucleotide reduced affinity in broken S49 lymphoma cells (Insel and Stoolman 1978; Ross et al. 1978). Differential removal of endogenous nucleotides with various homogenization and washing protocols may account for the difference in the magnitude of the dopamine K_i shift described for the anterior pituitary (i.e. Beach et al. 1979, 4× increase; Sibley and Creese 1979, 11× increase; versus Caron 1979, 40–80× increase). Furthermore, this could explain why the apparent K_i for dopamine in homogenates of porcine anterior pituitary is roughly an order of magnitude higher affinity than we had observed in steer anterior pituitary (Table 6.3). When these porcine anterior pituitary receptors are studied in the presence of Gpp(NH)p, there is a 20-fold decrease in dopamine's affinity, from an apparent K_i of 310 nM to 6200 nM (Cronin, unpublished observation). This is unlike the 4-fold shift we observed in steer anterior pituitary glands (Beach et al. 1979), but reminiscent of Caron's (1979) 40–80 fold shift of agonist affinity in the bovine anterior pituitary.

(2iv). *Calcium ionophore and antagonist effects.* Both calcium ionophores and calcium antagonists are now popular tools being used to construct a mechanistic scheme for dopamine inhibition of prolactin release in vitro. The removal of extracellular calcium produces a marked reduction in prolactin secretion from the anterior pituitary (Thorner et al. 1980a) and action potentials with a calcium component have been recorded in cells of anterior pituitary origin (Taraskevich and Douglas 1978; Dufy et al. 1979). Recently, it was demonstrated that dopamine inhibition of prolactin release could be blocked by calcium ionophores (Tam and Dannies 1980; Thorner et al. 1980a), and that the calcium channel blockers manganese and D-600 cause a reversible inhibition of prolactin release (Thorner et al. 1980a).

We tested calcium ionophores and channel blockers for their ability to interact with dopamine receptor binding, and some surprising results were produced. In the case of the ionophores A23187 and X537A, it was expected that there would be no interaction, since A23187 stimulated prolactin release in GH_3 cells (Tam and Dannies 1980), a prolactin-secreting clone that does not have detectable dopamine receptors (Cronin et al. 1980e). However, both ionophores dramatically increase the specific binding of [^{3}H]spiperone in the presence of anterior pituitary homogenates. This is entirely accounted for by enhanced binding to the GF/C filters in a dose-dependent manner (1–100 μM) (Cronin, unpublished observation). This artifact could have easily been interpreted as a specific ionophore-dopamine receptor interaction without a homogenate-free control experiment.

The calcium antagonist effect on dopamine receptor binding is more confusing at this point. We have found that both D-600 and verapamil compete for [^{3}H]spiperone binding to homogenates of the anterior pituitary, with apparent K_i values of 4100 nM ($n = 3$) and 1800 nM ($n = 2$), respectively. The potassium channel blocker tetraethyl ammonium chloride had no effect on binding up to 0.01 M ($n = 2$). Furthermore, both D-600 and verapamil significantly reduce [^{3}H]spiperone binding to GF/C filters by roughly 30–50%. Filter binding of [^{3}H]spiperone is less than 10% of tissue binding, so that the effect of these antagonists on the filter can not account for the 80% reduction in binding to the homogenate (Table 6.5; Cronin, unpublished observations). This finding is not unique to the dopamine receptor of the anterior pituitary. In both brain and heart, D-600 competitively blocked binding to the alpha$_1$ and alpha$_2$ adrenergic receptor, while potassium antagonists interact noncompetitively for alpha$_2$ but not alpha$_1$ adrenergic receptors in rat brain (Glossman and Hornung 1980). It is tempting to speculate from these data that the dopamine receptor may

Table 6.5

THE EFFECT OF ION CHANNEL ANTAGONISTS ON [^{3}H]SPIPERONE BINDING TO FILTER AND ANTERIOR PITUITARY HOMOGENATES

	Filter binding (fm per filter)	n	Anterior pituitary homogenate binding (fm per tube)	n
Total binding	2.01 ± 0.05	4	18.77 ± 0.25	7
d-Butaclamol (2 μM)	1.89 ± 0.28	4	3.31 ± 0.19	4
D-600 (0.1 mM)	1.10 ± 0.04	4	not measured	
Verapamil (0.1 mM)	1.24 ± 0.04	3	3.69	2
Tetraethylammonium chloride	not measured		18.63 ± 0.83	3

Values expressed as means ± SEM: 0.58 nM [^{3}H]spiperone with porcine anterior pituitary homogenates.

be structurally associated with calcium channels in the mammotroph, but this must await more rigorous experimentation.

(2v). *Multiple binding sites*. Various arguments have been recruited to support the hypothesis that multiple dopamine receptor types exist in the anterior pituitary. Among these are the following.

Biphasic binding and biological response. The observation of nonlinear Scatchard plots of saturation isotherms has been noted above. One of several interpretations of these data is that this represents more than one class of dopamine receptors in the anterior pituitary. In terms of prolactin secretion, while it has been exhaustively demonstrated that dopamine inhibits prolactin release at concentrations usually ranging from 1 nM to 1 μM, prolactin release is stimulated by lower dopamine concentrations in vitro (Cheung and Weiner 1978; Denef et al. 1980). Multiple receptor types or an allosteric shift in one dopamine receptor class can be invoked to explain this phenomenon.

Pharmacological differences. Pharmacological probes may indeed be able to elucidate multiple dopamine receptor types in the anterior pituitary. The fact that benzamide binding is sodium dependent (Stefanini et al. 1980a) and that guanine nucleotides do not reduce the affinity of the dopamine receptor for the agonist bromocriptine as well as antagonists (Beach et al. 1979; Sibley and Creese 1979) may be strong clues that multiple receptors or multiple subsites on a dopamine receptor complex do exist. Alternatively, these phenomena may be based on perturbations that alter the relationship between a universal class of dopamine receptor and the second messenger(s).

Some pharmacological disparities which have been exploited to distinguish a so-called D-1 and D-2 dopamine receptor (Kebabian and Calne 1979) may be artifacts of the assays used. Maguire, Ross and Gilman's edict states that if one is to compare binding and biological response (e.g. adenyl cyclase activity) quantitatively, "...experiments must be performed under identical conditions... Disparities (between binding and response)... can be far more complex and may be exquisitely dependent on incubation condition or on the identity of the individual competing ligand used." (Maguire et al. 1977). In all studies of dopaminergic binding and response to date, especially the measurement of dopamine-sensitive adenylate cyclase, the conditions of the two types of measurements differ. For example, a discrepancy exists between benzamide (e.g. sulpiride and metoclopramide) binding to dopamine receptors and benzamides' potency to block dopamine-sensitive adenylate cyclase in the corpus striatum. This difference is used to support the hypothesis of a D-1 (i.e. benzamide non-sensitive) and a D-2 (i.e. benzamide sensitive) receptor population (Kebabian and Calne 1979). The observation is that although benzamides are dopamine antagonists in the anterior pituitary and brain, they do not antagonize striatal dopamine-stimulated adenylate cyclase (referenced in Kebabian and Calne 1979). What was not recognized was that benzamide binding to the dopamine receptor of the anterior pituitary (Stefanini et al. 1980a) and the corpus striatum (Stefanini et al. 1980c) is sodium dependent. The non-cyclase dopamine antagonistic properties of benzamides in the anterior pituitary (e.g. reversal of prolactin inhibition) and striatum were tested in sodium replete conditions, while the ability of the benzamides to block dopamine-stimulated adenylate cyclase in the corpus striatum was tested in a sodium-free buffer system. Thus, one would expect to observe no interaction because the benzamides could not bind in the sodium-free environment.

This author also believes that it may be dangerous to make a major issue out of the absolute numbers gained with competition studies in the anterior pituitary and the response of prolactin secretion. Indeed, Fig. 6.3 shows that the binding of [^{3}H]dihydroergocriptine is shifted by about an order of magnitude from the prolactin response. This may be based on the species used (i.e. bovine in binding and rat in prolactin release), assay protein content differences (Brown et al. 1976), guanine nucleotide differences, etc. Inhibitory constants are now characteristically termed 'apparent K_i' because of such uncontrolled variables as the true free [^{3}H]spiperone concentration (Hartley and Seeman 1978). Variation between laboratories can be appreciated from Table 6.3. Finally, with the multiple mechanisms between binding and secretion, along with the possibility of different gains or sensitivities on each of these steps, one might be surprised if there was a simple relationship between stimulus and response in the mammotroph.

Adenylate cyclase linked and unlinked dopamine receptors. The existence of dopamine receptors which do or do not interact with adenylate cyclase is not strong grounds for proposing two types of dopamine receptor. The same receptor species could cause many effects depending on which second messenger is expressed in a given cell (e.g. adenylate cyclase, calcium channel control). The anterior pituitary dopamine receptor is the exemplar of the so-called D-2 type dopamine receptor because (in part) it is considered to be unlinked to adenylate cyclase (Kebabian and Calne 1979). In fact, the current evidence does not support this classification because the dopamine receptor may be linked to adenylate cyclase, but as an inhibitor of the adenylate cyclase activity (Hill et al. 1976; Barnes et al. 1978; Markstein et al. 1978; DeCamilli et al. 1979; Labrie et al. 1980a).

Ascorbate effects. Ascorbic acid preferentially destroys dopamine agonist (i.e. ADTN and apomorphine) but not dopamine antagonist (i.e. spiperone and haloperidol) binding in the corpus striatum (Kayaalp and Neff 1980). This has not been tested in the anterior pituitary. The observation suggests that multiple receptor types or multiple subsites on a receptor species exist in the corpus striatum.

Thermal effects. Differential thermal sensitivity suggests that multiple dopamine receptor types are present in the striatum. A brief exposure of striatal membranes to a high temperature decreases the affinity of agonists (i.e. dopamine and apomorphine) but has no effect on antagonist (i.e. spiperone and haloperidol) competitions for the dopamine receptor (Goldstein et al. 1980). This also has not been tested in the anterior pituitary.

To conclude this section, it is unassailable that dopamine receptors exist in the mammalian anterior pituitary as shown by direct radioligand binding studies. The ability to label the dopamine receptor directly should encourage investigators not only to become more quantitative in probing the mechanisms of prolactin inhibition, but also to further characterize the nature of the receptor complex itself. Because there are no presynaptic terminals in the anterior pituitary, the anterior pituitary could provide a utilitarian prototype of the postsynaptic species of dopamine receptor. Finally, in order to legitimately compare binding with another activity of the cell (e.g. adenylate cyclase activity), the conditions of the assays should be identical if at all possible.

3. *Binding properties of altered prolactin secreting cells*. Once the radioligand binding assay had been reasonably well validated in the normal anterior pituitary, it was envisioned that its application to altered prolactin secreting cells like those in human prolactinomas could shed some light on the level of failure in these abnormally behaving cells. For example, is the inability of dopamine to inhibit prolactin secretion in some tumor cells based on a loss of that cell's expression of the dopamine receptor? In addition, the presence of dopamine receptors in established prolactin secreting tumors or cell cultures would be productive in that massive numbers of a homogenous or near-homogenous cell type could be grown and studied. Thus, detailed quantification of receptors per prolactin cell, the measurement of intact cell binding characteristics and the search for second messenger(s) may be more readily accomplished with this approach than by starting with the heterogenous cell types of the anterior pituitary. The following discussion surveys the results of such studies to date, and Table 6.6 lists the apparent inhibition constants of selected competitors in normal anterior pituitary, a prolactin-secreting clone (GH_3) and a prolactin-secreting hard tumor (7315a).

(3i). *GH_3 Clone*. Some of the prolactin and growth hormone secreting GH_3 clones (Tashjian et al. 1968) express functional thyrotropin releasing hormone (Hinkel and Tashjian. 1973), somatostatin (Schonbrun and Tashjian. 1978) and epidermal growth factor (Schonbrun et al. 1979) receptors. However, the GH_3 clone was demonstrated to be hyporesponsive or unresponsive to dopamine or dopamine agonist inhibition of prolactin release in most cases (Dannies and Tashjian 1973; Bang and Gautvik 1977; Malarkey et al. 1977; Faure et al. 1980; Melmed et al. 1980; Tam and Dannies 1980). On the contrary, 16 nM dopamine inhibited prolactin secretion by 30% from GH_3B_6 cells (Dufy et al. 1979) and 10 μM dopamine reduced prolactin release by 30% in solid GH_3 tumors grown in rats (Melmed et al. 1980). Based on the majority of the evidence, we hypothesized that the GH_3 cells either lost the expression of the dopamine receptor or harbored a defect distal to a

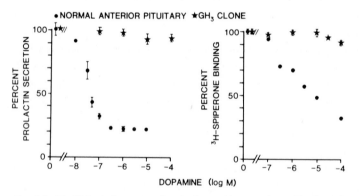

Fig. 6.5. The biological response of prolactin secretion to an increasing dopamine concentration is shown in the left graph for the normal anterior pituitary (Caron et al. 1978) and GH_3 clone (Faure et al. 1980). The right box graphs the potency with which dopamine competes for the [³H]spiperone binding site in the porcine anterior pituitary (Cronin, unpublished observation) and the GH_3 clone (Cronin et al. 1980e). It is clear that the biological response and dopamine receptor binding in the GH_3 clone has been compromised when compared to the normal anterior pituitary.

Table 6.6

APPARENT K_i VALUES WITH [^{3}H]SPIPERONE BINDING TO PROLACTIN-SECRETING CELLS

	Normal pituitary[A]	n	GH$_3$ Clone[B]	n	7315a Tumor[C]	n
Agonists						
Bromocriptine	19 ± 15	3	$5\,000 \pm 500$	3	10 ± 4	4
Apomorphine	220 ± 80	7	$14\,000 \pm 2\,500$	4	250 ± 70	4
Dopamine	$1\,300 \pm 40$	3	$>40\,000$	2	$2\,900 \pm 1\,200$	4
Epinephrine	$22\,000 \pm 10\,000$	3	$>40\,000$	2	$17\,000 \pm 1\,000$	3
Serotonin	$>40\,000$	2	$>40\,000$	2	$>40\,000$	2
Histamine	$>40\,000$	2	$>40\,000$	2	$>40\,000$	2
Antagonists						
Spiperone	0.8 ± 0.4	4	$1\,500 \pm 300$	5	0.12 ± 0.03	3
d-Butaclamol	1.6 ± 0.5	5	$1\,200 \pm 240$	4	0.7 ± 0.3	3
Haloperidol	12 ± 3	4	680 ± 120	3	4.1 ± 0.6	4
Chlorpromazine	16 ± 6	3	170 ± 70	5	7.8 ± 2.4	3
l-Butaclamol	$17\,000 \pm 5\,000$	3	$1\,300 \pm 250$	3	$8\,600 \pm 1\,000$	5

K_i values are expressed as mean (nM) $\pm$ SEM with n independent experiments.

[A] from Cronin and Weiner (1979).

[B] from Cronin et al. (1980e).

[C] from Cronin, Valdenegro, Perkins and MacLeod (unpublished observations).

normal dopamine receptor population. Using the dopamine antagonist [^{3}H]spiperone, we were unable to measure high affinity binding in both broken and intact cells (Table 6.4), and we concluded that the major lesion is at the level of the dopamine receptor itself (Cronin et al. 1980e). Fig. 6.5 illustrates the biological and binding refractoriness of the GH$_3$ clone compared to normal anterior pituitary glands.

Although no high affinity binding can be measured in the GH$_3$ cells, low affinity binding is saturable but not stereoselective. Both d- and l-butaclamol are equipotent at the [^{3}H]spiperone binding sites (Cronin et al. 1980e; Table 6.6) and in inhibiting prolactin release from the GH$_3$D$_6$ cells at high concentrations (Faure et al. 1980). In the normal anterior pituitary, binding and biological activity of low concentrations of these isomers of butaclamol differ by roughly three orders of magnitude (Table 6.3; Creese et al. 1977b; Caron et al. 1978; Denef and Folleboukt 1978; Cronin and Weiner 1979b). The high pharmacological concentrations of dopamine antagonists, which may be chaotropic in the membrane or may antagonize calcium fluxes (Denef et al. 1979), also reduce prolactin release from normal anterior pituitary glands in a nonstereoselective manner, while lower concentrations cause no biological effect alone but reverse dopamine agonist inhibition of prolactin release (MacLeod and Lamberts 1978; West and Dannies 1979). The mechanism of this rather non-specific phenomenon remains to be disclosed.

In the hyperplastic GH$_3$D$_6$ clone, which actively secretes prolactin and growth hormone, the expression of high affinity dopamine receptors has been silenced or muted. This in turn compromises the ability of dopamine agonists to reduce prolactin release. There exists low affinity binding and biological responsiveness to dopamine antagonists which is not related to the dopamine receptor and may be present normally in the anterior pituitary. Whether the absence of measurable high affinity dopamine receptors is based on a genotypic and phenotypic dominance of the somatotroph in this hybrid cell, is a property of rapidly

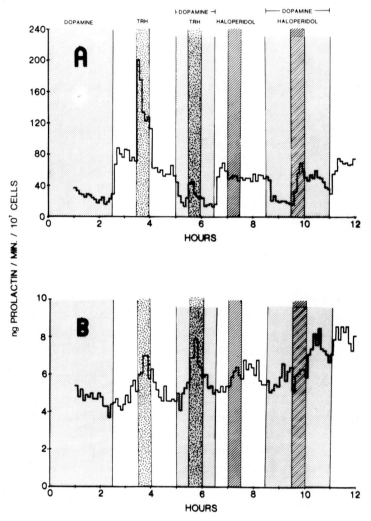

Fig. 6.6. The response of dispersed 7315a transplantable pituitary cells (B) or dispersed normal anterior pituitary cells (A) of female rats to a variety of agents is shown. Both kinds of cells were treated simultaneously in parallel columns of an isolated cell column perfusion apparatus. The 7315a tumor was unresponsive to 500nM pulses of dopamine, whereas the normal mammotroph was inhibited briskly. The dopamine antagonist haloperidol appears to have stimulated prolactin release from tumor cells, but in other tumor column experiments, no change in secretion was observed during haloperidol (50 nM) perfusion in the presence or absence of dopamine. Haloperidol had no effect on uninhibited prolactin release from the normal mammotroph, but reversed the dopamine inhibited release. Thyrotropin releasing hormone (TRH, 25 ng ml^{-1}) clearly stimulated prolactin release from both tumor and normal mammotroph cells in this and several other studies.

dividing cells or is a true functional lesion, the resolution of this issue should be actively pursued.

(3ii). *7315a Transplantable AP tumor.* The prolactin and ACTH secreting 7315a transplantable tumor was originally induced in the anterior pituitary by 2,4,6-trimethylaniline (Bates et al. 1966). As with the GH_3 clone, the 7315a cells are relatively (De Quijada et al. 1980) or absolutely (Cronin and MacLeod, unpublished observation; Fig. 6.6) refractory to dopamine agonist inhibition of prolactin release. Furthermore, chronic bromocriptine treatment of tumor-bearing rats has no impact on plasma prolactin or tumor size (Lamberts and MacLeod 1979). On the other hand, chronic treatment with the dopamine antagonist haloperidol doubles circulating prolactin levels (Login et al. 1981).

Because of our experience with the GH_3 clone, we expected to find no measurable dopamine receptors in the 7315a tumor. We were surprised to discover substantial binding of [^{3}H]spiperone to homogenates of the tumor. This binding is high affinity, low capacity (Table 6.4), stereoselective (Table 6.6) and reversible. The rank order of potency of a large variety of agonists and antagonists is appropriate for a dopaminergic interaction, and the apparent K_i values are similar to those previously observed in normal anterior pituitary homogenates (Fig. 6.7). Finally, the guanine nucleotide analogue Gpp(NH)p selectively lowers the affinity of the binding sites for the agonists dopamine, apomorphine and 6,7 ADTN while having no impact on the binding of the antagonists haloperidol, d-butaclamol, l-sulpiride and the agonist bromocriptine. Therefore, regarding the biochemical parameters measured, there is no obvious difference between the receptors in the 7315a tumor and the normal anterior pituitary. This finding stands in contrast to the situation in the GH_3 clone.

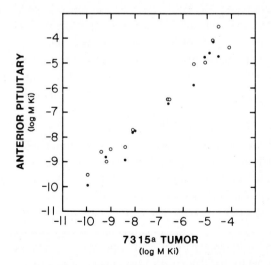

Fig. 6.7. The apparent K_i values of various agents competing for [^{3}H]spiperone binding to homogenates of the 7315a tumor are compared to the apparent K_i values of the same agents competing for [^{3}H]spiperone binding to homogenates of the normal anterior pituitary. A strong correlation exists suggesting that the dopamine receptors of the 7315a tumor are normal. Open circles are normal anterior pituitary values from the work of Creese and coworkers (1977b) and closed circles are values from the work of Cronin and Weiner (1979b).

Several hypotheses can be put forward to reconcile this dilemma of biological refractoriness in the presence of apparently normal receptors. (1) The number of dopamine receptors per tumor cell may be less than that of normal mammotrophs. This may limit or entirely compromise the inhibitory response. The resolution of this must await a pure preparation of tumor cells and normal mammotrophs so that receptors per cell can be enumerated. (2) A functional lesion lateral or distal to the dopamine receptor may exist. This would not set a precedent, since hybrid S49 lymphoma cells can exhibit normal beta-adrenergic receptor binding but have a compromised biological response due to a reduction in adenylate cyclase activity (Maguire et al. 1977). Other S49 lymphoma hybrids are deficient in beta-adrenergic receptors (Maguire et al. 1977; Johnson et al. 1979). The second messenger(s) for dopamine in the normal mammotroph must be elucidated before this hypothesis can be tested directly. (3) These 7315a tumor cells may be chronically locked into an inhibitory state. The many tumor cells secreting so-called 'transformed' (Grosvenor et al. 1980) or 'uninhibitable' prolactin may be adequate to increase blood prolactin to the extraordinary levels measured. In this case, little or no further inhibition could be imposed on the cells by dopamine agonists, although normal dopamine receptors are present. The observation that dispersed 7315a tumor cells release less prolactin than dispersed female anterior pituitary glands (Fig. 6.6) would mildly support this position, especially considering that only 20–30 % of the cells in the female rat anterior pituitary are mammotrophs. The 7315a cells are not panhyporesponsive, since both thyrotropin-releasing hormone (Fig. 6.6) and estradiol treatment (R.M. MacLeod, personal communication) stimulate prolactin release.

(3iii). *MtTW15 transplantable AP tumor.* Preliminary studies have also been performed on the prolactin- and growth hormone-secreting MtTW15 tumor which was originally induced by stilbestrol (Furth et al. 1956). As with the 7315a tumor, the MtTW15 is relatively (MacLeod et al. 1980a) or absolutely (Cronin, Valdenegro and MacLeod, unpublished observation) refractory to dopamine agonist inhibition of prolactin release. There also appears to be high affinity, saturable, reversible and stereoselective binding sites for [^{3}H]spiperone, which implies that these cells are more akin to the 7315a cells than the GH$_3$ cells.

Regarding the in situ anterior pituitary of the MtTW15 tumor-bearing rats, it is well documented that hyperprolactinemia increases dopamine activity in the tuberoinfundibular dopamine neurons (Moore et al. 1980). This in turn results in reduced anterior pituitary wet weight (MacLeod et al. 1966; Cronin and MacLeod, unpublished observation) and an enhanced inhibition of newly synthesized prolactin (MacLeod and Abad 1968) and prolactin content (MacLeod et al. 1966) of the anterior pituitary. These effects are reversed by haloperidol treatment (MacLeod and Lehmeyer 1974), indicating that they are dependent on dopaminergic mechanisms. [^{3}H]Spiperone binding in these anterior pituitary glands has also been measured in preliminary experiments, and there is no gross change in affinity or site number (M.J. Cronin, J. Ramsdell and R.M. MacLeod, unpublished observation).

(3iv). *Human prolactin secreting pituitary adenomas.* The prolactin secreting adenoma is the most common tumor in the human anterior pituitary (Faglia et al. 1980). This is generally a locus of mammotrophs (50–80 % mammotroph; Peake et al. 1969; Zimmerman et al. 1974; Hymer et al. 1976) which can be visualized and surgically removed. The majority of patients with prolactinomas respond to treatment with the potent dopamine agonist bromocriptine, and their circulating prolactin concentrations return to normal. Recently, several human prolactinomas attached to a basement membrane have been studied in vitro. There is no apparent difference in the potency of dopamine-inhibited prolactin release when human anterior pituitary glands are compared to the prolactinomas (Bethea et al. 1981). This implies that the dopamine receptor may be intact on many of these adenomatous cells. In support of this claim, we were able to measure high affinity and saturable binding of [3H]spiperone in several human prolactinomas. There are more binding sites per protein in the prolactinomas than in control anterior pituitary glands which were from patients with prostate or breast cancer. This is rationalized on the basis of the greater density of mammotrophs in the adenomas than in the control anterior pituitary glands. Thus, one would expect more binding per protein because the cell type expressing the dopamine receptor (i.e. mammotroph) was enriched (Cronin et al. 1980). Bression and colleagues (1980) have recently reported on the binding of the dopamine antagonist [3H]domperidone to human prolactinomas. A nonlinear Scatchard plot was generated, which they interpreted to indicate that two independent binding sites were present, and dopamine was capable of competing for the [3H]domperidone binding in the micromolar range. The agonist [3H]dihydroergocriptine has also been used to define a single class of high affinity, saturable and stereoselective sites in human prolactinomas (J. Ramsdell and R.I. Weiner, personal communication). These initial studies do indicate that a gross dopamine receptor affinity deficit is not present in the adenomas studied. Unfortunately, the availability of these adenomas for receptor binding study is now drastically reduced because of the efficacy of bromocriptine treatment over surgery. Thus, animal models must be developed in order to probe the range of mechanisms which may have failed in a hypersecretory mammotroph. Indeed, some human prolactinomas are hyporesponsive to bromocriptine, which indicates that a variety of lesions may exist in the population of prolactinomas (Thorner et al. 1980b).

(3v). *Estrogen treated anterior pituitaries.* Estradiol can decrease the sensitivity of mammotrophs to dopamine inhibition of prolactin release while stimulating prolactin synthesis and release (Herbert et al. 1978; Cronin et al. 1980a; Labrie et al. 1980b; MacLeod et al. 1980c). In a series of competition studies in the anterior pituitary, DiPaolo and colleagues (1979) find no effect of estradiol treatment on the affinity of the dopamine receptor for spiperone, dihydroergocriptine, apomorphine, clonidine or phentolamine. Chronic estradiol treatment of ovariectomized rats either has no effect on maximal [3H]spiperone binding per weight (estradiol injection, twice daily for 7 days, DiPaolo et al. 1979) or decreases [3H]spiperone binding from 10.2 fm per mg wet weight to 5.3 fm per mg wet weight (10 days, estradiol silastic implant, Cronin et al. 1980a)*. If these measurements

* Unfortunately, DiPaolo and colleagues (1979) defined specific [3H]spiperone binding with an excess of spiperone itself. Spiperone will compete for more [3H]spiperone sites than any other dopaminergic agent. This implies the presence of sites which have no relationship to monoaminergic receptors. We find saturable, high affinity [3H]spiperone binding to monkey placenta which can only be displaced by nonradioactive spiperone (Cronin et al. unpublished observations).

are expressed per mammotroph surface area, one might expect a significant decrease in dopamine receptors in the estrogen treated anterior pituitary. Indeed, mammotroph density increases significantly from 15% of the total gland in the anterior pituitary of the ovariectomized rat to 31% of the total gland in the anterior pituitary of the randomly cycling rat (Cronin et al. 1980c), presumably due to estrogen stimulation of the mammotrophs.

Although this initial work is provocative, the definitive studies will require measurements of dopamine receptors per mammotroph surface area, per mammotroph second messenger units, etc. Thus, starting with a homogenous cell type or controlling for the status of the cell type of interest becomes a requirement in many experiments of the future. Hopefully, a technology for harvesting large numbers of pure mammotrophs can be developed soon.

(3vi). *Medial basal hypothalamic lesion and the anterior pituitary*. Blockage of dopaminergic transmission in the nigral-striatal pathway induces a behavioral supersensitivity in the striatum to dopamine and dopamine agonists (Creese et al. 1977a; Martres et al. 1977). This phenomenon is correlated with a modest, but significant increase in the number of striatal dopamine receptors measured by dopamine ligands (Creese et al. 1977a; Müller and Seeman 1978). It was proposed that the increased receptor density contributed directly to the enhanced responsiveness of the postsynaptic elements of the striatum. Lesions which destroy the tuberoinfundibular dopamine neurons (Cheung and Weiner 1976; Cheung and Weiner 1978), chronic treatment with either a dopamine receptor blocker (Lal et al. 1977) or a dopamine synthesis blocker (Annunziato and Moore 1977), or time in culture (C. Bethea and R. Weiner, personal communication) renders the anterior pituitary supersensitive to the inhibitory action of dopamine on prolactin release. With parallel reasoning, it was surprising to find that the dopamine receptor of the anterior pituitary responds differently than the dopamine receptor of the striatum to chronic interruption of the dopamine input. Rather than an increase in total binding, a significant decrease not only in [^{3}H]spiperone binding after a chronic hypothalamic lesion (Cronin et al. 1980b) but also in [^{3}H]haloperidol and [^{3}H]apomorphine binding after chronic haloperidol treatment (Friend et al. 1978) is measured in the anterior pituitary. In the same experiments, significantly increased binding is measured in the neurointermediate lobe of the pituitary (Cronin et al. 1980b), indicating that denervation of the tuberoinfundibular tract to the posterior pituitary may induce an increase in dopamine receptors. In addition, increased binding is present in the striatum (Friend et al. 1978), suggesting that the reduction of dopamine receptors in the anterior pituitary of the haloperidol treated animals is not due to haloperidol occupancy of the dopamine receptors. This is a particularly curious finding, especially in light of the significant increase in the density of immunostained mammotrophs after the same hypothalamic lesion (Cronin et al. 1980c). One might have expected an increased number of sites if mammotrophs are the exclusive or even the majority domain of the dopamine receptor in the anterior pituitary. Several hypotheses come to mind to explain these observations: (1) Dopamine receptors exist on cells other than mammotrophs. These other cell types would atrophy or die after destruction of their releasing hormone neurons, and this may conceal an increased number of mammotroph receptors. Unfortunately, the haloperidol-induced decrease in binding cannot be explained this way. (2) The total complement of receptors is not available for binding in homogenates of the anterior pituitary from lesioned rats. (3) The elements responsible for the supersensitivity are distal to the receptor and are not limited by a decreased receptor pool. None of these possibilities are as valuable as a few more well designed experiments. Again, the dilemma may continue until a pure population of mammotrophs can be probed.

Immunocytochemistry

Another method of localizing dopamine receptors in the anterior pituitary is that of visualizing the binding of antibodies which are specific for dopaminergic ligands. What this technique loses in quantitative speed, it gains in resolution in terms of determining where in/on the cell and on which cell type the binding sites exist. Goldsmith and associates (1979) were the first to apply the immunocytochemical labelling technique to the dopamine receptor of the anterior pituitary. Briefly, an antibody (Clark et al. 1977) to the dopamine antagonist haloperidol is applied to enzymatically dispersed anterior pituitary cells that had been incubated in haloperidol. This binding is visualized at the ultrastructural level after the deposition of an electron-dense product formed by attached peroxidase molecules. Substitution of buffer for any of the antibodies and the haloperidol, absorption of the anti-haloperidol antibody with excess haloperidol, and the addition of a hundredfold excess of *d*-butaclamol results in sparse, nonspecific staining of all of the cell types. This suggests that the substantial staining above this background level may indeed represent the sites of the dopamine receptor (Goldsmith et al. 1979). An attractive feature of this approach is that one has every anterior pituitary cell type in each preparation. Due to ultrastructural features that are characteristic of certain of the anterior pituitary cell types, especially the mammotroph and somatotroph, as well as the ability to immunostain the secretory granules for their hormone content, one can identify which cell types show specific binding.

An example of a positive and negative cell is shown in Fig. 6.8. As tabulated in Table 6.7, nearly 80% of the positively identified mammotrophs show specific binding of haloperidol and, by inference, dopamine receptors on their plasma membranes. Only 10% and 20% of the thyrotrophs and corticotrophs (respectively) exhibited specific binding, although there were few of these cell types actually sampled. It is of interest to note that a substantial percentage of somatotrophs and gonadotrophs have specific binding, even though the scattered complexes are never like the dense patches seen on mammotrophs. The specific staining of non-mammotrophs may result from an underestimation of what constitutes specific binding or may actually represent a smaller complement of dopamine receptors on these cell types. The observation that only mammotrophs internalize the binding complex attached to membrane may indicate that this process is simply the recycling of plasma membrane in the hypersecretory mammotroph rather than some specific internal transfer of a message. Surface receptors would be recycled with the membrane. Other cell types, which are not stimulated by their particular releasing hormone in this in vitro preparation, would not be expected to show this internalization phenomenon if this interpretation is correct.

200

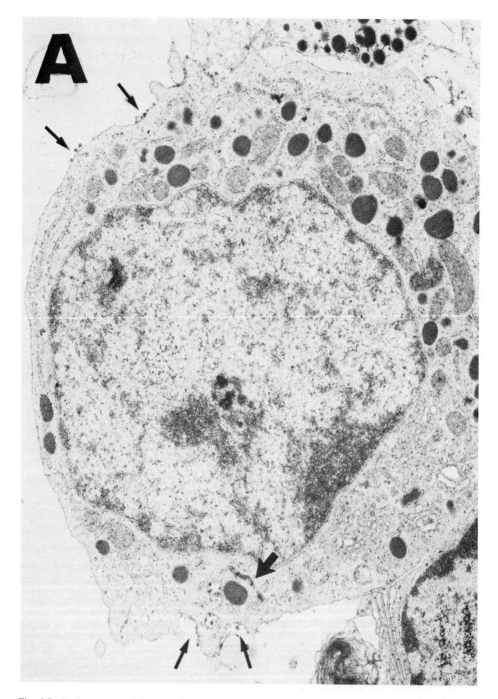

Fig. 6.8. A. A mammotroph is shown from a dispersed rat anterior pituitary gland preparation, stained immuno-cytochemically for the presence of dopamine receptor sites. Incubation in 1 µM haloperidol for 60 min., followed by 1:100 rabbit antiserum against haloperidol and the PAP technique. PAP complexes (arrows) indicate the location of dopamine receptors which appear concentrated in clusters and patches on the mammotroph plas-malemma. PAP labelled invaginations in receptor-rich portions of the plasmalemma may give rise to labelled

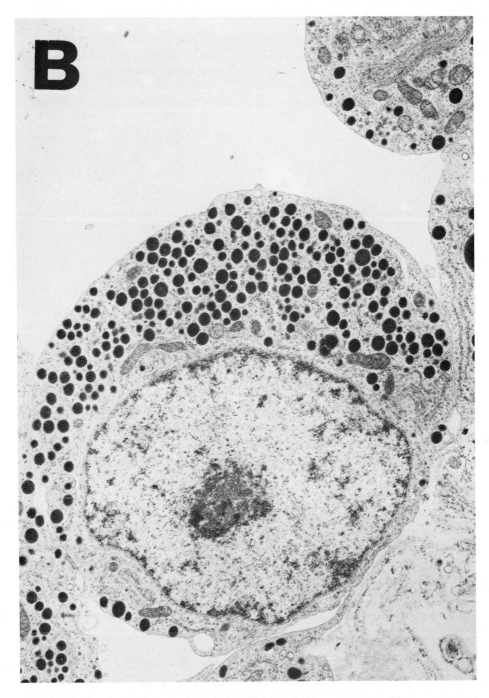

endocytotic vesicles, since PAP complexes are attached to the inner surface of the vesicle membrane. A tubular inclusion (large arrow) also contains numerous PAP complexes. Some cytoplasmic processes appear to lack limiting membrane due to the angle of the section. ×18 825. B. A somatotroph from the same cell pellet (preparation) as in A is shown. No PAP complexes are visible on the plasmalemma or within vesicles in the cytoplasm. ×13 390.

Table 6.7

HALOPERIDOL IMMUNOSTAINING OF DISPERSED RAT ANTERIOR PITUITARY CELLS

Cell type	Number of cells observed	Percent of cell type	
		Positive	Negative
Mammotroph	59	76	24
Somatotroph	58	34	66
Gonadotroph	21	52	48
Corticotroph	10	20	80
Thyrotroph	8	13	87
	156 total		

Table extracted from Goldsmith et al. 1979.

CONCLUSIONS

Dopamine is a physiological prolactin inhibitory hormone. The receptors for dopamine in the mammalian anterior pituitary can now be measured directly. Radioligand binding assays are the most popular technique to assess these dopamine receptors, but there are many uncontrolled and untested variables included in the present-day assay. The standardization of this methodology ought to be based on results from an exhaustive survey of the relevant variables before the method becomes routine. It would probably be wise to aim for conditions that mimic the physiological state (e.g. physiological concentration of ions), rather than aim for the simplest conditions that allow specific binding or the optimal conditions for maximal binding.

Once the dopamine receptor assay is routine, it is important to determine the normal complement of receptors per cell type in the anterior pituitary, especially per mammotroph. There is little doubt that the mammotrophs possess dopamine receptors which can inhibit prolactin secretion. The status of the dopamine receptor in the other cell types remains controversial because so few studies have been directed at this possibility. Further immunochemistry or autoradiographic studies of the dopamine receptor at the ultrastructural level may aid in resolving the cellular distribution dilemma. The ability to purify large numbers of the different anterior pituitary cell types will be required before the radioligand filtration assay for the dopamine receptor will be able to resolve dopamine receptors per cell type. An alternative approach is to study prolactin secreting clones or tumors derived from the anterior pituitary in the hope that at least one line of cells continues to express dopamine receptors. The difficulty of this approach is that one is dealing with an altered cell. Therefore, it is the researcher's burden to compare the measurement in the transformed cell to the same measurement in the normal cell. Again, the path points to the study of pure, normal mammotrophs.

ACKNOWLEDGMENTS

The majority of the author's data were produced in the laboratory of Richard Weiner at the University of California, San Francisco. The author is grateful for Dr Weiner's constant tutelage and encouragement. Other key collaborators include Dr Paul Goldsmith (University of California, San Francisco) as well as Drs Robert MacLeod, Michael Thorner and Ivan Login (University of Virginia). Invaluable technical assistance was performed by Lisa Dabney and Carlos Valdenegro (University of Virginia). Support for these studies include grants 5-F32-NS-05506 and USPHS/UVA 523537 (MC), HD-08924 (RW), CA-07535-17 (RM) and the Rockefeller Foundation.

REFERENCES

Ahlquist, R.P. (1948) A study of the adrenotropic receptors. Am. J. Physiol. 153, 586-600.

Annunziato, L. and Moore, K.E. (1977) Increased ability of apomorphine to reduce serum concentrations of prolactin in rats treated chronically with alpha-methyltyrosine. Life Sci. 21, 1845-1850.

Annunziato, L. (1979) Regulation of the tuberoinfundibular and nigrostriatal systems. Neuroendocrinology 29, 66-76.

Bang, S. and Gautvik, K.M. (1977) Inhibition of prolactin secretion and synthesis by dopamine, noradrenaline and pilocarpine in cultured rat pituitary tumor cells. Acta Pharmacol. Toxicol. (Copenhagen) 41, 317-327.

Barnes, G.D., Brown, B.L., Gard, T.G., Atkinson, D. and Elkins, R.P. (1978) Effect of TRH and dopamine on cyclic AMP levels in enriched mammotroph and thyrotroph cells. Mol. Cell Endocrinol. 12, 273-284.

Bates, R.W., Garrison, M.M. and Morris, H.P. (1966) Comparison of two different transplantable mammotropic pituitary tumors. Hormone content and effect on host. Proc. Soc. Exp. Biol. Med. 123, 67-70.

Beach, J.E., Cronin, M.J. and Weiner, R.I. (1979) Effect of guanine nucleotides on agonist binding to anterior pituitary dopamine receptors. 95th Annual Meeting of the Soc. Neuroscience, p. 548.

Ben-Jonathan, N., Oliver, C., Weiner, H.J., Mical, R.S. and Porter, J.C. (1977) Dopamine in hypophyseal portal plasma of the rat during the estrus cycle and throughout pregnancy. Endocrinology 100, 452-458.

Bethea, C., Wilson, C., Jaffe, R. and Weiner, R. (1981) Sensitivity to dopamine of human prolactin secreting cells cultured on extracellular matrix. Soc. Gynecol. Invest. Annual Meeting (in press).

Björklund, A. and Nobin, A. (1973) Fluorescence histochemistry and microspectrofluorometric mapping of dopamine and noradrenaline cell groups in the rat diencephalon. Brain Res. 51, 193-205.

Bression, D., Brandi, A.M., Martres, M.P., Nousbaum, A., Cesselin, F. and Peillon, F. (1980) Dopaminergic receptors in human prolactin-secreting adenomas: a quantitative study. J. Clin. Endocrinol. Metab. 51, 1037-1043.

Briley, M. and Langer, S.Z. (1978) Two binding sites for ^{3}H-spiroperidol on rat striatal membranes. Eur. J. Pharmacol. 50, 283-284.

Brown, E.M., Rodbard, D., Fedak, S.A., Woodard, C.J. and Aurbach, G.D. (1976) Beta-adrenergic receptor interactions: Direct comparison of receptor interaction and biological activity. J. Biol. Chem. 251, 1239-1246.

Brown, G.M., Seeman, P. and Lee, T. (1976) Dopamine/neuroleptic receptors in basal hypothalamus and pituitary. Endocrinology 99, 1407-1410.

Burt, D.R., Enna, S., Creese, I. and Snyder, S.H. (1975) Dopamine receptor binding in the corpus striatum of mammalian brain. Proc. Natl. Acad. Sci. USA 72, 4655-4659.

Calabro, M.A. and MacLeod, R.M. (1978) Binding of dopamine to bovine anterior pituitary gland membranes. Neuroendocrinology 25, 32-46.

Carlsson, A. (1959) The occurrence, distribution and physiological role of catecholamines in the nervous system. Pharmacol. Rev. 11, 490-493.

Caron, M.G., Beaulieu, M., Raymond, V., Gagne, B., Drouin, J., Lefkowitz, R.J. and Labrie, F. (1978) Dopaminergic receptors in the anterior pituitary gland. J. Biol. Chem. 253, 2244-2253.

204

Caron, M.G. (1979) Guanine nucleotides modulate the affinity of the dopamine receptor for agonists in bovine anterior pituitary. 61st Annual Meeting of the Endocrine Society, p. 81.

Cheung, C.Y. and Weiner, R.I. (1976) Supersensitivity of anterior pituitary dopamine receptors involved in the inhibition of prolactin secretion following destruction of the medial basal hypothalamus. Endocrinology 99, 914-917.

Cheung, C.Y. and Weiner, R.I. (1978) In vitro supersensitivity of the anterior pituitary to dopamine inhibition of prolactin secretion. Endocrinology 102, 1614-1620.

Cheung, C.Y., Kuhn, R.W. and Weiner, R.I. (1981) Increased responsiveness of the dopamine mediated inhibition of prolactin synthesis following destruction of the medial basal hypothalamus. Endocrinology 108, 747-751.

Clark, B.R., Tower, B.B. and Rubin, R.T. (1977) Radioimmunoassay of haloperidol in human serum. Life Sci. 20, 319-325.

Creese, I., Burt, D.R. and Snyder, S.H. (1977a) Dopamine receptor binding enhancement accompanies lesion-induced behavioral supersensitivity. Science 197, 596-598.

Creese, I., Schneider, R. and Snyder, S.H. (1977b) ^{3}H-Spiroperidol labels dopamine receptors in pituitary and brain. Eur. J. Pharmacol. 46, 377-381.

Creese, I. and Snyder, S.H. (1978a) ^{3}H-Spiroperidol labels serotonin receptors in rat cerebral cortex and hippocampus. Eur. J. Pharmacol. 49, 201-202.

Creese, I. and Snyder, S.H. (1978b) Dopamine receptor binding of ^{3}H-ADTN (2-amino-6, 7-dihydroxyl-1,2,3,4-tetrahydronapthalene) regulated by guanyl nucleotides. Eur. J. Pharmacol. 50, 459-461.

Creese, I., Padgett, L., Fazzini, E. and Lopez, F. (1979a) ^{3}H-N-n-propylnorapomorphine: a novel agonist ligand for central dopamine receptors. Eur. J. Pharmacol. 56, 411-412.

Creese, I., Stewart, K. and Snyder, S.H. (1979b) Species variation in dopamine receptor binding. Eur. J. Pharmacol. 60, 55-66.

Creese, I. (1980) Central nervous system dopamine receptors. In: Receptors for Neurotransmitters and Peptide Hormones (Pepeu, G., Kuhar M.J. and Enna, S.J. eds), pp. 235-242, Raven Press, New York.

Cronin, M.J., Roberts, J.M. and Weiner, R.I. (1978) Dopamine and dihydroergocriptine binding to the anterior pituitary and other brain areas of the rat and sheep. Endocrinology 103, 302-309.

Cronin, M.J. and Weiner, R.I. (1979a) Two high affinity binding sites in striatum and anterior pituitary for spiperone. 61st Annual Meeting of the Endocrine Society (Abstract 265), p. 139.

Cronin, M.J. and Weiner, R.I. (1979b) ^{3}H-Spiroperidol (spiperone) binding to a putative dopamine receptor in sheep and steer pitutary and stalk median eminence. Endocrinology 104, 307-312.

Cronin, M.J., Cheung, C.Y., Beach, J.E., Faure, N., Goldsmith, P.C. and Weiner, R.I. (1980a) Dopamine receptors on prolactin secreting cells. In: Central and Peripheral Regulation of Prolactin Function, (MacLeod, R.M. and Scapagnini, U. eds), pp. 43-58, Raven Press, New York.

Cronin, M.J., Cheung, C.Y. and Weiner, R.I. (1980b) Dopamine receptors in the pituitary and medial basal hypothalamic lesioned rats. 6th Int. Congress of Endocrinol (Abstract 871).

Cronin, M.J., Cheung, C.Y., Weiner, R.I. and Goldsmith, P.C. (1980c) Mammotroph density increases after medial basal hypothalamic lesion. 62nd Annual Meeting of the Endocrine Society, p. 181.

Cronin, M.J., Cheung, C.Y., Wilson, C.B., Jaffe, R.B. and Weiner, R.I. (1980d) ^{3}H-Spiperone binding to human anterior pituitaries and pituitary adenomas secreting prolactin, growth hormone and adrenocorticotropic hormone. J. Clin. Endocrinol. Metab. 50, 387-391.

Cronin, M.J., Faure, N., Martial, J.A. and Weiner, R.I. (1980e) Absence of high affinity dopamine receptors in GH_3 cells: a prolactin secreting clone resistant to the inhibitory action of dopamine. Endocrinology 106, 718-723.

Dale, H.H. (1906) On some physiological actions of ergot. J. Physiol. (London) 34, 163-206.

Dannies, P.S. and Tashjian Jr, A.H., (1973) Growth hormone and prolactin from rat pituitary tumor cells. In: Tissue Culture, (Kruse P.F. Jr, and Patterson, M.K. eds), pp. 561-569, Academic Press., New York

Dannies, P.S. and Rudnick, M.S. (1980) 2-Bromo-alpha-ergocriptine causes degradation of prolactin in primary cultures of rat pituitary cells after chronic treatment. J. Biol. Chem. 255, 2776-2781.

Davies, C., Jacobi, J., Lloyd, H.M. and Meares, J.D. (1974) DNA synthesis and the secretion of prolactin and growth hormone by the pituitary gland of the male rat: effects of diethylstiloestral and 2-bromo-alpha-ergocryptine methane-sulphate. J. Endocinol 61, 411-417.

De Camilli, P., Macconi, D. and Spada, A. (1979) Dopamine inhibits adenylate cyclase in human prolactin-secreting pituitary adenomas. Nature 278, 252-254.

de Greef, W.J. and Neill, J.D. (1979) Dopamine levels in hypophyseal stalk plasma of the rat during surges of prolactin secretion induced by cervical stimulation. Endocrinology 105, 1093-1099.

Denef, C. and Follebouckt, J. (1978) Differential effects of dopamine antagonists on prolactin secretion from cultured rat pituitary cells. Life Sci. 23, 431-436.

Denef, C., Van Nueten, J.M., Leysen, J.E. and Janssen, P.A.J. (1979) Evidence that pimozide is not a partial agonist of dopamine receptors. Life Sci. 25, 217-226.

Denef, C., Manet, D. and Dewals, R. (1980) Dopaminergic stimulation of prolactin release. Nature 285, 243-246.

De Quijada, M., Timmermans, H.A.T., Lamberts, S.W.J. and MacLeod, R.M. (1980) Tamoxifen enhances the sensitivity of dispersed prolactin-secreting pituitary tumor cells to dopamine and bromocriptine. Endocrinology 106, 702-706.

DiPaolo, T., Carmichael, R., Labrie, F. and Raynaud, J. (1979) Effects of estrogens on the characteristics of ^{3}H-spiroperidol and ^{3}H-RU24213 binding in rat anterior pituitary gland and brain. Mol. Cell. Endocrinol. 16, 99-112.

Dufy, B., Vincent, J.D., Fleury, H., Du Pasquier, P., Gourdji, D. and Tixier-Vidal, A. (1979) Dopamine inhibition of action potentials in prolactin secreting cell line is modulated by estrogen. Nature 282, 855-857.

Dunlap, C.E., Leslie, F.M., Rado, M. and Cox, B.M. (1979) Ascorbate destruction of opiate stereospecific binding in guinea pig brain homogenate. Mol. Pharmacol. 16, 105-119.

El-Refai, M.F. and Exton, J.H. (1980) Effects of trypsin on binding of ^{3}H-epinephrine and ^{3}H-dihydroergocryptine to rat liver membranes. J. Biol. Chem. 255, 5853-5858.

Enjalbert, A., Ruberg, M., Arancibia, S., Fiore, L., Priam, M. and Kordon, C. (1979a) Independent inhibition of prolactin secretion by dopamine and gamma-aminobutyric acid in vitro. Endocrinology 105, 823-826.

Enjalbert, A., Ruberg, M., Arancibia, S., Priam, M., Bauer, K. and Kordon, C. (1979b) Inhibition of in vitro prolactin secretion by histidyl-proline diketopiperazine, a degradation product of TRH. Eur. J. Pharmacol. 58, 97-98.

Ericson, L.E., Hakanson, R. and Lundquist, I. (1977) Accumulation of dopamine in mouse pancreatic beta-cells following injection of L-DOPA. Localization to secretory granules and inhibition of insulin secretion. Diabetologia 13, 117-124.

Faglia, G., Giovanelli, M.A. and MacLeod, R.M. (eds) (1980) Pituitary Microadenomas, Academic Press., New York.

Faure, N., Cronin, M.J., Martial, J.A. and Weiner, R.I. (1980) Decreased responsiveness of GH$_3$ cells to the dopaminergic inhibition of prolactin. Endocrinology 107, 1022-1026.

Fisher, J. and Moriarty, C. (1977) Control of bioactive corticotropin release from the neuro-intermediate lobe of the rat pituitary in vitro. Endocrinology 100, 1047-1054.

Friend, W.C., Brown, G.M., Jawhir, G., Lee, T. and Seeman, P. (1978) Effect of haloperidol and apomorphine treatment on dopamine receptors in pituitary and striatum. Am. J. Psychiat. 135, 839-841.

Furth, J., Gadsden, E.L., Clifton, K.H. and Anderson, E. (1956) Autonomous mammotropic pituitary tumors in mice, their somatotropic features and responsiveness to estrogens. Canc. Res. 16, 600-607.

Fuxe, K. (1964) Cellular localization of monoamines in the median eminence and the infundibular stem of some mammals. Z. Zellforsch. Mikrosk. Anat. 61, 710-724.

Glossman, H. and Hornung, R. (1980) Calcium and potassium channel blockers interact with alpha-adreno-receptors. Mol. Cell. Endocrinol. 19, 243-251.

Goldsmith, P.C., Cronin, M.J. and Weiner, R.I. (1979) Dopamine receptor sites in the anterior pituitary. J. Histochem. Cytochem. 27, 1205-1209.

Goldstein, M., Calne, D.B., Lieberman, A. and Thorner, M.O. (eds) (1980) Ergot compounds and brain function. In: Advances in Biochemical Pharmacology, Vol. 23, Raven Press, New York.

Grosvenor, C.E., Mena, F. and Whitworth, N.S. (1980) Evidence that the dopaminergic prolactin-inhibiting factor mechanism regulates only the depletion-transformation phase and not the release phase of prolactin secretion during suckling in the rat. Endocrinology 106, 481-485.

Gudelsky, G.A., Simkins, J. Mueller, G.P., Meites, J. and Moore, K.E. (1976) Selective actions of prolactin on catecholamine turnover in the hypothalamus and on serum LH and FSH. Neuroendocrinology 22, 206-215.

Gudelsky, G.A., Nansel, D.D. and Porter, J.C. (1979) Effects of 1-dopa and bromocriptine on the apparent association of dopamine with the prolactin secretory granule in the anterior pituitary gland of the rat. 61st Annual Meeting of the Endocrine Society, p. 201.

Haber, E. and Wrenn, S. (1976) Problems in identification of the betaadrenergic receptor. Physiol. Rev. 56, 317-338.

Hartley, E.J. and Seeman, P. (1978) The effect of varying ^{3}H-spiperone concentration on its binding parameters. Life Sci. 23, 513-518.

Herbert, D.C., Ishikawa, H., Shilno, M. and Rennels, E.G. (1978) Prolactin secretion from clonal pituitary cells following incubation with estradiol, progesterone, thyrotropin releasing hormone and dopamine. Proc. Soc. Expl. Biol. Med. 157, 605-609.

Hill, M.K., MacLeod, R.M. and Orcutt, P. (1976) Dibutyl cyclic AMP, adenosine and guanosine blockade of the dopamine, ergocryptine and apomorphine inhibition of prolactin release in vitro. Endocrinology 99, 1612-1617.

Hinkle, P.M. and Tashjian Jr, A.H. (1973) Receptors for thyrotropin-releasing hormone in prolactin-producing rat pituitary cells in culture. J. Biol. Chem. 248, 6180-6186.

Hoefer, M.T. and Ben-Jonathan, N. (1980) Prolactin inhibiting activity in rat hypothalamic extracts and effect of coincubation with dopaminergic and beta-adrenergic antagonists in vitro. 6th Int. Congress of Endocrinol. (Abstract 868).

Hökfelt, T. (1967) The possible ultrastructural identification of tuberoinfundibular dopamine-containing nerve endings in the median eminence of the rat. Brain Res. 5, 121-123.

Hökfelt, T. and Fuxe, K. (1972) Effects of prolactin and ergot alkaloids on the tuberoinfundibular dopamine neurons. Neuroendocrinology 9, 100-122.

Howlett, A.L., Sternweis, P.C., Macik, B.A., Van Arsdale, P.M. and Gilman, A.G. (1979) Reconstitution of catecholamine sensitive adenylate cyclase. J. Biol. Chem. 254, 2287-2295.

Hymer, W.C., Snyder, J., Willfinger, W., Bergland, R., Fisher, B. and Pearson, O. (1976) Characterization of mammotrophs separated from the human pituitary gland. J. Natl. Cancer Inst. 57, 995-1007.

Insel, P.A. and Stoolman, L.M. (1978) Radioligand binding to beta-adrenergic receptors of intact cultural S49 cells. Mol. Pharmacol. 14, 549-561.

Johnson, G.L., Bourne, H.R., Gleason, M.K., Coffino, P., Insel, P.A. and Melman, K.L. (1979) Isolation and characterization of S49 lymphoma cells deficient in beta-adrenergic receptors: relation of receptor number to activation of adenylate cyclase. Mol. Pharmacol. 15, 16-27.

Kalbermann, L.E., Szijan, I., Jahn, G.A., Krawiec, L. and Burdman, J.A. (1979) DNA synthesis in the pituitary gland of the rat. Neuroendocrinology 29, 42-48.

Kayaalp, S.O. and Neff, N.H. (1980) Differentiation by ascorbic acid of dopamine agonist and antagonist binding sites in striatum. Life Sci. 26, 1837-1841.

Kebabian, J.W. and Calne, D.B. (1979) Multiple receptors for dopamine. Nature 277, 93-96.

Labrie, F., Borgeat, P., Barden, N., Godbout, M., Beaulieu, M., Ferland, L. and Lavoie, M. (1980a) Mechanisms of action of hypothalamic hormones in the anterior pituitary. In: Polypeptide Hormones (Beers Jr, R.F. and Bassett, E.G. eds), pp. 235-251, Raven Press, New York.

Labrie, F., DiPaolo, T., Raymond, V., Ferland, L. and Beaulieu, M. (1980b) The pituitary dopamine receptor. In: Advances in Biochemical Psychopharmacology (Goldstein, M., Calne, D.B., Lieberman, A. and Thorner, M.O. eds), pp. 217-227, Vol. 23, Raven Press, New York.

Lal, H., Brown, W., Drawbaugh, R., Hynes, M. and Brown, G. (1977) Enhanced prolactin inhibition following chronic treatment with haloperidol and morphine. Life Sci. 20, 101-106.

Lamberts, S.W.J. and MacLeod, R.M. (1979) The inability of bromocriptine to inhibit prolactin secretion by transplantable rat pituitary tumors: observations on the mechanism and dynamics of the autofeedback regulation of prolactin secretion. Endocrinology 104, 65-70.

Langley, J.N. (1906) On nerve endings and on special excitable substances in cells. Proc. R. Soc. Lond. Ser. B78, 170-194.

Lautin, A., Wazer, D., Stanley, M., Rotrosen, J. and Gershon, S. (1980) Chronic treatment with metoclopramide induces behavioral supersensitivity to apomorphine and enhances specific binding of ^{3}H-spiroperidol to rat striata. Life Sci. 27, 305-316.

Lefkowitz, R.J., Limbird, L.E., Mukherjee, C. and Caron, M.G. (1976) The beta-adrenergic receptor and adenylate cyclase. Biochim. Biophys. Acta 457, 1-39.

Lew, J.Y. and Goldstein, M. (1979) Dopamine receptor binding for agonists and antagonists in thermal exposed membranes. Eur. J. Pharmacol. 55, 429-430.

Leysen, J.E., Gommeren, W. and Laduron, P.M. (1979) Distinction between dopaminergic and serotoninergic components of neuroleptic binding sites in limbic brain areas. Biochem. Pharmacol. 28, 447-448.

Login, I.S., Nagy, I. and MacLeod, R.M. (1981) Restoration of pituitary prolactin synthesis and release by the administration of morphine to rats bearing a transplanted prolactin-secreting tumor. Neuroendocrinology 33, 101-104.

MacLeod, R.M., Smith, M.C. and Dewitt, G.W. (1966) Hormonal properties of transplanted pituitary tumors and their relation to the pituitary gland. Endocrinology 79, 1149-1156.

MacLeod, R.M. and Abad, A. (1968) On the control of prolactin and growth hormone synthesis in rat pituitary glands. Endocrinology 83, 799-806.

MacLeod, R.M. and Lehmeyer, J.E. (1974a) Restoration of prolactin synthesis and release by the administration of monoaminergic blocking agents to pituitary tumor-bearing rats. Canc. Res. 34, 345-350.

MacLeod, R.M. and Lehmeyer, J.E. (1974b) Studies on the mechanism of the dopamine-mediated inhibition of prolactin secretion. Endocrinology 94, 1077-1085.

MacLeod, R.M. (1976) Regulation of prolactin secretion. In: Frontiers in Neuroendocrinology (Martini, L. and Ganong, W.F.eds), pp. 169-194, Vol. 4, Raven, New York.

Mac Leod, R.M. and Lamberts, S.W.J. (1978) The biphasic regulation of prolactin secretion by dopamine agonist-antagonists. Endocrinology 103, 200-203.

MacLeod, R.M., Lamberts, S.W.J., Nagy, I., Login, I.S. and Valdenegro, C.A. (1980a) Suppression of prolactin secretion by the physiological and pharmacological manipulation of pituitary dopamine receptors. In: Pituitary Microadenomas (Faglia, G., Giovanelli, M.A. and MacLeod, R.M. eds), pp. 37-54, Academic Press, New York.

MacLeod, R.M., Nagy, I., Login, I.S., Kimura, H., Valdenegro, C.A. and Thorner, M.O. (1980b) The roles of dopamine, cAMP and calcium in prolactin secretion. In: Central and Peripheral Regulation of Prolactin Function (MacLeod, R.M. and Scapagnini, U. eds), pp. 27-42, Raven Press, New York.

MacLeod, R.M., Cronin, M.J., Valdenegro, C.A., Login, I.S. and Thorner, M.O. (1980c) Neural and ovarian regulation of prolactin production. In: Progress in Psychoneuroendocrinology (Brambilla, F., Racagni, G. and De Wied, D. eds), pp. 63-74, Elsevier/North-Holland, New York.

Maguire, M.E., Ross, E.M. and Gilman, A.G. (1977) Beta-adrenergic receptor: ligand binding properties and the interaction with adenyl cyclase. In: Advances in Cyclic Nucleotide Research (Greengard, P. and Robison, G.A., eds), pp. 1-83, Vol. 8, Raven Press, New York.

Malarkey, W.B., Groshong, J.C. and Milo, G.E. (1977) Defective dopaminergic regulation of prolactin secretion in a rat pituitary tumor cell line. Nature 266, 640-641.

Markstein, R., Herrling, P. and Wagner, H. (1978) Bromocriptine mimics dopamine effects on the cyclic AMP system of rat pituitary gland. Proc. 7th Int. Cong. Pharmacol. (Paris) (Abstract 2632).

Martres, M.P., Costentin, J., Baudry, M., Marcais, H., Protais, P. and Schwartz, J.C. (1977) Long-term changes in the sensitivity of pre- and postsynaptic dopamine receptors in mouse striatum evidenced by behavioral and biochemical studies. Brain Res. 136, 319-337.

Maurer, R.A. (1980a) Bromoergocriptine-induced prolactin degradation in cultured pituitary cells. Biochemistry 19, 3573-3578.

Maurer, R.A. (1980b) Dopaminergic inhibition of prolactin synthesis and prolactin messenger RNA accumulation in cultured pituitary cells. J. Biol. Chem. 255, 8092-8097.

Meites, J., Kahn, R.H. and Nicoll, C.S. (1961) Prolactin production by rat pituitary in vitro. Proc. Soc. Exp. Biol. Med. 108, 440-443.

Melmed, S., Carlson, H.E., Briggs, J. and Hershman, J.M. (1980) Cell culture alters the hormonal response of rat pituitary tumors to dynamic stimulation. Endocrinology 107, 789-793.

Meltzer, H.Y., Goode, D.J. and Fang, V.S. (1978) The effects of psychotropic drugs on endocrine function. I.

Neuroleptics, precursors and agonists. In: Psychopharmacology. A Generation of Progress (Lipton, M.A., Di Mascio, A. and Killam, K.F. eds), pp. 509-529, Raven Press, New York.

Meltzer, H.Y., So, R., Miller, R.J. and Fang, V.S. (1979) Comparison of the effects of substituted benzamides and standard neuroleptics on the binding of ^{3}H-spiroperidol in the rat pituitary and striatum with in vivo effects on rat prolactin secretion. Life Sci. 25, 573-584.

Moore, K.E., Demarest, K.T. and Johnston, C.A. (1980) Influence of prolactin on dopaminergic neuronal systems in the hypothalamus. Fed. Proc. 39, 2912-2916.

Morgan, C.M. and Hadley, M.E. (1976) Ergot alkaloid inhibition of melanophore stimulating hormone secretion. Neuroendocrinology 21, 10-19.

Moriarty, C.M., Leuschen, M.P. and Cambell, G.T. (1978) Variations in the response of enzyme-dissociated rat pituitary cells to thyrotropin releasing hormone. Life Sci. 23, 2073-2078.

Müller, P. and Seeman, P. (1978) Dopaminergic supersensitivity after neuroleptics: time course and specificity. Psychopharmacology 60, 1-11.

Nansel, D.D., Gudelsky, G.A. and Porter, J.C. (1979) Subcellular localization of dopamine in the anterior pituitary gland of the rat: apparent association of dopamine with prolactin secretory granules. Endocrinology 105, 1073-1077.

Nansel, D.D., Gudelsky, G.A. and Porter, J.C. (1980) Dopamine-induced stimulation of lysosomal enzyme activity in the anterior pituitary. 62nd Annual Meeting of the Endocrine Society, p. 189.

Nikitovitch-Winer, M. and Everett, J.W. (1958) Functional restitution of pituitary grafts re-transplanted from kidney to median eminence. Endocrinology 63, 916-930.

O'Brien, R.D. (ed.) (1979) The Receptors, Vol. 1, Plenum Press, New York.

Pasteels, J.L. (1961) Secretion de prolactine par l'hypophyse en culture de tissus. C.R. Acad. Sci., Paris 253, 3074-3075.

Peake, G.T., McKell, D.W., Jarett, L. and Daughaday, W.H. (1969) Ultrastructural, histologic and hormonal characterization of a prolactin-rich human pituitary tumor. J. Clin. Endocrinol. Metab. 29, 1383-1393.

Pedigo, N.W., Reisine, T.D., Fields, J.Z. and Yamamura, H.T. (1978) ^{3}H-Spiroperidol binding to two receptor sites in both the corpus striatum and frontal cortex of rat brain. Eur. J. Pharmacol. 50, 451-453.

Perkins, N.A. and Westfall, T.C. (1978) The effect of prolactin on dopamine release from rat striatum and medial basal hypothalamus. Neuroscience 3, 59-63.

Perkins, N.A., Westfall, T.C., Paul, C.V., MacLeod, R.M. and Rogol, A.D. (1979) Effect of prolactin on dopamine synthesis in medial basal hypothalamus: evidence for a short loop feedback. Brain Res. 160, 431-444.

Plotsky, P.M., Gibbs, D.M. and Neill, J.D. (1978) Liquid chromatographic–electrochemical measurement of dopamine in hypophyseal stalk blood of rats. Endocrinology 102, 1887-1900.

Poirier, G., Delean, A., Pelletier, G., Lemay, A. and Labrie, F. (1974) Purification of adenohypophyseal plasma membranes and properties of associated adenylate cyclase. J. Biol. Chem. 249, 316-322.

Quijada, M., Illner, P., Krulich, L. and McCann, S.M. (1973) The effect of catecholamines on hormone release from anterior pituitaries and ventral hypothalami incubated in vitro. Neuroendocrinology 13, 151-163.

Ravitz, A.J. and Moore, K.E. (1977) Lack of effect of chronic haloperidol administration on the prolactin-lowering actions of piribedil. J. Pharm. Pharmacol. 29, 384-385.

Rick, J., Szabo, M., Payne, P., Kovathana, N., Cannon, J.G. and Frohman, L.A. (1979) Prolactin-suppressive effects of two amino tetralin analogs of dopamine: their use in the characterization of the pituitary dopamine receptor. Endocrinology 104, 1234-1242.

Ross, E.M., Maguire, M.E., Sturgill, T.W., Biltonen, R.L. and Gilman, A.G. (1977) The relationship between the beta-adrenergic receptor and adenylate cyclase: studies of ligand binding and enzyme activity in purified membranes of S49 lymphoma cells. J. Biol. Chem. 252, 5761-5775.

Ross, E.M., Howlett, A.C., Ferguson, K.M. and Gilman, A.G. (1978) Reconstitution of hormone-sensitive adenylate cyclase activity with resolved components of the enzyme. J. Biol. Chem. 253, 6401-6412.

Rotman, A., Daly, J.W. and Creveling, C.R. (1976) Oxygen-dependent reaction of 6-hydroxydopamine, 5,6 dihydroxytryptamine and related compounds with proteins in vitro. Mol. Pharmacol. 12, 887-899.

Saiani, L., Trabucchi, M., Tonon, G.L. and Spano, P.F. (1979) Bromocriptine and lisuride stimulate the accumulation of cyclic AMP in intact slices but not in homogenates of rat neostriatum. Neurosci. Lett. 14,

31-36.

Salih, H., Murthy, G.S. and Friesen, H.G. (1979) Stability of hormone receptors with fixation: implications for immunocytochemical localization of receptors. Endocrinology 105, 21-26.

Saner, A. and Thoenen, H. (1971) Model experiments on the molecular mechanism of action of 6-hydroxydopamine. Mol. Pharmacol. 7, 147-154.

Sato, G.H. and Ross, R. (eds) (1979) Hormones and Cell Culture, Cold Spring Harbor Laboratory.

Schaeffer, J.M. and Hsueh, J.W. (1979) 2-Hydroxyestradiol interaction with dopamine receptor binding in rat anterior pituitary. J. Biol. Chem. 254, 5606-5608.

Schonbrunn, A. and Tashjian, A.H. (1978) Characterization of functional receptors for somatostatin in rat pituitary cells in culture. J. Biol. Chem. 253, 6473-6483.

Schonbrunn, A., Krasnoff, A., Lomedico, M.A. and Tashjian Jr, A.H. (1979) Binding and biological actions of epidermal growth factor in cultured pituitary cells. 61st Ann. Meeting of the Endocrine Society p. 80).

Seeman, P., Chan-Wong, M. and Lee, T. (1974) Dopamine receptor block and nigral fiber impulse-blockade by major tranquilizers. Fed. Proc. 33 80.

Shaar, C.J. and Clemens, J.A. (1974) The role of catecholamines in the release of anterior pituitary prolactin 'in vitro'. Endocrinology 95, 1202-1212.

Sibley, D.R. and Creese, I. (1979) Guanine nucleotides regulate anterior pituitary dopamine receptors. Eur. J. Pharmacol. 55, 341-343.

Sibley, D.R. and Creese, I. (1980a) Dopamine receptor binding in bovine intermediate lobe pituitary membranes. Endocrinology 107, 1405-1409.

Sibley, D.R. and Creese, I. (1980b) Pseudo non-competitive agonist interactions with dopamine receptors. Eur. J. Pharmacol. 65, 131-133.

Smythies, J.R. and Bradley, R.J. (eds) (1978) Receptors in Pharmacology, Dekker, New York.

Stefanini, E., Clement-Cormier, Y., Vernaleone, F., Devoto, P., Marchisio, A.M. and Collu, R. (1980a) Sodium-dependent interaction of benzamides with dopamine receptors in rat and dog anterior pituitary gland. Neuroendocrinology 32, 103-107.

Stefanini, E., Devoto, P., Marchisio, A.M., Vernaleone, F. and Collu, R. (1980b) [^{3}H] Spiroperidol binding to a putative dopaminergic receptor in rat pituitary gland. Life Sci. 26, 583-587.

Stefanini, E., Marchisio, A.M., Devoto, P., Vernaleone, F., Spano, P.F. and Collu, R. (1980c) Sodium dependent interaction of benzamides with dopamine receptors. Brain Res. 198, 229-233.

Stepien, H., Wolaniak, A. and Pawlikowski, M. (1978) Effects of pimozide and bromocriptine on anterior pituitary cell proliferation. J. Neural Transmission. 42, 239-244.

Talwalker, P.K., Ratner, A. and Meites, J. (1963) In vitro inhibition of pituitary prolactin synthesis and release by hypothalamic extract. Am. J. Physiol. 205, 213-218.

Tam, S.W. and Dannies, P.S. (1980) Dopaminergic inhibition of ionophore A23187-stimulated release of prolactin from rat anterior pituitary cells. J. Biol. Chem. 255, 6595-6599.

Taraskevich, P.S. and Douglas, W.W. (1978) Catecholamines of supported inhibitory hypophysiotrophic function suppress action potentials in prolactin cells. Nature 276, 832-834.

Tashjian Jr, A.H., Yasamura, Y., Levine, L., Sato, G.H. and Parker, M.L. (1968) Establishment of clonal strains of rat pituitary tumor cells that secrete growth hormone. Endocrinology 82, 342-352.

Thorner, M.O., Hackett, J.T., Murad, F. and MacLeod, R.M. (1980a) Calcium rather than cyclic AMP as the physiological intracellular regulator of prolactin release. Neuroendocrinology 31, 390-402.

Thorner, M.O., Schran, H.F., Evans, W.S., Rogol, A.D., Morris, J.L. and MacLeod, R.M. (1980b) A broad spectrum of prolactin suppression by bromocriptine in hyperprolactinemic women: a study of serum prolactin and bromocriptine levels after acute and chronic administration of bromocriptine. J. Clin. Endocrinol. Metab. 50, 1026-1033.

Tilders, F.J. and Smelik, P.G. (1978) Effects of hypothalamic lesions and drugs interfering with dopaminergic transmission on pituitary MSH content of rats. Neuroendocrinology 25, 275-290.

Titeler, M., List, S. and Seeman, P. (1979a) High affinity dopamine receptors (D$_3$)in rat brain. Comm. Psychopharmacol. 3, 411-420.

Titeler, M. and Seeman, P. (1979b) Selective labeling of different dopamine receptors by a new agonist ^{3}H-ligand: ^{3}H-N-propylnorapomorphine. Eur. J. Pharmacol. 56, 291-292.

210

U'Prichard, D.C. and Snyder, S.H. (1978) Guanyl nucleotide influences on ^{3}H-ligand binding to alpha-noradrenergic receptors in calf membranes. J. Biol. Chem. 253, 3444-3452.

Usdin, T.B., Creese, I. and Snyder, S.H. (1980) Regulation by cations of ^{3}H-spiroperidol binding associated with dopamine receptors of rat brain. J. Neurochem. 24, 669-676.

Vogt, M. (1959) Catecholamines in brain. Pharmacol. Rev. 11, 483-489.

Weiner, R.I. and Ganong, W.F. (1978) Role of brain monoamines and histamine in regulation of anterior pituitary secretion. Physiol. Rev. 58, 905-976.

West, B. and Dannies, P.S. (1979) Antipsychotic drugs inhibit prolactin release from rat pituitary cells in culture by a mechanism not involving the dopamine receptor. Endocrinology 104, 877-880.

Williams, L.T. and Lefkowitz, R.J. (eds) (1978) Receptor Binding Studies in Adrenergic Pharmacology, Raven Press, New York.

Wirz-Justice, A., Kafka, M.S., Naber, D. and Wehr, T.A. (1980) Circadian rhythms in rat brain alpha- and beta-adrenergic receptors are modified by chronic imipramine. Life Sci. 27, 341-347.

Yamamura, H.I., Enna, S.J. and Kuhar, M.J. (eds.) (1978) Neurotransmitter Receptor Binding, Raven Press, New York.

Yeo, T., Thorner, M.O., Jones, A., Lowry, P.J. and Besser, G.M. (1979) The effects of dopamine, bromocriptine, lergotrile and metoclopramide on prolactin release from continuously perfused columns of isolated rat pituitary cells. Clin. Endocrinol. 10, 123-130.

York, D.H., Bakker, F.L. and Kraicer, J. (1973) Electrical changes induced in rat adenohypophysial cells, in vivo, with hypothalamic extract. Neuroendocrinoly 11, 212-228.

Zern, R.T., Foster, L.B., Blalock, J.A. and Feldman, J.M. (1979) Characteristics of the dopaminergic and noradrenergic systems of the pancreatic islets. Diabetes 28, 185-189.

Zimmerman, E.A., Defendini, R. and Frantz, A.G. (1974) Prolactin and growth hormone in patients with pituitary adenomas: a correlative study of hormone in tumor and plasma by immunoperoxidase technique and radioimmunoassay. J. Clin. Endocrinol. Metab. 38, 577-585.

E.E. Müller and R.M. MacLeod (eds) Neuroendocrine Perspectives Vol. 1
© Elsevier Biomedical Press, 1982

Chapter 7

Morphological, functional and electrical correlates in anterior pituitary cells

A. Tixier-Vidal, C. Tougard, B. Dufy, J.D. Vincent

INTRODUCTION

Anterior pituitary cells are endocrine cells that have become specialized for the synthesis and release of a variety of protein hormones, including polypeptide hormones of the pro-opiocortin series (β-lipotropin, α- and β-melanotropin, corticotropin and α- and β-endorphin), protein hormones (prolactin and somatotropin), and glycoprotein hormones (luteotropin, folliculotropin and thyrotropin). The synthesis and release of these secretory products are regulated either positively or negatively by a wide variety of agents which interact in a very complex manner. Schematically one may divide these regulating agents into three classes: neuropeptides having a hypophysiotropic activity, neurotransmitters and hormones of the anterior pituitary target glands, mostly steroids and thyroid hormones (see Table 7.1). The first two are carried by the portal veins at a short distance from the hypothalamus to the anterior pituitary (AP) cells, whereas the third group arises from the peripheral blood system. Complex interaction of these factors has led to multiple control mechanisms which may either stimulate or inhibit so that AP cell activity adapts rapidly and precisely to stimuli from the environment.

From a general point of view the functions of AP cells involve three types of basic mechanisms: (1) synthesis of specific gene products; (2) release of membrane-bound secretory proteins; and (3) responsiveness to peptide hormones, neurotransmitters, steroid and thyroid hormones. The biochemist must analyze these mechanisms in disrupted cells to reach the molecular level, but despite the necessity of such an approach, it cannot take into consideration the fact that a cell, and particularly a secretory cell, possesses a high degree of supramolecular organization. In contrast, both the morphological and electrophysiological approaches require study of the intact cell. Thus by offering an integrated view of AP cell function, they are complementary to biochemical studies.

The general scheme of structural organization of an anterior pituitary cell is the same as for other endocrine cells (Fig. 7.1). Electron microscopy has revealed three compartments in the cytoplasm: the rough endoplasmic reticulum (RER); the smooth endoplasmic reticulum including the Golgi zone; and the membrane-bound secretory granules. This

Table 7.1

SIMPLIFIED REGULATIONS OF ANTERIOR PITUITARY CELL ACTIVITY BY NEUROPEPTIDES, NEUROTRANSMITTERS AND PERIPHERAL HORMONES

Hormone and cell type	Direct inhibitory control	Direct stimulatory control	Modulating hormones
Gonadotrope LH-FSH	Inhibin	Gonadoliberin (GnRH or LH-RH)	Estrogens Androgens Substance P
Thyrotrope TSH	Somatostatin (SRIF)	Thyroliberin (TRH)	Estrogens Thyroid hormones
Lactotrope PRL	Dopamine (DA) Somatostatin SRIF GABA	Thyroliberin TRH Vasoactive intestinal peptide (VIP) PRL-releasing factor (PRF) Estrogens	Estrogens Glucocorticoids Opioids
Somatotrope GH	Somatostatin	Thyroliberin Growth hormone-releasing factor Glucocorticoids Thyroid hormones	
Corticotrope ACTH	Glucocorticoids	Corticotropin releasing factor (CRF) Vasopressin	

structural compartmentalization in fact involves the whole endoplasmic reticulum from the nuclear envelope to the plasma membrane. It offers a morphological basis for the intracellular pathway of secretory products proposed by Farquhar (Smith and Farquhar 1966; Farquhar 1977) according to Palade's concept (1975), i.e. (1) synthesis on attached polysomes and transfer into the RER; (2) concentration and packaging into secretory granules in the Golgi zone; (3) storage in mature secretory granules; and (4) extracellular discharge of secretory granules by exocytosis or, alternatively, intracellular fusion with lysosomes of secretory granules in excess.

The relations between structural organization and function of AP cells will be reviewed in mammals in this chapter. They will be considered from two points of view: firstly the biochemical specificity of the secretory products and then the variation of secretory activity in response to specific stimuli. Electrical correlates which have been studied in relation to secretory activity in a very few cell types will be reviewed in the third section.

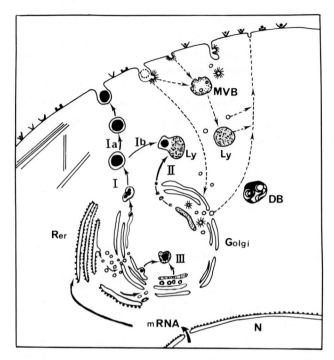

Fig. 7.1. Schematic representation of secretory process (solid arrows) and membrane traffic (broken arrows) in an ideal anterior pituitary cell. Route I represents the main pathway followed by AP hormones from synthesis on membrane-bound polysomes to storage in membrane-bound secretory granules via condensation in the Golgi zone. Route Ia leads to release by exocytosis whereas Route Ib leads to fusion with lysosomes. Route II represents the pathway of acid hydrolases from the GERL (Golgi-endoplasmic reticulum lysosomes) cisternae to lysosomes. Route III corresponds to the co-segregation within immature granules of secretory material (black areas) and acid hydrolases. The final fate of that membrane-bound material is not understood. As concerns membrane traffic, an outward route leads to the insertion in the plasma membrane of newly synthesized or reutilized membrane fragments. The inward route may follow several hypothetical pathways: re-insertion into Golgi saccule membrane, fusion with multivesicular bodies (MVB) or direct re-insertion into the plasma membrane dense bodies (DB). Ly and dotted areas: lysosomal hydrolases (modified from Tixier-Vidal 1980).

MORPHOLOGICAL CORRELATES OF BIOCHEMICAL SPECIFICITY OF AP CELLS

The cellular heterogeneity of anterior pituitary tissue was pointed out long ago by cytologists who discovered that AP cells display various tinctorial affinities related to the nature of secretory products stored within the cytoplasm. Further progress in the chemistry of AP hormones and in cytochemistry of AP cells has strengthened this concept (see review in Herlant 1964, 1975). A confirmation of the biochemical specialization of AP cells was obtained with the development of immunocytochemistry, first at the light microscope level (see review in Nakane 1970) and then at the electron microscope level by immunoenzyme techniques (Nakane 1970, 1975; Moriarty 1973). This procedure permitted the characterization of the ultrastructural organization of the cell types which secrete prolactin (PRL), growth hormone (GH), luteotropin (LH)/folliculotropin (FSH), thyrotropin (TSH) and adrenocorticotropin (ACTH) and led to the theory that for each anterior pituitary hormone, there is a corresponding type of pituitary cell. Within recent years, however, a better understanding of the chemistry of several anterior pituitary hormones, of antisera specificity and immunoelectron microscope methods have led researchers to reexamine that concept. At the same time, there emerged new insights into the understanding of the AP cell-secretory process. Rather than describing the ultrastructural features of immunocyto-chemically identified cell types, the present section will discuss two main problems raised by the bulk of recent immunocytochemical findings.

The one cell, one hormone concept

The one cell, one hormone concept has been tested for a number of different hormones.

Prolactin and growth hormone

The fact that PRL and GH are each secreted by a different cell type was first shown by conventional electron microscope studies (Herlant 1964) and then confirmed by immuno-cytochemical studies at both light microscope and electron microscope levels (Nakane 1975). Although PRL cells and GH cells display some common ultrastructural features, such as lamellar arrangement of the RER cisternae, conspicuousness of ribosomes, organization of the Golgi zone, and electron density of the secretory granules, they differ in the shape of their secretory granules, at least in several mammals (Herlant 1964). Briefly, secretory granules are large and rounded in GH cells instead of irregularly shaped as in PRL cells. This irregular shape is caused by the fusion in the Golgi zone of small rounded masses of newly condensed secretory material (Farquhar et al. 1978). It is well known, however, that in the case of hyperactive secretion the secretory granules become smaller and rounded. Hence, the distinction between PRL cells and GH cells may become difficult to define.

The situation is particularly critical for pituitary adenoma (Olivier et al. 1975) and for clonal, tumor-derived cell lines which secrete both PRL and GH (Tashjian et al. 1970). Recent investigations of the GH and PRL secreting rat MtTW15 mammosomatotropic tumor, using ultrastructural immunocytochemistry, support the hypothesis that GH and PRL are produced by separate cell types (Baskin et al. 1980). However, the authors did not rule out the possibility that some MtTW15 cells, which may contain both GH and PRL, escaped their immunoelectron microscope investigation. The existence of such dual cells, common precursors of GH and PRL cells, has been proposed in human 'acidophil stem' adenomas (Kovacs and Horvath 1980) but not unequivocally proven (see Duello and Halmi 1980).

'GH' cell lines, which were isolated (Tashjian et al. 1968) from the GH- and PRL-secreting rat mammosomatotropic tumor MtTW5, may offer an opportunity to solve that intriguing problem, but technical limitations have thus far precluded a clear answer. Theoretically repeated single-cell cloning operations should have produced clones derived from a single cell which produce either one hormone, or both hormones or no hormone at all. In fact it was found that an isolated single cell, whether or not it synthesizes PRL, gives rise to prolactin-producing cell colonies (Gautvik and Fossum 1976; Hoyt and Tashjian

1980). Most of the available 'GH' cell lines and their subclones produce both PRL and GH, although in very different ratios. These ratios moreover may vary with the number of subcultures, the 'quality' of the serum which participates in the composition of culture medium, the presence of steroid hormones, etc. Light microscope immunocytochemistry has also failed to solve the problem. When PRL was immunocytochemically localized the proportion of GH$_3$-stained cells varied from very low to 35% (Hoyt and Tashjian 1973, 1980a, 1980b). The same situation was observed when GH was immunocytochemically detected in GH$_1$ cells (Masur et al. 1974). Moreover a preliminary report on simultaneous localization of both hormones revealed that the parent GH$_3$ clone consists of PRL-positive cells, GH-positive cells and negative cells, while no individual cell containing more than one hormone was observed (Mazurkiewicz 1973). In conclusion, it still remains to be proven whether GH and PRL can be produced simultaneously by a single pituitary cell, and the concept of 'one hormone–one cell type' remains valid for both GH cells and PRL cells.

Cellular origin of ACTH, α-MSH and polypeptides of the pro-opiomelanocortin series

The immunocytochemical identification of ACTH-containing cells in both the pars distalis and the pars intermedia of mammalian and non-mammalian pituitary was definitively established through the use of antisera directed against several sequences of the C terminal part of the ACTH molecule which do not cross react with α-MSH (Baker et al. 1970; Moriarty and Halmi 1972a, 1972b; for review in mammals see Girod 1976). In contrast, α-MSH containing cells could be visualized in the pars intermedia only with the use of antisera directed against α-MSH which corresponds to the first 13 amino acids of the N terminal part of the ACTH molecule (Dubois 1972; Tramu and Dubois 1977). Simultaneously β-lipotropin (β-LPH) a 91 amino acid peptide discovered in sheep pituitaries by Li (1964) was also immunocytochemically localized in the pars distalis, in cells already shown to contain both ACTH and β-MSH and, in the pars intermedia, in cells already shown to contain α-MSH in addition to ACTH and β-MSH (Dessy et al. 1973; Dubois and Gráf 1973; Moon et al. 1973). The function of β-LPH was at that time not clearly understood, although the concept that it was a precursor molecule was already put forward (see review Chrétien et al. 1979).

Within the past 5–6 years, the considerable progress made in the knowledge of the chemistry and processing of the polypeptide hormones of the 'pro-opiomelanocortin' series has led to a reexamination of the peptides which are contained in ACTH and α-MSH cells. Briefly it is now well established that ACTH, and β-LPH, come from a common precursor

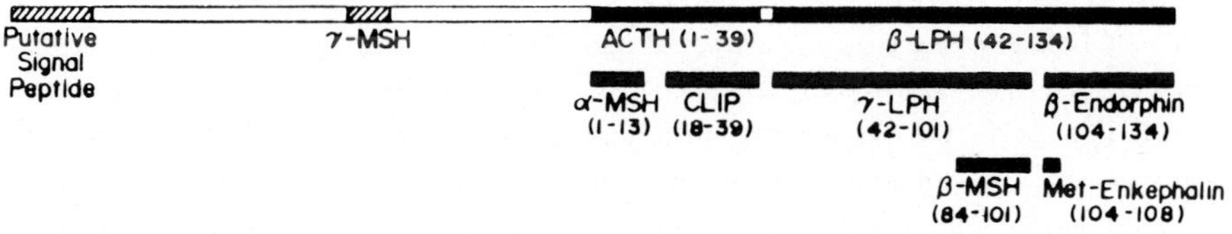

Fig. 7.2. Schematic representation of the structure of bovine ACTH-β-LPH precursor. Simplified from Nakanishi et al. (1979).

of mol.wt $\simeq$ 31 000. β-LPH is located at the C terminus of the precursor and contains the sequences of γ-LPH (N terminus), β-MSH and β-endorphin (C terminus). ACTH is adjacent to the N terminus of β-LPH. The N terminal part of the precursor is a glycopeptide (Fig. 7.2) (Chrétien et al. 1979; Herbert et al. 1980; Crine et al. 1980). Moreover the processing of the precursor has been followed in cultured AP cells, both tumoral (AtT–20 line) and normal, as well as in cells of the intermediate lobe. This clearly shows that β-LPH is an important and transient intermediary in the processing of β-endorphin. Moreover it has been found that products of enzymatic cleavages of the precursor are released from the cells (Vale et al. 1978, see also Chapter 5).

The availability of antibodies directed against several components of the mol.wt 31 000 precursor has made possible their immunocytochemical localization. Staining with anti-α-endorphin and anti-β-endorphin revealed all the ACTH cells in the pars distalis and the pars intermedia in several mammals (Bloom et al. 1977; Weber et al. 1978; Tramu and Beauvillain, 1980). Although these antibodies did not differentiate between β-LPH and β- or α-endorphin this result is consistent with the biochemical evidence for β-LPH being a precursor of endorphin. Most interestingly the mol.wt 16 000 fragment of the mol.wt 31 000 common precursor, which is present neither in ACTH nor in β-LPH, has also been localized in ACTH cells of both the pars distalis and the pars intermedia (Guy et al. 1980). Morevoer, co-existence within the same cells of ACTH, β-LPH, β-endorphin and the mol.wt 16 000 fragment of their common precursor has been correlated at the electron microscope level to their co-existence within the same secretory granules (Pelletier et al. 1977; Weber et al. 1978; Guy et al. 1980). This is in very good agreement with biochemical studies suggesting that the glycosylation and processing of polypeptides of the pro-opiomelanocortin series occur during their transit within the endoplasmic reticulum from the RER to the membrane-bound secretory granules (Herbert et al. 1980). However, the exact localization of the various enzymatic cleavages along the endoplasmic reticulum remains to be determined.

The present concept of the processing of the precursor of pro-opiomelanocortin does not account, however, for all the immunocytochemical findings concerning the cellular localization of components such as α-MSH and Met-enkephalin (Met-enk). It is now generally accepted that ACTH of the intermediate lobe is a precursor of α-MSH (Crine et al. 1979). However in some mammals, the cells of the intermediate lobe do not react with antisera specific to ACTH sequences (Tramu and Beauvillain 1980). Moreover, there is no explanation yet for the presence of α-MSH immunoreactivity only in cells of the pars intermedia. Met-enk, the N terminal pentapeptide of β-endorphin, has been localized in cells of both the anterior and intermediate lobes thanks to the use of antisera specific for Met-enk or for Leu–enk (Rossier et al. 1977). However, a further identification of the stained cells led to unexpected findings. The ACTH cells are only slightly stained in the rat and even less so in the guinea pig, whereas the thyrotropes in the rat and both the thyrotropes and the gonadotropes in the guinea pig are strongly stained (Tramu and Leonardelli 1979). Other authors have localized this activity in somatotropes of the rat pituitary (Weber et al. 1978). The hypothesis that this localization may correspond to binding sites for Met- or Leu-enk of brain origin in pituitary target cells has been put forward (Tramu and Leonardelli 1979). However, one cannot exclude an endogeneous synthesis, since cultured GH_3 cells have been found also to contain immunoreactive Met-enk (Gourdji et al. unpublished results).

On the whole, this 'natural history' of the ACTH cell represents an impressive example of a pituitary cell which secretes several hormones, some of them at least related by a common affiliation.

Cellular origin of glycoprotein hormones

The cellular origin of the three glycoprotein hormones FSH, LH and TSH has been, for many years, the subject of controversy.

(i) A separate origin for thyrotropin was, at first, rather convincingly suggested by cytochemical studies with the help of the Alcian blue PAS method applied to several vertebrate species (Herlant 1964). Immunocytology was not immediately successful in identifying thyrotropic cells because of cross reactivities between antisera directed against gonadotropins and thyrotropins. This has now been solved, in mammals at least, following progress in understanding the biochemistry of glycoprotein hormones in this vertebrate class. Indeed it is now well established that these hormones consist of two subunits: the α subunit, which is common to the three hormones, at least in a given species: and the β subunit, which determines the specificity of the biological activity of the corresponding hormone. Antibodies directed against purified α or β subunits from several mammalian species (rat, ovine, porcine, human being) were soon applied to the rat pituitary (Tougard et al 1971, 1973: Baker et al. 1972). As could be expected, antisera against LH-α stained both presumptive gonadotropes and thyrotropes. Besides, antiserum specific for TSH-β definitely demonstrated the existence of a separate cell type for TSH secretion (Moriarty 1976: Moriarty and Tobin 1976: Tougard et al. 1980a). The ultrastructure of the immunochemically identified TSH cells was identical to that previously described by Farquhar and

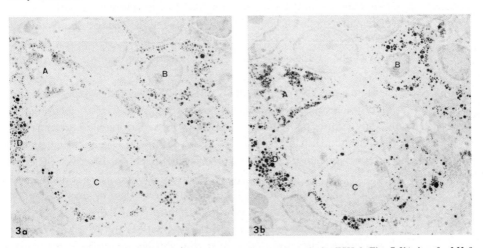

Fig. 7.3. Four type I gonadotropes (A, B, C, D) stained more intensely for FSH-β (Fig. 7.3b) than for LH-β (Fig. 7.3a). Cell A is stained only for FSH-β. In cells B, C, D, the secretory granules stained for LH-β are far less numerous than those stained for FSH-β (Courtesy of G.W. Childs) (× 3250).

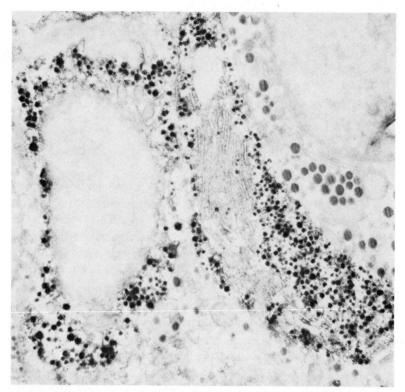

Fig. 7.4. Two type B gonadotropes from a male rat pituitary immunochemically stained with antiserum against ovine LH (pre-embedding method). They display the ultrastructural features of Kurosumi's 'LH cell' or Moriarty's type II gonadotrope (× 10 000).

Rinehart using conventional electron microscopy (1954a), that is with a polygonal or stellate shape, very small secretory granules (100–150 nm) and flattened or slightly dilated RER cisternae (Moriarty and Tobin 1976: Tougard et al. 1980a: Tougard 1980). In conclusion, at present one can consider that in the case of thyrotropin the concept 'one hormone-one cell type' remains valid.

(ii) A separate origin for the two gonadotropins, LH and FSH was long ago postulated on the basis of histophysiological correlations, using cytochemistry as well as electron microscopy (Herlant 1964). In the rat, where many studies were performed, Kurosumi and Oota (1968) defined the ultrastructural features of 'FSH cells' and 'LH cells' which served as a reference for further immunoelectron microscope identifications. Briefly, FSH cells possess two classes of secretory granules (approx. 200 nm and 300–700 nm diam.) and dilated RER cisternae (Fig. 7.3) whereas LH cells contain one class of small secretory granules (200–250 nm diameter) and flattened RER cisternae (Fig. 7.4).

The earliest immunocytochemical studies in rats showed that LH and FSH were contained in the same cells. Since they were performed with antisera directed against whole hormones, this result could be the consequence of cross reaction between the two hormones due to their common subunit. However, the use of antisera specific for the β subunits led again to the conclusion that both hormones are present in the same cells. At present this has been shown at both the light and the electron microscopic levels in several mammalian species: the rat (Nakane 1970, 1975: Tougard et al. 1980a: Tougard 1980: Moriarty 1973, 1975, 1976: Herbert 1975: Bugnon et al. 1977), the human being (Phifer et al. 1973: Pelletier et al. 1976), the monkey (Herbert 1976), the dog (El Etreby and Fath El Bab 1977), the mouse (Baker and Gross 1978), and the pig (Dacheux 1978). However, some of these authors found that a small proportion of the gonadotropes contained one hormone only, either FSH or LH, in the rat, the human being, the dog and the pig (Childs et al. 1980).

Electron microscope immunocytochemistry demonstrated moreover that the coexistence of LH and FSH within the same cell is associated with their coexistence within the same granules as revealed by post-embedding staining on serial thin sections (Moriarty 1976: Tougard et al. 1980).

The finding that LH and FSH coexist in the same cells and the same secretory granules raised two important questions: (1) What is the biochemical significance of the structural duality of the gonadotropes, as above reported in the rat for example? (2) How can we correlate the immunocytochemical findings with the many physiological data showing that LH and FSH are not released in a parallel manner? Regarding the first question, it should be emphasized that at the electron microscope level both Kurosumi's LH cell and FSH cell

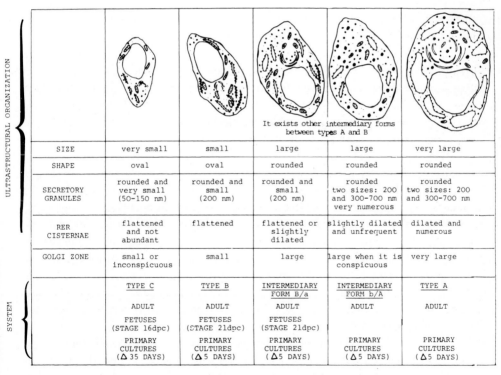

			It exists other intermediary forms between types A and B		
SIZE	very small	small	large	large	very large
SHAPE	oval	oval	rounded	rounded	rounded
SECRETORY GRANULES	rounded and very small (50-150 nm)	rounded and small (200 nm)	rounded and small (200 nm)	rounded two sizes: 200 and 300-700 nm very numerous	rounded two sizes: 200 and 300-700 nm
RER CISTERNAE	flattened and not abundant	flattened	flattened or slightly dilated	slightly dilated and unfrequent	dilated and numerous
GOLGI ZONE	small or inconspicuous	small	large	large when it is conspicuous	very large
	TYPE C	TYPE B	INTERMEDIARY FORM B/a	INTERMEDIARY FORM b/A	TYPE A
	ADULT	ADULT	ADULT	ADULT	ADULT
	FETUSES (STAGE 16dpc)	FETUSES (STAGE 21dpc)	FETUSES (STAGE 21dpc)		
	PRIMARY CULTURES (Δ 35 DAYS)	PRIMARY CULTURES (Δ5 DAYS)	PRIMARY CULTURES (Δ5 DAYS)	PRIMARY CULTURES (Δ5 DAYS)	PRIMARY CULTURES (Δ5 DAYS)

(left margin, vertical: ULTRASTRUCTURAL ORGANIZATION / SYSTEM)

Fig. 7.5. Diagrammatic representation of the different ultrastructural forms of the gonadotropic cells (reproduced from Tougard 1980).

contain both LH and FSH, and that, in addition, a large variety of intermediate forms are also immunochemically stained (Tixier-Vidal et al. 1975; Tougard et al. 1980a; Tougard 1980) (Fig. 7.5). Moreover, even when LH only or FSH only could be localized in 19 % of the gonadotropes, there was no clear cut ultrastructural distinction between cells containing both hormones and cells containing only one (Childs et al. 1980). It is clear therefore that the structural duality, or rather heterogeneity, of the gonadotropes does not reflect a biochemical specialization. Progress in the knowledge of the mechanism of biosynthesis of LH and FSH is nevertheless needed to confirm this conclusion, which is based on cytochemistry only. By analogy with the pro-opiocortin series, one might imagine the existence of a common precursor to LH and FSH which remains to be biochemically proven.

As an answer to the second question, it has been proposed that the structural heterogeneity of the gonadotropes may reflect several stages of the secretory cycle of one single cell type capable of storing or releasing LH and FSH in different proportions depending on the physiological situations (Fig. 7.5) (Tougard 1980). The structural heterogeneity would thus reflect a functional heterogeneity, which has also been suggested for other cell types. However, according to Childs et al. (1980), the 'presence of a significant number of cells containing only one of the hormones ... may be one mechanism for non-parallel release of gonadotropins'.

Conclusion

In the light of present immunocytochemical findings, the one cell–one hormone theory is still valid for GH, PRL and TSH. The fact that several hormones of the pro-opiomelanocortin series are stored within the same cells and the same granules does not represent a fundamental objection to the theory since all of these hormones derive from a common precursor. The only remaining exception therefore concerns the case of LH and FSH which are mostly stored within the same cells. But again, there are biochemical similarities between these two hormones. In terms of biochemical specialization one assists therefore to a reduction in number of specific cell types.

It should be pointed out nevertheless that immunocytochemistry has several limits, since it visualizes mostly cellular sites of storage. In most endocrine cells, the capacity of storage is associated with the capacity of synthesis. However this is not always the case. The material which is stored may represent exogenous molecules accumulated in target cells. This was proposed to explain the presence of a Met-enk-like immunoreactivity in thyrotropes and gonadotropes (Tramu and Leonardelli 1979). Similarly, the hypothalamic peptide, luliberin (GnRH) was visualized in secretory granules of gonadotropes using the post-embedding staining (Sternberger and Petrali 1975). The presence in secretory granules of ACTH-like reactivity together with reactivity for FSH-β in some gonadotropes may also reveal a multipotential capacity of these cells, either to produce or to store these hormones (Moriarty and Garner 1977; Childs et al. 1980). Conversely, the capacity to synthesize is not necessarily accompanied by a high storage capacity and thus the cells may escape immunocytochemical detection. This is the case of small granular, or poorly granulated cells which have been considered as multipotent stem cells (Shiino et al. 1978). Another limitation of immunocytochemistry resides in the fact that granulated cells may also be unstained, even with post-embedding staining on thin sections where problems with the penetration of antibodies are completely overcome (Childs et al. 1980). In spite of these limitations, immunocytochemistry remains a powerful tool and one can conclude that it led to a revision but not to destruction of the 'one cell–one hormone' concept.

Contribution of electron microscope immunocytochemistry to the present concept of the AP cell secretory process

The present concept of the intracellular pathway of AP cell secretory products, as reviewed in the introduction, received confirmation from quantitative autoradiographic studies of pulse chase experiments performed in GH cells (Howell and Whitfields 1973: Farquhar et al. 1975) and in PRL cells (Tixier-Vidal and Picart 1967: Farquhar et al. 1978). This demonstrated convincingly that the newly synthesized proteins undergo a transit from the RER cisternae to the Golgi zone where they undergo concentration and may stay for varying time intervals before being stored within membrane-bound secretory granules. However, this does not permit identification of the chemical nature of the transferred labelled proteins, which would enable us to follow the path of the specific secretory product within a given cell.

Theoretically, electron microscope immunocytochemistry should have satisfied that requirement, and thus should have brought information complementary to that of biochemistry, which also uses the immunological tool to identify nascent hormones in cell-free systems. In fact, the results vary greatly depending on the method (post-embedding versus pre-embedding staining), the fixative or the cell type. They will be examined at the successive steps of the secretory cycle.

RER cisternae

The presence of an immunostainable material within the RER cisternae, which could be expected, was in fact observed in some cases only and almost exclusively with the pre-embedding method. In the rat gonadotropic cells, dilated RER cisternae were sometimes seen filled with material antigenic for an anti-rLH-β in normal rat (Tougard 1980: Tougard et al. 1980a) (Fig. 7.6) or an anti-oLH-β in highly vacuolized cells of castrated rats (Tougard et al. 1973). In thyrotropic cells of thyroidectomized rats a positive reaction within dilated RER could be observed with the post-embedding method (Moriarty and Tobin 1976). In PRL cells the presence of an antigenic material within RER cisternae could be visualized with the pre-embedding method only and required permeabilizing the cells with saponin following fixation with glutaraldehyde with or without paraformol (Tougard et al. 1980b). Under these conditions almost all RER cisternae, including the perinuclear cisternae, were filled with reaction product in highly active PRL cells in primary cultures (Fig. 7.7). It seems therefore that the staining of an antigenic material within RER cisternae should be possible for any cell type provided the right conditions for fixation and immunostaining are selected. It is facilitated in highly active cells and with high title antisera.

222

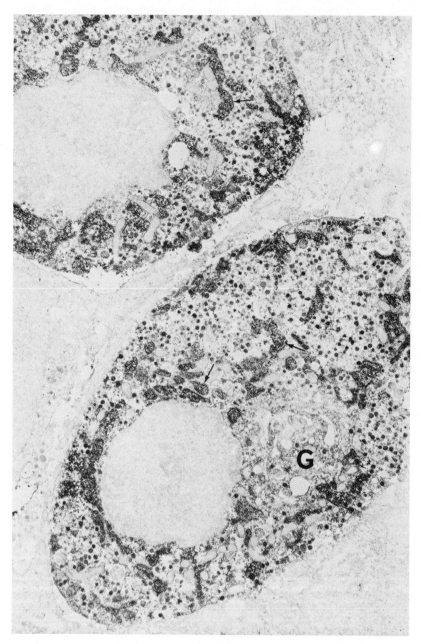

Fig. 7.6. Two gonadotropes from a male rat pituitary immunochemically stained with antiserum against rat LH-β (pre-embedding method). Their ultrastructural organization is very close to that of Kurosumi's 'FSH cells' or Moriarty's type I, excepted that they have a smaller amount of large secretory granules as compared to Fig. 7.3. One notes that the RER cisternae are filled with reaction product (arrow) whereas the Golgi cisternae (G) are negative (× 8000).

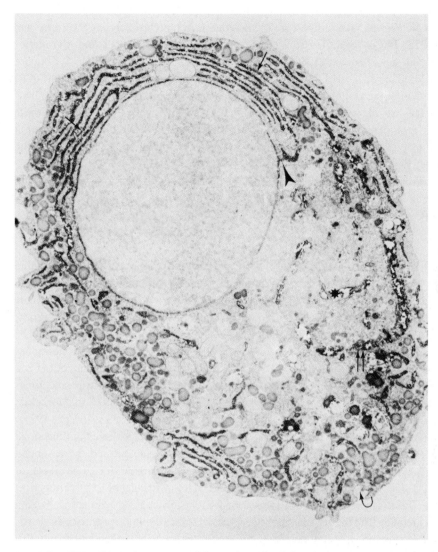

Fig. 7.7. A PRL cell in a primary culture of dispersed rat AP cells immunochemically stained with an antiserum against rat PRL using the pre-embedding method and permeabilization with saponin according to Tougard et al. (1980b). This method permits visualization of PRL within: 1, the perinuclear cisternae, sometimes in continuity (curved arrowhead) with the parallel RER cisternae (single arrow), 2, the most outer Golgi saccules (double arrows) and 3, a cisterna located in the core of the Golgi zone (asterisk) which may correspond to the GERL (Novikoff and Novikoff 1977). With this method secretory granules are only outlined with reaction product (the semicircular arrow marks a profile of granule exocytosis) (× 10 000).

Golgi zone

In most cases, the Golgi zone escaped immunostaining, with the exception of some positive secretory granules in the core of the zone in some corticotropes (Moriarty and Halmi 1972a: Bacsy et al. 1976: Weber et al. 1978c), gonadotropes and thyrotropes (Tougard et al. 1973: Tougard 1980) and PRL cells (Parsons and Erlandsen 1974: Tougard et al. 1980b). This suggested that the antigenicity of the hormone was masked during its movement within the Golgi saccules and vesicles. However, progress was recently obtained with the use of saponine, as noted above (Tougard et al. 1980b). Under these conditions, the inner faces of the outer Golgi cisternae were clearly underlined with reaction product. Inner saccules were also sometimes stained, depending on the extension of the Golgi zone (Fig. 7.7).

In GH$_3$ clonal prolactin cells the same fixative permitted the localization of PRL within cisternae and vesicles of the Golgi zone as well as within RER cisternae (Tougard et al. in press) (Fig. 7.8).

Secretory granules

Regardless of the technical procedure, secretory granules display the strongest staining intensity. This was observed for all pituitary cell types in complete agreement with fractionation data showing a maximal hormonal concentration in the secretory granule fraction. Moreover, in the case of hormones such as those of the pro-opiocortin series, which are derived from the sequential splitting of a large common precursor, most could be localized simultaneously in the same secretory granule. Similarly, in the case of hormones which display a quaternary structure, such as the gonadotropins, both subunits of LH and FSH were localized in the same secretory granule. Differential staining was sometimes reported for the two classes of secretory granules present in gonadotropes of Moriarty's type I, Tougard's type A, or Kurosumi's FSH type (Tougard et al. 1973: Moriarty 1975). With the post-embedding method, the large granules were more positive than the small ones, which suggested that they might be specific for the β subunit and the α subunit respectively (Moriarty 1975). However, this hypothesis was ruled out since both classes of secretory granules were stained with an anti-LH-α as well as with an anti-LH-β (Tougard et al. 1980a). There is therefore no conclusive evidence for a different subcellular localization of the two subunits. The finding that hormones derived from a common precursor as well as that hormone subunits are simultaneously present in the same granules is of theoretical importance because it suggests that there is no sorting of the secretory proteins at the level of the Golgi zone and no biochemical compartmentalization within the post-Golgi secretory granule population.

Cytoplasm

A slight cytoplasmic staining was always observed with the pre-embedding method only, for any cell type: gonadotropes and thyrotropes (Tougard et al. 1973, 1980a: Beauvillain et al. 1975), corticotropes (Bacsy et al. 1976: Weber et al. 1978a) and lactotropes (Tougard et al. 1980b). In some cases the distribution of the staining seemed to follow the ribosomal localization. The possibility that this staining represents an artifact, caused by a displace-

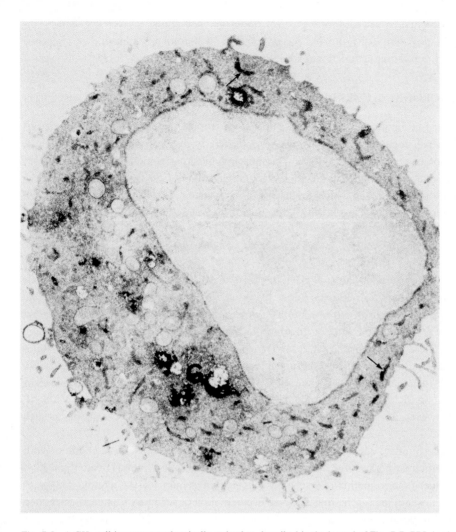

Fig. 7.8. A GH₃ cell immunocytochemically stained as described in the legend of Fig. 7.7. PRL is visualized within discontinuous RER cisternae (arrows) as well as in the perinuclear cisternae. The Golgi zone (G) displays a greater concentration of reaction product. A specific deposit also is found in the cytoplasm, likely associated to polysomes. As compared to normal PRL cells in culture the GH₃ cells differ by the extreme paucity and small size of secretory granules (which are not visible in this picture) and the different organization of RER and Golgi zone (× 12 000).

ment from other antigenic sites as a consequence of the fixation, cannot be completely ruled out. However, the fact that it was observed in cells with very few or no secretory granules such as clonal PRL cells (Tixier-Vidal et al. 1976) suggests that it may also reflect an intrinsic localization, at least under some conditions.

In conclusion, it appears from recent progress in the fixatives used with the pre-embedding method that electron microscopic immunostaining of the main subcellular steps delineating the pathway of the secretory products within AP cells is now possible, provided the right fixative is selected for a given hormone and sometimes a given organelle. This opens the possibility of following the progression of hormones within the endoplasmic reticulum in relation to functional stimuli (Tougard et al. in press).

MORPHOLOGICAL CORRELATES OF FUNCTIONAL REGULATION IN AP CELLS

As noted in the introduction to this chapter, the complex interactions of the numerous factors which regulate the activity of AP cells finally result in either an inhibition or stimulation of the secretory activity. The morphological correlations of these regulatory activities may be considered at several levels of organization, from the individual cell to the adenohypophysial tissue which represents a non-random association of different cell populations. These two levels will be examined separately.

Morphological correlates of individual cell response to inhibitory agents

Since the pioneering, and now classical, work of Farquhar (Smith and Farquhar 1966: Farquhar 1969) demonstrating the role of lysosomes in regulating secretion of AP cells, no further progress seems to have been made, at least up to 1981. Studying the lactating rat following removal of the litter or the thyroidectomized rat treated with thyroid hormone, Farquhar clearly showed that large numbers of secretory granules fuse with lysosomes where they are degraded. This is a fundamental mechanism which is also most probably involved when the inhibition of secretion is rapidly induced by a neurotransmitter, such as dopamine on PRL cells, or by an inhibiting peptide, such as somatostatin on several AP cells. However, to our knowledge, only a few observations have been made in such situations.

In human pituitary adenomas, treatment with L-dopa in vitro (Cesselin and Peillon 1980) or long-term treatment in vivo with 2-Br-α-ergocriptine (bromocriptine) (Beauvillain et al. 1976) induced the formation of lysosomes. Incubation of human GH-secreting adenomas with somatostatin led for the first 2 h to an accumulation of secretory granules which then decreased in number (Cesselin and Peillon 1980). In cultured GH_3 tumor rat PRL cells exposed for several days to high doses of bromocriptine an increased number of dense bodies was reported, together with a reduction in the size of the Golgi zone (Gourdji et al. 1980).

In normal PRL cells in primary cultures, bromocriptine treatment for a period ranging from 4 to 24 h induced the accumulation of large secretory granules and the formation of dense bodies and autophagic vacuoles. This was correlated with a transient increase of the cell immunoreactivity, which then decreased after several days of treatment. This result is consistent with a progressive, slow decrease in PRL cell content (Antakly et al. 1980). Biochemical studies have shown that this decrease results at least in part from degradation of the hormone (Dannies and Rudnick 1980), but it is not yet possible to tell whether PRL synthesis is affected as well (MacLeod et al. 1979). Moreover, a stimulation of lysosomal enzyme activity occurs rapidly in the anterior pituitary following exposure to dopamine in vivo as well as in vitro (Nansel et al. 1981).

Morphological correlates of individual cell response to stimulating agents

The secretion of AP hormones is stimulated primarily by neuropeptides. Steroids and thyroid hormones interfere with that stimulation through either facilitating or inhibiting effects (Labrie et al. 1980). Moreover, estrogens exert a direct stimulating action of their own, mostly on PRL cells. However this effect requires days of exposure and is classically considered to occur at the genomic level. In contrast, the effect of stimulating neuropeptides on hormonal secretion is biphasic. It involves first the rapid release of a previously formed hormonal pool and then a long–term delayed effect on hormone synthesis. The first phase occurs within minutes, whereas the second one lasts for hours and days (Vale et al. 1977; Tixier-Vidal and Gourdji 1981). Although there is a progressive transition from the first phase to the second, their respective ultrastructural correlates may be considered separately.

Ultrastructural correlates of rapid release

A rapid and massive extrusion of secretory granules via exocytosis occurs within a few minutes in TSH cells and GH cells in response to intravenous injection of TRH (Wilbur et al. 1978: Okino et al. 1979: Wilbur and Spicer 1980) and in LH cells in response to GnRH (Shiino et al. 1972: Mendoza et al. 1973). Morphometric studies in TSH cells showed that the number of granules released reaches its maximum after 10 min (Okino et al. 1979). Rapid hormonal release is not always so clearly correlated with granule exocytosis. In primary cultures of dispersed AP cells exposed to GnRH for 15–30 min, classical profiles of granule extrusion were not found in LH cells, but many granules were seen lining the plasma membrane, and after immunocytochemical staining they displayed structural changes. This suggests that GnRH simultaneously induced a rapid migration of secretory granules toward the plasma membrane and a structural reorganization of their matrix, leading to a decrease of its electron density before or during exocytosis (Tixier-Vidal et al. 1975). In cultured GH_3 cells, which have very few small secretory granules, the rapid release of PRL following exposure to TRH was not correlated with the classical profiles of granule extrusion. However, when present, small secretory granules were seen beneath the plasma membrane, which suggests their migration within the cytoplasm. Moreover, numerous vesicles and canaliculi were seen in close proximity to the plasma membrane (Tixier-Vidal et al. 1975).

Another morphological correlate of rapid hormonal release concerns ultrastructural signs of an increased mobility of the plasma membrane. This has been observed mostly in cultured cells, which offer a favorable model. Cell thin sections prepared in a direction parallel to the monolayer revealed in normal gonadotropes exposed to GnRH, as well as in clonal GH_3 cells exposed to TRH, a stretching of the plasma membrane, formation of microvilli and branched cytoplasmic processes (Gourdji et al. 1972; Tixier-Vidal et al. 1975). Under the phase contrast microscope, the cells were seen spread over their substrate and enlarged (Gourdji et al. 1972; Tashjian and Hoyt 1972). Scanning electron microscope observations also revealed the formation of blebs at the surface of GH_3 cells exposed to TRH (Tashjian and Hoyt 1972) and of blebs and microvilli at the surface of normal PRL cells cultured in the presence of estradiol or TRH (Antakly et al. 1980). An effect of TRH on the mobility of membrane components has also been demonstrated in another PRL cell line, SD$_1$, using binding of Concanavalin A as a quantitative tool (Brunet et al. 1977). These modifications in the mobility of plasma membrane strongly suggest a role of the cytoskeleton which, however, has not yet been morphologically documented. They also suggest that exposure to a stimulating agent enhances endocytosis either as a consequence of exocytosis, in order to retrieve membrane granules inserted in the plasma membrane, or as a direct effect of the ligand on the plasma membrane (Tixier-Vidal et al. 1976; Tixier-Vidal and Gourdji 1980).

The Golgi zone also undergoes rapid modifications concomitantly with acute stimulation of hormone release. These occur almost simultaneously with granule exocytosis and signs of increased membrane mobility, and consist of the accumulation of small vesicles, coated or smooth, the flattening of Golgi saccules and the appearance of newly formed secretory granules. A progressive extension of the Golgi zone also occurs. This was reported in clonal GH$_3$ cells (Gourdji et al. 1972) in normal LH cells in culture (Tixier-Vidal et al. 1975), and in LH cells and TSH cells in vivo (Okino et al. 1979; Wilbur and Spicer 1980).

Taken together, these observations suggest that an acute hormonal release is rapidly correlated with a rehandling of the entire smooth reticulum from the plasma membrane to the Golgi zone.

In contrast, an extension of the RER cisternae was reported primarily after chronic treatment (see next section). However, rapid alterations have also been reported in a few cases. Morphometric studies on TSH cells following injection of TRH revealed that the surface of the RER reached a maximum at 20 min, i.e., 10 min later than that of the Golgi zone (Okino et al. 1979). After infusion of TRH or GnRH into the portal vessels, the extension of the RER even preceded that of the Golgi zone (Wilbur and Spicer 1980).

The visualization of the hormonal content of the cell endoplasmic reticulum, both rough and smooth, would permit us to follow the progression of secretory product during acute release. Such an attempt has recently been made in our laboratory, using GH$_3$ cells exposed to TRH. This revealed that both the RER cisternae and the Golgi cisternae became empty of immunoreactive prolactin after 1 h of treatment. Within the following hour, their immunoreactive content was restored above control level simultaneously in both compartments. This re-loading of the endoplasmic reticulum is completely abolished in the presence of cycloheximide (Tougard et al. in press). These observations complement those obtained by immunocytochemistry at the light microscope level in GH$_3$ cells showing that TRH induces an initial loss of intracellular hormone (0–4 h), overlapped, beginning at 3–4 h, by a progressive increase of intracellular hormone (Hoyt and Tashjian 1980b). Taken together, these immunocytochemical findings offer a convincing morphological correlate to the biphasic effect of stimulating neuropeptides.

Ultrastructural correlates of chronic stimulation

Morphological studies on chronic stimulation with GnRH or TRH have been performed in vitro in organ cultures of rat pituitary exposed for up to 24 h (Zambrano et al. 1974; Cuerdo-Rocha and Zambrano 1974) or for up to 10 days (Shiino 1979). In vivo the effects of continuous infusion through the femoral vein with GnRH, or TRH, or both, for up to 72 h in young male rats have also been reported (Soji 1978a, 1978b). In spite of some differences in the results or in their interpretations, all of these works reveal similar features of the continuously stimulated cells: extreme extension of the Golgi zone, development and dilatation of RER cisternae, and a decrease in the size and number of secretory granules. At the same time, both gonadotropes and thyrotropes are hypertrophied. The pictures finally become quite similar to those previously described in gonadectomized or thyroidectomized rats (Farquhar and Rinehart 1954a, 1954b). Indeed, so-called 'castration' cells or 'thyroidectomy' cells may appear in cultures exposed to GnRH or TRH, respectively. However, the authors disagree on the rapidity of appearance of these cells, which would require 3–6 h for Zambrano's group, instead of the several days according to Shiino (1979), who used lower doses and pituitaries of younger rats. In young rats continuously infused with TRH or GnRH, thyroidectomy cells and castration cells appear after 48 h (Soji 1978a, 1978b). However, this author, in agreement with Yoshimura's theory (Yoshimura et al. 1974) of the secretory cycle of anterior basophils, considers that TRH, as well as GnRH, acts by progressive changes along the secretory cycle of a single basophil type which would be involved in the secretion of TSH, FSH and LH. This theory was based on electron microscopic observations in order to account for the extreme difficulty of differentiating gonadotropes and thyrotropes after prolonged stimulation of their activity. It hypothesized the conversion of one cell 'subtype' into another. However, with progress in immunocytochemistry it has become difficult to accept this theory in its totality (see previous section).

Chronic treatment of primary cultures of AP cells with GnRH (2 µg ml^{-1}) for 1 month also induced cell hypertrophy and degranulation of a single cell type, although castration cells were never found (Tixier-Vidal et al. 1975). Indeed, in such cultures GnRH failed to maintain the structural heterogeneity of the gonadotropes which evolve toward a single cell type in culture (Tougard et al. 1977a). Neither did it increase the number of immunoreactive gonadotropic cells (Tixier-Vidal et al. 1975). A similar observation was made in pituitary autografts whether or not the host was treated with GnRH, and whether in conjunction or not with estradiol or progesterone (Shiino et al. 1980).

Structural and functional heterogeneity of AP cells

The ultrastructural correlates of individual cell response to stimulating agents, as reported above, are never observed simultaneously in the totality of the cell population for a given cell type. This is true not only for the pituitary gland in vivo but also for primary cultures of dispersed pituitary cells in vitro and even for clonal cell lines like the GH$_3$ PRL cells. One is faced in fact with a heterogeneous population of cells which differ more or less from their archetype in the relative development of the three cytoplasmic compartments, RER, Golgi zone and secretory granules (Herlant 1975). This certainly represents one of the greatest difficulties in analyzing the ultrastructural correlates of pituitary cell function. Indeed in most experiments, the measured hormonal response represents the averaged response of individual cells which are not working in a synchronized fashion. Due to technical limitations, it is not yet possible to correlate ultrastructure and secretory activity at the single cell level. However, the recent development of a cell-separation technique by velocity sedimentation at unit gravity (Hymer 1975; Hymer et al. 1980) has permitted not only the isolation of cell populations enriched in a specific cell type, but also the separation according to size and density of cell subpopulations belonging to the same cell type. Functional and morphological studies on cell subpopulations have now been performed for PRL cells, GH cells, TSH cells and gonadotropes. These studies were not planned with the same purpose and have not yet led to common conclusions. They will be reviewed for each cell type.

PRL cells

The first indication of a link between structural heterogeneity and functional heterogeneity of PRL cells came from the finding that maximum cell PRL content was not found in cells of the same size density, depending on the physiological state of the donor. Moreover, the cell fractions which displayed maximum PRL content also displayed the maximum ability to secrete after 14 days in culture (Snyder et al. 1976). Further convincing evidence for a functional heterogeneity of PRL cells has been recently obtained by Walker and Farquhar (1980) using a different approach. Primary cultures of dispersed AP cells were submitted to pulse-chase experiments with [³H]leucine and then treated for electron microscope autoradiography. Analysis of the distribution of total grains per cell in mammotropes revealed the presence of several functional populations which differed in the rapidity of loss of autoradiographic grains during the chase period. This suggests that some cells have a faster turnover time of PRL than others and would be responsible for the rapid release of newly synthesized PRL observed after 15–30 min of chase. Such cells would not be responsive to TRH, which releases an older PRL pool in these primary cultures, a feature previously observed in PRL cell lines (Dannies and Tashjian 1973; Morin et al. 1976). In their light microscope immunocytochemical study, Hoyt and Tashjian (1980a) also established a functional diversity of these cloned cells.

GH cells

The separation of two classes of somatotropes by discontinuous density gradient centrifugation has been clearly demonstrated by Snyder et al. (1977). Type I somatotropes have few secretory granules and extensive Golgi zone and RER, whereas type II store many secretory granules. Type I cells produce more GH in culture and give better response to hormones than type II cells. However, after 6 days in culture, the ultrastructural differences between type I and type II cells were no longer visible.

TSH cells

Some evidence for a structural and functional heterogeneity in thyrotropes has been reported from separation experiments (Leuschen et al. 1978). In contrast to PRL cells, but like somatotropes, the thyrotrope fractions which contained the lowest content of TSH displayed the highest ability to secrete TSH in culture.

Gonadotropic cells

Strong evidence for a functional significance of the morphological heterogeneity of the gonadotropic cell population has been obtained from cell separation experiments by Denef and his colleagues (1978a, 1978b, 1980). Working with pituitaries of 14-day-old rats, male or female, they separated gonadotropes according to size and found that irrespective of cell size the majority of the cells contained both FSH and LH, but that FSH and, to a lesser extent, LH were also stored in separate cells. Moreover the FSH/LH ratio changed with cell size and the pattern was highly characteristic for each fraction (Denef et al. 1978a). When the secretory potential of five subfractions was measured in culture, a characteristic pattern of LH and FSH release was found for each of them. This pattern was related to the cell size rather than to the initial hormonal content. Moreover, in all fractions GnRH released both FSH and LH (Denef et al. 1978b). A differential modulation of FSH and LH release by androgens in response to GnRH was also found among gonadotrope subpopulations from 14-day-old female rats (Denef et al. 1980). Taken together, these findings strongly suggest that the selective modulations of FSH or LH release in vivo result from the functional heterogeneity of the gonadotropes. Variations in the number of cells in the different subpopulations may account for non-parallel release of FSH and LH in response to various hormones. The link between this functional heterogeneity and the structural heterogeneity previously demonstrated by electron microscope immunocytochemistry appears most likely. Preliminary electron microscopic observations have shown that the lightest fraction consists mostly of small cells belonging to Tougard's type B or Kurosumi's LH type, whereas the heaviest fraction mostly consists of large cells belonging to Tougard's type A or Kurosumi's FSH type. However, cells displaying numerous intermediate forms were also found in both fractions. When put in culture for 6 days both fractions evolved toward a single cell type with small secretory granules (Tougard and Denef, unpublished results). Thus, as already reported for long-term cultures of the total cell population (Tougard et al. 1977a), the structural heterogeneity of the gonadotropes disappear in culture whereas the functional heterogeneity persists (Denef 1980).

Conclusion

For the time being the studies available on separate cell subpopulations do not permit a common rule to be formulated for any cell type as concerns the exact link between structural and functional heterogeneity. The most important new finding is the discovery that a functional heterogeneity of the cells may account for selective hormonal responses. One of the most intriguing questions concerns the possibility of interconversion between the subpopulations of a same cell type. Are they the expression of a permanent situation or of different phases of a secretory cycle along which the cells would move in response to stimuli? The latter hypothesis seems the most probable. This is suggested for example by the fact that the structural heterogeneity of gonadotropes is established only after birth, whereas during fetal life a single cell type accounts for the secretion of both gonadotropes (Tougard et al. 1977b).

The mechanisms which are responsible for the structural and functional diversification of AP cells are certainly multiple. Among them hypothalamic peptides and peripheral hormones most probably play an important role. In addition, the influence of cell-to-cell communication between cells secreting different hormones has been recently put forward by a very promising finding of Denef (1980). This author showed that co-culture of gonadotropes with an acidophile–chromophobe fraction potentiated LH release. This effect required direct cell contact. This hypothesis is strongly supported by the morphological features of the pituitary gland, where homologous cells always form clusters closely associated with clusters of heterologous cells, sometimes through differentiated local junctions.

Regulation of pituitary cell number

The variation in the number of cells belonging to a specific cell type in response to hormonal triggering is another classical feature of the AP gland. It is well known, for example, that during gestation, as well as after castration or thyroidectomy, the number of PRL cells, gonadotropes or thyrotropes, is increased. This causes gland hyperplasia. The mechanism involved in such an adaptation of the AP tissue has received relatively scant attention since the review of Olivier et al. (1975). According to this review, the existence of mitosis in the AP tissue is no longer questioned, since this was demonstrated by the presence of mitotic figures as well as by autoradiography using labelled thymidine. To explain the recruitment of new cells within a specific cell type, several theories have been proposed: 1. The existence of stem cells which are not functionally determined, but are able to divide and then to differentiate into functionally specific cells. 2. The existence of stem cells is questioned and mitosis is held to occur in fully differentiated cells. 3. In addition to mitosis, another mechanism participates in hyperplasia: the conversion of fully differentiated cells from one cell type to another (Olivier et al. 1975). All of these theories are based on indirect evidence obtained from physiological situations which reflect complex hormonal regulations. It was of interest therefore to look for a direct mitogenic effect of specific agents which regulate hormonal secretion. This has been the subject of very few studies thus far.

Estrogens stimulate DNA synthesis in PRL cells (Stevens and Helfenstein 1966), whereas castration diminishes DNA replication in gonadotropes (Hymer et al. 1970) and bromocriptine does the same in PRL cells (Dannies et al. 1974). According to Kalbermann et al. (1979), these drugs or hormones regulate DNA replication indirectly. The signal responsible for the induction of DNA replication would be an acute transitory depletion of PRL cell content. Since all of these studies were performed in vivo, it should be mentioned that direct action of estrogens on glandular cell proliferation has never been found in vitro, which suggested to Sirbasku that they act in vivo by inducing a specific growth factor (Sirbasku 1978).

An effect of hypophysiotropic neuropeptides on cell mitosis has been reported in organ cultures of the male rat. Exposure for several days to high doses of TRH (10^{-6} M) increased the number of mitoses in basophiles, an effect which was antagonized by thyroxine (Pawlikowki et al. 1979) and by SRIF (Pawlikowski et al. 1978). TRH was also found to stimulate the proliferation of clonal GH_3 cells on serum-free medium (Wu and Sato 1978), but in the presence of serum it inhibited the proliferation of the same cells (Brunet et al.

1981). It should be mentioned however that to our knowledge no effect of TRH or GnRH, at physiological doses, on cell mitosis has been reported in primary culture of dispersed AP cells.

ELECTROPHYSIOLOGICAL CORRELATES OF AP CELL FUNCTION

From the early electrophysiological studies on AP cells, it was concluded that these cells have a very low transmembrane potential (Milligan and Kraicer 1970; Martin et al. 1973) and do not display action potentials either spontaneously or when stimulated by hypothalamic extracts (York et al. 1973). More recent studies of both tumoral and non-tumoral pituitary cells have demonstrated that these cells are able to generate action potentials spontaneously or in response to membrane depolarization (Vincent et al. 1980). Furthermore, it has been shown that substances which influence hormonal release from these cells also have an effect on their electrical membrane properties. This agrees with the suggestion that it may be through the initiation or modulation of action potentials that the brain, through the hypophysiotropic factors, regulates releasing activities in the anterior pituitary (Taraskevitch and Douglas 1977).

Passive electrical membrane properties

Different values of the mean resting membrane potential of AP cells have been reported, varying with the cell type and the technical conditions. Using slices of rat pituitary glands, Ozawa and Sand (1978) found resting potentials ranging from −20 to −65 mV. In the rat pituitary pars intermedia, the cells which yielded action potentials in response to depolarization had a resting potential of −66 ± 2.8 mV. Cells with lower resting potentials had probably been damaged by electrode penetration, since spikes either failed to appear or could be evoked only by determining a hyperpolarizing pulse (Douglas and Taraskevich 1978). A large range of values of mean resting potential has also been obtained from tumoral pituitary cells. In early studies of GH_3 cells, Kidokoro (1975) found a value of −41 ± 4 mV, which was lower than the −57 ± 3.1 mV obtained by Taraskevich and Douglas (1980) and by Biales et al. (1977). Using GH_4C_1 cells, a subclone of GH_3, Taraskevich and Douglas obtained a mean value of −40 ± 2 mV, close to Kidokoro's values. In our studies of GH_3/B_6, another subclone of GH_3, we found different values of resting potentials in successive experiments: −49 ± 8 mV, Dufy et al. 1979a; −45 ± 3 mV, Dufy et al. 1979b; −40 ± 5 mV, Vincent et al. 1980a; −44 ± 3 mV, Vincent et al. 1980b. Furthermore, we observed that the excitable cells had a mean resting potential (−50 ± 2 mV) which was significantly higher than that of the nonexcitable cells (−31 ± 6 mV) (Israel et al. 1981). The significance of these discrepancies is a matter of discussion. The lower values may be due to damage of the cell membrane. Because impalement of small cells usually causes more damage, the size of the cells may be a determining factor. The type of the electrode may also interfere with the value of resting potential; in GH_3/B_6, it was more polarized when using K_2SO_4 pipettes than with KCl pipettes (−55 ± 1.8 mV against −45 ± 2 mV). Nevertheless, the possibility cannot be ruled out that differences in resting potentials reflect variations in the cells that were used, including differences between sublines (GH_3/B_6, GH_4C_1) or variations in the same subline.

The input resistances of the pituitary cells which have been studied exhibit such discrepancies that they can hardly be compared one with the other: $42 \pm 15 M\Omega$ in rat adenohypophysis in vivo (York et al. 1971) against $1112 \pm 456 M\Omega$ in rat pituitary slices in vitro (Osawa and Sand 1978). Differences were also observed among tumoral cells. Taraskevich and Douglas (1980) found an input resistance ranging from 69 to 480 MΩ for GH_4C_1 cells, and from 320 to 880 MΩ for GH_3. These last values are within the range observed by others (Kidokoro 1975; Biales et al. 1977) in GH_3, but are higher than those we usually observed in GH_3/B_6: 169 ± 58 MΩ (Dufy et al. 1979a). Furthermore, the excitable cells had a mean value which was significantly higher than those of non-excitable cells ($280 \pm 80 M\Omega$ against $115 \pm 35 M\Omega$) (Israel et al. 1981). It is difficult to assign a functional significance to such discrepancies, since technical conditions may play an important role in determining the value of the input resistance. Conditions can vary from normal pituitary cells to tumoral ones; they can also vary from one culture to another. Even in the same culture, differences can be due to an asynchronism of mitosis in the cell population (Vincent et al. 1980).

The current voltage relation has been established for both normal pituitary cells in vitro (Ozawa and Sand 1978) and GH_3/B_6 (Vincent et al. 1980). In both cases, AP cells display the property of outward rectification seen in most of the excitable cells.

Very few data exist concerning the resting membrane properties of AP cells in relation to the cell type. With the exception of recordings from dissociated rat pituitary cells (Taraskevich and Douglas 1979) or from slices of rat adenohypophysis (Ozawa and Sand 1978), in which the type could not be determined, most experiments have been done on PRL-secreting cells. Recently, the electrophysiological properties of a clonal mouse pituitary cell line secreting ACTH and endorphin have been studied (Adler et al. 1980). These cells exhibited a low resting potential (-33 ± 22 mV) which did not seem to be linked with cell injury. We have studied the electrophysiological properties of cells cultured from four types of human adenoma (Dufy et al. 1981, unpublished data). The mean resting potential was usually low and differed only slightly from one type of pituitary tumor to the other. Cells secreting PRL and those derived from tumors secreting ACTH were less polarized (-26 ± 7 mV with a resistance of 66 ± 44 MΩ for PRL and -22 ± 5 mV with a resistance of 63 ± 30 MΩ for ACTH) than those recorded from tumors which released growth hormone (-35 ± 8 mV; 78 ± 41 MΩ). The most polarized cells (-40 ± 10 mV) which also had the higher resistance (82 ± 70 MΩ) were those cultured from a patient with a 'non-functioning' pituitary tumor, with no detectable hormone secretion. It is not possible to determine whether the differences in passive membrane characteristics among tumor cells reflect an intrinsic, in vivo property or variations in behavior due to culture conditions.

Electrophysiological activities

Regenerative voltage-dependent conductance changes have been described in different types of AP cells. They consist of all-or-none, high-amplitude phenomena (action potentials) and low-amplitude potential fluctuations.

Action potentials

Different groups have recently reported the occurrence of action potentials in pituitary cells from normal or tumoral origin. Electrical activity consisting of large amplitude spikes has been described in normal adenohypophysial cells (pars distalis) obtained from adult rat by tissue dissociation and maintained in culture (Taraskevich and Douglas 1977). The extracellular action potentials fired spontaneously or were initiated by depolarization. Since spiking persisted in the presence of tetrodotoxin (TTX) and in the absence of sodium, but was inhibited by Ca^{2+} blockers, such action potentials appeared to be calcium spikes, but contributions to spiking by other ions could not be excluded. The fact that only about one in three of the cells showed spontaneous or evoked action potentials does not mean that electrical activity and excitability is a property only of some categories of adenohypophysial cells; others may have lost excitability as a result of dissociation, i.e. trypsinisation, or of the culture conditions. Using intracellular recording from slices of non-dissociated pituitary glands of normal rats, Ozawa and Sand (1978) showed that most cells were electrically excitable either during an outward current pulse or at the cessation of an inward current pulse, but they never observed any spontaneous spiking activity. After studying the electrical activity of the pituitary cells in Na^+- and Ca^{2+}-free solutions, they concluded that the membranes of most adenohypophysial cells are able to generate calcium-dependent regenerative responses and that some cells have a sodium component in addition. Conversely in cells of rat pituitary pars intermedia, the major portion of the action potential was sodium dependent, with a small Ca^{2+} component (Douglas and Taraskevich 1978). This calcium component appeared to make a more important contribution to spiking activity in pars intermedia of the lizard (Taraskevich and Douglas 1979) and in PRL-secreting cells of the pars distalis in the fish (Taraskevich and Douglas 1978). The relative importance of the sodium component versus calcium in the generation of action potentials depending on the cell type suggests that some of them may have membrane features closer to those of neurons.

The electrical behavior of AP cells from tumoral origin has now been extensively studied. In an earlier attempt to record from rat tumoral anterior pituitary cells of the GH_3 line, which secrete prolactin spontaneously, Kidokoro (1975) observed spontaneously occurring spikes and concluded that the inward action current was exclusively carried by Ca^{2+}. This was confirmed by Dufy et al. (1979a, 1979b) and by Taraskevich and Douglas (1980). Biales et al. (1977) have also reported that GH_3 cells generated action potentials which were calcium dependent but with an additional sodium component.

Using GH_3/B_6, a subclone of the GH_3 rat prolactin cell line, we have shown that 50% of the cells were electrically excitable, in that they displayed action potentials during a depolarizing intracellular current injection (Fig. 7.9). Spikes were also obtained during depolarization induced by the application of KCl close to the cell using a pneumatic ejection system. 28% of all cells were spontaneously active with a firing rate which never exceeded 2 Hz. The observation that only half of the cells were excitable is puzzling. The possibility that the membrane of non-excitable cells was damaged cannot be excluded. But it is also possible that this difference was due to asynchronism of mitosis in the cell population.

The all-or-none action potential had a positive overshoot and a prominent after-potential

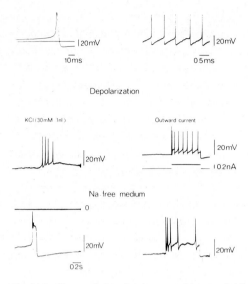

Fig. 7.9. Characteristics of action potentials recorded from GH₃/B₆ cells. Top two traces: spontaneous action potentials; centre traces: action potentials induced by the pressure administration of KCl directly on the cell and by an outward current pulse; bottom traces: spontaneous action potentials and action potentials triggered by an outward current in sodium free medium.

(Fig. 7.9). Furthermore, it was reduced or totally abolished by D-600, a blocker of calcium channels (Fig. 7.10A). Action potentials were suppressed by replacing Ca^{2+} by Mn^{2+} in the bathing solution or by directly applying Co^{2+} close to the cell (Fig. 7.10B). Addition of tetraethylammonium (TEA), which is a blocker of potential-dependent potassium conductance, prolonged the duration of the regenerative calcium potential (Fig. 7.10C). This result was in agreement with the delayed rectification which one observes in GH₃ cells. Exposure to TTX (2×10^{-6} M) or replacement of Na^+ in the bathing solution with choline chloride did not suppress the action potentials but decreased their amplitude by preventing the overshoot (Fig. 7.9). These findings clearly indicate that opening of potential-dependent calcium channels is responsible for a major part of the action potentials.

At present, most of the observations from tumoral pituitary cells concern PRL-secreting cells. In a preliminary report, Adler et al. (1980) have described a rhythmic electrical activity in an AP cell line secreting ACTH and endorphin. Single events consisted of several brief Na^+ spikes superimposed on the rising phase of a slow Ca^{2+}-dependent spike; events repeated periodically with a frequency varying from 2 Hz to 8 Hz.

In our studies of human adenomas, cells cultured from prolactinomas and those derived from ACTH-secreting tumors were rarely excitable and did not show any spontaneous activity. Conversely, a majority of cells recorded from GH-secreting and 'non-functioning' pituitary tumors were excitable and were spontaneously active. The action potentials were calcium dependent since they were observed in sodium-free medium and were completely blocked by Co^{2+}.

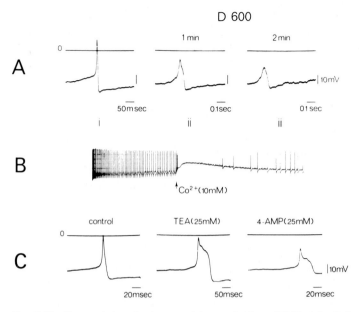

Fig. 7.10. Characteristics of action potentials recorded from GH_3/B_6 cells. Before being used for electrophysiological studies cells were grown for 5–7 days in Ham's F10 solution supplemented with 15 % horse serum and 2.5 % fetal calf serum. Recordings were taken using a bathing solution of the following composition (in mmol l^{-1}): NaCl, 142.6; KCl, 5.6; $CaCl_2$, 10.0; glucose, 5.0; Hepes buffer (pH, 7.4), 5.0. Substances to be tested were dissolved in the bathing solution and ejected, in the proper concentration, by a pressure ejection system directly onto the cell membrane. A: Effect of D-600, a blocker of Ca^{2+} channels, on the shape of action potentials of a spontaneously firing cell. B: Effects of Co^{2+} on a spontaneously firing cell. It should be noted that Co^{2+} completely suppressed action potentials and depolarized the cell, which is consistent with an involvement of Ca^{2+} in the spiking activity and also the resting membrane polarization. C: Effects of tetraethylammonium (TEA) and 4-amino-pyridine (4-AMP) on the shape of action potentials of a spontaneously firing cell. Lengthening of the phase of repolarization is to be noted.

Fluctuations of the membrane potential

In normal rat pituitary cells from slice preparations, Ozawa and Sand (1978) described spontaneous depolarizing potentials of less than 5 mV amplitude. In GH_3 cells, prominent fluctuations of the membrane potential of about 4 mV amplitude were observed (Kidokoro 1975). These fluctuations appeared as an increase in base line noise (Taraskevich and Douglas 1980) and occasionally initiated action potentials. In human pituitary adenomas, all recorded cells showed important fluctuations of membrane potentials. These fluctuations ranged from 1 to 6 mV and were voltage dependent since they increased with the level of depolarization. This voltage-dependent increase of membrane fluctuations was not due to a non-specific increase in K^+ permeability since they occurred at membrane potential values for which the voltage–current relationship was linear and the membrane input resistance was not affected by depolarization. Moreover, these fluctuations involved a calcium component since their amplitude was greatly reduced by Co^{2+}. Cells derived from prolactinomas or ACTH-secreting tumors which were not spontaneously spiking, displayed only this type of calcium-dependent active process. Since these cells released large amounts of hormone spontaneously in the recording medium, it is tempting to speculate that spontaneous calcium-dependent potential fluctuations were involved in the secretory process.

To summarize, these results demonstrate that pituitary cells from normal and tumor origin are able to generate active electrical membrane phenomena consisting of action potentials and/or low amplitude fluctuations of potential which are both at least partially calcium dependent. Since calcium is intimately related with release mechanisms during secretion, it is worthwhile to examine whether factors which influence secretion also have an effect on the calcium-dependent electrical activity of the pituitary cells.

Effects on electrical activity of substances which stimulate hormonal secretion

Thyroliberin

Kidokoro (1975) found that the mean rate of action potential firing in a population of GH_3 cells exposed to 30 nM TRH was higher than when TRH was absent. Taraskevich and Douglas (1980) confirmed that application of TRH (10–100 nM) close to the membrane increases the frequency of extracellularly recorded action potentials within a few seconds. On the other hand, TRH failed to increase action potential activity in GH_4C_1 cells, a clonal line which had lost their TRH receptors as determined by binding studies.

We have studied the effect of TRH on GH_3/B_6 cells by intracellular recording of their electrical activity (Dufy et al. 1979). TRH (25–125 nM) added to the bathing solution increased the percentage of cells displaying action potentials, as previously shown by extracellular recording of GH_3 (Kidokoro 1975) and of normal rat AP cells (Taraskevich and Douglas 1977). Application of TRH (50 nM, 2 nl) close to the cell evoked a train of

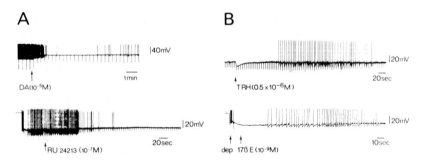

Fig. 7.11. Effects of inhibitory and excitatory substances on the membrane electrical activity of GH_3/B_6 cells. (A) inhibitory substances. Upper trace, ejection of DA directly onto the membrane of a cell grown in estrogen-free medium. Lower trace, ejection of RU-24213, a DA analog in similar conditions. (B) excitatory substances. Upper trace, ejection of TRH (50 nM, 2 nl) into the proximity of the cell membrane elicits a precocious hyperpolarization followed within 1 min by a sustained spiking activity. Lower trace, ejection of 17-βE directly onto the membrane induces an early depolarization followed by the firing of action potentials. A measure of the membrane resistance (vertical bars) is obtained by injecting constant hyperpolarizing pulses.

action potentials within 1 min (Fig. 7.11B). This spiking activity was preceded by a progressive increase of the input resistance without any detectable change in the resting membrane polarization apart from an early hyperpolarization. This early TRH-induced hyperpolarization has been demonstrated to be due to an increase in the membrane permeability to K^+ (Ozawa and Kimura 1979). This transient phenomenon appeared less consistently in our preparations and did not seem to be directly involved in the spiking activity. Furthermore, since this early phenomenon was not affected by Co^{2+}, which blocked both spiking activity and hormonal release, it did not appear to be closely related to the TRH-stimulated hormone release. The TRH-induced spiking activity was also accompanied by an increase in the membrane noise (unpublished). After 1 to 10 min the cells stopped firing as the resistance and the membrane noise returned to the resting level. Repeated administration of TRH at less than 10-min intervals showed a desensitization of the response. The electrical response was reduced or totally abolished by D-600 and by introduction of Co^{2+} in the medium.

The fact that TRH induces a change in membrane resistance without a corresponding change in membrane potential remains puzzling. This observation has been confirmed by Ozawa and Kimura (1979), who showed that (i) the enhancement of spike generation was not due to a membrane depolarization, (ii) the response also occurred in Na^+-free solution, which indicated that a change in Na^+ conductance was not indispensable for the initiation of spike facilitation, and (iii) the input resistance increased during the facilatory period. The mechanism by which TRH induces spiking without changing the resting potential remains to be determined. TRH may possibly increase the excitability through lowering the spike threshold by changing the voltage at which activation of the calcium conductance underlying the spikes occurs. Such a direct effect of a peptide in changing the action potential threshold and hence the excitability has already been observed in spinal cord neurons (Barker et al. 1979). Other examples of the action of peptides on voltage-dependent conductances have also been described for invertebrate neuronal systems (Barker and Smith 1977).

Besides the increase in the frequency of calcium-dependent action potentials, another electrophysiological mechanism by which TRH may affect the entry of Ca^{2+} into the cell has been reported (Sand et al. 1980). Intracellular recordings from the same GH_3 cell before and during TRH stimulation showed this peptide to prolong the duration of the action potential. This effect was mimicked by 4-amino-pyridine (Fig. 7.10) which inhibited the repolarizing K^+ current. It has been suggested that TRH may act in a similar way. Conversely, we have not been able to observe any effect of TRH on spike duration in our GH_3/B_6 preparation.

TRH, which is remarkably effective in causing GH release in acromegalic patients, has also been applied to cells cultured from pituitary fragments of an acromegalic patient (Dufy et al. unpublished results). Cells responded to TRH by depolarization accompanied by an increase in the size of membrane fluctuations. Some of the cells also showed a prolonged burst of action potentials during depolarization. Since TRH was highly effective in augmenting GH secretion these observations suggest that membrane fluctuations and not just action potentials may be involved in the secretory process.

Estrogens

When 17-β-estradiol (17-βE) was added to the bathing solution (50 pg l⁻¹) of GH_3/B_6 cells, the percentage of spontaneously firing cells was greater than in a non-treated control group. Furthermore, ejection of 17-βE ($10^{-10}–10^{-8}$ M) in the close vicinity of the cell elicited two different effects (Fig. 7.11B). The first one, observed in all the excitable cells, consisted of a brief depolarization triggering a burst of action potentials. This effect could be repeated several times in the same cell. It did not appear to be calcium dependent, since administration of Co^{2+} did not significantly modify the depolarization. This transient response, which never exceeded 20 s duration, was followed 1 min later by a second effect which was a prolonged discharge of action potentials accompanied by an increase in membrane resistance without any change in membrane potential. The spiking activity lasted 3–30 min after application of 17-βE and was reduced or almost totally suppressed by application of D-600. The discharge of spikes in response to 17-βE was observed in only about 30% of the excitable cells. Furthermore, when an application of 17-βE was successful in eliciting spikes, a subsequent ejection was totally ineffective although the cell remained excitable. 17-αE had a much weaker effect even at higher doses but prevented the effect of 17-βE. Progesterone and testosterone were not able to induce spiking activity. This indicates a high degree of stereospecificity for the effects of estrogen on the electrical activity of pituitary cells (Dufy et al. 1979a). The spiking effect of 17-βE was similar in time course, passive membrane-property changes and Ca^{2+} dependence to that induced by TRH. The rapid and specific effect of 17-βE on membrane properties implies recognition sites for the steroid at the membrane surface and most probably reflects conformational changes in membrane components. The physiological implication of such early effects of estrogen on the membrane properties of GH_3/B_6 remains unclear. The possibility that PRL release is stimulated within minutes after 17-βE ejection, which would be consistent with the Ca^{2+}-dependent electrical effect, has been suggested (Dufy et al., unpublished results). It is also possible that Ca^{2+} is required to initiate the long-term effect of 17-βE in PRL synthesis. Finally, the changes in ionic permeability may also initiate other unknown intracellular processes triggered by the steroid.

Effects on electrical activity of substances which inhibit hormonal secretion

The secretion of PRL by the anterior pituitary is primarily controlled by the brain through inhibitory substances released from nerve endings in the median eminence of the hypothalamus and carried by the adenohypophysial portal blood system to the PRL-secreting cells. These inhibitory substances are commonly referred to as prolactin-inhibiting factors (PIFs). Among them dopamine (DA) is one of the most potent in vivo as well as in vitro (MacLeod 1969). It has been suggested that DA may represent the major PIF (MacLeod et al. 1970; Meites 1977). However, evidence has been presented recently (Schally et al. 1977; Racagni et al. 1979; Enjalbert et al. 1979) that γ-aminobutyric acid (GABA) may also have an important PIF activity. We shall consider here the effects of both these inhibitory substances on the electrical activity of AP cells.

Catecholamines

Douglas and Taraskevich (1978) have demonstrated that the action potentials in pars intermedia cells of rat were suppressed by DA and norepinephrine (NE), both of which are inhibitors of secretory activity of the pars intermedia in the rat (Tilders and Smelik 1977). Similar inhibitory action of catecholamines on electrical activity has also been directly recorded from frog neurointermediate lobe (Davis and Hadley 1978). DA and NE have also been observed to inhibit electrical activity of cultured PRL cells obtained from the fish pars distalis (Taraskevich and Douglas 1978).

In our studies of GH_3/B_6, we have observed that the firing of 40% of the spontaneously active cells was inhibited by an application of DA close to the cells (Dufy et al. 1979b). This inhibitory action was concomitant with a rapid decrease in input resistance without any detectable change in resting membrane polarization (Fig. 7.11A). In addition, DA inhibited the TRH-induced action potentials. The DA agonist RU-24213 (Roussel UCLAF) mimicked the effect of DA. Conversely, the DA antagonists haloperidol and chlorpromazine suppressed the inhibitory effect of DA on action potentials. We observed also that the inhibitory effect of DA on PRL secretory cells was modulated by estrogen. The percentage of cells inhibited by DA was different according to the presence or absence of estrogen in the medium in which the cells were grown: in the cells grown for at least 24 h in an estrogen-depleted medium, the percentage of DA-inhibited cells reached 80%, instead of 40% in normal medium.

We have also tested the effects of DA on human tumor GH-secretory cells. The DA agonist RU-24213, when applied close to the cell, induced a hyperpolarization with a decrease in the input resistance of the membrane. A reduction or cessation of spiking activity accompanied the hyperpolarization. It was also possible to demonstrate that RU-24213 inhibits the release of GH in the same preparation.

Finally, the fact that DA inhibits the firing and hormone release once again supports the hypothesis that Ca^{2+}-dependent electrical activity is involved in the mechanism of release of AP hormones.

GABA

Local application of this amino acid was able to alter the electrophysiological properties of GH_3/B_6 cells (Israel et al. 1980). The effects of GABA on these cells were: (i) decrease in membrane conductance, (ii) hyperpolarization of 5–10 mV, and (iii) inhibition or suppression of the spontaneous spiking activity. GABAergic receptor antagonists such as picrotoxin and bicuculline prevented the effect of GABA, whereas dopaminergic receptors antagonists such as haloperidol had no effect. Recently, a partial inhibition of PRL secretion by GABA has been observed in GH_3/B_6 cells (Gourdji et al. unpublished data). It is possible, therefore, to conclude that the inhibitory effect of GABA on the electrical activity of PRL cells may correspond to an inhibitory effect of this substance on PRL secretion.

In conclusion there are an increasing number of data showing that pituitary cells are electrically excitable. A similar property has also been found for β cells of the pancreas (Matthews and Sakamoto 1975) and adrenal chromaffin cells (Biales et al. 1976; Brandt et al. 1976). These findings challenge the classical division between electrically excitable neurons and non-excitable gland cells. It has been claimed that excitable endocrine cells may belong to Pearse's 'APUD' series (amine precursor uptake decarboxylase) which shares with neurons a common affiliation from neuroectoderm (Pearse 1969; Takor-Takor and Pearse 1975). Even though one may question the application of this concept to endocrine cells of the gut and the pancreas (Fontaine and Le Douarin 1977), it may still be relevant to adenohypophysial cells since they differentiate from the hypophysial placode and so share a common ectodermal origin with neural crest derivatives (Le Douarin 1978).

The presently available data on electrophysiological properties of pituitary cells would barely permit the definition of electrical characteristics common to any pituitary cell type. Indeed a large heterogeneity in input resistance and mean resting membrane potential as well as in the features of the spontaneous action potentials has been reported either from cell to cell or between cell types. Moreover, there is no proof so far of a direct link between the presence of action potentials and the releasing capacity of the cell. Whether action potentials represent a physiological mean for coupling the stimulus to the hormonal release is still to be demonstrated. In fact such a conclusion is also dependent on progress in understanding the sequences of events triggered by the recognition of a ligand to specific sites on the cell membrane. In that respect, the electrophysiological response which occurs within 1 min or less appears to be the most rapidly detectable. Its exact link with intracellular calcium movement, metabolism of cyclic nucleotides, exocytosis of secretory granules and membrane endocytosis is completely unknown. One of the major difficulties in correlating various aspects of the cell response resides in the heterogeneity of the cell response and in the technical limits of measuring these various parameters at the level of a single cell.

GENERAL CONCLUSIONS

The morphological and electrophysiological approaches, by providing information obtained on intact cells and at the single cell level, complement those obtained on broken cell preparations by the biochemists or on the whole gland in vivo by the physiologists. The morphological and electrophysiological correlates of anterior pituitary cell functions have been examined here in relation to the biochemical specialization of the various cell types and the regulation, either stimulatory or inhibitory, of their secretory activity.

Within the last 5 years, progress in both the immunocytochemistry and chemistry of AP hormones have led to a reexamination of the 'one hormone, one cell type' theory and to a simplification of the number of specific cell types. From the classical seven cell types, five still remain as specific for GH, PRL, TSH, FSH plus LH and pro-opiomelanocortin, respectively. Nevertheless, it remains possible that under particular conditions, such as hyperfunction or tumorigenesis, GH and PRL on the one hand, and TSH, FSH and LH on the other hand, may be secreted by the same cell. This remains to be unequivocally proved. In addition, progress in electron microscope immunocytochemistry has permitted new insight into two aspects of the AP cell function: the structural heterogeneity versus functional heterogeneity and the intracellular transport of immunochemically identifiable secretory products. Further progress in these two directions may be hoped for in the near future.

The morphological correlates of functional regulations have been examined at two levels of organization from single cells to cell populations. In the case of inhibition of hormone release, some progress has been made and the link between a decrease in hormonal release and an apparent decrease in the number of the corresponding cell type is not understood. In the case of stimulation of hormonal secretion, the numerous available data have permitted observers to analyze separately the morphological correlates of rapid hormonal release and those of chronic stimulation of hormone secretion. A rapid hormonal release is correlated with a concomitant modification of both the plasma membrane (formation of microvilli, of blebs, increased exposure of some sugar residues) and the Golgi zone (accumulation of vesicles, flattening of Golgi cisternae). Typical profiles of granule exocytosis have been reported only for some cell types, whereas a stimulation of membrane endocytosis has been demonstrated in some cases in the absence of visible granule exocytosis. A chronic stimulation of hormone secretion is correlated with a dramatic change in the relative size of the intracellular compartments of secretory products. The enlargement of both the RER and the Golgi zone is accompanied by a decrease in number and size of secretory granules. Little attention has been paid to the ultrastructure of cell nuclei which should also undergo dramatic changes in relation to the increase in protein synthesis and mRNA transcription. A relationship between stimulation of hormone synthesis and cell proliferation has been studied in a few experiments. Promising evidence obtained in culture should permit progress in the future. The recent development of cell-separation techniques has provided new insights into the understanding of cellular mechanisms involved in pituitary cell response to stimulation. This clearly shows that within a given cell type, and for any cell type except the corticotropes, the cells are functionally heterogenous. This heterogeneity may also account for selective hormonal response. Neither the exact link between functional and structural heterogeneity, however, nor the mechanisms which control this heterogeneity are clearly understood. Finally, the possibility of an interaction through cell to cell communication between cell clumps made of different cell types has recently been proposed. This offers a fascinating opportunity to integrate individual cell responses and pituitary tissue response.

In the last several years, research in the field of electrophysiological correlates of AP cell function has increased rapidly. It is clear now that endocrine pituitary cells are electrically excitable and able to respond to specific stimuli, stimulatory as well as inhibitory, by a modification of their electrical properties. This offers a fascinating approach to the analysis of rapid membrane events triggered by specific ligands. The exact correlation with other intracellular events, biochemical or structural, which are triggered at the same time remains to be understood. Further progress may be expected in the near future from this rapidly growing field.

ACKNOWLEDGMENTS

We are grateful to Mrs Renée Picart and M.C. Pennarun for their skillful assistance in the

244

preparation of illustrations and to Miss A. Bayon and Mrs C. Scalbert for typing the manuscript.

REFERENCES

Adler, M., Busis, N., Higashida, H., Sabol, B., Rotter, A. and Nirenberg, M. (1980) Modulation of rhytmic electrical activity in an anterior pituitary cell line. 10th Neuroscience Meeting, Vol. 6, pp. 107-111, Society for Neuroscience, Bethesda, MD.

Antakly, T., Pelletier, G., Zeytinoglu, F. and Labrie, F. (1980) Changes in cell morphology and prolactin secretion induced by 2-Br-α-Ergocryptine, estradiol and thyrotropin-releasing hormone in rat anterior pituitary cells in culture. J. Cell. Biol. 86, 377-387.

Bacsy, E., Tougard, C., Tixier-Vidal, A., Marton, J. and Stark, E. (1976) Corticotroph cells in primary cultures of rat adenohypophysis. A light and electron microscope immunocytochemical study. Histochemistry 50, 161-174.

Baker, B.L. and Drummond, T. (1972) The cellular origin of corticotropin and melanotropin as revealed by immunochemical staining, Am. J. Anat. 134, 395-410.

Baker, B.L. and Gross, D.S. (1978) Cytology and distribution of secretory cell types in the mouse hypophysis as demonstrated with immunocytochemistry. Am. J. Anat. 153, 193-215.

Baker, B.L., Pierce, J.G. and Cornell, J.S. (1972) The utility of antiserum to subunits of TSH and LH for immunochemical staining of the rat hypophysis. Am. J. Anat. 135, 251-268.

Barker, J.L. and Smith, T.G. (1977) Peptides as neurohormones. In: Biological Approaches to Neurons, Neuroscience Symposia, Vol. II (Cawan, W.M. and Ferrendelli, J.A eds), pp. 340-373, Society for Neuroscience, Bethesda M.D.

Barker, J.L., Gruol, D.L., Huang, L.M., Neale, J.H. and Smith, T.G. (1978) Enkephalin: pharmacologic evidence for diverse functional roles in the neurons system using primary cultures of dissociated spinal neurons. In: Characteristics and Functions of Opioids (Terenius, L. ed.), pp. 87-98, Elsevier/North-Holland, Amsterdam.

Baskin, D.G., Erlandsen, S.L. and Parsons, J.A. (1980) Functional classification of cell types in the growth hormone and prolactin secreting rat MtTW15, mammosomatotropic tumor with ultrastructural immunocytochemistry. Am. J. Anat. 158, 455-461.

Beauvillain, J.C., Tramu, G. and Dubois, M.P. (1975) Characterization by different techniques of adrenocorticotropin and gonadotropin producing cells in Lerot pituitary (Eliomys quercinus L.) Cell Tissue Res. 158, 301-317.

Beauvillain, J.C., Tramu, G., Mazzuca, M., Christiaens, J.L., L'Hermite, M., Asfour, M., Fossati, P. and Linquette, M. (1976). Etude morphologique d'un adénome à prolactine après traitement par la 2-bromo-ergocryptine (CB-154). Ann. Endocrinol. (Paris) 37, 117-118.

Biales, B., Dichter, M. and Tischler, A. (1976) Electrical excitability of cultured adrenal chromaffin cells. J. Physiol. (Lond.), 262, 743-753.

Biales, B., Dichter, M.A. and Tischler, A. (1977) Sodium and calcium action potential in pituitary cells. Nature 267, 172-174.

Bloom, F., Battenberg, E., Rossier, J., Ling, N., Leppaluoto, J., Vargo, T.M. and Guillemin, R. (1977) Endorphins are located in the intermediate and anterior lobes of the pituitary gland, not in the neurohypophysis. Life Sci. 20, 43-48.

Brandt, B.L., Magiwara, S., Kidokoro, Y. and Miyazaki, S. (1976) Action potentials in the rat chromaffin cell and effects of acetylcholine. J. Physiol. (Lond.) 263, 417-439.

Brunet, N. and Tixier-Vidal, A. (1977). Modifications de surface induites par le TRH sur les cellules à Prolactine (lignées SD$_1$). Mise en évidence d'une augmentation du nombre de sites de liaison de la concanavaline A. IIe colloque du Cercle Français de Biologie Cellulaire. Biol. Cell. 30, p. A.

Brunet, N., Rizzino, A., Gourdji, D. and Tixier-Vidal, A. (1981) Effects of thyroliberin (TRH) on cell proliferation and prolactin secretion by GH3/B6 rat pituitary cells: a comparison between serum-free and rat serum-supplemented media. J. Cell Physiol. 109, 363-372.

Bugnon, C., Fellmann, D., Lenys, D. and Bloch, B. (1977) Etude cytoimmunologique des cellules gonadotropes et des cellules thyréotropes de l'adénohypophyse du Rat, C.R. Soc. Biol. 4, 907-913.

Cesselin, F. and Peillon, F. (1980) In vitro studies on the secretion of human prolactin and growth hormone. In: Synthesis and Release of Adenohypophyseal Hormones (Jutisz, M. and McKerns, K.W. eds), pp. 677-722, Plenum Press, New York, NY.

Childs, G.V. (Moriarty), Ellison, D.G. and Garner, L.L. (1980) An immunocytochemist's view of gonadotropin storage in the adult male rat: Cytochemical and morphological heterogeneity in serially sectioned gonadotropes. Am. J. Anat. 158, 397-409.

Chretien, M., Benjannet, S., Gossard, F., Gianoulakis, C., Crine, P., Lis, M. and Seidah, N.G. (1979) From β-lipotropin to β-endorphin and 'pro-opiomelanocortin'. Canad. J. Biochem. 57, 1111-1121.

Crine, P., Gossard, F., Seidah, N.G., Blanchette, L., Lis, M. and Chretien, M. (1979) Concomitant synthesis of β-endorphin and α-melanotropin from 2 forms of pro-opiomelanocortin in the rat pars intermedia, Proc. Natl. Acad. Sci. USA 76, 5085-5089.

Crine, P., Gossard, F., Seidah, N.G., Gianoulakis, C., Lis, M. and Chretien, M. (1980) Biosynthesis of β-endorphin in the rat pars intermedia. In: Synthesis and Release of Adenohypophyseal Hormones (Jutisz, M. and McKerns, K.W. eds), pp. 263-284, Plenum Press, New York, NY.

Cuerdo-Rocha, S. and Zambrano, D. (1974) The action of protein synthesis inhibitors and thyrotropin releasing factor on the ultrastructure of rat thyrotrophs. J. Ultrastr. Res. 48, 1-16.

Dacheux, F. (1978) Ultrastructural localization of gonadotrophic hormones in the porcine pituitary using the immunoperoxidase technique. Cell Tissue Res. 191, 219-232.

Dannies, P.S. and Rudnick, M.S. (1980) 2-Bromo-α-ergocryptine causes degradation of prolactin in primary cultures of rat pituitaries cells after chronic treatment. J. Biol. Chem. 255, 2776-2781.

Dannies, P.S. and Tashjian Jr, A.H. (1973) Effects of thyrotropin-releasing hormone and hydrocortisone on synthesis and degradation of prolactin in a rat pituitary cell strain. J. Biol. Chem. 248, 6174-6179.

Davies, C., Jacobi, J., Lloyd, H.M. and Meares, J.D. (1974) DNA synthesis and the secretion of prolactin and growth hormone by the pituitary gland of the male rat. Effects of diethylstilboestrol and 2-bromo-ergo-cryptine methane sulphonate. J. Endocrinol, 61, 411-417.

Davis, M.D. and Haddley, M.E. (1976) Spontaneous electrical potentials and pituitary hormone secretion. Nature 261, 422-423.

Denef, C. (1980) Functional heterogeneity of separated dispersed gonadotropic cells. In: Synthesis and Release of Adenohypophyseal Hormones (Jutisz, M. and McKerns, K.W. eds), pp. 659-676. Plenum Press, New York, NY.

Denef, C., Hautekeete, E., De Wolf, A. and Vanderschueren, B. (1978a) Pituitary basophils from immature male and female rats: Distribution of gonadotrophs and thyrotrophs as studied by unit gravity sedimentation. Endocrinology 103, 724-735.

Denef, C., Hautekeete, E. and Dewals, R. (1978b) Monolayer cultures of gonadotrophs separated by velocity sedimentation: Heterogeneity in response to luteinizing hormone-releasing hormone. Endocrinology 103, 736-747.

Denef, C., Hautekeete, E., Dewals, R. and De Wolf, A. (1980) Differential control of luteinizing hormone and follicle-stimulating hormone secretion by androgens in rat pituitary cells in culture: functional diversity of subpopulations separated by unit gravity sedimentation. Endocrinology 106, 724-729.

Dessy, C., Herlant, M. and Chretien, M. (1973) Detection par immunofluorescence des cellules synthetisant la lipotropine. C.R. Acad. Sci. Paris 276, 335-338.

Douglas, W.W. and Taraskevich, P.S. (1978) Action potentials in gland cells of rat pituitary pars intermedia: inhibition by dopamine, an inhibitor of MSH secretion. J. Physiol. (Lond.) 285, 171-184.

Dubois, M.P. (1972) Localization cytologique par immunofluorescence des secretions corticotropes, α- et β-mélanotropes au niveau de l'antehypophyse des bovins, ovins et porcins. Z. Zellforsch. 125, 200-209.

Dubois, M.P. and Gráf, L. (1973) Demonstration by immunofluorescence of the lipotropic hormone/LPH in bovine, ovine and porcine adenohypophysis. Horm. Metabol. Res. (abstr.) 5, 229.

Duello, T.M. and Halmi, N.S. (1980) Immunocytochemistry of prolactin-producing human pituitary adenomas. Am. J. Anat. 158, 463-470.

Dufy, B. and Vincent, J.D. (1980) Effects of sex steroids on cell membrane excitability: a new concept for the

246

action of steroids on the brain. In: Hormones and the Brain (de Wied, D. and Van Keep, P.A. eds), pp. 29-42, M.T.P. Press, Lancaster.

Dufy, B., Vincent, J.D., Fleury, H., Du Pasquier, P., Gourdji, D. and Tixier-Vidal, A. (1979) Membrane effects of thyrotropin-releasing hormone and estrogen shown by intracellular recording from pituitary cells. Science, 204, 509-511.

Dufy, B., Vincent, J.D., Fleury, H., Du Pasquier, P., Gourdji, D. and Tixier-Vidal, A. (1979) Dopamine inhibition of action potentials in a prolactin secreting cell line is modulated by estrogen. Nature, 282, 855-857.

El Etreby, M.F. and Fath El Bab, M.R. (1977) Localization of gonadotropic hormones in the dog pituitary gland. A study using immunoenzyme histochemistry and chemical staining. Cell Tissue Res. 183, 167-175.

Farquhar, M.G. (1969) Lysosome function in regulating secretion. Disposal of secretory granules in cells of the anterior pituitary gland. In: Lysosomes in Biology and Pathology. Vol. 2 (Dingle, J.T. and Fell, H.B. eds),, 462-482, North-Holland, Amsterdam.

Farquhar, M.G. (1977) Secretion and crinophagy in prolactin cells. In: Comparative Endocrinology of Prolactin (Dellman, H.D., Johnson, J.A. and Klachko, D.M. eds), pp. 37-91, Plenum Press, New York, NY.

Farquhar, M.G. and Rinehart, J.F. (1954a) Cytologic alterations in the anterior pituitary gland following thyroidectomy: An electron microscopic study. Endocrinology 55, 857-876.

Farquhar, M.G. and Rinehart, J.F. (1954b) Electron microscope studies of the anterior pituitary of castrated rats. Endocrinology 54, 516-541.

Farquhar, M.G., Skutelsky, E.H. and Hopkins, C.R. (1975) Structure and function of the anterior pituitary and dispersed pituitary cells: in vitro studies. In: The Anterior Pituitary (Tixier-Vidal, A. and Farquhar, M.G. eds), pp. 83-135, Academic Press, New York.

Farquhar, M.G., Reid, J.J. and Daniell, L.W. (1978) Intracellular transport and packaging of prolactin: A quantitative electron microscope autoradiographic study of mammotrophs dissociated from rat pituitaries. Endocrinology 102, 296-311.

Fontaine, J. and Le Douarin, N. (1977) Analysis of endoderm formation in the avian blastoderm by the use of the quail-chick chimeras. The problem of the neurectodermal origin of the cells of the APUD series. J. Embryol. Exp. Morphol. 41, 209-222.

Gautvik, K.M. and Fossum, S. (1976) Basal and thyroliberin-stimulated prolactin synthesis in single-cell cultures and in populations of rat pituitary cells. Biochem. J. (Cellular Aspects) 158, 119-125.

Girod, C. (1976) Histochemistry of the adenohypophysis. In: Handbuch der Histochemie (Graumann, W. and Neumann, K. eds), Vol. VIII, pp. 205-224. Gustav Fischer Verlag, Stuttgart.

Gourdji, D. (1980) Characterization of thyroliberin (TRH) binding sites and coupling with prolactin and growth hormone secretion in rat pituitary cell lines. In Synthesis and Release of Adenohypophyseal Hormones (Jutisz, M. and McKerns, K.W. eds), pp. 463-494, Plenum Press, New York, NY.

Gourdji, D., Kerdelhué, B. and Tixier-Vidal, A. (1972) Ultrastructure d'un clone de cellules hypophysaires secrétant de la prolactine (clone GH3). Modifications induites par l'hormone hypothalamique de libération de l'hormone thyréotrope (TRF). C.R. Acad. Sci. Ser. D. 274, 437-440.

Gourdji, D., Dufy, B., Vincent, J.D. and Tixier-Vidal, A. (1980) Effets de la dopamine et de la bromocriptine sur les cellules à prolactine de rat en culture cellulaire. In: La Bromocriptine, Sandoz Symposium Ed. Paris, pp. 45-47.

Guy, J., Leclerc, R. and Pelletier, G. (1980) Localization of a 16 000-dalton fragment of the common precursor of adrenocorticotropin and β-lipotropin in the rat and human pituitary gland. J. Cell Biol. 86, 825-830.

Herbert, D.C. (1975) Localization of antisera to LHβ and FSHβ in the rat pituitary gland. Am. J. Anat. 144, 379-385.

Herbert, D.C. (1976) Immunocytochemical evidence that luteinizing hormone (LH) and follicle stimulating hormone (FSH) are present in the same cell type in the rhesus monkey pituitary gland. Endocrinology 98, 1554-1557.

Herbert, E., Phillips, M., Hinman, M., Roberts, J.L., Buderf, M. and Paquette, T.L. (1980) Processing of the common precursor to ACTH and endorphin in mouse pituitary tumor cells and monolayer cultures from mouse anterior pituitary. In: Synthesis and Release of Adenohypophyseal Hormones (Jutisz, M. and McKerns, K.W. eds), pp. 237-262, Plenum Press, New York, NY.

Herlant, M. (1964) The cells of the adenohypophysis and their functional significance. Internat. Rev. Cytol. 17,

299-381.

Herlant, M. (1975) Introduction. In: The Anterior Pituitary (Tixier-Vidal, A. and Farquhar, M.G. eds), pp. 3-15, Academic Press, New York, NY.

Howell, S.L. and Whitfield, M. (1973) Synthesis and secretion of growth hormone in the rat anterior pituitary. I. The intracellular pathway, its time course and metabolic requirements. J. Cell Sci. 12, 1-21.

Hoyt Jr, R.F. and Tashjian Jr, A.H. (1973) Immunocytochemical localization of prolactin in clonal strains of rat anterior pituitary tumor cells in monolayer culture. Anat. Rec. 175, 347 (Abstract).

Hoyt Jr, R.F. and Tashjian Jr, A.H. (1980a) Immunocytochemical analysis of prolactin production by monolayer cultures of GH_3 rat anterior pituitary tumor cells. I. Long-term effects of stimulation with thyrotropin-releasing hormone (TRH). Anat. Rec. 196, 153-162.

Hoyt Jr, R.F. and Tashjian Jr, A.H. (1980b) Immunocytochemical analysis of prolactin production by monolayer cultures of GH_3 rat anterior pituitary tumor cells: II. Variation in prolactin content of individual cell colonies, and dynamics of stimulation with thyrotropin-releasing hormone (TRH). Anat. Rec. 196, 163-181.

Hymer, W.C. (1975) Separation of organelles and cells from the mammalian adenohypophysis. In: The Anterior Pituitary (Tixier-Vidal, A. and Farquhar, M.G. eds), pp. 137-180, Academic Press, New York, NY.

Hymer, W.C., Mastro, A. and Griswold, E. (1970) DNA synthesis in the anterior pituitary of the male rat. Effect of castration and photoperiod. Science 167, 1629-1630.

Hymer, W.C., Page, R., Kelsey, R.C., Augustine, E.C., Wilfinger, W. and Ciolkosz, M. (1980) Separated somatotrophs: their use in vitro and in vivo. In: Synthesis and Release of Adenohypophyseal Hormones (Jutisz, M. and McKerns, K.W. eds), pp. 125-166, Plenum Press, New York, NY.

Israel, J.M. and Dufy, B. (1980) Effects of GABA on the electrical properties of a clonal pituitary cell line, 10th Neuroscience Meeting Abstracts, Vol. 6, pp. 289-296, Society for Neuroscience, Bethesda, MD.

Kalberman, L.E., Szijan, I., Jahn, G.A., Krawiec, L. and Burdman, J.A. (1979) DNA synthesis in the pituitary gland of the rat. Effect of sulpiride and postnatal maturation. Neuroendocrinology 29, 42-48.

Kidokoro, Y. (1975) Spontaneous calcium action potentials in a clonal pituitary cell line and their relationship to prolactin secretion. Nature 258, 741-742.

Kovacs, K. and Horvath, E. (1980) Pituitary adenomas associated with hyperprolactinemia: morphological and immunocytological aspects. In: Pituitary Microadenomas (Faglia, G., Giovanelli, M.A. and MacLeod, R.M. eds), pp. 123-135, Academic Press, London.

Kunert-Radek, J. (1974) The effect of synthetic thyrotropin releasing hormone (TRH) on cell proliferation of the anterior pituitary gland in organ culture. Endokrynologia Polska 25, 21-24.

Kurosumi, K. and Oota, Y. (1968) Electron microscopy of two types of gonadotrophs in the anterior pituitary of persistent estrous and diestrous rats. Z. Zellforsch. Mikrosk. Anat. 85, 34-46.

Labrie, F., Borgeat, P., Godbout, M., Barden, N., Beaulieu, M., Lagacé, L., Massicotte, J. and Veilleux, R. (1980) Mechanism of action of hypothalamic hormones and interactions with sex steroids in the anterior pituitary gland. In: Synthesis and Release of Adenohypophyseal Hormones (Jutisz, M. and McKerns, K.W. eds), pp. 415-440, Plenum Press, New York, NY.

Le Douarin, N. (1978) The embryological origin of the endocrine cells associated with the digestive tract. In: Gut Hormones (Bloom, S.R. ed.), pp. 49-56, Churchill Livingstone, Edinburgh.

Leuschen, P.M., Tobin, R.B. and Moriarty, M.C. (1978) Enriched populations of rat pituitary thyrotrophs in monolayer culture. Endocrinology 102, 509-518.

Li, C.H. (1964) Lipotropin, a new active peptide from pituitary glands. Nature 201, 924.

MacLeod, R.M. (1969) Influence of norepinephrine and catecholamine depleting agents on the synthesis and release of prolactin and growth hormone. Endocrinology 85, 916-923.

MacLeod, R.M., Fontham, E.H. and Lehmeyer, J.E. (1970) Prolactin and growth hormone production as influenced by catecholamines and agents that affect brain catecholamines. Neuroendocrinology 6, 283-294.

MacLeod, R.M., Nagy, I., Valdenegro, C.A., Login, I.S. and Thorner, M.O. (1980) Studies on the control of prolactin synthesis and release: differential effects of bromocriptine and lisuride. In: Growth Hormone and Other Biologically Active Peptides (Pecile, A. and Müller, E.E. eds), pp. 224-233, Excerpta Medica, Amsterdam.

Martin, S., York, D.M. and Kraicer, H. (1979) Alterations in transmembrane potential of adenohypophysial cells in elevated and Ca-free media. Endocrinology, 92, 1084-1087.

248

Masur, S.K., Holtzmann, E. and Bancroft, F.C. (1974) Localization within cloned rat pituitary tumor cells of material that binds antigrowth hormone antibody. J. Histochem. Cytochem. 22, 385-394.

Matthews, E.K. and Sakamoto, Y. (1975) Electrical characteristics of pancreatic islet cells, J. Physiol. (Lond.) 246, 421-437.

Mazurkiewicz, J.E. (1973) Differentiation of rat anterior pituitary tumor cells in tissue culture. Anat. Rec. 175, 387 (Abstr.).

Meites, J. (1977) Catecholamines and prolactin secretion. In: Nonstriatal Dopaminergic Neurons (Costa, E. and Gessa, G.L. eds), Vol. 16, pp. 139-146, Adv. Biochem. Psychopharmacol., Raven Press, New York, N.Y.

Mendoza, D., Arimura, A. and Schally, A.V. (1973) Ultrastructural and light microscopic observations of rat pituitary LH containing gonadotrophs following injection of synthetic LH-RH. Endocrinology 92, 1153-1160.

Milligan, J.V. and Kraicer, J. (1970) Adenohypophysial transmembrane potentials: polarity reversal by elevated external potassium ion concentration. Science 167, 182-184.

Moon, H.D., Li, C.H. and Jennings, B.M. (1973) Immunohistochemical and histochemical studies of pituitary β-lipotrophs. Anat. Rec. 175, 529-537.

Morin, A., Tixier-Vidal, A., Gourdji, D., Kerdelhue, B. and Grouselle, D. (1975) Effect of thyrotrope releasing hormone (TRH) on prolactin turnover in culture. Mol. Cell. Endocrinol. 3, 351-373.

Moriarty, G.C. (1973) Adenohypophysis: ultrastructural cytochemistry. A review. J. Histochem. Cytochem. 21, 855-892.

Moriarty, G.C. (1975) Electron microscopic immunocytochemical studies of rat pituitary gonadotrophs. A sex difference in morphology and cytochemistry of LH cells. Endocrinology 97, 1215-1225.

Moriarty, G.C. (1976) Immunocytochemistry of the pituitary glycoprotein hormones. J. Histochem. Cytochem. 24, 846-863.

Moriarty, G.C. and Garner, L.L. (1977) Immunocytochemical studies of cells in the rat adenohypophysis containing both ACTH and FSH. Nature 265, 356-358.

Moriarty, G.C. and Halmi, N.S. (1972a) Adrenocorticotropin production by the intermediate lobe of the rat pituitary. An electron microscopic-immunohistochemical study. Z. Zellforsch. 132, 1-14.

Moriarty, G.C. and Halmi, N.S. (1972b): Electron microscopic study of the adrenocorticotropin producing cell with the use of unlabelled antibody and the soluble peroxidase-antiperoxidase complex. J. Histochem. Cytochem. 20, 590-603.

Moriarty, G.C. and Tobin, R.B. (1976). An immunocytochemical study of TSHβ storage in rat thyroidectomy cells with and without D or L thyroxine treatment. J. Histochem. Cytochem. 24, 1140-1149.

Nakane, P.K. (1970) Classifications of anterior pituitary cell types with immunoenzyme histochemistry, J. Histochem. Cytochem. 18, 9-20.

Nakane, P.K. (1975) Identification of anterior pituitary cells by immunoelectron microscopy. In: The Anterior Pituitary (Tixier-Vidal, A. and Farquhar, M.G. eds), pp. 45-61, Academic Press, New York, NY.

Nakanishi, S., Inoue, A., Kita, T., Nakamura, M., Chang, A.C.Y., Cohen, S.N. and Numa, S. (1979) Nucleotide sequence of cloned cDNA for bovine corticotropin β-lipotropin precursor. Nature 278, 423-427.

Nansel. D.D., Gudelsky, G.A., Reymond, M.J., Neaves, W.B. and Porter, J.C. (1981) A possible role for lysosomes in the inhibitory action of dopamine on PRL release. Endocrinology 108, 896-902.

Novikoff, A.B. and Novikoff, P.M. (1977) Cytochemical studies on Golgi apparatus and GERL. Histochem. J. 9, 525-535.

Okino, H., Matsui, S., Shioda, S., Nakai, Y. and Kurosumi, K. (1979) Ultrastructural and morphometric studies on the rat pituitary thyrotrophs and thyroid follicular cells following administration of thyrotropin releasing hormone. Archivium Histologicum Japonicum 42, 489-505.

Olivier, L., Vila-Porcile, E., Racadot, O., Peillon, F. and Racadot J. (1975), Ultrastructure of pituitary tumor cells: a critical study. In: The Anterior Pituitary (Tixier-Vidal, A. and Farquhar, M.G. eds), pp. 231-276, Academic Press, New York, NY.

Ozawa, S. and Sand, O. (1978) Electrical activity of rat anterior pituitary cells in vitro. Acta Physiol. Scand. 102, 330-341.

Ozawa, S. and Kimura, N. (1979) Membrane potential changes caused by thyrotropin-releasing hormone in the clonal GH$_3$ cell and their relationship to secretion of pituitary hormone. Proc. Natl. Acad. USA 76, 6017-6020.

Palade, G.E. (1975) Intracellular aspects of the process of protein secretion. Science 189, 347-358.

Parsons, J.A. and Erlandsen, S.L. (1974) Ultrastructural immunocytochemical localization of prolactin in rat anterior pituitary by use of the unlabelled antibody enzyme method. J. Histochem. Cytochem. 22, 340-351.

Pawlikowski, M., Stepien, H. and Kunert-Radek, J. (1975) Thyroxine inhibition of the proliferative response of the anterior pituitary to thyrotropin releasing hormone in vitro. Neuroendocrinology 18, 277-280.

Pawlikowski, M., Kunert-Radek, J. and Stepien, H. (1978) Somastostatin inhibits the mitogenic effect of thyroliberin. Experientia 34, 271-272.

Pearse, A.G.E. (1969) The cytochemistry and ultrastructure of polypeptide hormone-producing cells of the APUD series and the embryologic, physiologic and pathologic implications of the concept. J. Histochem. Cytochem. 17, 303-313.

Pelletier, G., Leclerc, R. and Labrie, F. (1976) Identification of gonadotropic cells in the human pituitary by immunoperoxidase technique, Mol. Cell. Endocrinol. 6, 123-126.

Pelletier, G., Leclerc, R., Labrie, F., Cote, J., Chretien, M. and Lis, M. (1977). Immunohistochemical localization of β-lipotropic hormone in the pituitary gland. Endocrinology 100, 770-776.

Phifer, R.F., Midgley, A.R. and Spicer, S.S. (1973) Immunohistologic evidence that follicle-stimulating and luteinizing hormones are present in the same cell types in the human pars distalis. J. Clin. Endocrinol. Metab. 36, 125-142.

Racagni, G., Apud, J.A., Locatelli, V., Cocchi, D., Nisticò, G., Di Giorgio, R.M. and Müller, E.E. (1979) GABA of CNS origin in the rat anterior pituitary inhibits prolactin secretion. Nature 281, 575-578.

Rossier, J., Vargo, T.M., Minick, S., Ling, N., Bloom, F.E. and Guillemin, R. (1977) Regional dissociation of β-endorphin and enkephalin contents in rat brain and pituitary. Proc. Natl. Acad. Sci. USA 74, 5162-5165.

Sand, O., Hang, E. and Gautvik, K.M. (1980) Effects of thyroliberin and 4-aminopyridine on action potentials and prolactin release and synthesis in rat pituitary cells in culture. Acta Physiol. Scand. 108, 247-252.

Shiino, M. (1979) Morphological changes of pituitary gonadotrophs and thyrotrophs following treatment with LH-RH or TRH in vitro. Cell Tissue Res. 202, 399-406.

Shiino, M., Arimura, A., Schally, A.V. and Rennels, E.G. (1972) Ultrastructural observations of granule extrusion from rat anterior pituitary cells after injection of LH-releasing hormone. Z. Zellforsch. Mikrosk. Anat. 128, 152-161.

Shiino, M., Ishikawa, H. and Rennels, E.G. (1978) Specific subclones derived from a multipotential clone of rat anterior pituitary cells. Am. J. Anat. 153, 81-96.

Shiino, M., Fujihara, N. and Rennels, E.G. (1980) Maintenance of gonadotrophs in pituitary autographs under the kidney capsules of female rats given sex hormones or LRH. Am. J. Anat. 158, 433-444.

Sirbasku, D.A. (1978) Estrogen induction of growth factors specific for hormone-responsive mammary, pituitary and kidney tumor cells. Proc. Natl. Acad. Sci. USA 75, 3786-3790.

Smith, R.E. and Farquhar, M.G. (1966) Lysosome function in the regulation of the secretory process in cells of the anterior pituitary gland. J. Cell. Biol. 31, 319-347.

Snyder, J., Wilfinger, W. and Hymer, W.C. (1976) Maintenance of separated rat pituitary mammotrophs in cell culture. Endocrinology 98, 25-32.

Snyder, G., Hymer, W.C. and Snyder, J. (1977) Functional heterogeneity in somatotrophs isolated from the rat anterior pituitary. Endocrinology 101, 788-799.

Soji, T. (1978a) Cytological changes of the pituitary basophils in rats slowly infused with thyrotropin-releasing hormone (TRH), Endocrinol. Jpn. 25, 245-258.

Soji, T. (1978b) Cytological changes of the pituitary basophils in rats slowly infused with LRH and with LRH and TRH in combination. Endocrinol. Jpn. 25, 259-274.

Sternberger, L.A. and Petrali, J.P. (1975) Quantitative immunocytochemistry of pituitary receptors for Luteinizing hormone-releasing hormone. Cell Tissue Res. 162, 141-176.

Stevens, E. and Helfenstein, J.E. (1966) Some effects of certain naturally occuring oestrogens on the anterior pituitary glands of rats. Nature 211, 879-880.

Takor-Takor, T. and Pearse, A.G.E. (1975) Neurectodermal origin of avian hypothalamo hypophyseal complex: the role of the ventral neural ridge. J. Embryol. Exp. Morphol. 31, 311-325.

Taraskevich, P.S. and Douglas, W.W. (1977) Action potentials occur in cells of the normal anterior pituitary gland and are stimulated by the hypophysiotropic peptide thyrotropin-releasing hormone. Proc. Natl. Acad. Sci. USA 74, 4064-4067.

Taraskevich, P.S. and Douglas, W.W. (1978) Catecholamines of supposed inhibitory hypophysiotropic function suppress action potentials in prolactin cells. Nature 276, 831-834.

Taraskevich, P.S. and Douglas, W.W. (1979) Stimulant effect of 5-hydroxytryptamine on action potential activity in pars intermedia cells of the lizard anolis carolinensis: contrasting effects in pars intermedia of rat and rostral pars distalis of fish (*Alosa pseudoharengus*). Brain Res. 178, 584-588.

Taraskevich, P.S. and Douglas, W.W. (1980) Electrical behavior in a line of anterior pituitary cells (GH cells) and the influence of the hypothalamic peptide, thyrotropin releasing factor. Neuroscience 5, 421-431.

Tashjian Jr, A.H. and Hoyt Jr, R.F. (1972) Transient controls of organ-specific functions in pituitary cells in culture. In: Molecular Genetics and Developmental Biology (Sussmann, M. ed.), pp. 353-387, Prentice Hall Inc., Englewood Cliffs, NJ.

Tashjian Jr, A.H., Yasumura, Y., Levine, L., Sato, G.H. and Parker, M.L. (1968) Establishment of clonal strains of rat pituitary tumor cells that secrete growth hormone. Endocrinology 82, 342-352.

Tashjian Jr, A.H., Bancroft, F.C. and Levine, L. (1970) Production of both prolactin and growth hormone by clonal strains of rat pituitary tumor cells. J. Cell Biol. 47, 61-70.

Tischler, A.S., Dichter, M.A., Biales, B., Delellis, R.A. and Wolfe, H. (1976) Neural properties of cultured human endocrine tumors of proposed neural crest origin. Science 192, 902-904.

Tixier-Vidal, A. (1980) Structural basis of adenohypophyseal secretory processes. In: Synthesis and Release of Adenohypophyseal Hormones (Jutisz, M. and McKerns, K.W. eds), pp. 1-14, Plenum Press, New York, NY.

Tixier-Vidal, A. and Gourdji, D. (1980) Endocytosis in cultured prolactin cells. In: Central and Peripheral Regulation of Prolactin Function (MacLeod, R.M. and Scapagnini, U. eds), pp. 125-139, Raven Press, New York, NY.

Tixier-Vidal, A. and Gourdji, D. (1981) Mechanism of action of synthetic hypothalamic peptides on anterior pituitary cells. Physiol. Rev. 61, 974-1011.

Tixier-Vidal, A. and Picart, R. (1967) Etude quantitative par radioautographie au microscope électronique de l'utilisation de la DL-leucine-^{3}H par les cellules de l'hypophyse du canard en culture organotypique. J. Cell Biol. 35, 501-519.

Tixier-Vidal, A., Tougard, C., Kerdelhué, B. and Jutisz, M. (1975a) Light and electron microscopic studies on immunocytochemical localization of gonadotropic hormones in rat pituitary using antisera against ovine FSH, ovine LH and its two subunits. Ann. N.Y. Acad. Sci. USA 254, 433-461.

Tixier-Vidal, A., Gourdji, D. and Tougard, C. (1975b) A cell culture approach to the study of the anterior pituitary. International Review of Cytology. Vol. 41, pp. 173-239.

Tixier-Vidal, A., Tougard, C. and Picart, R. (1976a) Subcellular localization of some protein and glycoprotein hormones of the hypothalamo-hypophyseal axis as revealed by the peroxidase-labelled antibody method. In: Immunoenzymatic Techniques (Feldmann, G., Druet, P., Bignon, J. and Avrameas, S. eds), pp. 307-321, North-Holland, Amsterdam.

Tixier-Vidal, A., Moreau, M.F. and Picart, R. (1976b) Endocytose et secretion dans les cellules antehypophysaires en culture. Action des hormones hypothalamiques. J. Microscop. Biol. Cell. 25, 159-172.

Tougard, C. (1980) Immunocytochemical identification of LH and FSH secreting cells at the light and electron-microscope levels. In: Synthesis and Release or Adenohypophyseal Hormones (Jutisz, M. and McKerns, K.W. eds), pp. 15-38, Plenum Press, New York, NY.

Tougard, C., Kerdelhué, B., Tixier-Vidal, A. and Jutisz, M. (1971) Localisation par cytoimmunoenzymologie de la LH, de ses sous-unités α et β, et de la FSH dans l'adénohypophyse de la ratte castrée. C.R. Acad. Sci. 273, 897-900.

Tougard, C., Kerdelhué, B., Tixier-Vidal, A. and Jutisz, M. (1973) Light and electron microscope localization of binding sites of antibodies against ovine luteinizing hormone and its two subunits in rat adenohypophysis using peroxidase-labelled antibody technique J. Cell Biol. 58, 503-521.

Tougard, C., Tixier-Vidal, A., Kerdelhué, B. and Jutisz, M. (1977a) Etude immunocytochimique de l'évolution des cellules gonadotropes dans des cultures primaires de cellules antéhypophysaires de rat: Aspects quantitatifs et ultrastructuraux. Biol. Cell. 28, 251-260.

Tougard, C., Picart, R. and Tixier-Vidal, A. (1977b) Cytogenesis of immunoreactive gonadotropic cells in the fetal rat pituitary at the light and electron microscope levels. Dev. Biol. 58, 148-163.

Tougard, C., Picart, R. and Tixier-Vidal, A. (1980a) Immunocytochemical localization of glycoprotein hormones in the rat anterior pituitary. A light and electron microscope study using antisera against rat β subunits: a comparison between preembedding and postembedding methods. J. Histochem. Cytochem. 28, 101-114.

Tougard, C., Picart, R. and Tixier-Vidal, A. (1980b) Electron-microscopic cytochemical studies on the secretory process in rat prolactin cells in primary culture. Am. J. Anat. 158, 471-490.

Tramu, G. and Beauvillain, J.C. (1980) Pituitary polypeptide secreting cells: immunocytochemical identification of ACTH, MSH and peptides related to LPH. In: Synthesis and Release of Adenohypophyseal Hormones (Jutisz, M. and McKerns, K.W. eds), pp. 39-66. Plenum Press, New York, NY.

Tramu, G. and Dubois, M.P. (1977) Comparative cellular localization of corticotropin and melanotropin in lerot adenohypophysis (Eliomys quercinus): An immunohistochemical study. Cell Tissue Res. 183, 457-462.

Tramu, G. and Leonardelli, J. (1979) Immunohistochemical localization of enkephalins in median eminence and adenohypophysis. Brain Res. 168, 457-471.

Vale, W., Rivier, C. and Brown, M. (1977) Regulatory peptides of the hypothalamus. Annu. Rev. Physiol. 39, 473-527.

Vale, W., Rivier, C., Yang, L., Monick, S. and Guillemin, R. (1978) Effects of purified hypothalamic corticotropin releasing factor and other substances on the secretion of adrenocorticotropin and β-endorphin-like immunoreactivities in vitro. Endocrinology 103, 1910-1915.

Vincent, J.D., Dufy, B., Gourdji, D. and Tixier-Vidal, A. (1980) Electrical correlates of prolactin secretion in cloned pituitary cells. In: Central and Peripheral Regulation of Prolactin Function (MacLeod, R.M. and Scapagnini, U. eds), pp. 141-157. Raven Press, New York, NY.

Vincent, J.D., Dufy, B., Israel, J.M., Zyzeck, E., Dufy-Barbe, L., Guerin, J., Gourdji, D. and Tixier-Vidal, A. (1980) Neurohormonal communication: an electrophysiological study of the membrane properties of anterior pituitary cells. In: Progress in Psychoneuroendocrinology (Brambilla, F., Racagni, G. and de Wied, D. eds), pp. 25-37, Elsevier North Holland, Amsterdam.

Walker, A.M. and Farquhar, M.G. (1980) Preferential release of newly synthesized prolactin granules is the result of functional heterogeneity among mammotrophs. Endocrinology 107, 1095-1104.

Weber, E., Voigt, K.H. and Martin, R. (1978a) Concomitant storage of ACTH and endorphin-like immunoreactivity in the secretory granules of anterior pituitary corticotrophs. Brain Res. 157, 385-390.

Weber, E., Voigt, K.H. and Martin, R. (1978b) Pituitary somatotrophs contain Met-enkephalin-like immunoreactivity. Proc. Natl. Acad. Sci. USA 75, 6134-6138.

Weber, E., Voigt, K.H. and Martin, R. (1978c) Granules and golgi vesicles with differential reactivity to ACTH antiserum in the corticotroph of the rat anterior pituitary. Endocrinology 102, 1466-1474.

Wilbur, D.L. and Spicer, S.S. (1980) Pituitary secretory activity and endocrinophagy. In: Synthesis and Release of Adenohypophyseal Hormones (Jutisz, M. and McKerns, K.W. eds), pp. 167-186, Plenum Press, New York, NY.

Wilbur, D.L., Yee, J.A. and Raigue, S.E. (1978) Hypophysial portal vascular infusion of TRH in the rat: an ultrastructural and radioimmunoassay study. Am. J. Anat. 151, 277-294.

Wu, R. and Sato, G. (1978) Replacement of serum in cell culture by hormones: a study of hormonal regulation of cell growth and specific gene expression. J. Toxicol. Environm. Health 4, 427-448.

Zambrano, D., Cuerdo-Rocha, S. and Bergmann, I. (1974) Ultrastructure of rat pituitary gonadotrophs following incubation of the gland with synthetic LH-RH. Cell Tiss. Res. 150, 179-192.

York, D.H., Baker, F.L. and Kraicer, J. (1973) Electrical changes induced in rat adenohypophysial cells, in vivo, with hypothalamic extract. Neuroendocrinology 11, 212-228.

Yoshimura, F., Soji, T., Yachi, H. and Ishikawa, H. (1974) Life stage and secretory cycle of anterior pituitary basophils. Endocrinol. Jpn. 21, 217-249.

Chapter 8

Neuroendocrine regulation of the renin–angiotensin–aldosterone system

Robert M. Carey

INTRODUCTION

The renin–angiotensin–aldosterone system is a coordinated hormonal cascade intimately involved in the homeostasis of peripheral vascular resistance and the volume and composition of body fluids. The proteolytic enzyme, renin, the octapeptide, angiotensin II, and the mineralocorticoid, aldosterone, have been the centers of interest and investigation of the physiologic and/or pathophysiologic importance of this intricate system. During the past twenty years, our knowledge of the control of renin and aldosterone secretion has increased progressively, aided greatly by the availability of assays for measuring renin activity, the angiotensin peptides and aldosterone in plasma and tissues. A vast literature has accumulated on the regulation of renin secretion by neurohormonal factors, as well as by other mechanisms, including angiotensin itself. Recently, preliminary evidence has indicated that aldosterone secretion also may be controlled by neuroendocrine determinants. To review critically the evidence for and against neuroendocrine factors regulating the renin-angiotensin-aldosterone system is the principal purpose of this chapter.

GENERAL PHYSIOLOGY OF THE
RENIN–ANGIOTENSIN–ALDOSTERONE SYSTEM

Renin secretion

Renin is a proteolytic enzyme with a molecular weight of approximately 40 000 (Inagami and Murakami 1977). Renin is synthesized and stored by specialized cells, the juxtaglomerular cells, of the renal afferent arteriole adjacent to the macula densa (Edelman and Hartroft 1961; Robertson et al. 1965; Cook 1967; Johnston et al. 1973; Silverman and Barajas 1974; Davis and Freeman 1976). The juxtaglomerular cells are thought to be modified smooth muscle cells (Latta 1973). The macula densa consists of an elongated group of columnar epithelial cells situated in the distal convoluted tubule as it passes the

254

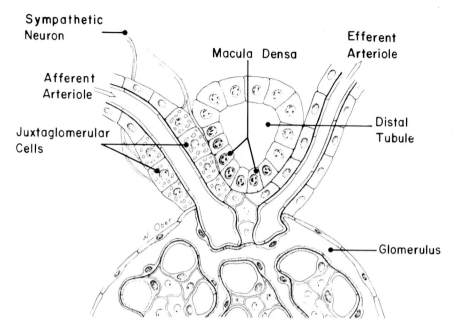

Fig. 8.1. A diagramatic representation of the renal juxtaglomerular apparatus. Reproduced from Levens et al. Circ. Res. 48, 157-167, 1981c.

glomerulus after it ascends from the medulla (Latta 1973). Together, the juxtaglomerular cells, the afferent glomerular arteriole and the macula densa are designated as the juxtaglomerular apparatus (Fig. 8.1).

Renin activity has been found in a number of extrarenal tissues such as adrenal cortex, large arteries and veins, brain, uterus and submaxillary gland (Peach 1977; Ganten et al. 1978). It is uncertain whether any of these renin-like enzymes, or isorenins, are identical to renin of renal origin, and their physiologic relevance remains in question. After bilateral nephrectomy, plasma renin activity decreases to low or undetectable levels, indicating that the kidney is the principal source of renin (Michelakis and Mizukoshi 1971; Laragh and Sealey 1973).

In the kidney, renin secretion is controlled by at least four major independent mechanisms: the renal baroreceptor, the macula densa, angiotensin negative feedback, and neuroendocrine influences; neuroendocrine mechanisms will be discussed in detail in subsequent sections.

Renin secretion increases in response to decreased perfusion pressure or stretch of the afferent arteriole and decreases with increased stretch. The large body of evidence in support of this concept has been reviewed thoroughly by Davis and Freeman (1976). The most definitive evidence supporting the baroreceptor mechanism was obtained in the non-filtering kidney model, in which reduction in renal perfusion pressure increased renin secretion in the absence of nervous system and tubular influences (Blaine et al. 1970; Blaine et al. 1971). This increased renin secretion was blocked by paralysis of the renal vasculature with papaverine (Witty et al. 1971), further substantiating the renal barorecep-tor as a major control mechanism.

The composition of the renal tubular fluid at the macula densa also modulates renin secretion (Davis et al. 1976). Intrarenal infusion of sodium and potassium chloride or lactate inhibits secretion in the filtering but not the non-filtering kidney (Shade et al. 1972; Stephen et al. 1978). Sodium chloride-induced volume expansion has a greater inhibitory effect than comparable volume expansion with dextran, suggesting that sodium chloride itself is sensed by the macula densa (Tuck et al. 1974). Sodium chloride transport rather than load seems to be the signal received by the macula densa (Davis et al. 1976), although recent evidence suggests that chloride transport also may inhibit renin release (Kotchen et al. 1978). Although much investigation has been performed, the precise signal perceived and the cellular mechanisms for the control of renin secretion by the macula densa remain unknown.

Renin secretion is inhibited by angiotensin II, and also by its heptapeptide derivative, (des-aspartyl[1])-angiotensin II (Vandongen et al. 1974; Freeman et al. 1976; Carey et al. 1978). This effect appears to be directly on the juxtaglomerular cells (Naftilan and Oparil 1978).

A number of other substances also affect renin secretion. Calcium inhibits renin secretion in both the filtering and the non-filtering kidney, indicating a direct effect of calcium on the juxtaglomerular apparatus independent of tubular flow (Watkins et al. 1976). Renin release from isolated perfused kidneys seems to be inversely proportional to calcium concentration of the perfusate (Fray 1977; Lester and Rubin 1977; Baumbach and Leyssac 1977). The intracellular calcium concentration may influence renin secretion in response to other control mechanisms as well (Park and Malvin 1978).

Arachidonic acid, prostaglandin endoperoxides and prostacyclin stimulate renin sec-retion in vivo and in vitro (Larsson et al. 1974; Bolger et al. 1976; Weber et al. 1976; Whorton et al. 1977; Gerber et al. 1979). Indomethacin, an inhibitor of prostaglandin synthetase, decreases basal renin secretion and inhibits the renin response to low sodium diet, diuretics, vasodilators, upright posture, hemorrhage and aortic constriction (Rumpf et al. 1975; Donker et al. 1976; Frolich et al. 1976; Romero et al. 1976; Speckart et al. 1977; Norbiato et al. 1978, Glasson et al. 1979, Henrich et al. 1979, Campbell et al. 1979, Berl et al. 1979). Prostaglandin synthetase inhibition with aspirin or indomethacin reduces exces-sive renin secretion in Bartter's syndrome (McGiff 1977). Inhibition of renin release with blockers of prostaglandin synthesis is independent of sodium retention and renal tubular factors, since it occurs in the non-filtering kidney (Data et al. 1978; Frolich et al. 1979). Reduction of the renin response to the wide variety of stimuli by inhibition of prostaglandin production suggests that prostaglandins may be a common intermediary factor in the baroreceptor and macula densa mechanisms. Recent evidence also suggests that pros-taglandins stimulate renin secretion directly at the juxtaglomerular apparatus independent of the other control mechanisms, since arachidonic acid stimulates renin release in the non-filtering, denervated, maximally vasodilated kidney (Seymour and Zehr 1979). The precise cellular mechanism whereby renal prostaglandins may influence renin secretion are unknown.

Positive control mechanisms
1. Baroreceptor mechanism
   Decreased pressure (decreased stretch of juxtaglomerular cells)
2. Macula densa mechanism
   Decreased sodium reabsorption across the macula densa
3. Neuroendocrine factors
   Renal sympathetic nerve activity and circulating catecholamines
4. Calcium
5. Prostaglandins

Negative control mechanism
1. Angiotensin II
2. Angiotensin III

Fig. 8.2. Control of renin secretion.

Present knowledge of the control mechanisms for renin secretion is summarized in Fig. 8.2. Although many fundamental mechanisms have been described, their relative physiologic and pathophysiologic roles still require definition. The underlying bases, especially at the cellular level, of these factors regulating renin secretion remain a fruitful area of future investigation.

Generation of the angiotensins

After release from the juxtaglomerular cells, renin enters the renal interstitial space, lymphatics, tubular fluid and urine and the systemic circulation (Peach 1977; Levens et al. 1981c). Renin cleaves the leucyl–leucine bond of renin substrate, an alpha$_2$ globulin synthesized by the liver, to form the decapeptide, angiotensin I. Renin substrate has a molecular weight of 66 000–110 000, and its plasma concentration is increased by glucocorticoids, estrogens, angiotensin II, bilateral nephrectomy and hypoxia (Laragh and Sealey 1973; Oparil and Haber 1974; Peach 1977; Reid et al. 1978). The enzymatic activity of renin may be inhibited or enhanced by plasma circulating factors (Smeby et al. 1967, Kotchen et al. 1975; Sambhi 1977), but this concept requires further verification (Poulsen 1971). Renin is metabolized principally by the liver, and the half-life of circulating renin is 10–20 min (Heacox et al. 1967; Schaechtelin et al. 1964).

Different molecular forms of renin have been identified in renal tissue and plasma. Renin's enzymatic activity increases after acidification of plasma or prolonged incubation of plasma at cold temperatures (Day et al. 1976; Derkx et al. 1976; Sealey et al. 1976; Leckie et al. 1976; Weinberger et al. 1977; Boyd 1977; Millar et al. 1978). Acid activation converts a large molecular weight form of renin (63 000) to a smaller (40 000), more active form (Boyd 1974; Leckie and McConnell 1975; Morris and Johnston 1976; Derkx et al. 1976; Boyd 1977). Circulating renin is also activated by trypsin, pepsin and urinary kallikrein (Cooper et al. 1977; Shulkes et al. 1978; Sealey et al. 1978). Plasma contains proteinase inhibitors, which limit the effect of proteolytic enzymes on renin (Tewksbury and Premeau 1976). Thus, acid and cold activation may decrease the plasma content of a neutral serine protease inhibitor with the liberated protease converting inactive to active renin (Atlas et al. 1978). In addition to the different molecular forms of renin, different affinities for renin may also exist in plasma (Eggena et al. 1978).

Angiotensin II, an octapeptide, is formed by the action of converting enzyme which cleaves histidyl–leucine from the C-terminus of angiotensin I (Erdos 1975; Peach 1977; Oparil 1979). Converting enzyme activity is dependent upon chloride and divalent cations and is inhibited by EDTA (Erdos 1975; Oparil 1979). Converting enzyme is distributed in plasma and in the endothelium of vascular beds in tissues such as lung and kidney. Converting enzyme purified from human lung has a molecular weight of approximately 200 000 (Erdos 1975). Changes in pulmonary hemodynamics and hypoxia reduce pulmonary converting enzyme activity (Stalcup et al. 1979). Angiotensin II production, however, is not thought to be limited by physiologic alterations in converting enzyme activity, because of the widespread distribution and large capacity of the enzyme. Angiotensin converting enzyme also inactivates bradykinin, a vasodilator substance (Erdos 1975). Thus, the same enzyme forms the potent vasopressor hormone, angiotensin II, while at the same time inactivating vasodepressor kinins.

Angiotensin II is degraded by angiotensinases, proteolytic enzymes present in plasma and tissues (Peach 1977; Khairallah and Hall 1977). Angiotensin III (des-aspartyl[1])-angiotensin II, the C-terminal heptapeptide fragment of angiotensin II, is the initial product of aminopeptidase action, and is the only fragment of angiotensin II with significant biologic activity (Peach 1977). However, the heptapeptide is metabolized more readily by proteolytic enzymes than is angiotensin II (Mendelsohn and Kachel 1980). Aminopeptidases also convert angiotensin II to the nonapeptide, (des-aspartyl[1])-angiotensin I, and converting enzyme then converts the nonapeptide to angiotensin III. This is an alternate pathway for angiotensin III production which does not involve angiotensin II formation (Vaughan et al.

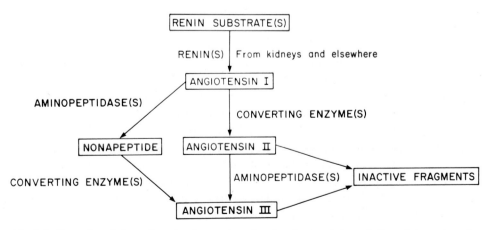

Fig. 8.3. Generation of the angiotensins from renin and renin substrate, and metabolism of the angiotensin peptides.

1977). Because angiotensinases are ubiquitous, changes in their activities are unlikely to affect the activity of the renin–angiotensin–aldosterone system.

Fig. 8.3 depicts the generation of angiotensins from renin and renin substrate and summarizes the routes of metabolism of the angiotensin peptides.

Aldosterone secretion

In comparison with the myriad of factors regulating renin release, the control of aldosterone secretion is less complex. Four trophic stimuli are universally accepted as stimulating aldosterone biosynthesis and secretion: the renin-angiotensin system, ACTH, the plasma potassium concentration, and under certain circumstances the plasma concentration of sodium. The majority of the evidence suggests that the renin-angiotensin system is predominant, but other factors may also be important in certain situations (Davis 1975; Fraser et al. 1979; Coghlan et al. 1979; Reid and Ganong 1979).

Angiotensin II stimulates both the early and late phases of aldosterone biosynthesis. Angiotensin stimulates the early phase by a calcium-dependent mechanism (Fakunding and Catt 1980). The mechanism(s) by which angiotensin stimulates the late phase is unknown. Several studies have demonstrated parallel changes in plasma renin activity and aldosterone under a variety of physiological and pathophysiological conditions, suggesting that the renin-angiotensin system is the principal regulator of aldosterone secretion (Davis 1975; Fraser et al. 1979; Coghlan et al. 1979; Reid and Ganong 1979; Swartz et al. 1980). Plasma aldosterone concentration decreases in response to blockade of the renin-angiotensin system with angiotensin II antagonists or converting enzyme inhibitors (Williams et al. 1978; Fraser et al. 1979) Angiotensin III also stimulates aldosterone secretion, but is not as efficacious as angiotensin II, primarily because of the shorter half-life of angiotensin III in plasma (Peach 1977; Mendelsohn and Kachel 1980).

ACTH is an important factor in the control of aldosterone secretion (Davis 1975; Fraser et al. 1979; Coghlan et al. 1979; Reid and Ganong 1979). ACTH stimulates aldosterone biosynthesis proximally by stimulation of the conversion of cholesterol to pregnenolone. ACTH stimulates steroidogenesis predominantly by activation of adenylate cyclase and elevation of intracellular cyclic AMP concentration (Fujita et al. 1979), but calcium is required for ACTH-stimulated cyclic AMP production and the aldosterone steroidogenic response (Fakunding et al. 1979). Variations in aldosterone secretion are not mediated by ACTH because suppression of ACTH secretion with dexamethasone does not alter the circadian rhythm of aldosterone (Katz et al. 1975; Fraser el al. 1979). Infusion of ACTH increases plasma aldosterone concentrations in sustained fashion, suggesting that ACTH may mediate acute increases in aldosterone secretion physiologically (Nicholls et al. 1975; Kem et al. 1975). Chronic regulation of aldosterone secretion is not ACTH dependent, however, because plasma aldosterone concentrations are normal in hypophysectomized animals and ACTH-deficient man (Himathongham et al. 1975; McKenna et al. 1978). Sodium depletion enhances the aldosterone responses to ACTH, but chronic ACTH deficiency reduces the aldosterone response to sodium depletion (Kem et al. 1975; Fraser et al. 1979).

Positive control mechanisms
1. Angiotensins II and III
2. ACTH
3. Potassium
4. Hyponatremia

Negative control mechanisms
Neuroendocrine factors
　? dopamine

Fig. 8.4. Control of aldosterone secretion.

Potassium stimulates aldosterone secretion and potassium depletion inhibits aldosterone secretion (Davis 1975; Himathongham et al. 1975; Fraser et al. 1979; Coghlan et al. 1979; Reid and Ganong 1979). Potassium stimulates both early and late steroid metabolic pathways in the adrenal zona glomerulosa (McKenna et al. 1978). The early phase is stimulated by a calcium-dependent mechanism (Fakunding and Catt 1980), but the mechanism of late phase stimulation by potassium is unknown. In man, an increase of as little as 0.1 meq l^{-1} in plasma potassium concentration increases plasma aldosterone concentration significantly (Himathongham et al. 1975). In the rat, low potassium diet decreases and high potassium diet enhances angiotensin II-induced aldosterone secretion (Campbell and Schmitz 1978; Douglas 1980). During sodium depletion, potassium may assume a role of equal importance with angiotensin in the acute regulation of aldosterone secretion (Dluhy et al. 1977). Since aldosterone increases potassium excretion, inhibition of its secretion by potassium depletion may be regarded as a protective mechanism.

Hyponatremia can increase aldosterone secretion. However, very large decreases in serum sodium concentration (10–20 meq l^{-1}) are necessary to stimulate aldosterone secretion, so that the physiological role of hyponatremia is minimal (Davis 1975; Fraser et al. 1979; Coghlan et al. 1979; Reid and Ganong 1979).

In the anephric state, aldosterone secretion does not increase with upright posture, indicating that a functioning renin–angiotensin system is necessary for this stimulus (Fraser et al. 1979). However, acute sodium depletion by hemodialysis stimulates aldosterone secretion in the anephric state without alteration of other known factors which stimulate aldosterone secretion. Thus, as yet unidentified factors also may contribute to control of aldosterone secretion. A pituitary factor other than ACTH may increase aldosterone secretion in response to chronic sodium depletion (McCaa et al. 1975; Fraser et al. 1979), and an aldosterone stimulating glycoprotein has been extracted from urine (Sen et al. 1977).

Fig. 8.4 shows the various stimulating and inhibitory factors responsible for the control of aldosterone secretion from the adrenal zona glomerulosa.

Physiologic actions of the components of the renin–angiotensin–aldosterone system

Renin itself has no direct physiologic actions, and its indirect biologic effects are due to angiotensin production (Laragh and Sealey 1973; Oparil and Haber 1974; Peach 1977;

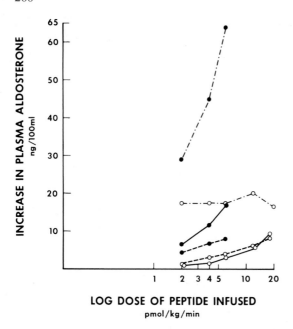

Fig. 8.5. Effect of angiotensin II (●) and angiotensin III (○) on plasma aldosterone concentration in normal human subjects ($n = 6$) on 10 meq (dashed and dotted lines), 150 meq (solid lines) and 300 meq (dashed lines) sodium balance. Low sodium intake increases sensitivity of the adrenal cortex to both angiotensins II and III. However, with low sodium intake, the dose–response curve for angiotensin II is steep, and for angiotensin III it is flat. High sodium intake renders the angiotensin II– and III–aldosterone dose–response curves more nearly parallel, but angiotensin II is more efficacious than angiotensin III at all levels of sodium intake.

(Figure axis labels: INCREASE IN PLASMA ALDOSTERONE ng/100ml; LOG DOSE OF PEPTIDE INFUSED pmol/kg/min)

Goodfriend and Peach 1979). Angiotensin vascular smooth muscle and adrenal receptors differ from each other, as do receptors for angiotensins II and III (Devynek and Meyer 1978; Carey et al. 1978b; Goodfriend 1979). Angiotensins I and II stimulate catecholamine release from the adrenal medulla, act at the level of the central nervous system to induce thirst, salt appetite and vasopressin release and to increase systemic blood pressure, and may redistribute renal blood flow from the outer cortex to the inner zones of the kidney.

Angiotensin II is a potent vascular constrictor. In addition, angiotensin II releases norepinephrine at sympathetic nerve terminals, activates tyrosine hydroxylase, and decreases norepinephrine reuptake by sympathetic neurons, thus increasing sympathetic nervous system activity by increasing the availability of norepinephrine at vascular smooth muscle receptors. Conversely, angiotensin III decreases norepinephrine release and reuptake (Campbell and Jackson 1979). In the kidney, angiotensin II in low physiologic quantities has a primary antidiuretic action independent of changes in glomerular filtration rate or vasopressin (Levens et al. 1981a; Levens et al. 1981b). In low physiologic quantities, angiotensin II is antinatriuretic but at high doses natriuresis ensues. Angiotensin II also increases absorption of salt and water across transporting epithelia in the kidney and intestine (Harris and Young 1977; Levens et al. 1981c; Levens et al. 1981d). Angiotensin II increases heart rate and myocardial contractility, but in vivo infusion is associated with a decrease in cardiac output mediated by the baroreceptor reflex. Angiotensins II and III stimulate adrenal aldosterone secretion, but angiotensin II is the more effective agent (Fig. 8.5) (Carey et al. 1978). Angiotensin II is approximately four times as pressor as angiotensin III. Angiotensin II and III are equally effective suppressors of renin release (Fig. 8.6), elicit comparable central pressor responses and release prostaglandins from peripheral

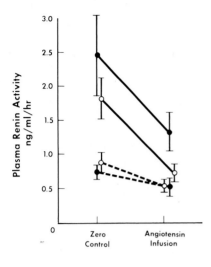

Fig. 8.6. Responses of plasma renin activity to angiotensin II (●) and angiotensin III (○) in normal subjects (n = 6) on 10 meq (solid lines) and 150 meq (dashed lines) sodium intake. Angiotensin II and III were equally efficacious in suppressing plasma renin activity at both levels of sodium intake.

blood vessels. Angiotensin II increases vascular permeability and alters peripheral vascular blood flow.

Physiologic responses to angiotensins depend on target organ sensitivity as well as plasma and tissue concentrations (Laragh and Sealey 1973; Peach 1977). Pressor responses are reduced with sodium depletion and are enhanced when the renin–angiotensin system is supressed. Tachyphalaxis with continued angiotensin administration is related to decreased receptor number and/or affinity, or to production of prostaglandins.

Aldosterone stimulates sodium transport across epithelia in the kidney, salivary and sweat glands, and the gastrointestinal tract (Sharp and Leaf 1973; Nelson 1980). This action relies upon DNA-dependent synthesis of RNA and new proteins. In the kidney, the primary site of action of aldosterone is the distal tubule. Continuous administration of aldosterone in vivo causes escape from the initial sodium retention, and whether or not this natriuresis is related to a humoral factor is unknown. Aldosterone also promotes potassium and hydrogen ion secretion into the distal tubular lumen. Potassium and hydrogen ion

---

1. Vasoconstriction
2. Stimulation of aldosterone biosynthesis and secretion
3. Increase sympathetic nervous system activity
4. Direct renal effects
    Antinatriuresis
    Antidiuresis
5. Cardiac effects
    Increase heart rate
    Increase myocardial contractility
6. Stimulation of thirst, salt appetite and vasopressin release
7. Increase salt absorption across gastrointestinal epithelia
8. Negative feedback to suppress renin release

Fig. 8.7. Physiological actions of angiotensin II.

1. Stimulation of sodium transport across epithelia in the kidney, salivary and sweat glands, and the gastrointestinal tract.
2. Stimulation of secretion of potassium and hydrogen ion across epithelia in the kidney.

Fig. 8.8. Physiological actions of aldosterone.

transport are not necessarily coupled with tubular sodium transport, because the negative lumen potential created by increased sodium reabsorption may facilitate secretion of potassium and hydrogen ion.

Fig. 8.7 depicts the physiologic actions of the angiotensins, and Fig. 8.8 the actions of aldosterone.

NEUROENDOCRINE CONTROL OF RENIN SECRETION

Neuroanatomical considerations

As a background to a discussion of the role of neuroendocrine mechanisms in the control of renin secretion, it is important to be familiar with the innervation of the renal juxtaglomerular apparatus, including the afferent arteriole and the juxtaglomerular cell. A large body of evidence from many different research groups has accumulated indicating that the juxtaglomerular cells are innervated with sympathetic fibers (Barajas 1964; Nilsson 1965; Biava and West 1965; Wagermark et al. 1968). Noradrenergic nerve terminals have been identified in the walls of the afferent arterioles in approximation to the juxtaglomerular cells by means of specific stains for juxtaglomerular cell granules and fluorohistochemical techniques (Wagermark et al. 1968). These noradrenergic nerve terminals are located within about 1200–2000 Å of the juxtaglomerular cells, and a basement membrane lies between the two structures (Barajas 1964; Hartroft 1966; Barajas and Müller 1973; Barajas et al. 1977). The noradrenergic neurons supplying the juxtaglomerular apparatus consist of axons and varicosities surrounded by Schwann cells (Barajas and Müller 1973). The close anatomic relationships between the sympathetic nervous system and the renal juxtaglomerular apparatus have been reviewed in detail by Barajas (1972). Taken together, these investigations (Barajas 1964; Nilsson 1965; Biava and West 1966; Hartroft 1966; Wagermark et al. 1968; Barajas 1972; Barajas and Müller 1973; Barajas et al. 1977) strongly support the concept that the renal arterioles and juxtaglomerular apparatus are innervated by noradrenergic sympathetic nerves.

In contrast, cholinergic innervation of the renal arterioles and juxtaglomerular apparatus is not well-defined. The afferent arterioles may receive cholinergic innervation from renal hilar ganglion cells, but these nerve fibers were not affected by destruction of nerves associated with the renal artery, indicating that any cholinergic innervation is independent of noradrenergic nerve supply (McKenna and Angelakos 1968). Whether or not the juxtaglomerular apparatus receives a cholinergic nerve supply is unknown.

Sympathetic nervous system

Direct stimulation of the renal nerves

Early studies by Vander in anesthetized dogs demonstrated that electrical stimulation of the renal artery with its surrounding sympathetic nerves released renin into the circulation (Vander 1965). However, renal nerve stimulation decreased renal blood flow, glomerular filtration rate and urinary sodium excretion, and it was possible that mechanisms other than direct noradrenergic influences could have increased renin secretion (Vander 1965; Assaykeen and Ganong 1971). Thus, renin secretion might have been caused by (1) afferent arteriolar constriction with activation of the baroreceptor mechanism, (2) decreasing glomerular filtration rate resulting in decreased sodium load to the macula densa or (3) direct action on the juxtaglomerular cells. However, in later studies in anesthetized dogs with a single non-filtering kidney to eliminate the macula densa mechanism, stimulation of isolated renal nerves increased renin secretion associated with an approximate 20% decrease in renal blood flow (Johnson et al. 1971). In these experiments, prior infusion of the vasodilator, papaverine, prevented the decrement in renal blood flow, but not the increment in renin secretion produced by renal nerve stimulation. These studies strongly suggested a direct action of noradrenergic nerve stimulation on renin release at the juxtaglomerular cell, independent of baroreceptor or macula densa mechanisms.

Renin release engendered by renal nerve stimulation was characterized pharmacologically by a number of investigators. In one study, the 2–4 fold increase in plasma renin activity resulting from renal nerve stimulation was totally abrogated by pretreatment with the beta-adrenergic antagonist, propranolol (Loeffler et al. 1972). Administration of phenoxybenzamine, an alpha-adrenergic antagonist, increased basal plasma renin activity by 3-fold and decreased blood pressure by 30%, but did not attenuate the increase in plasma renin activity in response to renal nerve stimulation. Simultaneous administration of propranolol and phenoxybenzamine, while not affecting the phenoxybenzamine-induced hypotension, completely abolished the increment in basal plasma renin activity produced by phenoxybenzamine and the increase in plasma renin activity produced by renal nerve stimulation. These results indicate that nerve-stimulated and alpha-adrenergic antagonist-induced renin secretion are mediated by an action at beta-adrenergic receptors.

In another study, *d,l*-propranolol prevented the increase in plasma renin activity elicited by renal nerve stimulation, but *d*-propranolol, which possesses only 1% of the beta-adrenergic receptor antagonist activity of *l*-propranolol, did not alter nerve-stimulated renin release (Johns and Singer 1974). Renal vasoconstriction was increased similarly by both *d*-propranolol and *d,l*-propranolol. Neither *d,l*-propranolol nor phentolamine altered the increase in plasma renin activity due to renal vasoconstriction (Coote et al. 1972; Johns and Singer 1974). The authors concluded that nerve-stimulated renin release is caused by a direct action of norepinephrine on juxtaglomerular cell beta-adrenergic receptors independent of renal blood flow (Johns and Singer 1974).

Other investigators have shown that renal nerve stimulation can raise plasma renin activity without changing renal blood flow, glomerular filtration rate or renal sodium excretion (Taher et al. 1976). Nerve-stimulated renin secretion was blocked by *l*- and *d,l*-propranolol but not by *d*-propranolol. Thus, nerve-stimulated renin secretion was mediated by an action of norepinephrine at beta-adrenergic receptors independent of the baroreceptor and macula densa mechanisms.

Central nervous system stimulation

It is recognized that the source of physiologic stimulation of the renal nerves is located within the central nervous system, and numerous studies have elucidated the effects of electrical stimulation of various central neuronal tracts on renin secretion. Stimulation of the mesencephalic pressor area in the dorsal part of the central gray stratum produces an increase in plasma renin activity associated with a marked increase in blood pressure and a decrease in renal blood flow (Ueda et al. 1967). The increase in plasma renin activity could be prevented by renal denervation, although renal blood flow was still slightly depressed. It was not possible to be certain that the increase in renin secretion was related to increased renal sympathetic activity, because alterations in renal blood flow and/or renal sodium metabolism also could have contributed. Stimulation of the medullary pressor area also increased plasma renin activity and markedly elevated blood pressure (Passo et al. 1971a). This form of central stimulation of renin release can be blocked by propranolol or by renal denervation, but the effects on renal hemodynamics and sodium excretion are unknown (Passo et al. 1971b).

Stimulation of the hypothalamus decreases plasma renin activity in conscious dogs (Zehr and Feigl 1973; Richardson et al. 1974). Renal blood flow is unchanged, but blood pressure is increased and heart rate is lowered. Renal denervation and propranolol lower basal plasma renin activity and prevent any further decrement in plasma renin activity as a result of hypothalamic stimulation. This study provided evidence that renin secretion could be stimulated tonically by the central nervous system, and that activation of neural tracts in the hypothalamus could inhibit this stimulatory effect. Other studies have shown that stimulation of the dorsolateral pons increases plasma renin activity and decreases renal blood flow, effects which can be prevented unilaterally by ipsilateral renal denervation or can be prevented by propranolol pretreatment (Blair and Feigl 1968). Further, electrical stimulation of the defense area near the superior colliculus increases plasma renin activity, blood pressure and heart rate, and stimulation of the supramamillary part of the hypothalamus increases plasma renin activity, which is blocked by renal denervation (Natchoff et al. 1977).

From this discussion, it is evident that renin secretion can be altered by the central nervous system by means of changes in the level of renal nerve activity. These neural influences on renin secretion are transmitted via intrarenal beta-adrenergic receptors and do not depend on changes in renal blood flow. Most remarkably, these changes in renin secretion are opposite to those which would be predicted on the basis of changes in blood pressure, indicating that the predominant stimulus is mediated by direct beta-adrenergic activity at the level of the juxtaglomerular cell.

The concept that neural mechanisms originating in the central nervous system are responsible for physiologic regulation of renin secretion is difficult to prove, because experiments such as those cited above are invariably associated with hemodynamic responses. However, enough indirect evidence exists to suggest that at least some of basal renin secretion is under tonic influence of the sympathetic nervous system. Chronic renal denervation is associated with suppression of plasma renin activity (Magil et al. 1969; Zehr and Feigl 1973; Reid et al. 1975). Beta-adrenergic blockade reduces plasma renin activity (Assaykeen and Ganong 1971; Johnson et al. 1971; Weber et al. 1974). Stimulation of the hypothalamus reduces renin secretion, an effect mediated by renal nerves (Zehr and Feigl 1973; Richardson et al. 1974). Clonidine, a centrally acting alpha-adrenergic agonist, suppresses sympathetic outflow and reduces renin secretion despite a decrease in blood pressure (Onesti et al. 1971; Reid et al. 1975). Thus, at least a fraction of basal renin secretion is mediated by the central nervous system, and the rate of renin secretion may be modulated by various peripheral reflex mechanisms.

Peripheral reflex mechanisms

(i) *Cardiopulmonary reflex mechanism.* Evidence from several sources has shown that low pressure cardiopulmonary receptors may modulate renin secretion as a function of volume homeostatic mechanisms. Studies employing cardiac autotransplantation, in which atrial volume receptors remain innervated but ventricular receptors are denervated, documented that the increase in plasma renin activity with non-hypotensive hemorrhage was greatly reduced (Thames et al. 1971). Cardiopulmonary receptors in the atria, ventricles and lungs were found to reduce the rate of depolarization of adrenergic nerves, innervating the renal vascular bed (Mancia et al. 1973). Subsequently, cardiopulmonary receptors associated with the vagus nerve were discovered to inhibit renin release (Mancia et al. 1975a). In a dog preparation with constant control of aortic and carotid baroreflex activity, it was demonstrated that inhibition of vagal afferent impulses by cooling produced a 5-fold increase in plasma renin activity (Mancia et al. 1975b). This increase in plasma renin activity was prevented by renal denervation. These results suggest that cardiopulmonary vagal afferent fibers tonically inhibit renin secretion by attenuating efferent renal nerve activity. Consistent with these results was the suppression of plasma renin activity with right atrial stretch and its interruption by bilateral cervical vagotomy (Annat et al. 1976). Distention of the superior vena cava at the junction with the right atrium produced stepwise decreases in right atrial pressure and progressive increases in plasma renin activity but no alteration of blood pressure or renal blood flow (Brosnihan and Bravo 1978). A decrease in right atrial pressure of as little as 1 mm Hg could increase renin secretion. Mechanical distention of the left atrium and adjacent pulmonary veins rapidly suppressed renin secretion without alteration of central venous pressure, blood pressure or renal blood flow (Zehr et al. 1976). This decrease in renin secretion could be prevented by renal denervation and by bilateral cervical vagotomy. Ventricular receptors with vagal afferents capable of reflexly suppressing renin secretion also have been identified (Thames 1977).

The increase in renin secretion attendant to very moderate degrees of non-hypotensive hemorrhage (Claybaugh and Share 1973; Weber et al. 1974) suggested that low pressure cardiopulmonary receptors might sense relatively small decrements in blood volume and consequently increase renin secretion. Renal denervation, ganglionic blockade or pretreatment with beta-adrenergic antagonists prevented the renin response to non-hypotensive hemorrhage (Zehr and Feigl 1973; Weber et al. 1974), supporting the concept that neural reflex pathways are important in this response.

All studies are not in complete agreement that cardiopulmonary receptors may play a role in the control of renin secretion. Thus, studies in man have shown that an acute 10% reduction in blood volume sufficient to decrease right atrial pressure did not increase renin secretion (Hesse et al 1978). Several investigators have shown that phlebotomy of 400–600 ml of blood in man did not increase plasma renin activity (Brown et al. 1966; Bull et al. 1970; Goetz et al. 1974; Hesse et al. 1975). Recent studies using graded lower body suction in man and experimental animals have indicated that the cardiopulmonary volume receptors express their maximal effect on renin secretion only if the activity of the arterial barorecep-tors in the carotid sinus and aortic arch is held constant (Mark et al. 1978; Thames et al. 1978). Mild degrees (− 10 to − 20 mm Hg) of lower body suction which decreased central venous pressure, thus reducing low pressure baroreceptor inhibition, did not stimulate renin secretion (Mark et al. 1978). When lower body suction was increased to −40 mmHg, central venous and arterial pulse pressures were reduced and heart rate increased, indicative of a decrease in sympathetic inhibition by both low- and high-pressure receptors. The resultant increase in heart rate was abolished with propranolol (Mark et al. 1978). These results are consistent with the failure of plasma renin activity to increase after mild reduction in blood volume. On the contrary, when venous return to the heart is obstructed in man by lower extremity tourniquets, cardiopulmonary volume receptors are activated (Kiowski and Julius 1978). Plasma renin activity increases, but not in the presence of propranolol. Thus, the presence of cardiopulmonary receptors remains controversial.

(ii) *Carotid sinus and aortic arch baroreceptor reflex mechanism.* Since renin secretion is closely associated with intravascular volume and blood pressure regulation and is modulated by the sympathetic nervous system, numerous investigators have studied the role of arterial baroreceptors in the control of renin secretion. Again, as with cardiopul-monary volume receptors, the influence of arterial baroreceptors is controversial.

Initially, studies in vagotomized, anesthetized dogs failed to demonstrate an increase in plasma renin activity with bilateral carotid occlusion (Skinner et al. 1964), but later renin release was increased if renal perfusion pressure was held constant (Bunag et al. 1966; McPhee and Lakey 1971). Other investigators demonstrated that carotid sinus hypotension produced a rapid, sustained increase in sodium-depleted, vagotomized, anesthetized dogs with aortic pressure held constant (Cunningham et al. 1978). Denervation of the carotid sinuses prevented the increase in plasma renin activity engendered by bilateral carotid occlusion.

On the other hand, studies in vagotomized or intact animals have demonstrated no relationship between carotid sinus pressure and plasma renin activity even with constant renal perfusion pressure (Brennan et al. 1974). Similarly, in saline-infused anesthetized cats, bilateral carotid occlusion failed to increase renin secretion (Brosnihan and Travis 1976).

(iii) *Interrelationships between neural reflex arcs mediating renal sympathetic stimula-tion.* The most recent studies have indicated that if cardiopulmonary neural input and renal perfusion pressure are controlled, carotid sinus hypotension produces consistent increases in renin secretion (Reid and Jones 1976; Thames et al. 1978; Cunningham et al. 1978; Jarecki et al. 1978). Further study of the interrelationship of arterial baroreceptor with cardiopulmonary volume receptor mechanisms has shown that cardiopulmonary receptors with vagal afferent pathways tonically inhibit renin release even when arterial baroreceptors are intact. Additionally, cardiopulmonary receptors appear to be more sensitive to small decreases in central blood volume than arterial baroreceptors. However, arterial baroreceptor activity can prevent the increase in renin secretion which results from complete blockade of vagal afferent activity from cardiopulmonary receptors (Thames et al. 1978). Similarly, the cardiopulmonary receptors act to counterbalance renal arterial constriction resulting from carotid sinus hypotension (Mancia et al. 1975).

In summary, conclusive evidence has been presented that the renal sympathetic nerves play a role in the control of renin secretion and that renal nerve activity is modulated by several different neural reflex arcs. Several recent reports have implicated the renal sympathetic nerves in the increased renin secretion observed with psychosocial stimuli (Clamage et al. 1976), acoustical stimuli (Vander et al. 1977), electrical shock (Leenen and Shapiro 1974) and excercise (Leon et al. 1973) in rats; immobilization stress in rabbits (Tsukiyama et al. 1973); heat stress (Eisman and Rowell 1977) and avoidance operant conditioning in baboons (Balir et al. 1976); and heat stress (Kosunen et al. 1976), exercise (Kosunen and Pakarinen 1976), mental arithmetic (Kosunen 1977), psychosocial stimuli (Clamage et al. 1977), operant conditioning (Young et al. 1976), ethanol intoxication and hangover (Linkola et al. 1976), passive head-up tilt (Oparil et al. 1970; Esler and Nestil 1973), upright posture (Cohen et al. 1966), cold pressor tests (Gordon et al. 1967), insulin hypoglycemia (Lowder et al. 1975), and high renin essential hypertension (Esler et al. 1977) in man. In none of these studies was data presented to indicate that activation of central nervous system mechanisms was the underlying cause for increased renin secretion. Nevertheless, it is reasonable to believe that central neuronal mechanisms mediate renin secretion by means of renal sympathetic stimulation in many of these stressful situations.

Effects of catecholamines on renin secretion

(i) *Effects of catecholamines on renin secretion in vivo.* In 1965, Vander discovered that norepinephrine and epinephrine stimulated renin secretion in anesthetized dogs with constant baseline renal perfusion pressure (Vander 1965). Since glomerular filtration rate and renal sodium excretion decreased in these experiments, and since mannitol-induced osmotic diuresis attenuated catecholamine-induced renin secretion, it was thought that norepinephrine and epinephrine probably were acting by means of the macula densa mechanism, although a direct effect on the juxtaglomerular cells could not be excluded. In the same year, Wathan et al. (1965) found that intrarenal infusions of norepinephrine and epinephrine increased renin secretion in anesthetized dogs. The increase in renin secretion with intrarenal norepinephrine was accompanied by a rise in intrarenal vascular resistance, a fall in renal blood flow, glomerular filtration rate and urine volume and no significant change in blood pressure. When norepinephrine was infused systemically, blood pressure increased and renin secretion was suppressed. Thus, it appeared that norepinephrine-induced renin secretion was related to renal arteriolar vasoconstriction which could be overridden by an increase in systemic blood pressure. Subsequent studies in anesthetized dogs confirmed that intrarenal norepinephrine infusion increased renin secretion, and intrarenal isoproterenol administration was reported to have no effect on renin release (Bunag et al. 1966). Nash et al. (1968) later showed that the decrease in renal blood flow probably was not the stimulus for norepinephrine-induced renin secretion because simultaneous intrarenal volume expansion with saline did not attenuate the effect of norepinephrine on renin release. Johnson et al. (1971) demonstrated convincingly that norepinephrine and epinephrine stimulated renin secretion independent of the macula densa mechanism, since both of these agents release renin in anesthetized dogs with non-filtering kidneys. Further, papaverine-induced renal vasodilatation did not affect norepinephrine-induced renin secretion, indicating a direct stimulatory effect at the level of the juxtaglomerular cell independent of the baroreceptor mechanism controlling renin release. Norepinephrine and epinephrine administered intravenously were shown to increase plasma renin activity as well as blood pressure in man (Gordon et al. 1967).

Studies in the early 1970s demonstrated that norepinephrine and epinephrine increase renin secretion by a direct effect at beta-adrenergic receptors on juxtaglomerular cells. Intravenous norepinephrine infusion in anesthetized dogs increased renal venous plasma renin activity as blood pressure increased and renal blood flow, glomerular filtration rate and sodium excretion fell (Ueda et al. 1970). The alpha adrenergic antagonist, dibenamine, completely blocked the effects of norepinephrine on renal hemodynamics and sodium excretion, but did not alter the increase in renin secretion, which was blocked by propranolol. Small quantities of intravenous isoproterenol increased renin secretion without changing renal blood flow, glomerular filtration rate or sodium excretion. Isoproterenol-induced renin release was prevented by propranolol but not by renal denervation. Further investigations in anesthetized dogs showed that elevation of plasma epinephrine concentrations following insulin hypoglycemia were associated with a rise in plasma renin activity without change in blood pressure (Assaykeen et al. 1970; Otsuka et al. 1970). Unilateral adrenalectomy and denervation of the contralateral adrenal gland decreased the renin response to insulin hypoglycemia, which was not affected by renal denervation. Renin release induced by hypoglycemia or by infusion of epinephrine to approximate the same plasma epinephrine concentration was blocked by propranolol and potentiated by phenoxybenzamine. All of these studies strongly supported beta-adrenergic stimulation of renin secretion.

However, Winer et al. (1971) reported that in anesthetized dogs norepinephrine- and isoproterenol-induced renin release was blocked with the alpha-adrenergic antagonist, phentolamine, in addition to propranolol. These conflicting results were not substantiated in later studies, as the increase in plasma renin activity elicited by norepinephrine, epinephrine or isoproterenol was blocked by propranolol, but not by phentolamine or phenoxybenzamine (Tanigawa et al. 1972; Assaykeen et al. 1974).

Although some of the early work suggested that the relatively specific beta-adrenergic agonist, isoproterenol, did not increase renin secretion, numerous investigators now have documented that isoproterenol is a potent stimulator of renin release in a variety of experimental animals and man. Isoproterenol stimulates renin release in anesthetized dogs

(Ueda et al. 1970; Winer et al. 1971; Tanigawa et al. 1972; Chokski et al. 1972; Reid et al 1972; Assaykeen et al. 1974), conscious dogs (Gutman et al. 1973; Ayers et al. 1981), anesthetized rats (Peskar et al. 1970; Myer et al. 1971), conscious rats (Pettinger et al. 1972; Leenen and McDonald 1974) and man (Kuchel et al. 1972; Leenen et al. 1975; Davies et al. 1977). Further, propranolol blocks isoproterenol-induced renin secretion in anesthetized and conscious dogs (Ueda et al. 1970; Winer et al. 1971; Tanigawa et al. 1972; Chokski et al. 1972; Assaykeen et al. 1974; Ayers et al. 1981), anesthetized and conscious rats (Myer et al. 1971; Leenen and McDonald 1974) and man (Leenen et al. 1975). Although some investigators have not been able to demonstrate increased renin secretion with intrarenal isoproterenol (Reid et al. 1972a), almost all studies have demonstrated that intrarenal isoproterenol stimulates renin secretion (Winer et al. 1971; Tanigawa et al. 1972; Chokski et al. 1972; Assaykeen et al. 1974; Ayers et al. 1981).

Recent studies (Katholi et al. 1977; Ayers et al. 1981) from our laboratory in conscious dogs have indicated that chronic administration of intrarenal norepinephrine or isoproterenol is associated with an initial 3-fold increase in plasma renin activity followed by a decline to control levels within 24 h despite continuous infusion. On the eleventh day of chronic intrarenal isoproterenol infusion, a 4-fold increase in the dose was not associated with an increase in renin. However, when isoproterenol was given intermittently for 7 h on 4 consecutive days, an increase in plasma renin activity was observed each day. These data argue strongly that beta-adrenergic receptors on juxtaglomerular cells become refractory with continuous stimulation, and that chronic elevations of beta-adrenergic agonists do not necessarily lead to sustained increases in renin secretion. This refractoriness of the beta-adrenergic mechanism for renin secretion may be related to decreased juxtaglomerular cell beta-adrenergic receptor number (Mukherjee et al. 1975; Shear et al. 1976; Mukherjee et al. 1976).

(ii) *Effects of catecholamines on renin secretion in vitro.* Vandongen et al. (Vandongen et al. 1973; Vandongen 1974) were the first to demonstrate that catecholamines stimulate renin secretion in the isolated, perfused kidney preparation. Isoproterenol increased renin secretion from the perfused rat kidney in the absence of any alteration in pressure or flow, and this effect was blocked by *d,l*-propranolol, but not by *d*-propranolol or phenoxybenzamine. Norepinephrine also increased renin secretion in association with a 60% increase in perfusion pressure; this response to norepinephrine was blocked by *d,l*-propranolol and was potentiated by phenoxybenzamine, which nullified the increase in renal perfusion pressure. Non-vasoconstrictor quantities of norepinephrine and epinephrine also stimulated renin release, which again was blocked by *d,l*-propranolol and potentiated by phenoxybenzamine (Vandongen and Greenwood 1975). These results now have been confirmed by several groups of investigators using isolated perfused kidney preparations from rats (Sinaika and Mirkin 1978), rabbits (Viskoper et al. 1977) and cats (Harada and Rubin 1978).

Renin secretion has been examined in renal slice preparations to exclude hemodynamic, tubular, hormonal and neurogenic determinants. Michelakis et al. (1969) first demonstrated that norepinephrine (2.7 μM) and epinephrine (5.4 μM) increased renin secretion from dog renal cell suspensions. Two later studies (Rosset and Veyrat 1971; Johns et al.

1975) showed that norepinephrine increased renin secretion from human renal slices and that norepinephrine, epinephrine and isoproterenol stimulated renin release from cat renal cortical cells. Perhaps the best pharmacologic study was by Nally et al. (1974) who found that *l*-norepinephrine produced a dose-related increase in renin secretion which was blocked by *l*-propranolol and potentiated by phentolamine and phenoxybenzamine. This observation was totally consistent with the results of previous studies in vivo (Assaykeen et al. 1970; Otsuka et al. 1970) and in isolated perfused kidneys (Vandongen et al. 1973; Vandongen 1974). Subsequently, it was shown that prevention of oxidation of catecholamines in vitro with ascorbate allowed norepinephrine, epinephrine and isoproterenol to be effective inducers of renin release at physiologic concentrations (1 – 100 nM) (Weinberger et al. 1975). Renin secretion in response to norepinephrine, epinephrine and isoproterenol also has been demonstrated in superfused isolated rat glomeruli which contain juxtaglomerular but not renal tubular cells (Morris et al. 1976).

(iii) *Mediation of the beta-adrenergic response.* From the antecedent discussion, it is established conclusively that renal nerve stimulation and circulating norepinephrine and epinephrine increase renin secretion by means of a direct action at juxtaglomerular cell beta-adrenergic receptors. Beta-adrenergic receptors have been subdivided into two distinct types (Lands et al. 1967). Beta$_1$-adrenergic receptors mediate cardiac stimulation and lipolytic activity; beta$_2$-adrenergic receptors mediate peripheral vascular and bronchial responses. Evidence now has accumulated that the intrarenal beta-adrenergic receptors controlling renin secretion are of the beta$_2$ subtype. Beta-adrenergic antagonists with affinity predominantly for the beta$_1$ receptor have little influence on plasma renin activity, whereas beta$_2$ antagonists block the increase in renin secretion produced by beta-adrenergic agonists (Allison et al. 1972; Reid et al. 1972; Lopes et al. 1978). However, recent studies in vivo in conscious dogs resulted in oppositie conclusions. Himori et al. (1980) have shown that the selective beta$_1$ antagonist, atenolol, inhibits isoproterenol-induced increases in plasma renin activity in a fashion similar to the non-selective beta-adrenergic antagonist, propranolol. In contrast, the selective beta$_2$ antagonist, IPS-399, was entirely ineffective in inhibiting isoproterenol-induced increases in plasma renin activity. In this study, there was a good correlation between inhibition of isoproterenol-induced tachycardia and suppression of isoproterenol-induced increases in plasma renin activity, but a poor correlation between inhibition of isoproterenol-induced hypotension and suppression of isoproterenol-induced increases in plasma renin activity. Thus the results of this study, showing that renin secretion is mediated by beta$_1$ receptors, are in contradistinction to most of the other literature, and this area remains controversial.

The exact intracellular mechanism by which catecholamines stimulate the secretion of renin is unknown. In many tissues, beta-adrenergic events are mediated intracellularly by activation of adenylate cyclase and the formation of cAMP. There is some evidence suggesting that catecholamine-induced renin secretion is mediated by cAMP. Dibutyryl cAMP administered intrarenally in dogs stimulated renin secretion (Allison et al. 1972) and cAMP increased net renin production in canine renal cortical cell suspensions (Michelakis et al. 1969). Also, theophylline, a phosphodiesterase inhibitor, inhibits degradation of cAMP and increases plasma renin activity in the dog (Reid et al. 1972). Theophylline also potentiates the increase in renin secretion elicited by norepinephrine in renal slice preparations (Nally et al. 1974). Further, the renin response to norepinephrine is associated with accumulation of cAMP in the medium (Lopez et al. 1978).

On the other hand, there is recent mounting evidence that catecholamines may stimulate renin secretion by hyperpolarizing the juxtaglomerular cell membrane with associated extrusion of calcium from the cytoplasm. Epinephrine has been shown to hyperpolarize isolated juxtaglomerular cells in vitro (Fishman 1976) and norepinephrine extrudes calcium from the perfused kidney (Harada and Rubin 1978). Epinephrine also hyperpolarizes vascular smooth muscle cells, and juxtaglomerular cells are modified smooth muscle cells (Scheid et al. 1979). Catecholamine-induced renin secretion can be blocked by high extracellular potassium concentrations, which depolarize the juxtaglomerular cell membrane, and by lanthanum, a blocker of calcium efflux (Fishman 1976; Logan et al. 1977; Fray 1978). Increasing extracellular calcium or decreasing extracellular sodium suppresses catecholamine-induced renin secretion (Fray and Park 1979). These findings are consistent with an action of catecholamines to lower cytoplasmic calcium in smooth muscle (Scheid et al. 1979).

Thus, the indications for one or more processes mediating the catecholamine response at the juxtaglomerular cell are unsettled, but current evidence would favor a calcium-dependent mechanism (Fray 1980).

(iv) *Possible role of the alpha-adrenergic receptor*. The potentiation of norepinephrine-induced renin release with alpha-adrenergic blocking agents cited above (Assaykeen et al. 1970; Otsuka et al. 1970; Vandongen et al. 1973; Vandongen 1974) has suggested the possibility that alpha-adrenergic stimulation might suppress renin release. Several investigators now have addressed this problem, but the role of alpha-adrenergic receptors in the control of renin release remains controversial.

Pettinger et al. (1972), studying dose–response curves of catecholamines on plasma renin activity in conscious rats, observed that norepinephrine at low doses suppressed renin and at high doses stimulated renin, while isoproterenol stimulated renin at all doses employed. This biphasic norepinephrine response indicated that alpha-adrenergic stimulation might suppress renin release. Also, clonidine appeared to suppress renin release by an agonist activity at alpha-adrenergic receptors (Reid et al. 1975; Pettinger et al. 1976). Other authors (Vandongen and Peart 1974; Weinberger et al. 1975) reported that the relatively specific alpha-adrenergic agonist, methoxamine, blocked isoproterenol-induced renin release in the isolated perfused kidney and in renal slice preparations. This observation could have been related either to alpha-adrenergic stimulation or to beta-adrenergic blockade to suppress renin release (Vandongen and Peart 1974; Weinberger et al. 1975).

The concentration of norepinephrine necessary to stimulate postganglionic alpha$_1$ receptors is 30–100 fold that required to activate post-ganglionic beta-adrenergic receptors (Adler-Graschinsky and Langer 1975). Thus, if an alpha-adrenergic receptor is involved in suppressing renin release at the level of the juxtaglomerular cell, norepinephrine should stimulate renin release at low doses and inhibit renin release at high doses. Although in vivo observations (Pettinger et al. 1972) were not consistent with this concept, in vitro studies tended to support it. That is, in renal cortical slice preparations, low concentrations of norepinephrine (1 pM–100 nM) stimulated but high concentrations (10 µM) inhibited renin release (Desaulles et al. 1975; Capponi and Valloton 1976; Lopez et al. 1978). Further, phentolamine and phenoxybenzamine reversed the inhibitory effect of norepinephrine on renin secretion (Desaulles et al. 1975; Lopez et al. 1978). These results suggest that alpha-adrenergic stimulation suppresses renin release directly at renin-secreting cells.

Vandongen et al. (1979) have performed careful studies of alpha-adrenergic mechanisms in the isolated, perfused kidney, and have concluded that alpha receptor stimulation suppresses renin secretion directly at the juxtaglomerular cell, independent of vascular mechanisms. Suppression of renin release to isoproterenol by the alpha agonist, phenylephrine, was demonstrated even with maximal renal vasodilatation with dihydralazine. However, since renal tubular function was not studied, phenylephrine-induced changes in macula densa sodium transport influencing renin secretion could not be excluded entirely.

Recent studies from our laboratory in conscious dogs indicate that, while alpha-adrenergic mechanisms may suppress renin release directly at the juxtaglomerular cell, alpha-adrenergic activity may stimulate renin secretion in vivo by an indirect, possibly vascular, mechanism (Ayers et al. 1981). Intrarenal infusion of methoxamine increased plasma renin activity by 2- to 7-fold and blood pressure by 25–36% and decreased renal blood flow by 40%. These effects were abolished by phentolamine, and also by indomethacin, suggesting mediation by prostaglandins (Ayers et al. 1978). Chronic intrarenal methoxamine infusion was associated with a return of plasma renin activity to control levels by 24 h, suggesting the possibility of alpha receptor refractoriness (Ayers et al. 1981).

Although much work remains to be done on the role of alpha-adrenergic receptors in the control of renin secretion, current evidence suggests the possibility of two different alpha receptor-mediated effects: (1) intrarenal alpha receptor stimulation (low concentrations of alpha agonist) inhibiting renin release directly at the juxtaglomerular cell and (2) intrarenal alpha receptor stimulation (high concentrations of alpha agonist) large enough to cause marked renal vasoconstriction stimulating renin release, perhaps via increased renal prostaglandin production. In any event, it is important to remember that increased renal sympathetic nerve activity is associated uniformly with increased renin secretion.

Parasympathetic nervous system

While the sympathetic nervous system is an established modulator of renin secretion, the parasympathetic nervous system has not been demonstrated to influence renin release. Intrarenal infusion of acetylcholine has no effect on renin secretion in anesthetized or conscious dogs (Bunag et al. 1966; Ayers et al. 1969; Abe et al. 1973). Further, acetylcholine does not affect renin release in a renal slice preparation (Devito et al. 1970). Thus, although acetylcholine may alter renal hemodynamics and sodium excretion (Tagawa and Vander 1969), the parasympathetic nervous system does not appear to play a significant role in the control of renin secretion.

Dopaminergic mechanisms in the control of renin secretion

The role of dopamine, if any, in the control of renin secretion is not well defined. Several in vivo studies in conscious and anesthetized dogs have shown intrarenal dopamine infusion to be without effect on plasma renin activity (Ayers et al. 1969; Chokski et al. 1972). On the other hand, some investigators have reported that intravenous or intrarenal dopamine administration increases renin secretion associated with renal vasodilatation (Otsuka et al. 1970; Imbs et al. 1975; Dzau et al. 1978). In the latter two studies, the renal vasodilatation and increase in renin secretion was suppressed by haloperidol, a relatively nonspecific dopamine receptor blocking agent (Imbs et al. 1975; Dzau et al. 1978).

In man, dopamine has no consistent effect on renin secretion. Intravenous infusions of dopamine usually do not alter plasma renin activity (Atuk et al. 1968; Carey 1981a). One investigator (Wilcox et al. 1974) has reported that pressor doses of dopamine increased plasma renin activity in normal human subjects, while another group (Barnardo et al. 1970) found that subpressor amounts of dopamine decreased plasma renin activity in patients with hepatic cirrhosis.

With regard to the effects of dopamine on renin release in vitro, Henry et al. (1977) observed a significant elevation of renin release at dopamine concentrations of 10 nM to 10 µM in a renal slice preparation. However, this effect of dopamine was blocked with d,l-propranolol, and it was concluded that dopamine stimulated renin release by an effect at beta-adrenergic receptors. In the isolated perfused rat kidney, dopamine at 4 µM increased renin secretion, but again this effect was antagonized by propranolol (Quesada et al. 1979).

In summary, dopamine appears not to affect renin secretion directly by a dopamine-specific mechanism and also does not seem to play a role in the physiologic regulation of renin by indirect mechanisms. However, the effects of dopamine on renin secretion have not been studied extensively and probably need further characterization.

Serotoninergic mechanisms in the control of renin secretion

The effects of serotonin (5-hydroxytryptamine) on renin secretion are largely unknown. Intrarenal infusion of serotonin initially was reported to have no effect in anesthetized dogs (Meyer et al. 1974). However, later studies showed that serotonin in anesthetized rats elevated plasma renin concentration (Bunag et al. 1966). Methysergide, a serotonin antagonist, but one which also affects the dopaminergic system, completely blocked this response without affecting basal plasma renin concentration. Pretreatment with propranolol and camphidonium, a ganglionic blocker, reduced the renin response to serotonin by 50 and 40%, respectively. Thus, the increase in renin release caused by serotonin may well have been related to serotonin-induced vasodepression with consequent activation of the sympathetic nervous system and the baroreceptor mechanisms for renin release, but other mechanisms are possible.

Tryptophan, a metabolic precursor of serotonin, has been administered to normal human subjects (Modlinger et al. 1979). Oral tryptophan increased plasma renin activity without any consistent alteration of blood pressure, and this was attributed to a central serotoninergic mechanism (Modlinger et al. 1979). Also, cyproheptadine, a serotonin antagonist, inhibited furosemide-induced renin release in normal man (Epstein and Hamilton 1977).

However, cyproheptadine also has antihistamine and anticholinergic properties, so that these findings must be interpreted with caution.

In summary, the possible role of serotonin in the control of renin secretion requires much further investigation.

NEUROENDOCRINE CONTROL OF ALDOSTERONE SECRETION

Dopaminergic mechanisms in the control of aldosterone secretion

Dopamine, a precursor of the sympathetic neurotransmitter norepinephrine, is well established as a neurotransmitter in the central nervous system (Hornykiewicz 1966). Dopamine also may have transmitter function in the peripheral autonomic nervous system (Goldberg 1972; Thorner 1975; Costa and Gesa 1977; Van Loon and Sole 1980). Dopamine inhibits prolactin secretion directly at the pituitary gland (MacLeod 1976) and increases blood flow in the renal and mesenteric vascular beds by means of its vasodilator action (Goldberg 1975).

Recent evidence has suggested that aldosterone secretion may be inhibited by dopaminergic mechanisms. Administration of metoclopramide, a dopamine antagonist, in vivo increases plasma aldosterone concentration independent of known aldosterone regulating factors (Norbiato et al. 1977; Carey et al. 1979). Support for the concept that dopamine inhibits aldosterone secretion was provided by in vitro studies showing that angiotensin II-induced aldosterone production is diminished by dopamine (McKenna et al. 1979). The observation that metoclopramide increases plasma aldosterone concentration, together with the finding that the dopamine agonists, dopamine and bromocriptine, do not modify basal plasma aldosterone concentration, has led to the hypothesis that aldosterone secretion may be under maximum tonic dopaminergic inhibition (Carey et al. 1979; Carey et al. 1980; Noth et al. 1980).

Dopamine antagonists

(i) *Metoclopramide.* Metoclopramide (N-diethylaminoethyl-2-methoxy-4-amino-5-chlorobenzamide) is a procaineamide derivative with well-established dopamine antagonist properties (Jenner and Marsden 1979). Metoclopramide is a competitive antagonist of dopamine in the central nervous system (Dolphin et al. 1975; Jenner et al. 1975; Peringer et al. 1976; Jenner et al. 1978), gastrointestinal tract (Valenzuela 1976) and cardiovascular system (Day and Blower 1975). Metoclopramide stimulates prolactin secretion from the pituitary gland in vivo in experimental animals and man (Delitala et al. 1975; McCallum et al. 1976; Sowers et al. 1976; Sowers et al. 1977; Carlson et al. 1977; Healy and Burger 1978; Aona et al. 1978) and antagonizes the inhibitory effect of dopamine on prolactin secretion in vitro (Yeo et al. 1978).

Of the dopamine antagonists currently available in the United States, metoclopramide appears to be the most specific (Goldberg 1978; Goldberg and Weder 1981). However, some of the effects of metoclopramide may be related to its antiserotoninergic properties (Pinder et al. 1976; Fozard and Mobarok 1978; Niemegeers and Janssen 1979). In addition, metoclopramide may stimulate the release of pancreatic polypeptide (Spitz et al. 1979) and motilin (Byrnes et al. 1980). Metoclopramide increases gastroesophageal tone and motility; whether or not these effects are related to metoclopramide's antagonist properties at dopamine receptors is uncertain (Hay 1975; Valenzuela 1976; Goldberg 1978).

Recently, Kebabian and Calne (1979) have emphasized the diversity of dopamine receptors in various tissues. Evidence exists for at least two different classes of dopamine receptors on the basis of biochemical criteria. One type of dopamine receptor, designated as the D-1 receptor, is linked to adenylate cyclase; stimulation of this receptor results in accumulation of intracellular cAMP. Postsynaptic nigrostriatal and renal vascular dopamine receptors are examples of D-1 receptors. The other type of dopamine receptor, termed the D-2 receptor, is not adenylate cyclase linked; pituitary lactotrophs are prototype cells containing D-2 receptors (see also Chapter 6). Metoclopramide has been proposed as a specific antagonist of D-2 receptors.

Although the initial study with metoclopramide (Ogihara et al. 1977) reported no effect on plasma aldosterone concentration in man, all subsequent studies have documented an

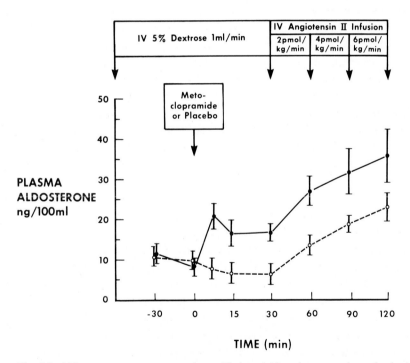

Fig. 8.9. Aldosterone responses to metoclopramide (●—●) 10 mg intravenously or placebo (o——o) in normal subjects (*n* = 6) in sodium and potassium balance. 30 min after metoclopramide or placebo administration, the subjects received cumulative doses of angiotensin II by continuous intravenous infusion for 90 min. Metoclopramide increased plasma aldosterone concentration, but the aldosterone response to angiotensin II was not influenced by prior metoclopramide administration. Reproduced from Carey et al. J. Clin. Invest. 63, 727-735, 1979.

increase in plasma aldosterone concentration as a result of metoclopramide administration (Norbiato et al. 1977; Carey et al. 1979; Carpenter et al. 1979; Carey et al. 1980; Noth et al. 1980; Sowers et al. 1980). An intravenous bolus dose of 10 mg of metoclopramide produces an increase in plasma aldosterone concentration within 5 min with a peak of 2–3 fold increase at 10–15 min and return to baseline over 1–3 h in man (Fig. 8.9) (Norbiato et al. 1977; Carey et al. 1979; Carpenter et al. 1979; Carey et al. 1980; Noth et al. 1980; Sowers et al. 1980), the rat (Sowers et al. 1980c) and the sheep (Coghlan et al. 1980). In contrast, 10 mg of metoclopramide orally increased plasma aldosterone concentration in only two of five human subjects (Noth et al. 1980). However, oral metoclopramide resulted in 60% lower plasma levels of metoclopramide than intravenous metoclopramide (Noth et al. 1980). Since oral metoclopramide did increase serum prolactin concentrations in these studies, the threshold for metoclopramide-induced prolactin secretion is lower than for metoclopramide-induced increases in plasma aldosterone concentration. The increase in plasma aldosterone concentration engendered by metoclopramide is associated with an increase in urinary aldosterone excretion (Carey et al. 1979). Metoclopramide does not affect aldosterone metabolic clearance (Carpenter et al. 1979), so that the increases in plasma and urinary aldosterone represent an increase in adrenal aldosterone secretion.

During studies with metoclopramide, none of the known stimuli for aldosterone secretion were altered. Metoclopramide-induced increases in plasma aldosterone concentration were not accompanied by any changes in blood pressure, pulse rate, plasma renin activity or plasma concentrations of sodium, 11-hydroxycorticosteroids or cortisol (Norbiato et al. 1977; Carey et al. 1979; Carpenter et al. 1979; Carey et al. 1980; Noth et al. 1980; Pratt et al. 1979; Sowers et al. 1980a; Sowers et al. 1980b; Coghlan et al. 1980). Bevilacqua et al. reported that metoclopramide produces a significant decrease in serum potassium concentration 10 and 20 min after intravenous administration, but all other carefully controlled studies have shown no change in serum potassium (Norbiato et al. 1977; Carey et al. 1979; Carpenter et al. 1979; Carey et al. 1980; Noth et al. 1980; Sowers et al. 1980a; Sowers et al. 1980b; Coghlan et al. 1980). Recent studies by Sowers et al. (Sowers et al. 1980a; Sowers et al. 1980b; Sowers et al. 1981) in experimental animals and man have shown that dopaminergic modulation of aldosterone secretion is independent of renin and ACTH secretion. In the rat, metoclopramide-induced aldosterone secretion is not affected by bilateral nephrectomy or by blockade of the renin-angiotensin system with an angiotensin competitive antagonist, saralasin, or a converting enzyme inhibitor, SQ14, 225 (Sowers et al. 1980a; Sowers et al. 1980c). In man, metoclopramide-induced aldosterone secretion in not blocked by saralasin or by dexamethasone (Sowers et al. 1981).

Taken together, these results strongly suggest that metoclopramide stimulates aldosterone secretion independent of known aldosterone-regulating mechanisms.

Metoclopramide-induced aldosterone secretion is probably not related to pituitary factors. Plasma aldosterone concentration is increased in response to metoclopramide in hypopituitary subjects in whom serum prolactin concentrations remained undetectable or unchanged by metoclopramide (Pratt et al. 1979). Dexamethasone administration at doses which completely suppress plasma cortisol, and presumably ACTH, has no effect on metoclopramide-induced aldosterone secretion (Carpenter et al. 1979; Sowers et al. 1981).

Also, metoclopramide increases plasma aldosterone concentration in at least some hypophysectomized patients (Norbiato et al. 1977).

Previous studies have suggested that prolactin may increase plasma aldosterone concentration or aldosterone secretion (McCaa et al. 1974; Solyom 1974; Lichtenstein et al. 1976; Carroll et al. 1980). Since metoclopramide increases prolactin secretion, it was possible that prolactin secondarily was increasing aldosterone secretion. However, this is not the case as ovine prolactin administration to normal subjects does not alter plasma aldosterone concentration (Fig. 8.10) (Carey et al. 1977). Further, administration of TRH to normal human subjects acutely raises serum prolactin concentration but has no effect on aldosterone secretion (Bauman and Loriaux 1976). Finally, glucocorticoid administration significantly depresses prolactin responses to metoclopramide without altering metoclopramide-induced aldosterone secretion (Sowers et al. 1981) The site of metoclopramide's action to increase aldosterone secretion is unknown. Recent studies by Brown et al. (1979) have suggested that metoclopramide acts directly at the adrenal cortex, because metoclopramide (10 nM–10μM) stimulated aldosterone-producing adenomas and nodular hyperplastic adrenal tissue from patients with primary aldosteronism to produce aldosterone in vitro. Whether metoclopramide acts at specific dopamine receptors to antagonize the effects of dopamine in these tissues is unknown.

(ii) *Sulpiride.* Sulpiride is a substituted benzamide which is structurally related to metoclopramide. Sulpiride is the most specific antagonist of dopamine receptors thus far studied (Goldberg et al. 1979a). The R enantiomer of sulpiride is more potent than the S enantiomer at the renal vascular dopamine receptor (Goldberg et al. 1979b). Many of the biologic effects of sulpiride are similar to those of metoclopramide (Jenner et al. 1975; Trabucchi et al. 1976; Roufogalis et al. 1976; Elliot et al. 1977; Meltzer et al. 1979;

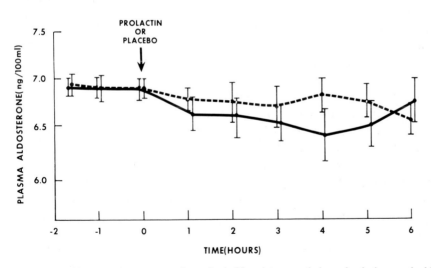

Fig. 8.10. Aldosterone responses to ovine prolactin 25 mg intramuscularly or placebo in normal subjects (*n* = 6) in sodium and potassium balance. Prolactin did not alter plasma aldosterone concentration over a 6 h experimental period.

Niemegeers and Janssen 1979). However, sulpiride possesses antipsychotic effects, and metoclopramide does not (Bratfos and Huang 1979).

Mori et al. (1980) have reported that 50 mg of sulpiride intramuscularly failed to increase plasma aldosterone concentration in normal human subjects. However, in some dopaminergic systems sulpiride is considerably less potent than metoclopramide (Niemegeers and Janssen 1979). Since the aldosterone response to metoclopramide is dependent upon dose and route of administration, it is important that higher doses of sulpiride administered intravenously be studied to determine the effect of sulpiride on aldosterone secretion.

(iii) *Chlorpromazine.* Chlorpromazine is a phenothiazine with a relatively narrow range of specificity for dopamine receptors compared with sulpiride or metoclopramide (Goldberg et al. 1978). Chlorpromazine possesses central and peripheral dopamine antagonist properties as well as alpha-adrenoceptor blocking activity (Brotzu 1970; Greese et al. 1976; Caron et al. 1978). Chlorpromazine causes a delayed increase at 60 min in plasma aldosterone concentration when given intravenously to schizophrenic patients (Szalay 1973). The aldosterone elevation was preceded by a rise in plasma renin activity in this study. However, chlorpromazine 1–10 μM did not affect aldosterone production, and 100 μM chlorpromazine decreased aldosterone production in rat adrenal cell suspensions (Szalay 1973).

Dopamine agonists

(i) *Bromocriptine.* Bromocriptine (2-brom-alpha-ergocriptine) was developed originally as a specific inhibitor of prolactin secretion by Fluckiger and Wagner (1968). Only later was bromocriptine recognized as a dopamine agonist (Corrodi et al. 1973; Fuxe et al. 1974). Bromocriptine acts as a dopamine agonist in the central nervous system (Fluckiger and Wagner 1968; Corrodi et al. 1973) and at the pituitary gland to inhibit prolactin release in vivo and in vitro (Besser et al. 1972; Fluckiger et al. 1976; Yeo et al. 1979) and at peripheral vascular dopamine receptors to produce vasodilatation of renal and mesenteric arteries (Clarke et al. 1978). Bromocriptine has been demonstrated to act directly at dopamine receptors by means of receptor assays in membranes from brain tissue using tritiated dopamine or tritiated haloperidol as ligands (Goldstein et al. 1978). In addition to its agonist activity at dopamine receptors, bromocriptine interacts with central alpha-adrenergic and serotonin receptors (Fuxe et al. 1974; Lew et al. 1977), but its order of potency is much greater for dopamine receptors (Fuxe et al. 1974). The action of bromocriptine at central presynaptic alpha-adrenergic receptors may decrease peripheral sympathetic nervous system activity (DiChiara et al. 1977; Judy et al. 1978; Hertting et al. 1979; Van Loon et al. 1979, Ziegler et al. 1979), which may at least partially account for the hypotensive action of this compound (Judy et al. 1978). Further, peripheral effects of bromocriptine may contribute to inhibition of norepinephrine release from sympathetic neurons (Steinsland and Hieble 1978; Gibson and Samini 1978).

Edwards et al. (1975) initially reported that bromocriptine inhibited the increase in plasma aldosterone concentration in response to furosemide in normal man. However, interpretation of this report is problematic because of the small number of subjects studied, the acute increase of plasma aldosterone concentration immediately following bromoc-

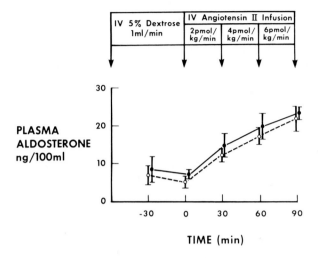

IV 5% Dextrose 1ml/min	IV Angiotensin II Infusion		
	2pmol/ kg/min	4pmol/ kg/min	6pmol/ kg/min

PLASMA ALDOSTERONE ng/100ml

TIME (min)

Fig. 8.11. Aldosterone responses to bromocriptine (●—●) 2.5 mg 8 h for 1 day or placebo (o— — —o) in normal subjects ($n = 6$) in sodium and potassium balance. Bromocriptine did not alter basal or angiotensin II-induced plasma aldosterone concentration. Reproduced from Carey et al. J. Clin. Invest. 63, 727-735, 1979.

riptine, and the widely fluctuating plasma renin activity values.

Recent investigations almost uniformly have documented bromocriptine to be without effect on aldosterone secretion. Administration of bromocriptine did not alter basal plasma aldosterone concentration (Fig. 8.11) (del Pozo et al. 1977; Carey et al. 1979; Birkhauser et al. 1979; Carey et al. 1980), the circadian rhythm of plasma aldosterone concentration (Uberti et al. 1979), urinary excretion of aldosterone (Birkhauser et al. 1979) or the plasma aldosterone response to upright posture (del Pozo et al. 1977; Birkhauser et al. 1979) or dietary sodium depletion (Semple and Mason 1978; Carey et al. 1981a). Additionally, bromocriptine did not inhibit the increase in plasma aldosterone concentration in patients with renal failure between dialyses (Olgaard et al. 1977) or plasma aldosterone concentration in acromegalic patients (Nilsson and Hökfelt 1978).

Birkhauser et al. (1979) reported that bromocriptine partially inhibited the plasma aldosterone response to intravenous angiotensin II infusion and to ACTH injection. Whitfield et al. (1980) reported that bromocriptine 2.5 mg t.i.d. orally for 5 days significantly inhibited the responses of plasma aldosterone concentration to upright posture, isometric hand grip and graded angiotensin II infusions, but did not alter the plasma aldosterone response to ACTH. In marked contrast, we were unable to find any inhibitory effect of bromocriptine on angiotensin II-induced aldosterone secretion despite suppression of serum prolactin concentration to undetectable levels in well-controlled studies at our Clinical Research Center (Carey et al. 1979). Furthermore, bromocriptine, at a dose which suppressed basal serum prolactin concentration and completely prevented the prolactin response to metoclopramide, had no effect on aldosterone responses to metoclopramide (Fig. 8.12) (Carey et al. 1980).

Taken together, this evidence strongly suggests that bromocriptine does not affect aldosterone secretion. This finding indicates that any putative dopamine receptors mediating the adrenal response to metoclopramide are not D-2, because bromocriptine has been tendered as a prototype D-2 dopamine receptor agonist (Kebabian and Calne 1979).

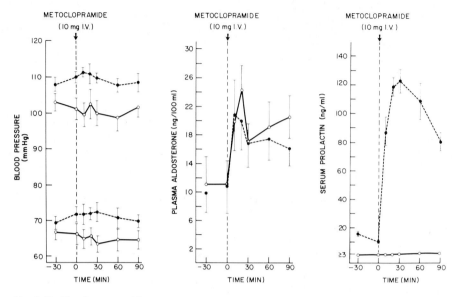

Fig. 8.12. Blood pressure, aldosterone and prolactin response to metoclopramide 10 mg intravenously in normal human subjects ($n = 6$) pretreated with bromocriptine 2.5 mg three times for 1 day (o—o) or placebo (●- - -●). Bromocriptine did not alter the aldosterone response to metoclopramide but lowered blood pressure and suppressed prolactin secretion to undetectable levels. Reproduced from Carey et al. J. Clin. Invest. 66, 10-18, 1980.

Some of the ergot derivatives have been described as possessing antagonist properties at the D-1 receptor. However, bromocriptine could not be acting in this manner because bromocriptine does not stimulate basal aldosterone secretion.

(ii) *Dopamine*. Dopamine interacts with specific receptors in the central nervous system and in peripheral tissues. In the periphery, dopamine interacts at specific dopaminergic neuronal receptors. Stimulation of presynaptic dopamine receptors on sympathetic ganglia or postganglionic nerve terminals inhibits norepinephrine release (Goldberg and Weder 1981). Stimulation of postsynaptic dopamine receptors in various vascular beds produces vasodilatation (Goldberg and Weder 1981). In addition to its agonist effects at dopamine receptors, dopamine also possesses agonist activity at $beta_1$- and alpha-adrenergic receptors (Goldberg 1972). However, Lorenzi et al. (1979) have demonstrated that effective alpha- and beta-adrenergic receptor blockade with phentolamine and propranolol, respectively, does not block inhibition of prolactin secretion by 1.5 $\mu g\ kg^{-1}\ min^{-1}$ of dopamine in man. Thus dopamine acts preferentially at its own receptor to suppress prolactin secretion.

We (Carey et al. 1980) have shown that intravenous infusion of dopamine in normal human subjects at doses (2 and 4 $\mu g\ kg^{-1}\ min^{-1}$) which suppress basal serum prolactin concentration to a non-detectable level does not alter basal plasma aldosterone concentration (Fig. 8.13). However, intravenous dopamine infusion blocks metoclopramide-induced

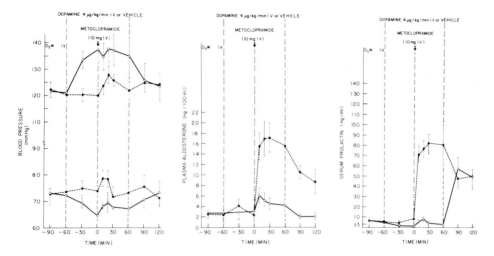

Fig. 8.13. Blood pressure, aldosterone and prolactin responses to metoclopramide 10 mg intravenously in normal human subjects ($n = 6$) treated with dopamine 4 μg kg^{-1} min^{-1} intravenously (o—o) or vehicle (●- - -●). Dopamine inhibited aldosterone and prolactin responses to metoclopramide. Reproduced from Carey et al. J. Clin. Invest. 66, 10-18, 1980.

increases in plasma aldosterone concentration in a dose-dependent manner (Fig. 8.13) (Carey et al. 1980). Although this effect could be related to an indirect effect of dopamine, this possibility seems unlikely. None of the known mediators of aldosterone secretion (renin secretion as reflected by plasma renin activity, ACTH secretion as reflected by plasma cortisol concentration, or serum sodium or potassium concentrations) changed as a result of metoclopramide or dopamine administration alone or in combination. Although there was a slight increase in pulse pressure with the administration of dopamine, it is unlikely that this represents significant alpha-adrenergic receptor stimulation at the dose level employed in these studies (Lorenzi et al. 1979). Further, there is no precedent for suppression of aldosterone secretion by sympathomimetic agents. These results, then, strongly suggest that the aldosterone response to metoclopramide is mediated by an antagonist activity at dopamine receptors (Carey et al. 1980).

Dopamine administration also inhibited metoclopramide-induced increases in serum prolactin concentration (Fig. 8.13) (Carey et al. 1980). After cessation of the dopamine infusion, serum prolactin concentration increased markedly above control values, but plasma aldosterone concentration continued to decrease toward baseline levels (Fig. 8.13). These findings could be related to (1) increased sensitivity of pituitary lactotrophs compared with aldosterone-secreting cells to dopamine's acute inhibitory activity, (2) prolonged interaction of dopamine with dopamine receptors influencing aldosterone secretion, or (3) other homeostatic mechanisms as yet undiscovered controlling aldosterone secretion.

The observation that dopamine inhibits metoclopramide-induced aldosterone secretion without influencing basal aldosterone secretion in man now has been confirmed by two other groups of investigators (Noth et al. 1980; Sowers et al. 1981). In addition, Sowers et al. (1980a; 1980b) have demonstrated in the rat that pretreatment with L-dopa inhibits the increase in plasma aldosterone concentration engendered by metoclopramide. Thus, the evidence to date is in agreement with the concept that the aldosterone response to meto-clopramide is related to dopamine antagonism rather than to a nonspecific pharmacologic effect of the drug.

McKenna et al. (1979) have performed in vitro studies of the effects of dopamine on aldosterone production in bovine adrenal glomerulosa cells in suspension. Dopamine did not alter basal aldosterone production, but significantly inhibited angiotensin II-induced aldosterone production, probably by inhibiting late steps (deoxycorticosterone to aldoste-rone) in the aldosterone biosynthetic pathway. Inhibition of aldosterone production stimu-lated by grossly supraphysiologic doses of angiotensin II (10 µM) by dopamine was dose-dependent. Inhibition of 50% was observed at 10 µM dopamine, and 20% at 10 nM dopamine (McKenna et al. 1979).

We (Carey 1981a) have studied in vivo responses of plasma aldosterone concentration to angiotensin II and ACTH in the presence and absence of dopamine in man. Aldosterone responses to graded doses of angiotensin II (2,4 and 6 pmol kg^{-1} min^{-1}) each administered intravenously for 30 min were not altered by infusion of dopamine 4 µg kg^{-1} min^{-1} given 1 h prior and during the angiotensin infusion (Fig. 8.14). This dose of dopamine resulted in approximately 70% attenuation of the aldosterone response to metoclopramide. In ad-dition, dopamine 4 µg kg^{-1} min^{-1} failed to inhibit ACTH-induced aldosterone secretion in vivo (Fig. 8.15). These observations are consistent with our previous findings that meto-clopramide does not modify the aldosterone response to angiotensin II in sodium replete normal man (Carey et al. 1979). Thus, the weight of the evidence, taken largely from

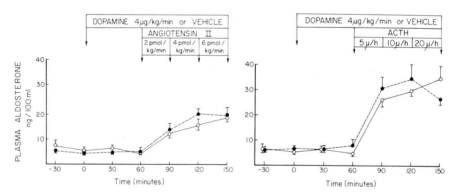

Fig. 8.14. (Left) Aldosterone responses to cumulative doses of angiotensin II intravenously in the presence of dopamine 4 µg kg^{-1} min^{-1} (●– – –●) or vehicle (o—o). Dopamine did not decrease basal plasma aldosterone concentrations or alter the aldosterone response to angiotensin II.

Fig. 8.15. (Right) Aldosterone response to cumulative doses of ACTH intravenously in the presence of dopamine 4 µg kg^{-1} min^{-1} (●– – –●) or vehicle (o—o). Dopamine did not decrease basal plasma aldosterone concentrations or alter the aldosterone response to ACTH.

carefully controlled in vivo studies, suggests that metoclopramide acts on aldosterone secretion by dopamine mechanisms, and not by nonspecific effects mediated by the renin-angiotensin system or by ACTH.

In the studies demonstrating that dopamine inhibits metoclopramide–induced aldosterone secretion, it is possible that dopamine increased aldosterone metabolic clearance by increasing hepatic blood flow (Innes and Nickerson 1975). However, the failure of dopamine to alter the increase in plasma aldosterone concentration or urinary aldosterone excretion in response to angiotensin II or ACTH argues against this point (Carey 1981a). Nevertheless, a formal study of the effect of dopamine on aldosterone metabolic clearance would be necessary to exclude this possibility.

Dopamine is an agonist at both D-1 and D-2 receptors, but dopamine may have a differential effect on D-1 and D-2 receptors based on quantitative considerations (Kebabian and Calne 1979). Relatively large amounts (micromolar concentrations) of dopamine are required to stimulate D-1 receptors, but relatively smaller quantities (nanomolar concentrations) are required for stimulation of D-2 receptors.

Inhibition of metoclopramide-induced aldosterone secretion by dopamine does not indicate conclusively which class of dopamine receptors is involved. However, on the basis of the dose-related inhibitory effect of dopamine to suppress prolactin secretion, we postulated that we were dealing with nanomolar quantities of dopamine (Carey et al. 1980). We gave almost enough dopamine to maximally suppress prolactin secretion, and thus for stimulation of D-2 receptors. This quantity of dopamine would be insufficient to stimulate D-1 receptors (Kebabian and Calne 1979).

On the basis of the foregoing discussion, it is evident that the dopamine receptors modulating aldosterone secretion cannot be characterized exclusively as D-1 or D-2. It is possible, therefore, that another type of dopamine receptor may inhibit aldosterone secretion. This hypothesis is consistent with the suggestion of Kebabian and Calne (1979) that new categories or subcategories of dopamine receptors may be identified on the basis of pharmacological evidence. Studies of the effects of treatment with a wide range of dopamine agonists and antagonists will be required to define more clearly the specific dopamine receptor mechanism involved in the control of aldosterone secretion.

Site of dopaminergic inhibition of aldosterone secretion.

If aldosterone secretion is modulated by a dopaminergic inhibitory mechanism, it is important to identify the site of this mechanism. At present, no conclusive information is available, but the two most likely possibilities are the adrenal cortex and the central nervous system.

Regarding an adrenal site for this mechanism, the concentration of dopamine in the zona glomerulosa is unknown. Histochemical studies of normal and transplanted sheep adrenal cortex show sparse postganglionic aminergic innervation entering the gland with the adrenal arteries (Innes and Nickerson 1975; Robinson et al. 1977). Whether or not these are dopaminergic neurons as described for a variety of other tissues such as the renal cortical juxtaglomerular vessels, the retina, glomus cells of the carotid body and sympathetic ganglia, is unknown (Ungerstedt 1978; Bell and Lang 1979; Dinerstein et al. 1979).

According to some investigators, dopamine may constitute only 1–2 % of the total adrenal catecholamine content, most of it being located in the medulla (Almgren et al. 1979). According to others, however, a sizeable portion of adrenal dopamine may be present in the adrenal cortex. After adrenal medullectomy in rats, total adrenal norepinephrine and epinephrine were reduced by over 98 %, but total adrenal dopamine was decreased by only 50 % (Kvetňanský et al. 1979). Renal clearance studies have established that dopamine is formed in the kidney (Christensen et al. 1976; Unger et al. 1978; Ball et al. 1978). The adrenal glands appear to receive blood supply from the subarcuate arteries of the kidney, which could contribute to adrenal cortical dopamine levels (Dempster 1978; Katholi et al. 1979).

Circulating plasma levels of free dopamine are low, in the range of 40–70 pg ml^{-1} (Peuler and Johnson 1976; Da Prada and Zurcher 1976; Ben-Jonathan and Porter 1976; Carey et al. 1981). Higher values for plasma free dopamine reported earlier (Callingham and Barrand 1976; Sole and Hussain 1977; Romoff et al. 1979) may have been artifactual and related to contaminant aromatic amino acid decarboxylase activity in the COMT preparations employed in the assay (Da Prada and Zurcher 1976; Kuchel et al. 1980). Similar to norepinephrine and epinephrine, dopamine is present in plasma in both conjugated and free forms (Peuler and Johnson 1976; Kuchel et al. 1979a; Kuchel et al. 1979b). However, in contrast to norepinephrine and epinephrine, the sources of plasma free dopamine have not been defined satisfactorily. In addition to the adrenal gland and sympathetic neurons, a number of other tissues may provide a source for circulating dopamine (Peuler and Johnson 1976). The kidney is one important potential source of plasma dopamine. Furthermore, some plasma dopamine could derive from plasma conversion of dihydroxyphenylalanine by dopa decarboxylase. It also is possible that a small fraction of dopamine enters the circulation from the brain. Finally, both conjugated dopamine and dopa are present in high quantities in plasma, and both are potential sources of free circulating dopamine (Louis and Sampson 1974; Johnson et al. 1978; Da Prada and Zurcher 1979). Conjugated dopamine and dopa have been implicated in peripheral nonneuronal dopaminergic processes (Van Loon et al. 1977; Johnson et al. 1978; Unger et al. 1979; Buu and Kuchel 1979; Baines and Chan 1980).

Plasma dopamine concentrations may be influenced by a variety of physiologic and pathophysiologic situations (Peuler and Johnson 1976). For example, stress, exercise, hypovolemic shock and increased intracranial pressure have been demonstrated to increase plasma dopamine concentrations. Plasma concentrations of dopamine and its metabolites change following administration of certain drugs, including dopamine agonists and antagonists (Cuche et al. 1972). However, the factors which influence plasma dopamine concentration are not understood clearly at the present time.

From the above discussion, it is apparent that much remains to be learned about the sources and regulation of circulating dopamine. Whether or not the adrenal cortex is exposed to a sufficient quantity of dopamine and whether or not physiologic changes in circulating dopamine would be sufficient to alter aldosterone secretion remains to be determined by future studies. However, since peripherally administered dopamine blocks metoclopramide-induced aldosterone secretion and since dopamine crosses the blood-brain barrier poorly, the current data favor a peripheral site of action for dopamine in the control of aldosterone secretion.

Physiologic relevance of dopamine in the control of aldosterone secretion.

We recently have demonstrated a consistent decrease in urinary dopamine excretion and a variable decrease in plasma dopamine concentration during the course of dietary sodium depletion in normal human subjects (Fig. 8.16) (Ben-Jonathan and Porter 1976). In contrast, other authors have reported that plasma dopamine concentrations increase with dietary sodium deprivation (Romoff et al. 1979). However, a number of methodological difficulties, including relatively short time of venous cannulation and supine rest prior to collection of blood specimens, render interpretation of this study difficult. Cuche et al. (1972) reported that normal subjects on sodium restricted diets experienced a decrease in urinary dopamine and sodium excretion with assumption of erect posture. Alexander and colleagues (1974) found that normal subjects in balance at 209 meq per day sodium intake have significantly higher urinary dopamine excretion than when the subjects were studied in balance at 9 meq per day sodium intake. Faucheux et al. (1977) and Ball et al. (1978) have reported that saline administration increases urinary dopamine excretion in the dog and the rat, respectively. Faucheux et al. (1970) also showed that albumin-induced volume expansion produces no alteration in urinary dopamine excretion, so that the increase in urinary dopamine cannot be attributed to the effect of simple volume expansion. Taken together, the data from the majority of these studies are consistent with a reciprocal decrease in urinary dopamine excretion and perhaps also plasma dopamine concentration during the course of dietary sodium depletion. It is possible, therefore, that the aldosterone response to sodium deprivation may be modulated by decreased dopaminergic activity. This proposed decrease in dopaminergic activity could occur by means of decreased activity of peripheral dopaminergic neurons or of nonneuronal dopamine-secreting cells, for example, in the kidney or adrenal gland.

If dopamine mechanisms are important modulators of the response of aldosterone to sodium depletion, one would expect that as dopaminergic activity decreased the aldosterone response to dopamine antagonists also might decrease. Such a study recently has been conducted by Coghlan et al. (1980), who studied the effects of metoclopramide in sodium replete and sodium deplete sheep. Although the absolute increase in plasma aldosterone concentration was greater in the sodium deplete sheep, the percent increase was less in the sodium deplete animals. Further studies of the effects of dopamine agonists and antagonists in experimental animals and man in response to variations in sodium status will be required to demonstrate whether changes in dopaminergic activity modulate aldosterone secretory patterns.

Serotoninergic mechanisms in the control of aldosterone secretion

The effects of serotonin on aldosterone secretion have not been studied extensively. Haning et al. (1970) originally reported that serotonin stimulates aldosterone production in dispersed rat adrenal cells in vitro. Albano et al. (1974) have confirmed this finding.

286

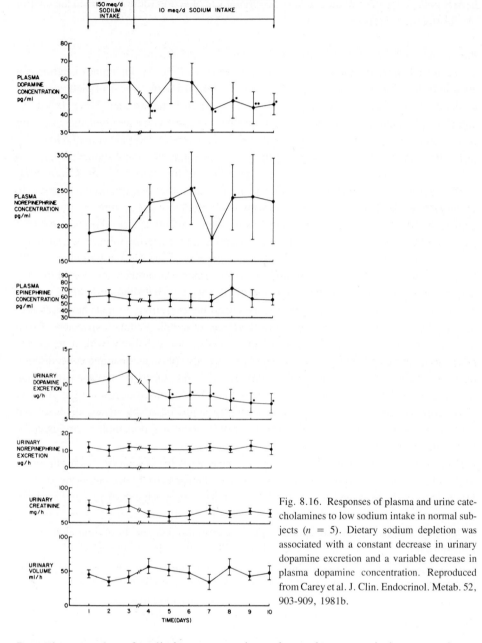

Fig. 8.16. Responses of plasma and urine catecholamines to low sodium intake in normal subjects ($n = 5$). Dietary sodium depletion was associated with a constant decrease in urinary dopamine excretion and a variable decrease in plasma dopamine concentration. Reproduced from Carey et al. J. Clin. Endocrinol. Metab. 52, 903-909, 1981b.

Recently, a number of preliminary reports have shown that serotonin increases plasma aldosterone concentration and serotonin antagonists decrease plasma aldosterone concentration in vivo in man and experimental animals (Al-Dujaili et al. 1980; Espiner et al. 1980; Gross et al. 1980; Mantero et al. 1980). Serotonin antagonists also have been demonstrated to decrease plasma aldosterone concentration in primary aldosteronism.

SUMMARY AND CONCLUSIONS

As discussed in some detail above, neuroendocrine mechanisms contribute substantially to the regulation of the renin–angiotensin–aldosterone system. In the control of renin secretion, the role of neurohormonal factors is well established, while in the mitigation of aldosterone secretion, neuroendocrine influences are relatively less well-defined. It is apparent that the coordination of the various neuroendocrine mechanisms relating to the components of the renin–angiotensin–aldosterone system is poorly understood. Further, the physiologic and pathophysiologic relevance of many of these mechanisms with regard to overall fluid, electrolyte and blood pressure homeostasis in the intact animal in many instances is not established.

During the past twenty years, a large body of information concerning the control of the renin–angiotensin–aldosterone system by neuroendocrine mechanisms has emerged. We now know that the central neural stimuli increase renin secretion via renal nerve excitation, and that renal nerve activity is tempered by the cardiopulmonary and baroreceptor reflex arcs in the periphery. Renal nerve stimulation increases renin secretion directly at beta-adrenergic receptors located on renal juxtaglomerular cells, but the exact type of beta receptor and the mediation of the beta-adrenergic response at the cellular level require further clarification. Alpha-adrenergic receptors appear to play a dual role in the regulation of renin secretion. Stimulation of alpha receptors on juxtaglomerular cells inhibits renin release, while stimulation of vascular alpha receptors appears to stimulate renin release, possibly by a prostaglandin-dependent mechanism. The parasympathetic nervous system and dopaminergic and serotoninergic mechanisms do not seem to be involved in the control of renin secretion, although information is scanty and further investigation may be required.

Recent evidence, taken largely from in vivo studies, suggests that dopaminergic mechanisms may play an inhibitory role in the modulation of aldosterone secretion. However, the site of these dopaminergic mechanisms and their physiologic relevance in the regulation of aldosterone secretion is presently obscure. There also is some preliminary evidence that serotonin may influence aldosterone secretion. These potentially important neuroendocrine mechanisms controlling aldosterone secretion should furnish a fruitful area for future investigation.

REFERENCES

Abe, Y., Okahara, T., Kishimoto, T., Yamamoto, K. and Ueda, J. (1973) Relationship between intrarenal distribution of blood flow and renin secretion. Am. J. Physiol. 225, 319-323.

Adler-Graschinskyy, E. and Langer, S.Z. (1975) Possible role of a β-adrenoceptor in the regulation of noradrenaline release by nerve stimulation through a positive feedback mechanism. Br. J. Pharmacol. 53, 42-50.

Al-Dujaili, E.S.A., Boscaro, M., Espiner, E.A. and Edwards, C.R.W. (1980) In vitro and in vivo effects of indolamines on aldosterone biosynthesis in the rat. Program and Abstracts, Sixth International Congress of Endocrinology, p. 409.

Albano, J.D.M., Brown, B.L., Ekins, R.P., Tait, S.A.S. and Tait, J.F. (1974) The effects of potassium, 5-hydroxytryptamine, adrenocorticotropin and angiotensin II on the concentration of adenosine 3'5'-cyclic monophosphate in suspensions of dispersed rat adrenal zona glomerulosa and zona faciculata cells. Biochem. J. 142, 391-400.

Alexander, R.W., Gill Jr, J.R., Yanake, H., Lovenberg, W. and Kaiser, H.R. (1974) Effects of dietary sodium and of acute saline infusion on the interrelationship between dopamine excretion and adrenergic activity in man. J. Clin. Invest. 54, 194-200.

Allison, D.J., Tanigawa, H. and Assaykeen, T.A. (1972) The effects of cyclic nucleotides on plasma renin activity and renal function in dogs. In: Control of Renin Secretion (Assaykeen, T.A. ed), pp. 33-47, Plenum Press, New York.

Almgren, O., Carlsson, A. and Snider, S. (1979) Tissue dopamine levels as an indicator of tyrosine hydroxylase activity. Adv. Biosci. 20, 29-40.

Annat, G., Gandjean, B., Vincent, M., Jarsaillon, E. and Sassard, J. (1976) Effects of right atrial stretch on plasma renin activity. Arch. Int. Physiol. Biochem. 84, 311-315.

Aona, T., Shioji, T., Kinugasa, T., Onishi, T. and Kurachi, K. (1978) Clinical and endocrinological analyses of patients with galactorrhea and menstrual disorders due to sulpiride or metoclopramide. J. Clin. Endocrinol. Metab. 47, 675-680.

Assaykeen, T.A., Clayton, P.L., Goldfien, A. and Ganong, W.F. (1970) Effect of alpha- and beta-adrenergic blocking agents on the renin response to hypoglycemia and epinephrine in dogs. Endocrinology 87, 1318-1322.

Assaykeen, T.A. and Ganong, W.F. (1971) The sympathetic nervous system and renin secretion. In: Frontiers in Neuroendocrinology (Martini, L. and Ganong, W.F. eds), pp. 67-102, Oxford University Press, New York.

Assaykeen, T.A., Tanigawa, H. and Allison, D.J. (1974) Effect of adrenoceptor blocking agents on the renin response to isoproterenol in dogs. Eur. J. Pharmacol. 26, 285-297.

Atlas, S.A., Sealey, J.E. and Laragh, J.H. (1978) 'Acid' and 'cryo' activated inactive plasma renin. Circ. Res. 43 (Suppl. I): I-128–I-133.

Atuk, N.O., Ayers, C.R. and Westfall, T. (1968) Effect of dopamine on blood pressure and urinary excretion of catecholamines in man. Clin. Res. 16, 90.

Ayers, C.R., Harris, Jr, R.H., and Lefer, L.G. (1969) Control of renin release in experimental hypertension. Circ. Res. 24/25 (Suppl. I), 103-113.

Ayers, C.R., Katholi, R.E., Carey, R.M., Yancey, M.R. and Morton, C.L., (1978) Acute and chronic intrarenal alpha and beta adrenergic receptor stimulation. Circulation 55/56 (Suppl. III)-213 (abstract).

Ayers, C.R., Katholi, R.E., Carey, R.M., Yancey, M.R. and Morton, C.L. (1981) Acute and chronic intrarenal alpha- and beta-adrenergic stimulation of renin release in the conscious dog. Hypertension 3, 615-622.

Baines, A.D. and Chan, W. (1980) Source of urine dopamine in natriuretic rats. Life Sci. 26, 253-259.

Ball. S.G., Oats, N.S. and Lee, M.R. (1978) Urinary dopamine in man and rat: effects of inorganic salts on dopamine excretion. Clin. Sci. Mol. Med. 55, 167-173.

Barajas, L. (1964) The innervation of the juxtaglomerular apparatus: an electron microscopic study of the innervation of the glomerular arterioles. Lab. Invest. 13, 916-929.

Barajas, L. (1972) Anatomical considerations in the control of renin secretion. In: Control of Renin Secretion (Assaykeen, T.A. ed.), pp. 1-16, Plenum Press, New York.

Barajas, L. and Müller, J. (1973) The innervation of the juxtaglomerular apparatus and surrounding tubules: a quantitative analysis by serial section electron microscopy. J. Ultrastruct. Res. 43, 107-132.

Barajas, L., Bennett, C.M., Connor, G. and Lindstrom, R.R. (1977) Structure of a juxtaglomerular cell tumor. The presence of neural components. A light and electron microscopic study. Lab. Invest. 37, 357-368.

Barnardo, D.E., Summerskill, W.H.J., Strong, C.G. and Baldus, W.P. (1970) Renal function, renin activity and endogenous vasoactive substances in cirrhosis. Digest. Dis. 15, 419-425.

Bauman, G. and Loriaux, D.L. (1976) Failure of endogenous prolactin to alter renal salt and water excretion and adrenal function in man. J. Clin. Endocrinol. Metab. 43, 643-649.

Baumbach, L. and Leyssac, P.P. (1977) Studies on the mechanism of renin release from isolated superfused rat glomeruli: effects of calcium, calcium ionophores and lanthanum. J. Physiol. (Lond.) 273, 745-764.

Bell, C. and Lang, W.J. (1979) Histochemical and biochemical estimations of dopamine in postganglionic autonomic nerves. Adv. Biosci. 20, 45-49.

Ben-Jonathan, N. and Porter, J.C. (1976) A sensitive radioenzymatic assay for dopamine, norepinephrine and epinephrine in plasma and tissue. Endocrinology 98, 1497-1507.

Berl, T., Henrich, W.L., Erickson, A.L. and Schrier, R.W. (1979) Prostaglandins in the beta adrenergic and baroreceptor mediated secretion of renin. Am. J. Physiol. 236, F472-F477.

Besser, G.M., Parke, L., Edwards, C.R.W., Forsyth, I.A. and McNeilly, A.S. (1972) Galactorrhea: successful treatment with reduction of plasma prolactin levels by brom-ergocryptine. Br. Med. J. 3, 669-672.

Bevilacqua, M., Norbiato, G., Raggi, U., Micossi, P., Baggio, E. and Prandelli, M. (1980) Dopaminergic control of serum potassium in man. Metabolism 29, 306-310.

Biava, C.G. and West, M. (1966) Fine structure of normal human juxtaglomerular cells. Am. J. Pathol. 49, 679-721.

Birkhauser, M., Riondel, A. and Vallotton, M.B. (1979) Bromocriptine-induced modulation of the plasma aldosterone response to acute stimulation. Acta Endocrinol. (Copenhagen) 91, 294-302.

Blaine, E.H., Davis, J.O. and Witty, R.T. (1970) Renin release after hemorrhage and after suprarenal aortic constriction in dogs without sodium delivery to the macula densa. Circ. Res. 27, 1081-1089.

Blaine, E.H., Davis, J.O. and Prewitt, R.L. (1971) Evidence for a renal vascular receptor in control of renin secretion. Am. J. Physiol. 220, 1593-1597.

Blair, C.S. and Feigl, E.O. (1968) Renin release from brain stimulation. Fed. Proc. 27, 629.

Blair, M.L., Feigl, E.O. and Smith, O.A. (1976) Elevation of plasma renin activity during avoidance performance in baboons. Am. J. Physiol. 231, 772-776.

Bolger, P.M., Eisner, G.M., Ramwell, P.W. and Slotkott, L.M. (1976) Effect of prostaglandin synthesis on renal function and renin in the dog. Nature 259, 244-245.

Boyd, G.W. (1974) A protein-bound form of porcine renal renin. Circ. Res. 35, 426-438.

Boyd, G.W. (1977) An inactive higher-molecular-weight renin in normal subjects and hypertensive patients. Lancet 1, 215-218.

Bratfos, O. and Huang, J.O. (1979) Comparison of sulpiride and chlorpromazine in psychoses. Acta Psychiatr. Scand. 60, 1-9.

Brennan, L.A., Henninger, A.L., Jochim, K.E. and Malvin, R.L. (1974) Relationship between carotid sinus pressure and plasma renin level. Am. J. Physiol. 227, 295-299.

Brosnihan, K.B. and Bravo, E.L. (1978) Graded reductions of atrial pressure and renin release. Am. J. Physiol. 235, H175-H181.

Brosnihan, K.B. and Travis, R.H. (1976) Influence of the vagus and carotid sinus nerves on plasma renin in the cat. J. Endocrinol. 71, 59-65.

Brotzu, G. (1970) Inhibition by chlorpromazine of the effects of dopamine on the dog kidney. J. Pharm. Pharmacol. 22, 662-667.

Brown, J.J., Davies, D.L., Lever, A.F., Robertson, J.I.S. and Verniory, A. (1966) The effect of acute hemorrhage in the conscious dog and man on plasma renin concentration. J. Physiol. London 182, 649-663.

Brown, R.D., Wisgerhof, M., Carpenter, P.C., Brown, G., Jiang, N.S., Kao, P. and Hagstad, R. (1979) Adrenal sensitivity to angiotensin II and undiscovered aldosterone stimulating factors in hypertension. J. Steroid Biochem. 11, 1043-1050.

Bull, M.B., Hillman, R.S., Cannon, P.J. and Laragh, J.H., (1970) Renin and aldosterone secretion in man as influenced by changes in electrolyte balance and blood volume. Circ. Res. 27, 953-960.

Bunag, R.O., Page, I.H. and McCubbin, J.W. (1966) Neural stimulation of release of renin. Circ. Res. 19, 851-858.

Buu, N.T. and Kuchel, O. (1979) Dopamine 3-0-sulfate, a direct precursor of free norepinephrine: an alternative biosynthetic pathway? Adv. Biosci. 20, 95-100.

Byrnes, D., Henderson, L., Meredith, C. and Borody, T. (1980) Release of motilin by metoclopramide. Aust. N.Z. J. Med. 10, 109.

Callingham, B.A. and Barrand, M.A. (1976) Catecholamines in blood. J. Pharmacol. 28, 356-360.

Campbell, W.B. and Jackson, E.K. (1979) Modulation of adrenergic transmission by angiotensins in the perfused rat mesentery. Am. J. Physiol. 236, H211-H217.

Campbell, W.B. and Schmitz, J.M. (1978) Effect of alterations in dietary potassium on the pressor and steroidogenic effects of angiotensins II and III. Endocrinology 103, 2098-2104.

Campbell, W.B., Graham, R.M. and Jackson, E.K. (1979) Role of renal prostaglandins in sympathetically mediated renin release in the rat. J. Clin. Invest. 64, 448-456.

Capponi, A.M. and Valloton, M.B. (1976) Renin release by rat kidney slices incubated in vitro: role of sodium, alpha- and beta-adrenergic receptors, and effect of vincristine. Circ. Res. 39, 200-203.

Carey, R.M. (1981) Acute dopaminergic inhibition of aldosterone secretion in man is independent of angiotensin II and ACTH. J. Clin. Endocrinol. Metab. (in press).

Carey, R.M., Johanson, A.J. and Sief, S.M. (1977) The effects of ovine prolactin on water and electrolyte excretion in man are attributable to vasopressin contamination. J. Clin. Endocrinol. Metab. 44, 85-88.

Carey, R.M., Peach, M.J., Vaughan Jr, E.D. and Ayers, C.R. (1978) Responses to angiotensin II and [des-aspartyl']-angiotensin II in man: are there different receptors? Circ. Res. 43 (Suppl. I), 1-63 – 1-69.

Carey, R.M., Vaughan, Jr. E.D., Peach, M.J. and Ayers, C.R., (1978) Activity of [des-aspartyl']-angiotensin II and angiotensin II in man. J. Clin. Invest. 61, 20-31.

Carey, R.M., Thorner, M.O. and Ortt, E.M. (1979) Effects of metoclopramide and bromocriptine on the renin-angiotensin-aldosterone system in man: dopaminergic control of aldosterone. J. Clin. Invest. 63, 727-735.

Carey, R.M., Thorner, M.O. and Ortt, E.M. (1980) Dopaminergic inhibition of metoclopramide-induced aldosterone secretion in man: dissociation of responses to dopamine and bromocriptine. J. Clin. Invest. 66, 10-18.

Carey, R.M., Thorner, M.O. and Van Loon, G.R. (1981a) Bromocriptine does not influence aldosterone responses to sodium deprivation. J. Clin. Endocrinol. Metab. (submitted).

Carey, R.M., Van Loon, G.R., Baines, A.D. and Ortt, E.M. (1981b) Decreased plasma and urinary dopamine during dietary sodium depletion in man. J. Clin. Endocrinol. Metab. 52, 903-909.

Carlson, H.E., Briggs, J.E. and McCallum, R.W. (1977) Stimulation of prolactin secretion by metoclopramide in the rat. Proc. Soc. Exp. Biol. Med. 154, 475-478.

Caron, M.G., Beaulieu, M., Raymond, V., Gagne, B., Drouin, J., Lefkowitz, R.J. and Labrie, F. (1978) Dopaminergic receptors in the anterior pituitary gland. Correlation of (H^3) dihydroergocryptine binding with the dopaminergic control of prolactin release. J. Biol. Chem. 253, 2244-2253.

Carroll, J.E., Campanile, C.P. and Goodfriend, T.L. (1980) Role of prolactin in aldosterone secretion. Clin. Res. 28, 772A.

Chokski, D.S., Yeh, B.K. and Samet, P. (1972) Effects of dopamine and isoproterenol on renin secretion in the dog. Proc. Soc. Exp. Biol. Med. 140, 54-57.

Christensen, N.J., Mathias, C.J. and Frankel, H.L. (1976) Plasma and urinary dopamine: studies of fasting and exercise in tetraplegic man. Eur. J. Clin. Invest. 6, 403-409.

Clamage, D.M., Sanford, C.S., Vander, A.J. and Mouw, D.R. (1976) Effects of psychosocial stimuli on plasma renin activity in rats. Am. J. Physiol. 231, 1290-1294.

Clamage, D.M., Vander, A.J. and Mouw, D.R. (1977) Psychosocial stimuli and human plasma renin activity. Psychosomatic Med. 39, 393-401.

Clarke, B.J., Scholtysik, G. and Flückiger, E. (1978) Cardiovascular actions of bromocriptine. Acta Endocrinol. (Copenhagen) (Suppl. 216) 188, 75-81.

Claybaugh, J.R. and Share, L. (1973) Vasopressin, renin and cardiovascular responses to continuous slow hemorrhage. Am. J. Physiol. 222, 519-523.

Coghlan, J.P., Blair-West, J.R., Denton, D.A., Fei, D.T., Fernley, R.T., Hardy, K.J., McDougall, J.G., Puy, R. Robinson, P.M., Scoggins, B.A. and Wright, R.D. (1979) Factors regulating aldosterone secretion. J. Endocrinol. 81, 55P-67P.

Coghlan, J.P., Blair-West, J.R., Butkus, A., Denton, D.A., Hardy, K.J., Leksell, L., McDougall, G.G., McKinley, M.J., Scoggins, B.A., Tarjan, E., Weisinger, R.S. and Wright, R.D., (1980) Factors regulating aldosterone secretion. In: Endocrinology 1980 (Cumming, I.A., Funder, J.W. and Mendelsohn, F.A.O. eds), pp. 385-388, Elsevier/North-Holland Biomedical Press, Amsterdam.

Cohen, E.L., Rovner, D.R. and Conn, J.W. (1966) Postural augmentation of plasma renin activity: importance in diagnosis of renovascular hypertension. J. Am. Med. Assoc. 197, 973-978.

Cook, W.F. (1967) The detection of renin in juxtaglomerular cells. J. Physiol. (Lond.) 194, 73-74.

Cooper, R.M., Gordon, E.M. and Osmond, D.H. (1977) Trypsin-induced activation of renin precursor in plasma of normal and anephric man. Circ. Res. 40 (Suppl. I) I-171-I-179.

Coote, J.H., Johns, E.J., MacLeod, V.H. and Singer, B. (1972) Effect of renal nerve stimulation, renal blood flow and adrenergic blockade on plasma renin activity in the cat. J. Physiol. (Lond.) 226, 15-36.

Corrodi, H., Fuxe, K., Hökfelt, T., Lidbrink, P. and Ungerstedt, U. (1973) Effect of ergot drugs on central catecholamine neurons. Evidence for stimulation of central dopamine neurons. J. Pharm. Pharmacol. 25, 409-411.

Costa, E. and Gessa, G.L. (eds) (1977) Nonstriatal Dopaminergic Neurons. Raven Press, New York.

Creese, I., Burt, D.R. and Synder, S.H., (1976) Dopamine receptor binding predicts clinical and pharmacological properties of antipsychotic drugs. Science 192, 481-483.

Cuche, J.L., Kuchel, O., Barbeau, A., Boucher, R. and Genest, J. (1972) Relationship between the adrenergic nervous system and renin during adaptation to upright posture; a possible role for 3,4-dihydroxyphenylethyla-mine (dopamine). Clin. Sci. 43, 481-489.

Cunningham, S.G., Feigl, E.O. and Scher, A.M. (1978) Carotid sinus reflex influence on plasma renin activity. Am. J. Physiol. 234, H670-H678.

Da Prada, M. and Zurcher, G. (1976) Simultaneous radioenzymatic determination of plasma and tissue adrena-line, noradrenaline and dopamine within the femtomole range. Life Sci. 19, 1161-1174.

Da Prada, M. and Zurcher, G. (1979) Radioenzymatic assay of plasma and urinary catecholamines in man and various animal species: physiological and pharmacological applications. In: Radioimmunoassay of Drugs and Hormones in Cardiovascular Medicine (Albertini, A., Da Prada, M. and Peskar, B.A. eds), pp. 175-198, Elsevier/North-Holland Biomedical Press, Amsterdam.

Data, J.L., Gerber, J.C., Crump, W.J., Frolich, J.C., Hollifield, J.W. and Nies, A.S. (1978) The prostaglandin system: a role in canine baroreceptor control of renin release. Circ. Res. 42, 454-458.

Davies, R., Slater, J.D.H., Rudolf, M. and Geddes, D.M. (1977) The effect of isoprenaline on plasma renin activity in man. Clin. Endocrinol. 6, 393-399.

Davis, J.O. (1975) Regulation of aldosterone secretion. In: Handbook of Physiology: Adrenal Physiology (Blascko, H., Sayers, G. and Smith, A.D. eds), pp. 77-106, American Physiological Society, Washington, D.C.

Davis, J.O. and Freeman, R.H. (1976) Mechanisms regulating renin release Physiol. Rev. 56, 1-56.

Day, M.D. and Blower, P.R. (1975) Cardiovascular dopamine receptor stimulation antagonized by metoclopra-mide. J. Pharm. Pharmacol. 27, 276-278.

Day, R.P., Luetscher, J.A. and Zager, P.G. (1976) Big renin identification, chemical properties and clinical implications. Am. J. Cardiol. 37, 667-674.

del Pozo, E., Darragh, A., Lancranjan, I., Ebling, D., Burmeister, P., Buhler, F., Marbach, P. and Braun, P. (1977) Effect of bromocriptine on the endocrine system and fetal development. Clin. Endocrinol. (Suppl.) 6, 47s-55s.

Delitala, G., Masala, A., Alagna, S. and Devilla, L. (1975) Metoclopramide and prolactin secretion in man: effects of pretreatment with L-DOPA and 2-brom-alpha-ergocriptine (CB-154). IRCS, Med. Sci. Libr. Compend. 3, 274.

Dempster, W.J. (1978) Renal-adrenal interrelationships. Jpn Heart J. 19, 426-433.

Deryx, F.H.M., Wenting, A.J., Man Int'T Veld, A.J., Van Gool, J.M.G., Verhoeven, R.P. and Schalekamp, M.A.D.H. (1976) Inactive renin in human plasma. Lancet 2, 496-498.

Desaulles, E., Forler, C., Velly, J. and Schwartz, J. (1975) Effect of catecholamines on renin release in vitro. Biomedicine 23, 433-439.

Devito, E., Gordon, S.B., Cabrera, R.R. and Fasciolo, J.C. (1970) Renin release by rat kidney slices. Am. J. Physiol. 219, 1036-1041.

Devynek, M.A. and Meyer, P. (1978) Commentary: angiotensin receptors. Biochem. Pharmacol. 27, 1-5.

Di Chiara, G., Vargiu, L., Porceddu, M.L. and Gessa, G.L. (1977) Bromocriptine: a rather specific stimulant of dopamine receptors regulating dopamine metabolism. Adv. Biochem. Psychopharmacol. 16, 443-446.

Dinerstein, R.J., Vannice, J., Hendersen, R.C., Roth, L.J., Goldberg, L.I. and Hoffman, P.C. (1979) His-tofluorescence techniques provide evidence for dopamine-containing neuronal elements in canine kidney. Science 205, 497-499.

Dluhy, R.G., Greenfield, M. and Williams, G.H. (1977) Effect of simultaneous potassium and saline loading on plasma aldosterone levels. J. Clin. Endocrinol. Metab. 45, 141-146.

Dolphin, A., Jenner, P., Marsden, C.D., Pycock, C. and Tarsy, D. (1975) Pharmacological evidence for cerebral

292

dopamine receptor blockade by metoclopramide in rodents. Psychopharmacologia 41, 133-138.

Donker, A.J., Arisz, L., Brentjens, J.R., Van Der Hem, G.K. and Hollemans, H.J. (1976) The effect of indomethacin on kidney function and plasma renin activity in man. Nephron 17, 288-296.

Douglas, J.G. (1980) Effects of high potassium diet on angiotensin II receptors and angiotensin-induced aldosterone production in rat adrenal glomerulosa cells. Endocrinology 106, 983-990.

Dzau, V.J., Siwek, L.G. and Barger, A.C. (1978) Intrarenal dopaminergic receptors in control of renin release in the conscious dog. Fed. Proc. 37, 901.

Edelman, R. and Hartroft, P.M. (1961) Localization of renin in juxtaglomerular cells of rabbit and dog through the use of the fluorescent antibody technique. Circ. Res. 9, 1069-1077.

Edwards, C.R.W., Thorner, M.O., Miall, P.A., Al-Dujaili, E.A.S., Hanker, J.P. and Besser, G.M. (1975) Inhibition of the plasma aldosterone response to frusemide by bromocriptine. Lancet 2, 903-905.

Eggena, P., Hiroshi, H., Barrett, J.D. and Sambhi, M.P. (1978) Multiple forms of human plasma renin substrate. J. Clin. Invest. 62, 367-372.

Eisman, M.M. and Rowell, L.B. (1977) Renal vascular response to heat stress in baboons-role of adrenocorticoid. J. Appl. Physiol. 43, 739-746.

Elliot, P.N.C., Jenner, P., Huizing, G., Marsden, C.D. and Miller, R. (1977) Substituted benzamides as cerebral dopamine antagonists in rodents. Neuropharmacology 16, 333-342.

Epstein, S. and Hamilton, S. (1977) Cyproheptadine inhibition of stimulated plasma renin activity. J. Clin. Endocrinol. Metab. 45, 1235-1237.

Erdos, E.G. (1975) Angiotensin I converting enzymes. Circ. Res. 36, 247-255.

Esler, M.D. and Nestel, P.J. (1973) Renin and sympathetic nervous system responsiveness to adrenergic stimuli in isolated hypertension. Am. J. Cardiol. 32, 643-649.

Esler, M., Julius, S., Zweifler, A., Randall, O., Harburg, R., Gardiner, H. and DeQuattro, V. (1977) Mild high-renin essential hypertension. New Engl. J. Med. 296, 405-411.

Espiner, E.A., Al-Dujaili, E.A.S., Martin, V.I. and Edwards, C.R.W. (1980) Indoleamines stimulate steroidogenesis in isolated human adrenal cells. Program and Abstracts, Sixth International Congress of Endocrinology, p. 507.

Fakunding, J.L., Chow, R. and Catt., K.J. (1979) The role of calcium in the stimulation of aldosterone production by adrenocorticotropin, angiotensin II and potassium in isolated glomerulosa cells. Endocrinology 105, 327-333.

Fakunding, J.L. and Catt, K.J. (1980) Dependence of aldosterone stimulation in adrenal glomerulosa cells on calcium uptake: effects of lanthanum and verapamil. Endocrinology 107, 1345-1353.

Faucheux, B., Buu, N.T. and Kuchel, O. (1977) Effects of saline and albumin on plasma and urinary catecholamines in dogs. Am. J. Physiol. 232, F123-F127.

Fishman, M.C. (1976) Membrane potential of juxtaglomerular cells. Nature (Lond.) 260, 542-544.

Flückiger, E., Markò, M., Doepfner, W. and Niederer, W. (1976) Effects of ergot alkaloids on the hypothalamo-pituitary axis. Postgrad. Med. J. 52 (Suppl. I), 57-61.

Flückiger, E. and Wagner, H.R. (1968) 2-Br-alpha-ergocriptine. Beeinflussung von Fertilität und Lactation bei der Ratte. Experimentia 24, 1130.

Fozard, J.R. and Mobarok Aki, A.T.M. (1978) Blockade of neuronal tryptamine receptors by metoclopramide. Eur. J. Pharmacol. 49, 109-112.

Fraser, R., Brown, J.J., Lever, A.F., Mason, P.A. and Robertson, J.I.S. (1979) Control of aldosterone secretion. Clin. Sci. Mol. Med. 56, 389-399.

Fray, J.C.S. (1977) Stimulation of renin release in perfused kidney by low calcium and high magnesium. Am. J. Physiol. 232, F377-F382.

Fray, J.C.S. (1978) Stretch receptor control of renin release in perfused rat kidney: effect of high perfusate potassium. J. Physiol. (Lond.) 282, 207-217.

Fray, J.C.S. (1980) Stimulus-secretion coupling: role of hemodynamic and other factors. Circ. Res. 47, 485-492.

Fray, J.C.S. and Park, C.S. (1979) Influence of potassium, sodium, perfusion pressure and isoprenaline on renin release induced by calcium deprivation. J. Physiol. (Lond.) 292, 363-372.

Freeman, R.H., Davis, J.O. Lohmeier, T.E. and Spielman, W.S. (1976) Evidence that des-asp'-angiotensin-II mediates the renin-angiotensin response. Circ. Res. 38 (Suppl. 2), 99-103.

Frolich, J.C., Hollifield, J.W., Dormois, J.C., Frolich, B.L., Seyberth, H., Michelakis, A.M. and Oates, J.A. (1976) Suppression of plasma renin activity by indomethacin in man. Circ. Res. 39, 447-452.

Frolich, J.C., Hollifield, J.W., Michelakis, A.M., Vesper, B.S., Wilson, J.P., Shand, D.G., Seyberth, H.J., Frolich, W.H. and Oates, J.A. (1979) Reduction of plasma renin activity by inhibition of the fatty acid cyclooxygenase in human subjects: independence of sodium retention. Circ. Res. 44, 781-787.

Fujita, K., Aguilera, G. and Catt, K.J. (1979) The role of cyclic AMP in aldosterone production by isolated zona glomerulosa cells. J. Biol. Chem. 254, 8567-8574.

Fuxe, K., Corrodi, H., Hökfelt, T., Lidbrink, P. and Ungerstedt, U. (1974) Ergocornine and 2-Br-alpha-ergocriptine. Evidence for prolonged dopamine receptor stimulation. Med. Biol. (Helsinki) 52, 121-132.

Ganten, D., Schelling, P., Hoffman, W.I., Phillips, M.I. and Ganten, U. (1978) The measurement of external isorenins. In: Radioimmunoassay: Renin-Angiotensin (Krause, D.K., Kumerich, W. and Poulsen, K. eds), pp. 144-150, George Thieme Publishers, Stuttgart.

Gerber, J.G., Keller, R.T. and Nies, A.S. (1979) Prostaglandins and renin release: the effect of PGI_2, PGE_2, and 13,14-dihydro PGE_2 on the baroreceptor mechanism of renin release in the dog. Circ. Res. 44, 796-799.

Gibson, A. and Samini, M. (1978) Bromocriptine is a potent alpha-adrenoceptor antagonist in the perfused mesenteric blood vessels of the rat. J. Pharm. Pharmacol. 30, 314-315.

Glasson, P., Gaillard, R., Riondel, A., Valloton, M.B. (1979) Role of renal prostaglandins and relationship to renin, aldosterone, and antidiuretic hormone during salt depletion in man. J. Clin. Endocrinol. Metab. 49, 176-181.

Goetz, K.L., Bond, G.C. and Smith, W.E. (1974) Effect of moderate hemorrhage in humans on plasma ADH and renin. Proc. Soc. Exp. Biol. Med. 145, 277-280.

Goldberg, L.I. (1972a) Cardiovascular and renal actions of dopamine: potential clinical applications. Pharmacol. Rev. 24, 481-495.

Goldberg, L.I. (1972b) Cardiovascular and renal actions of dopamine: potential clinical applications. Pharmacol. Rev. 24, 1-19.

Goldberg, L.I. (1975) The dopamine vascular receptor. Biochem. Pharmacol. 24, 651-643.

Goldberg, L.I. (1978) Characteristics of the vascular dopamine receptor: comparison with other receptors. Fed. Proc. 37, 2396-2402.

Goldberg, L.I., Kohli, J.D., Listinsky, J.J. and McDermed, J.D. (1979) Structure-activity relationships of the pre- and post-synaptic dopamine receptors mediating vasodilation. In: Catecholamines: Basic and Clinical Frontiers (Usdin, E., Kopin, I.J. and Barchas, J. eds), pp. 447-449, Pergamon Press. New York.

Goldberg, L.I., Musgrave, G.E. and Kohli, J.D. (1979) Antagonism of dopamine-induced renal vasodilatation in the dog by bulbocapnine and sulpiride. In: Sulpiride and Other Benzamides. (Spano, P.F., Trabucchi, M., Corsini, G.U. and Gessa, G.L. eds), pp. 73-81, Raven Press, New York.

Goldberg, L.I. and Weder, A.B. (1981) Connections between endogenous dopamine, dopamine receptors and sodium excretion: evidences and hypotheses. Rec. Adv. Clin. Pharmacol. (in press).

Goldberg, L.I., Volkman, P.H. and Kohli, J.D. (1978) A comparison of the vascular dopamine receptor with other dopamine receptors. Ann. Rev. Pharmacol. Toxicol. 18, 57-79.

Goldstein, M., Lieberman, A., Battista, A.F., Lew, J.Y. and Matsumoto, Y. Experimental and clinical studies on bromocriptine in the Parkinsonian syndrome. Acta Endocrinol. (Copenhagen) (Suppl. 216) 88, 57-66.

Goodfriend, T.L. (1979) Receptors for angiotensin. In: Hypertension (Genest, J., Koiw, E. and Kuchel, O. eds), pp. 173-179, McGraw-Hill, New York.

Goodfriend, T.L. and Peach, M.J. (1979) Specific functions of angiotensins I, II and III. In: Hypertension (Genst, J., Koiw, E. and Kuchel, O. eds), pp. 168-173, McGraw-Hill, New York.

Gordon, R.D., Kuchel, O., Liddle, G.W. and Island, D.P. (1967) Role of the sympathetic nervous system in regulating renin and aldosterone production in man. J. Clin. Invest. 46, 599-605.

Gross, M.D., Gniadek, T.C. and Grekin, R.J. (1980) Inhibition of aldosterone secretion by cyproheptadine in primary aldosteronism due to bilateral hyperplasia. Clin. Res. 28, 260A (abstract).

Gutman, F.D., Tagawa, H., Haber, E. and Barger, A.C. (1973) Renal arterial pressure, renin secretion and blood pressure control in trained dogs. Am. J. Physiol. 224, 66-72.

Hagstad, R. (1979) Adrenal sensitivity to angiotensin II and undiscovered aldosterone stimulating factors in hypertension. J. Steroid Biochem. 11, 1043-1050.

294

Haning, R., Tait, S.A.S. and Tait, J.F. (1970) In vitro effects of ACTH, angiotensins, serotonin and potassium on steroid output and conversion of corticosterone to aldosterone by isolated adrenal cells. Endocrinology 87, 1146-1167.

Harada, E. and Rubin, R.P. (1978) Stimulation of renin secretion and calcium efflux from the isolated perfused rat kidney by noradrenaline after prolonged calcium deprivation. J. Physiol. (Lond) 274, 367-379.

Harris, P.J. and Young, J.A. (1977) Dose-dependent stimulation and inhibition of proximal tubular sodium reabsorption by angiotensin II in the rat kidney. Pfleugers Arch. 367, 295-297.

Hartroft, P.M. (1966) Electron microscopy of nerve endings associated with juxtaglomerular cells and the macula densa. Lab. Invest. 15, 1127-1128.

Hay, A.M. (1975) The mechanism of action of metoclopramide. Gut 16, 403.

Heacox, R., Harvey, A.M. and Vander, A.J. (1967) Hepatic inactivation of renin. Circ. Res. 21, 49-52.

Healy, D.L. and Burger, H.G. (1978) Sustained elevation of serum prolactin by metoclopramide: a clinical model of idiopathic hyperprolactinemia. J. Clin Endocrinol. Metab. 46, 709-714.

Henrich, W.L., Schrier, R.W. and Berl, T. (1979) Mechanisms of renin secretion during hemorrhage in the dog. J. Clin. Invest. 64, 1-7.

Henry, D.P., Aoi, W. and Weinberger, M.H. (1977) The effects of dopamine on renin release in vitro. Endocrinology 101, 279-283.

Hertting, G., Reimann, W., Zumstein, A., Jackisch, R. and Starke, K. (1979) Dopaminergic feedback regulation of dopamine release in slices of caudate nucleus of the rabbit. Adv. Biosci. 18, 145-150.

Hesse, B., Nielsen, I., Ring-Larsen, H. and Hansen, J.F. (1978) The influence of acute blood volume changes on plasma renin activity in man. Scand. J. Lab. Clin. Invest. 38, 155-161.

Hesse, B., Nielson, K. and Hansen, J.F. (1975) The effect of reduction in blood volume on plasma renin activity in man. Clin. Sci. Mol. Med. 49, 515-517.

Himathongham, T., Dluhy, R.J. and Williams, G.H. (1975) Potassium–aldosterone–renin interrelationships. J. Clin. Endocrinol. Metab. 41, 153-159.

Himori, N., Izumi, N. and Tsutomu, I. (1980) Analysis of Beta-adrenoceptors mediating renin release produced by isoproterenol in conscious dogs. Am. J. Physiol. 238, F387-F392.

Hornykiewicz, O. (1966) Dopamine (3-hydroxytyramine) and brain function. Pharmacol. Rev. 18, 925-964.

Imbs, J.L., Schmidt, M. and Schwartz, J. (1975) Effect of dopamine on renin secretion in the anesthetized dog. Eur. J. Pharmacol. 33, 151-157.

Innes, I.R. and Nickerson, M. (1975) Norepinephrine, epinephrine, and the sympathomimetic amines. In: The Pharmacological Basis of Therapeutics, (Goodman, L.S. and Gilman, A. eds), pp. 477-513, McMillan Publishing Co., New York.

Jarecki, M., Thoren, P.N. and Donald, D.E. (1978) Release of renin by the carotid baroreflex in anesthetized dogs. Circ. Res. 42, 614-619.

Jenner, P. Elliott, N.C., Clow, A., Reavill, C. and Marsden, C.D. (1978) A comparison of in vitro and in vivo dopamine receptor antagonism produced by substituted benzamide drugs. J. Pharm. Pharmacol. 30, 46-48.

Jenner, P. and Marsden, C.D. (1979) The substituted benzamides - a novel class of dopamine antagonists. Life Sci. 25, 479-486.

Jenner, P., Marsden, C.D. and Perringer, E. (1975) Behavioral and biochemical evidence for cerebral dopamine receptor blockade by metoclopramide in rodents. Br. J. Pharmacol. 54, 275P-276P.

Johns, E.J. and Singer, B. (1974) Specificity of blockade of renal renin release by propranolol in the cat. Clin. Sci. Mol. Med. 47, 331-343.

Johns, E.J., Richards, H.K. and Singer, B. (1975) Effects of adrenaline, noradrenaline and isoprenaline and salbutamol on the production and release of renin by isolated renal cortical cells of the cat. Br. J. Pharmacol. 53, 67-73.

Johnson, G.A., Gren, J.M. and Kupiecki, R. (1978) Radioenzymatic assay of dopa (3,4-dihydroxyphenylalanine). Clin. Chem. 24, 1927-1930.

Johnson, J.A., Davis, J.O. and Witty, R.T. (1971) Effects of catecholamines and renal nerve stimulation on renin release in the non-filtering kidney. Circ. Res. 29 646-653.

Johnston, C.I., Mendelsohn, F.A.O., Hutchinson, J.H. and Morris, B. (1973) Composition of juxtaglomerular granules isolated from rat kidney cortex. In: Mechanisms of Hypertension (Sambhi, M.P.S. ed), pp. 238-248,

Excerpta Medica, Amsterdam.

Judy, W.V., Watanabe, A.M., Henry, D., Besch, H.R. and Aprison, B. (1978) Effect of L-dopa on sympathetic nerve activity and blood pressure in the spontaneously hypertensive rat. Circ. Res. 43, 24-28.

Katholi, R.E., Carey, R.M., Ayers, C.R., Vaughan, Jr, E.D., Yancey, M.R. and Morton, C.L. (1977) Production of sustained hypertension by chronic intrarenal norepinephrine infusion in conscious dogs. Circ. Res. 40 (Suppl. I), 118-126.

Katholi, R.E., Oparil, S., Urthaler, F. and James, T.N. (1979) Mechanism of postarrhythmic renal vasoconstriction in the anesthetized dog. J. Clin. Invest. 64, 17-31.

Katz, F.H., Romfh, P. and Smith, J.A. (1975) Diurnal variation of plasma aldosterone, cortisol and renin activity in supine man. J. Clin. Endocrinol. Metab. 40, 125-134.

Kebabian, J.W. and Calne, D.B. (1979) Multiple receptors for dopamine. Nature 277, 93-96.

Kem, D.C., Gomez-Sanchez, C. Kramer, N.J., Holland, O.B. and Higgins, J.R. (1975) Plasma aldosterone and renin activity in response to ACTH infusion in dexamethasone suppressed normal and sodium depleted man. J. Clin. Endocrinol. Metab. 40, 116-124.

Khairallah, P.A. (1971) Pharmacology of angiotensin. In: Kidney Hormones, (Fisher, J.W. ed), pp. 129-171, Academic Press, New York.

Khairallah, P.A. and Hall, M.M. (1979) Angiotensinases. In: Hypertension, (Genest, J., Koiw, E. and Kuchel, O. eds), 179-183, McGraw Hill, New York.

Kiowski, W. and Julius, S. (1978) Renin response to stimulation of cardiopulmonary mechanoreceptors in man. J. Clin. Invest. 62, 1656-1663.

Kosunen, K.J. (1977) Plasma renin activity, angiotensin II and aldosterone after mental arithmetic. Scand. J. Clin. Lab. Invest. 37, 425-429.

Kosunen, K.J. and Pakarinen, H.J. (1976) Plasma renin, angiotensin II and plasma and urinary aldosterone in running exercice. J. Appl. Physiol. 41, 26-29.

Kosunen, K.J., Pekarinen, A.J., Kuoppasalmi, K. and Aldercreutz, H. (1976) Plasma renin activity, angiotensin II and aldosterone during intense heat stress. J. Appl. Physiol. 41, 323-327.

Kotchen, T.A. and Guthrie, G.P. (1980) Renin-angiotensin-aldosterone and hypertension. Endocrinol Rev. 1, 78-99.

Kotchen, T.A., Talwalker, R.T., Kotchen, J.M. and Miller, M.C. (1975) Evidence for the existence of an acetone soluble renin inhibiting factor in normal human plasma. Circ. Res. 36-37 (Suppl. I), 17-27.

Kotchen, T.A., Galla, J.H. and Luke, R.G. (1978) Contribution of chloride to the inhibition of plasma renin by sodium chloride in the rat. Kidney Int. 13, 201-207.

Kuchel, O., Cuche, J.L., Hamet, P., Boucher, R., Barbeau, A. and Genest, J. (1972) The relationships between adrenergic nervous system and renin in labile hyperkinetic hypertension. In: Hypertension' 72 (Genest, J. and Kiow, E. eds), pp. 118-125, Springer-Verlag, New York.

Kuchel, O., Buu, N.T. and Unger, T. (1979) Free and conjugated dopamine: physiological and clinical implications. In: Peripheral Dopaminergic Mechanisms (Imbs, J.L. and Schwartz, J. eds), pp. 11-27, Pergamon Press, New York.

Kuchel, O., Buu, N.T. and Unger, T. (1979) Free and conjugated dopamine: physiological and clinical implications. Adv. Biosci. 20, 15-27.

Kuchel, O., Buu, N.T., Unger, T., Lise, M. and Genest, J. (1979) Free and conjugated plasma and urinary dopamine in human hypertension. J. Clin. Endocrinol. Metab. 48, 425-429.

Kvetňanský, R., Weise, V.K., Thoa, N.B. and Kopin, I.J. (1979) Effects of chronic guanethidine treatment and adrenal medullectomy on plasma levels of catecholamines and corticosterone in forcibly immobilized rats. J. Pharmacol. Exp. Ther. 209, 287-291.

Lands, A.M., Arnold, A., McAuliff, J.P., Ludeena, F.P. and Brown, T.G., Jr. (1967) Differentiation of receptor systems activated by sympathomimetic amines. Nature 214, 597-598.

Laragh, J.H. and Sealey, J.E. (1973) The renin-angiotensin-aldosterone hormonal system and regulation of sodium, potassium, and blood pressure homeostasis. In: Handbook of Physiology: Renal Physiology (Orloff, J. and Berliner, R.W. eds), pp. 831-908, American Physiological Society, Washington, D.C.

Larsson, C., Weber, P. and Anggard. F. (1974) Arachidonic acid increases and indomethacin decreases plasma renin activity in the rabbit. Eur. J. Pharmacol. 28, 391-394.

Latta, H. (1973) In: Handbook of Physiology: Renal Physiology (Orloff, J. and Berliner, R.W. eds), pp. 1-29, American Physiological Society, Washington, D.C.

Leckie, B.J. and McConnell, A. (1975) A renin inhibitor from rabbit kidney: conversion of a large inactive renin to a smaller active enzyme. Circ. Res. 36, 513-519.

Leckie, B.J., Brown, J.J., Lever, A.F., Morton, J.J. Robertson, J.I.S. and Tree, M. (1976) Inactive renin in human plasma. Lancet, 2, 748-749.

Leenen, F.H.H. and McDonald Jr, R.H., (1974) Effect of isoproterenol on blood pressure, plasma renin activity and water intake in rats. Effect of intermittent electric shock on plasma renin activity in rats. Eur. J. Pharmacol. 26, 129-135.

Leenen, F.H.H. and Shapiro, A.P. (1974) Effect of intermittent electrical shock on plasma renin activity in rats. Proc. Soc. Exp. Biol. Med. 146, 534-538.

Leenen, F.H.H., Redmond, D.P. and McDonald Jr, R.H. (1975) Alpha- and beta-adrenergic-induced renin release in man. Clin. Pharmacol. Ther. 18, 31-38.

Leon, A.S., Pettinger, W.A. and Saviano, M.A. (1973) Enhancement of serum renin activity in the rat. Med. Sci. Sports 5, 40-43.

Lester, G.E. and Rubin, R.P. (1977) The role of calcium in renin secretion from the isolated perfused cat kidney. J. Physiol. (Lond.) 269, 93-108.

Levens, N.R., Peach, M.J. Vaughan, Jr, E.D., and Carey, R.M., (1981a) Demonstration of a primary antidiuretic action of angiotensin II: effects of intrarenal converting enzyme inhibition in the dog. Endocrinology 107, 318-330.

Levens, N.R., Peach, M.J., Carey, R.M., Poat, J.A. and Munday, K.A. (1981b) Stimulation of intestinal sodium and water transport in vivo by angiotensin II and analogs. Endocrinology 107, 1946-1953.

Levens, N.R., Peach, M.J. and Carey, R.M. (1981c) Role of the intrarenal renin-angiotensin in the control of renal function. Circ. Res. 48, 157-167.

Levens, N.R., Peach, M.J. and Carey, R.M. (1981d) Interactions between angiotensin II and the sympathetic nervous system mediating intestinal sodium and water transport. J. Clin. Invest. 67, 1197-1207.

Lew, J.Y., Hata, F., Ohashi, T. and Goldstein, M. (1977) The interactions of bromocriptine and lergotrile with dopamine and β-adrenergic receptors. J. Neural Transmission 41, 109-121.

Lichtenstein, L.S., Colwell, J.A. and Levine, J.H. (1976) Prolactin stimulates aldosterone biosynthesis. Program and Abstracts of the Sixth International Congress of Endocrinology, p. 86.

Linkola, J., Fyhrquist, F., Neiminen, M.N., Weber, T.H. and Tontti, I. (1976) Renin-aldosterone axis in ethanol intoxication and hangover. Eur. J. Clin. Invest. 6, 191-194.

Loeffler, J.R., Stockigt, J.R. and Ganong, W.F. (1972) Effect of alpha- and beta-adrenergic blocking agents on the increase in renin secretion produced by stimulation of the renal nerves. Neuroendocrinology 10, 129-138.

Logan, A.G., Tenyi, I., Peart, W.S., Breathnoch, A.S. and Martin, B.G.H. (1977) The effect of lanthanum on renin secretion and renal vasoconstriction. Proc. R. Soc. Lond. Ser. Biol. 195, 327-342.

Lopez, G.A., Reid, I.A., Rose, J.C. and Ganong, W.F. (1978) Effect of norepinephrine on renin release and cyclic AMP content of rat kidney slices: modification by sodium deficiency and alpha-adrenergic blockade. Neuroendocrinology 127, 63-73.

Lorenzi, M., Karam, J.H., Tsalikian, E., Bohannon, N.V., Gerich, J.E. and Forsham, P. (1979) Dopamine during alpha- and beta-blockade in man. J. Clin. Invest. 63, 310-317.

Louis, W.J. and Sampson, R. (1974) Renal and vascular actions of dopamine and their clinical significance. Prog. Biochem. Pharmacol. 9, 22-28.

Lowder, S.C., Fraser, M.G. and Liddle, G.W. (1975) Effect of insulin-induced hypoglycemia upon plasma renin activity in man. J. Clin. Endocrinol. Metab. 41, 97-105.

Mac Leod, R.M. (1976) Regulation of prolactin secretion. In: Frontiers in Neuroendocrinology (Martini, L. and Ganong, W.F. eds), pp. 169-194, Raven, New York.

Mancia, G., Donald, D.E. and Shepherd, J.T. (1973) Inhibition of adrenergic outflow to peripheral blood vessels by vagal afferents from the cardiopulmonary region in the dog. Cir. Res. 33, 713-721.

Mancia, G. Romero, J.C. and Shepherd, J.T. (1975a) Continuous inhibition of renin release in dogs by vagally innervated receptors in the cardiopulmonary region. Circ. Res. 36, 529-535.

Mancia, G., Shepherd, J.T. and Donald, D.E. (1975b) Role of cardiac, pulmonary and carotid mechanoreceptors in the control of hind limb and renal circulation in dogs. Circ. Res. 37, 200-208.

Mantero, F., Boscaro, M., Opocher, G., Aramini, D. and Edwards, C.R.W. (1980) In vitro and in vivo effect of metergoline on aldosterone secretion. Program and Abstracts of the Sixth International Congress of Endocrinology, 405.

Marek, K.L. and Roth, R.H. (1980) Ergot alkaloids: interaction with presynaptic dopamine receptors in the neostriatum and olfactory tubercles. Eur. J. Pharmacol. 62, 137-146.

Mark, A.D., Abboud, F.M. and Fitz, A.E. (1978) Influence of low- and high-pressure baroreceptors on plasma renin activity in humans. Am. J. Physiol. 235, H29-H33.

McCaa, R.E., Young, D.B. and Guyton, A.C. (1974) Evidence of a role of an unidentified pituitary factor regulating aldosterone secretion during altered sodium balance. Circ. Res. (Suppl. I) 34-35, 15-25.

McCaa, R.E., McCaa, C.S. and Guyton, A.C. (1975) Role of angiotensin II and potassium in the long term regulation of aldosterone secretion in intact conscious dogs. Circ. Res. 36-37 (Suppl. I), 57-67.

McCallum, R.W., Sowers, J.R., Hershman, J.M. and Sturdevant, R.A.L. (1976) Metoclopramide stimulates prolactin secretion in man. J. Clin. Endocrinol. Metab. 42, 1148-1152.

McGiff, J.C. (1977) Bartter's syndrome results from an imbalance of vasoactive hormones. Am. Int. Med. 87, 369-372.

McKenna, O.C. and Angelakos, E.T. (1968) Acetylcholinesterase-containing fibers in the canine kidney. Circ. Res. 23, 645-651.

McKenna, T.J., Island, D.P., Nicholson, W.P. and Liddle, G.W. (1978) The effects of potassium on early and late steps in aldosterone biosynthesis in cells of the zona glomerulosa. Endocrinology 103, 1411-1416.

McKenna, T.J., Island, D.P., Nicholson, W.E. and Liddle, G.W. (1979) Dopamine inhibits angiotensin-stimulated aldosterone biosynthesis in bovine adrenal cells. J. Clin. Invest. 64, 287-291.

McPhee, M.S. and Lakey, W.H. (1971) Neurologic release of renin in mongrel dogs. Can. J. Surg. 14, 142-147.

Meltzer, H.Y., So, R., Miller, R.J. and Fang, V.S. (1979) Comparison of the effects of the substituted benzamides and standard neuroleptics on the binding of ^{3}H-spiroperidol in the rat pituitary and striatum with in vivo effects on rat prolactin secretion. Life Sci. 25, 573-584.

Mendelsohn, F.A.O. and Kachel, C.D. (1980) Action of angiotensins I, II and III on aldosterone production by isolated rat adrenal zona glomerulosa cells: importance of metabolism and conversion of peptides in vitro. Endocrinology 106, 1760-1768.

Meyer, D.K., Abele, M. and Hertting, G. (1974) Influence of serotonin on water intake and the renin-angiotensin system. Arch. Int. Pharmacodyn. Ther. 212, 130-140.

Michelakis, A.M. and Mizukoshi, H. (1971) Distribution and disappearance rate of renin in dog and man. J. Clin. Endocrinol. Metab. 33, 27-34.

Michelakis, A.M., Caudle, J. and Liddle, G.W. (1969) In vitro stimulation of renin production by epinephrine, norepinephrine and cyclic AMP. Proc. Soc. Exp. Biol. Med. 130, 748-753.

Millar, J.A., Leckie, B.J., Semple, P.F., Morton, J.J., Sonkodi, S. and Robertson, J.I.S. (1978) Active and inactive renin in human plasma. Circ. Res. 43 (Suppl. I), 120-127.

Modlinger, R.S., Schonmueller, J.M. and Arora, S.P. (1979) Stimulation of aldosterone, renin and cortisol by tryptophan. J. Clin. Endocrinol. Metab. 48, 599-603.

Mogil, R.A., Itskovitz, H.D., Russell, J.H. and Murphy, J.J. (1969) Renal innervation and renin activity in salt metabolism and hypertension. Am. J. Physiol 216, 693-697.

Mori, M., Kobayashi, I., Ohshima, K., Maruta, S., Shimomura, Y. and Fukuda, H. (1980) Potentiation of sulpiride-induced prolactin secretion by sodium deprivation in man. Acta Endocrinol. (Copenhagen), 94, 25-29.

Morris, B.J. and Johnston, C.I. (1976) Isolation of renin granules from rat kidney cortex and evidence for an inactive form of renin (prorenin) in granules and plasma. Endocrinology 98, 1466-1474.

Morris, B.J., Nixon, R.L. and Johnston, C.I. (1976) Release of renin from glomeruli isolated from rat kidney. Clin. Exper. Pharmacol. Physiol. 3, 37-47.

Mukherjee, C., Caron, M.G. and Lefkowitz, R.J. (1975) Catecholamine-induced subsensitivity of adenylate cyclase associated with loss of beta-adrenergic receptor bindig sites. Proc. Natl. Acad. Sci. USA 72, 1945-1949.

Mukherjee, C., Caron, M.G. and Lefkowitz, R.J. (1976) Regulation of adenylate cyclase coupled beta-adrenergic receptors by beta-adrenergic catecholamines. Endocrinology 99, 347-357.

Mulrow, P.J. and Goffinet, J.A. (1979) The renin-angiotensin system. In: Physiology of the Human Kidney (Wesson, G. ed), pp. 465-520, Grune and Stratton, New York.

Myer, D.K., Peskar, B., Tauchmann, U. and Hertting, G. (1971) Potentiation and abolition of the increase in plasma renin activity seen after hypotensive drugs in rats. Eur. J. Pharmacol. 116, 278-282.

Naftilan, A.J. and Oparil, S. (1978) Inhibition of renin release from rat kidney slices by the angiotensins. Am. J. Physiol. 235, F62-F68.

Nally, H.L., Reid, I.A. and Ganong, W.F. (1974) Effect of theophylline and adrenergic blocking drugs on the renin response to norepinephrine in vitro. Circ. Res. 35, 575-579.

Nash, F.D., Rosterfa, H.H., Bailin, M.D., Wathern, W.L. and Schneider, E.G. (1968) Renin release: relation to renal sodium load and dissociation from hemodynamic changes. Circ. Res. 22, 473-487.

Natcheff, N., Logofetov, A. and Tzaneva, V. (1977) Hypothalamic control of plasma renin activity. Pflugers Arch. 371, 279-283.

Nelson, D.H. (1980) Aldosterone and the mineralocorticoids. In: The Adrenal Cortex: Physiologic Function and Disease, pp. 89-101, W.B. Saunders, Philadelphia.

Nicholls, M.G., Espiner, E.A. and Donald, R.A. (1975) Plasma aldosterone response to low dose ACTH stimulation. J. Clin. Endocrinol. Metab. 41, 186-188.

Niemegeers, C.J.E. and Janssen, P.A.J. (1979) A systematic study of the pharmacological activities of the dopamine antagonists. Life Sci. 24, 2201-2216.

Nilsson, A. and Hökfelt, B. (1978) Effects of the dopamine agonist bromocriptine on blood pressure, catecholamines and renin activity in acromegalics at rest, following exercise and during insulin induced hypoglycemia. Acta Endocrinol. (Suppl.) (Copenhagen) 216, 83-96.

Nilsson, O. (1965) The adrenergic innervation of the kidney. Lab. Invest. 14, 1392-1395.

Norbiato, G., Bevilacqua, M., Raggi, U., Micossi, P., Moroni, C., and Fasoli, A. (1978) Effect of prostaglandin synthetase inhibitors on renin and aldosterone in man on a normal or low sodium diet. Acta Endocrinol. (Copenhagen) 87, 577-588.

Norbiato, G., Bevilacqua, M., Raggi, U., Micossi, P. and Moroni, C. (1977) Metoclopramide increases plasma aldosterone in man. J. Clin. Endocrinol. Metab. 45, 1313-1316.

Noth, R.H., McCallum, W., Contino, C. and Havelick, J. (1980) Tonic dopaminergic suppression of plasma aldosterone. J. Clin. Endocrinol. Metab. 51, 64-69.

Ogihara, T., Matsumera, S., Onishi, T., Miyai, K. Uozumi, T. and Kumahara, Y. (1977) Effect of metoclopramide-induced prolactin on aldosterone secretion in normal subjects. Life Sci. 20, 523-526. 38B.

Olgaard, K., Hagen, C., Madsen, S. and Hummer, L. (1977) Lack of effect of prolactin inhibition by alpha-bromergocriptine (CB154) on plasma aldosterone in anephric and non-nephrectomized patients on regular hemodialysis. Acta Endocrinol. (Copenhagen) 85, 587-594.

Onesti, G., Schwartz, A.B., Kim, K.E., Paz-Martinez, V. and Swartz, C. (1971) Antihypertensive effect of clonidine. Circ. Res. 28-19 (Suppl.), 53-69.

Oparil, S., Vassaux, C., Sanders, C.A. and Haber, E. (1970) Role of renin in acute postural homeostasis. Circulation 41, 89-95.

Oparil, S. and Haber, E. (1974) The renin-angiotensin system. New Engl. J. Med. 291, 389-401, 446-457.

Oparil, S. (1979) Angiotensin I converting enzyme and inhibitors. In: Hypertension (Genest, J., Koiw, E. and Kuchel, O. eds), pp. 156-167 McGraw-Hill, New York.

Otsuka, K., Assaykeen, T.A., Goldfien, A. and Ganong, W.F. (1970) Effect of hypoglycemia on plasma renin activity in dogs. Endocrinology 87, 1306-1317.

Page, I.H. and Bumpus, F.M. (1961) Angiotensin. Physiol. Rev. 41, 331-390.

Page, I.H. and Bumpus, F.M. (eds) (1974) Angiotensin. Handbook of Experimental Pharmacology, Vol. 37, Springer-Verlag, New York.

Park, C.S. and Malvin, R.L. (1978) Calcium in the control of renin release. Am. J. Physiol. 235, F22-F25.

Passo, S.S., Assaykeen, T.A., Otsuka, K., Wise, B.L., Goldfein, A. and Ganong, W.F. (1971a) Effect of stimulation of the medulla oblongata on renin secretion in dogs. Neuroendocrinology 7, 1-10.

Passo, S.S., Assaykeen, T.A., Goldfien, A. and Ganong, W.F. (1971b) Effect of alpha- and beta-adrenergic blocking agents on the increase in renin secretion produced by stimulation of the medulla oblongata in dogs.

Neuroendocrinology 7, 97-104.

Peach, M.J. (1977) Renin-angiotensin system: biochemistry and mechanisms of action. Physiol. Rev. 57, 313-370.

Peart, W.S. (1965) The renin-angiotensin system. Pharmacol. Rev. 17, 143-182.

Peringer, E., Jenner, P. Donaldson, I.M. and Marsden, C.D., (1976) Metoclopramide and dopamine receptor blockade. Neuropharmacology 15, 463-469.

Peskar, B., Meyer, D.K., Tauchmann, U. and Hertting, G. (1970) Influence of isoproterenol, hydralazine and phentolamine on renin activity of plasma and renal cortex of rats. Eur. J. Pharmacol. 9, 394-396.

Pettinger, W.A., Augusto, L. and Leon, A.S. (1972) Alteration of renin release by stress and adrenergic receptor and related drugs in anesthetized rats. In: Comparative Pathophysiology of Circulatory Disturbances (Bloor, C.M. ed), pp. 105-117, Plenum Press, New York.

Pettinger, W.A., Keeton, T.K., Campbell, W.B. and Harper, D.C. (1976) Evidence for a renal alpha-adrenergic receptor inhibiting renin release. Circ. Res. 38, 338-346.

Peuler, J.D. and Johnson, G.A. (1977) Simultaneous single isotope radioenzymatic assay of plasma norepinephrine, epinephrine and dopamine. Life Sci 21, 625-636.

Pinder, R.M., Brogden, R.M., Sawyer, P.R., Speight, T.M. and Avery, F.S. (1976) Metoclopramide: a review of its pharmacological properties and clinical use. Drugs 12, 81-131.

Poulsen, K. (1971) No evidence of active renin-inhibitors in plasma. Scand. J. Clin. Lab. Invest. 27, 37-46.

Pratt, J.H., Ganguly, A. and Weinberger, M.H. (1979) Metoclopramide-induced aldosterone stimulation: independence from pituitary and renal factors. Clin. Res. 27, 680A.

Quesada, T., Garcia-Torres, L., Alba, F. and Garcia del Rio, C. (1979) The effects of dopamine on renin release in the isolated perfused rat kidney. Experientia 35, 1205.

Regoli, D., Park, W.K. and Rioux, F. (1974) Pharmacology of angiotensin. Pharmacol. Rev. 26, 69-123.

Reid, I.A. and Ganong, W.F. (1979) Control of aldosterone secretion. In: Hypertension (Genest, J., Koiw, E. and Kuchel, O. eds), pp. 265-292, McGraw-Hill, New York.

Reid, I.A., Schrier, R.W. and Earley, L.E. (1972a) An effect of extrarenal beta-adrenergic stimulation on the release of renin. J. Clin. Invest. 51, 1861-1869.

Reid, I.A., Stockigt, J.R., Goldfien, A. and Ganong, W.F. (1972b) Stimulation of renin secretion in dogs by theophylline. Eur. J. Pharmacol. 17, 325-332.

Reid, I.A., McDonald, D.M., Pachnis, B. and Ganong, W.F., (1975) Studies concerning the mechanism of suppression of renin secretion by clonidine. J. Pharmacol. Exp. Ther. 192, 713-721.

Reid, I.A., and Jones, A. (1976) Effects of carotid occlusion and clonidine on renin secretion in anesthetized dogs. Clin. Sci. Mol. Med. 51, 109s-111s.

Reid, I.A., Morris, B.J. and Ganong, W.F. (1978) The renin-angiotensin–system. Annu. Rev. Physiol. 40, 370-410.

Richardson, D., Stella, A., Leonetti, G., Bartorelli, A. and Zanchetti, A. (1974) Mechanisms of renal release of renin by electrical stimulation of brainstem in the cat. Circ. Res. 34, 425-434.

Robertson, A.L., Smeby, R.R., Bumpus, F.M. and Page, I.H. (1975) Renin production by organ cultures of renal cortex. Science 149, 650-651.

Robinson, P.M., Perry, R.A., Hardy, K.J., Coghlan, J.P., and Scoggins, B.A. (1977) The innervation of the adrenal cortex in the sheep, ovis ovis. J. Anat. 124, 117-129.

Romero, J.C., Dunlap, C.L. and Strong C.G. (1976) The effect of indomethacin and other anti-inflamatory drugs on the renin-angiotensin system. J. Clin. Invest. 58, 282-288.

Romoff, M.S., Keusch, G., Campese, V.M., Wang, M-S. Friedler, R.M., Wiedmann, P. and Massry, S.G. (1979) Effect of sodium intake on plasma catecholamines in normal subjects. J. Clin. Endocrinol. Metab. 48, 26-31.

Rosset, E. and Veyrat, R. (1971) Release of renin by human kidney slices, in vitro effect of angiotensin II, norepinephrine and aldosterone. Rev. Eur. Etudes Clin. Biol. 16, 792-794.

Roufogalis, B.D., Thornton, M. and Wade, D.N. (1976) Specificity of the dopamine sensitive adenylate cyclase for antipsychotic antagonists. Life Sci. 19, 927-934.

Rumpf, K.W., Frenzel, S., Lowetz, H.D. and Scheler, F. (1975) The effect of indomethacin on plasma renin activity in man under normal conditions and after stimulation of the renin-angiotensin system. Prostaglandins

10, 641-648.

Sambhi, M.P. (1977) Activators and inhibitors of renin. In: Hypertension (Genest, J., Kiow, E. and Kuchel, O. eds), pp. 202-210, McGraw-Hill, New York.

Schaechtelin, G., Regoli, D. and Gross, F. (1964) Quantitative assay and disappearance rate of circulating renin. Am. J. Physiol. 206, 1361-1364.

Scheid, C.R., Honeyman, T.W. and Fay, F.S. (1979) Mechanism of Beta-adrenergic relaxation of smooth muscle. Nature (Lond.) 277, 32-26.

Sealey, J.E., Moon, C., Laragh, J.H. and Alderman, M. (1976) Plasma prorenin: cryoactivation and relationship to renin substrate in normal subjects. Am. J. Med. 61, 731-738.

Sealey, J.E., Atlas, S.A., Laragh, J.H., Oza, N.B., Ryan, J.W. (1978) Human urinary kallikrein converts inactive renin to renin: a possible physiological activator of renin. Nature (Lond.) 275, 144-145.

Semple, P.F. and Mason, P.A. (1978) Bromocriptine: lack of effect on the angiotensin II and aldosterone responses to sodium deprivation. Clin. Endocrinol. 9, 155-161.

Sen, S., Bravo, E.L. and Bumpus, F.M. (1977) Isolation of a hypertension producing compound from normal human urine. Circ. Res. 40 (Suppl. I), 5-10.

Seymour, A.A. and Zehr, J.E. (1979) Influence of renal prostaglandin synthesis on renin control mechanisms in the dog. Circ. Res. 45, 13-25.

Shade, R.D., Davis, J.O., Johnson, J.A., Witty, R.T. (1972) Effects of renal arterial infusion of sodium and potassium on renin secretion in the dog. Circ. Res. 31, 719-727.

Sharp, G.W.G. and Leaf, A. (1973) Effects of aldosterone and its mechanism of action on sodium transport. In: Handbook of Physiology: Renal Physiology (Orloff, J. and Berliner, R.W. eds), pp. 815-830, American Physiological Society, Washington, D.C.

Shear, M., Insel, P.A., Melman, K. and Coffino, P. (1976) Agonist-specific refractoriness induced by isoproterenol. J. Biol. Chem. 251, 7572-7576.

Shulkes, A.A., Gibson, R.R. and Skinner, S.L. (1978) The nature of inactive renin in human plasma and amniotic fluid. Clin. Sci. Mol. Med. 55, 41-50.

Silverman, A.J. and Barajas, L. (1974) Effect of reserpine on the juxtaglomerular granular cells and renal nerves. Lab. Invest. 30, 723-731.

Sinaiko, A.R. and Mirkin, B.L. (1978) Isoproterenol-evoked renin release from the in situ perfused kidney. Dose-response characteristics in spontaneously hypertensive and normotensive Wistar rats. Circ. Res. 42, 381-385.

Skinner, S.L., McCubbin, J.W. and Page, I.H. (1964) Control of renin secretion. Circ. Res. 15, 64-76.

Smeby, R.R., Sen, S. and Bumpus, F.M. (1967) A naturally occurring renin inhibitor. Circ. Res. 20-21 (Suppl. 2), II, 129-134.

Sole, M.J. and Hussain, M.N. (1977) A simple specific radioenzymatic assay for simultaneous measurement of picogram quantities of norepinephrine, epinephrine and dopamine in plasma and tissues. Biochem. Med. 18, 301-307.

Solyom, J. (1974) Anterior pituitary and aldosterone secretion. Lancet 2, 507.

Sowers, J.R., McCallum, R.W., Hershman, J.M., Carlson, H.E., Sturdevant, R.A.L. and Meyer, N. (1976) Comparison of metoclopramide with other dynamic tests of prolactin secretion. J. Clin. Endocrinol. Metab. 43, 679-681.

Sowers, J.R., Carlson, H.E., Brautbar, N. and Hershman, J.M. (1977) Effects of dexamethasone on prolactin and TSH responses to TRH and metoclopramide in man. J. Clin. Endocrinol. Metab. 44, 327-341.

Sowers, J.R., Sollars, E., Barrett, J.D. and Sambhi, M.P. (1980a) Effect of L-DOPA and bilateral nephrectomy on the aldosterone response to metoclopramide. Life Sci. 27, 497-501.

Sowers, J.R., Sollars, E., Tuck, M.L. and Asp, N. (1980b) Dopaminergic modulation of renin activity, aldosterone and prolactin secretion in the spontaneously hypertensive rat. Proc. Soc. Exp. Biol. Med. 164, 598-601.

Sowers, J.R., Tuck, M.L., Golub, M.S. and Sollars, E.G. (1980c) Dopaminergic control of aldosterone secretion is independent of alterations in renin secretion. Endocrinology 107, 937-941.

Sowers, J.R., Brickman, A.S., Sowers, D.K. and Berg, G. (1981) Dopaminergic modulation of aldosterone secretion in man is unaffected by glucocorticoids and angiotensin blockade. J. Clin. Endocrinol. Metab. (in press).

Speckart, P., Zia, P., Zipser, R. and Horton, R. (1977) The effect of sodium restriction and prostaglandin inhibition on the renin angiotensin systems in man. J. Clin. Endocrinol. Metab. 44, 832-837.

Spitz, I.M., Zylber, E., Jershky, J. and Leroith, D. (1979) Atropine suppression of basal and metoclopramide-induced human pancreatic polypeptide secretion in man. Metabolism 28, 527-530.

Stalcup, S.A., Lipset, J.S., Woan, J.M. and Leuenberger, P. (1979) Inhibition of angiotensin converting enzyme activity in cultured endothelial cells by hypoxia. J. Clin. Invest. 63, 966-976.

Steinsland, D.S. and Hieble, J.P. (1978) Dopaminergic inhibition of adrenergic neurotransmission as a model for study of dopamine receptor mechanisms. Science 199, 443-445.

Stephens, G.A., Davis, J.O., Freeman, R.H. and Watkins, B.E. (1978) Effects of sodium and potassium salts with anions other than chloride on renin secretion in the dog. Am. J. Physiol. 234, F10-F15.

Swartz, S.L., Williams, G.H., Hollenberg, N.K., Dluhy, R.G., and Moore, T.J. (1980) Primacy of the renin-angiotensin system in mediating the aldosterone response to sodium restriction. J. Clin. Endocrinol. Metab. 50, 1071-1074.

Szalay, K.S. (1973) In vitro aldosterone production: effect of ethacrynic acid, chlorpromazine and veratrine. Acta Physiol. Acad. Sci. Hung. 43, 275-279.

Tagawa, H. and Vander, A.J. (1969) Effect of acetylcholine on renin secretion in salt-depleted dogs. Proc. Soc. Exp. Biol. Med. 132, 1087-1090.

Taher, M.S., McLain, L.G., McDonald, K.M. and Schrier, R.W. (1976) Effect of beta-adrenergic blockage on the renin response to renal nerve stimulation. J. Clin. Invest. 57, 459-465.

Tanigawa, H., Allison, D.J. and Assaykeen, T.A. (1972) A comparison of the effects of various catecholamines on plasma renin activity alone and in the presence of adrenergic blocking agents. In: Hypertension '72 (Genest, J. and Koiw, E. eds), pp. 37-44, Springer-Verlag, New York.

Tewksburry, D.A. and Premeau, M.R. (1976) The effect of proteolytic activity on plasma renin activity assay. Clin. Chim. Acta 73, 67-70.

Thames, M.D., Ul-Hassan, Z., Brackett, N.C., Lower, R.R. and Kontos, H.A. (1971) Plasma renin responses to hemorrhage after cardiac autotransplantation. Am. J. Physiol. 221, 1115-1119.

Thames, M.D. (1977) Reflex suppression of renin release by ventricular receptors with vagal afferents. Am. J. Physiol. 233, H181-H184.

Thames, M.D., Jarecki, M. and Donald, D.E. (1978) Neural control of renin secretion in anesthetized dogs: interaction of cardiopulmonary and carotid baroreceptors. Circ. Res. 42, 237-245.

Thorner, M.O. (1975) Dopamine is an important neurotransmitter in the autonomic nervous system. Lancet 1, 662-665.

Trabucchi, M., Spano, P.F., Tonon, G.C., Frattola, L. (1976) Effects of bromocriptine on central dopamine receptors. Life Sci. 19, 225-232.

Tsukiyama, H., Otsuka, K., Lyusio, S., Fujishima, S. and Kijima, F. (1973) Influence of immobilization stress on blood pressure, plasma renin activity and biosynthesis of adrenocorticoid. Jpn Circ. J. 37, 1265-1269.

Tuck, M.L., Dluhy, R.G., Williams, G.T. (1974) A specific role for saline or the sodium ion in the regulation of renin and aldosterone secretion. J. Clin. Invest. 53, 988-995.

Uberti E.C., Fabbri, B.L., Margutti, A.R., Fersini, C.M. and Pansini, R. (1979) Effect of bromocriptine on the control of plasma aldosterone diurnal variation in normal supine man. Horm. Res. 10, 64-78.

Ueda, H., Yasuda, H., Takabatake, Y., Iizuka, M., Iizuka, T., Ihori, M., Yamamoto, M. and Sakamoto, Y. (1967) Increased renin release evoked by mesencephalic stimulation in the dog. Jpn Heart J. 8, 498-506.

Ueda, H., Yasuda, H., Takabatake, Y., Iizuka, T., Ihori, M. and Sakamoto, Y. (1970) Observations on the mechanism of renin release by catecholamines. Circ. Res. 26/27 (Suppl. I), 195-200.

Unger, T., Buu, N.T. and Kuchel, O. (1978) Renal handling of free and conjugated catecholamines following surgical stress in the dog. Am. J. Physiol. 235, F542-F547.

Unger, T., Buu, N.T. and Kuchel, O. (1979) Renal and adrenal dopamine balance: implications for the role of conjugated dopamine. Adv. Biosci. 20, 357-367.

Ungerstedt, U. (1978) The role of dopamine as a neurotransmitter in the central and the autonomic nervous system. Acta Endocrinol. (Copenhagen) [Suppl.] 216, 13-26.

Valenzuela, J.E. (1976) Dopamine as a possible neurotranmitter in gastric relaxation. Gastroenterology 71,

1019-1022.

Van Loon, G.R. and Sole, M.J. (1980) Plasma dopamine: source, regulation and significance. Metabolism 29, 1119-1123.

Van Loon, G.R., Sole, M.J., Bain, J. and Ruse, J.L. (1979) Effects of bromocriptine on plasma catecholamines in normal men. Neuroendocrinology 28, 425-434.

Vander, A.J. (1975) Effect of catecholamines and the renal nerves on renin secretion in anesthetized dogs. Am. J. Physiol. 209, 659-662.

Vander, A.J., Kay, L.L., Dugan, M.E. and Mouw, D.R. (1977) Effects of noise on plasma renin activity in rats. Proc. Soc. Exp. Biol. Med. 156, 24-26.

Vandongen, R. (1974) Adrenergic receptor mechanisms and renin secretion. Aust. N.Z. J. Med. 4, 237-242.

Vandongen, R. and Greenwood, D.M. (1975) The stimulation of renin secretion by non-vasoconstrictor infusions of adrenaline and noradrenaline in the isolated rat kidney. Clin. Sci. Mol. Med. 49, 609-612.

Vandongen, R. and Peart, W.S. (1974) The inhibition of renin secretion by alpha-adrenergic stimulation in the isolated rat kidney. Clin. Sci. Mol. Med. 47, 471-479.

Vandongen, R., Peart, W.S. and Boyd, G.W. (1973) Adrenergic stimulation of renin secretion in the isolated perfused rat kidney. Circ. Res. 32, 290-296.

Vandongen, R., Peart, W.S. and Boyd, G.W. (1974) Effect of angiotensin II and its non-pressor derivatives on renin secretion. Am. J. Physiol. 226, 227-232.

Vandongen, R., Strong, K.D., Poesse, M.H. and Birkenhajer, W.H. (1979) Suppression of renin secretion in the rat kidney by a non-vascular alpha-adrenergic mechanism. Circ. Res. 45, 435-439.

Vaughan, Jr, E.D., Peach, M.J., Ackerly, J.A., Tsai, B.S. and Larner, A. (1977) Pressor and steroidogenic actions of (des-Asp) angiotensin I. Dependency on conversion to angiotensin III. Circ. Res. 40 (Suppl. I), 94-97.

Viskoper, R.J., Maxwell, M.W., Lupu, A.N. and Rossenfield, S. (1977) Renin stimulation by isoproterenol and theophylline in the isolated perfused kidney. Am. J. Physiol. 232, F248-F253.

Wagermark, J., Ungerstedt, U. and Ljungqvist, A. (1968) Sympathetic innervation of the juxtaglomerular cells of the kidney. Circ. Res. 22, 149-153.

Wathan, R.L., Kingsberry, W.S., Stouder, D.A., Schneider, E.G. and Rostorfer, H.H. (1965) Effects of infusions of catecholamines and angiotensin II on renin release in anesthetized dogs. Am. J. Physiol. 209, 1012-1024.

Watkins, B.E., Davis, J.O., Lohmeier, T.E. and Freeman, R.H. (1976) Intrarenal site of action of calcium on renin secretion in dogs. Circ. Res. 39, 847-853.

Weber, M.A., Stokes, G.S. and Gain, M.J. (1974) Comparison of the effects on renin release of beta-adrenergic antagonists with differing properties. J. Clin. Invest. 54, 1413-1419.

Weber, M.A., Thornell, I.R. and Stokes, G.S. (1974) Effects of beta adrenergic blocking agents on plasma renin activity in the conscious rabbit. J. Pharmacol. Exp. Ther. 188, 234-240.

Weber, P.C., Larsson, C., Anggard, E., Hamberg, M., Carey, E.J., Nicolaou, K.C. and Samuelsson, B. (1976) Stimulation of renin release from rabbit renal cortex by arachidonic acid and prostaglandin endoperoxides. Circ. Res. 39, 868-873.

Weinberger, M. Aoi, W. and Grim, C. (1977) Dynamic responses of active and inactive renin in normal and hypertensive humans. Circ. Res. 41 (Suppl. 2), 21-25.

Weinberger, M.H., Aoi, W. and Henry, D.P. (1975) Direct effect of beta-adrenergic stimulation on renin release by the rat kidney slice in vitro. Circ. Res. 37, 318-324.

Whitfield, L. Sowers, J.R., Tuck, M.L. and Golub, M.S. (1980) Dopaminergic control of plasma catecholamines and aldosterone responses to acute stimuli in normal man. J. Clin. Endocrinol. Metab. 51, 724-729.

Whorton, A.R., Misono, K., Hollifield, J., Frolich, J.C., Inagami, T. and Oates, J.A. (1977) Prostaglandins and renin release: stimulation of renin release from rabbit renal cortical slices by PGI_2. Prostaglandins 14, 1095-1104.

Wilcox, C.S., Aminoff, M.J., Kurtz, A.B. and Slater, J.D.H. (1974) Comparison of the renin response to dopamine and noradrenaline in normal subjects. Clin. Sci. Mol. Med. 46, 481-488.

Williams, G.H., Hollenberg, N.K., Brown, C. and Mersey, J.H. (1978) Adrenal response to pharmacologic interruption of the renin-angiotensin system in sodium restricted normal man. J. Clin. Endocrinol. Metab. 47,

725-731.

Winer, N., Chokshi, D.S. and Walkenhorst, W.G. (1971) Effects of cyclic AMP, sympathomimetic amines and adrenergic receptor antagonists on renin secretion. Circ. Res. 29, 239-248.

Witty, R.T., Davis, J.O., Johnson, J.A. and Prewitt, R.L. (1971) Effect of papaverine and hemorrhage on renin secretion in the non-filtering kidney. Am. J. Physiol. 221, 1666-1671.

Yeo, T., Thorner, M.O., Jones, A., Lowry, P.J. and Besser, G.M. (1978) Release from continuous perfused columns of isolated rat pituitary cells. Clin Endocrinol, 10, 123-130.

Yeo, T., Thorner, M.O., Jones, A., Lowry, P.J. and Besser, G.M. (1979) The effects of dopamine, bromocriptine, lergotrile and metoclopramide on prolactin release from continuous perfused columns of isolated rat pituitary cells. Clin. Endocrinol. 10, 123-130.

Young, L.D., Langford, H.G. and Blanchard, E.G. (1976) Effect of operant conditioning of heart rate on plasma renin activity. Psychosomatic Med. 38, 278-281.

Zehr, J.E. and Feigl, E.O. (1973) Suppression of renin activity by hypothalamic stimulation. Circ. Re. 27-28 (Suppl. I), 17-26.

Zehr, J.E., Hasbargen, J.A. and Kurz, K.D. (1976) Reflex suppression of renin secretion during distention of cardiopulmonary receptor in dogs. Circ. Res. 38, 232-239.

Zehr, J.E., Kurz, K.D., Seymour, A.A. and Schultz, H.D. (1980) Mechanisms controlling renin release. In: The Renin-Angiotensin System (Johnson, J.A. and Anderson, R.R. eds), Advances in Experimental Medicine and Biology, Vol. 130, Plenum Press, New York.

Ziegler, M.G., Lake, C.R., Williams, A.S., Teychenne, P.F., Shonloon, I. and Steinsland, J. (1979) Bromocriptine inhibits norepinephrine release. Clin. Pharmacol. Ther. 25, 137-142.

E.E. Müller and R.M. MacLeod (eds) Neuroendocrine Perspectives Vol. 1
© Elsevier Biomedical Press, 1982

Chapter 9

The chronoendocrinology of endogenous depression

Robert T. Rubin and Russell E. Poland

INTRODUCTION

Major psychiatric illnesses have many biological components – genetic, neurophysiological, neurochemical and neuroendocrine. For decades, researchers have attempted to elucidate the biological correlates of psychiatric illnesses in order to understand better their etiologies and to adduce new information to aid in differential diagnosis and prediction of treatment response. Affective disorders, in particular depression, have been the focus of psychiatric investigations for several reasons. First, depression is a prominent illness; its lifetime incidence in the United States is about 10%. Second, depression is the only psychiatric illness that has a significant, and often preventable, mortality: as depicted in Fig. 9.1, the incidence of successful suicide in patients with affective disorder is about 15% (Avery and Winokur 1978). Third, major depressive illness often recurs episodically, so that patients may be at risk for much of their lives. And fourth, certain affective disorders often respond to somatic therapies, including antidepressants of several classes, antimanic agents such as lithium, and electroconvulsive treatment. Thus, the search for biologic markers in depressive illness, as clinical aids to diagnosis and prediction of treatment response, has a special importance.

Typology of depression

Depressive illness encompasses a heterogeneous group of disorders that have dissimilar features in clinical symptomatology and response to treatment, as well as, undoubtedly, in etiology. While any individual may suffer a depression, often precipitated by some identifiable major life stress, there is a certain type of depression that is characterized by a specific cluster of symptoms, a prolonged course, often a family history of similar illness, and generally a responsiveness only to somatic therapies (antidepressant medication or electroconvulsive treatment, ECT). This type of depression, called endogenous (Kendall 1976) or endogenomorphic (Klein 1974) depression, also may follow an identifiable

306

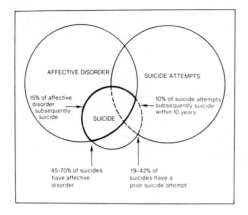

Fig. 9.1. Venn diagram of the interrelations among suicide, suicide attempts, and affective disorders in psychiatric patients. Figure reproduced, with permission, from Avery and Winokur (1978). Copyright 1978 by the American Medical Association.

precipitating stress and thus be 'reactive' in one sense. However, the particular symptom cluster and requirement for somatic therapy are the primary factors that characterize such a depression as endogenous. The signs and symptoms of endogenous or endogenomorphic depression have been codified in the Research Diagnostic Criteria (Spitzer et al. 1978) and in the DSM-III of the American Psychiatric Association (1980); they include anhedonia (inability to experience pleasure), lack of energy, fatigability, reduced sexual drive, anorexia, weight loss, sleep disturbance (especially early morning awakening), depression worse in the morning, self-reproach, excessive guilt, psychomotor agitation or retardation, lack of reactivity to the environment, etc. Delusions or hallucinations (often of a depressive, somatic nature) also may be present, giving an additional, psychotic dimension to the illness.

Severe endogenous depression not infrequently has concomitant neuroendocrine disturbances (Rubin et al. 1973; Rubin and Kendler 1977; Carroll et al. 1978; Rubin et al. 1979; Checkley 1980). These include abnormalities in the secretion patterns of the anterior pituitary polypeptide hormones and their peripheral target endocrine gland steroid hormones, the most clearly delineated being the hypersecretion of ACTH and cortisol; the resistance of ACTH and cortisol to suppression by the synthetic glucocorticoid, dexamethasone; the reduced responsiveness of pituitary thyrotropin (TSH) secretion to thyrotropin releasing hormone (TRH); and the reduced responsiveness of growth hormone (GH) secretion to several challenges, including amphetamine, desmethylimipramine, clonidine, and insulin-induced hypoglycemia. The regularity of some of these endocrine changes and their specificity to endogenous depression have already led to the proposal of endocrine testing as a laboratory adjunct to the differential diagnosis of this illness (Carroll et al. 1981). This paper will review the data published on endocrine changes in endogenous depression, with particular emphasis on the chronoendocrine aspects of these changes, including their relationship to the sleep–wake cycle.

Methodologic advances in psychoendocrine depression research

Several methodologic advances in the last 10 to 15 years have fostered a considerable increase in psychoneuroendocrine studies of depression (Rubin 1977; Poland and Rubin 1981). First, as mentioned above, a detailed and objective diagnostic schema has been developed; the Research Diagnostic Criteria (Spitzer et al. 1978). Under the heading of major depressive disorder, patients may be further subtyped along several dimensions: primary (de novo) vs secondary (following upon another major psychiatric or medical illness) depression; unipolar (depression only) vs bipolar (both manic and depressive episodes); endogenous (symptoms detailed above) vs non-endogenous; agitated vs retarded; psychotic (delusions and/or hallucinations) vs non-psychotic; etc. While these criteria do much to objectify the diagnostic process, they may be overinclusive (Nelson et al. 1978; Feinberg et al. 1979), highlighting the need for specific biological markers as additional diagnostic refinements.

A second methodologic advance has been the development and thorough validation of several depression rating scales, both rater scored and self (patient) administered, such as the Hamilton, Beck, and Zung scales (Carroll et al. 1973). These are useful for quantitating the severity of the depression and following its response to treatment.

Third, the development of very specific and sensitive, and relatively uncomplicated and inexpensive, radioimmunoassays (Yalow 1978) has permitted the measurement of low concentrations of many polypeptide and steroid hormones in the serum or plasma from both normal subjects and depressed patients. The automation of much of the radioimmunoassay procedure permits the analysis of hundreds of samples, in duplicate, in a single assay. Reliable enzymatic radioiodination schemes have been worked out for even the most delicate polypeptide hormones (Tower et al. 1977, 1978, 1980), and ever-purer polypeptide hormone preparations for standards and iodination are being supplied by the National Pituitary Agency.

These improvements in laboratory assay technique have made feasible the fourth methodologic advance, which is the recognition that frequent blood sampling is necessary over at least a 24-h period in order to characterize fully the patterns of hormone concentrations in blood. Frequent blood sampling paradigms have led to the recognition that most hormones are secreted episodically, several have prominent circadian (24 h) rhythms, and some of these rhythms are linked to the sleep–wake cycle.

Finally, the chemical characterization and synthetic preparation of several of the hypothalamo–hypophysiotropic hormones, including TRH, gonadotropin releasing hormone (LH-RH), and somatostatin, have permitted the testing of hormone dynamics by perturbation tests with these substances, in addition to the elucidation of hormone rhythms.

NORMAL SLEEP–ENDOCRINE RELATIONS

The presence of normally occurring hormone rhythms, some of which are closely linked to the sleep–wake cycle or to specific sleep stages within the sleep period itself; their alteration by experimental neurochemical and neuroanatomic manipulations of the central

308

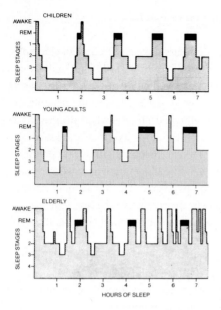

Fig. 9.2. Sleep cycles of normal subjects. Children and young adults have early appearance of stages 3 and 4 (slow wave) sleep, progressive lengthening of the first few rapid eye movement (REM) episodes, and infrequent awakenings. Elderly persons have reduced slow wave sleep, more uniform REM episodes, and frequent awakenings. Figure reproduced, with permission, from Kales (1968).

nervous system (CNS), such as hypothalamic deafferentation of experimental animals; and the responsiveness of many of these hormones to psychological stress, all provide supporting evidence for the importance of the CNS in endocrine function. They highlight the role of open loop mechanisms (CNS driving) in the control of pituitary hormone release, in addition to the more classical closed loop mechanisms (negative and positive feedback between target organ hormones and the hypothalamo-pituitary unit), and between the pituitary and the hypothalamus, perhaps by retrograde flow through the capillary portal plexus (Bergland and Page 1978, 1979).

The electrophysiology of sleep

The sleep–wake cycle and shifts between the stages of sleep are regularly occurring phenomena. The cycle in humans normally has a circadian rhythm, occurring once every 24 h. Electrophysiologic (electroencephalographic, electromyographic and electrooculographic) recordings of normal nocturnal sleep have shown that sleep is not a unitary state but consists of two distinct phases, rapid eye movement (REM) and non-REM sleep. Non-REM sleep can be subdivided further into four numbered stages (Rechtschaffen and Kales 1968; Anders et al. 1971).

In most normal adults, the waking electroencephalogram (EEG) is dominated by 8–12 Hz alpha activity. The transition from waking to sleep, stage 1, is characterized by the disappearance of more than 50% of this rhythm. The appearance of 12–14 Hz sleep spindles marks the onset of stage 2 sleep. Stages 3 and 4 (slow wave sleep, SWS) are defined by the onset of high amplitude, synchronized slow waves, which in moderate amount constitute stage 3 sleep and when occupying more than 50% of the EEG constitute stage 4 sleep. During these sleep stages there often are slow, rolling eye movements and slightly less muscle tone than during the awake state. Episodes of REM sleep are characterized by low amplitude, desynchronized EEG activity resembling the waking EEG; a clear, persistent decrease in muscle tone; and bursts of rapid eye movements. Although considerable mental activity can be elicited during non-REM sleep, the bulk of what is considered dreaming occurs during REM sleep.

Sleep staging within the hours of sleep demonstrates an ultradian rhythm of 80–110 min. Fig. 9.2 illustrates the 'architecture' of sleep; the regular alteration between REM episodes and non-REM sleep, including SWS (Kales 1968). Normally, individuals pass through stages 1 to 4 in the first one or two hours of sleep. A short REM episode then appears, and throughout the rest of the night REM and non-REM sleep alternate rhythmically. As sleep progresses, SWS occurs less and less, while REM sleep becomes more prominent. By the last one-third of the night, REM episodes occupy about half the sleep time, with stage 2 sleep comprising the other half. Under normal conditions, the relative amount of time spent in each of the stages of sleep is relatively constant from night to night and from subject to subject. In young adults, stage 1 occupies 4–5 % of total sleep time; stage 2, 50 %; stages 3 and 4 (SWS) 20–25 %; and REM sleep 20–25 %. Infants have relatively large amounts of REM sleep. By the age of one year, however, the amount of REM has decreased to the 20–25 % level, which remains about the same throughout the rest of life. SWS, on the other hand, declines throughout life, being occasionally absent in the elderly, as indicated in Fig. 9.2.

After so many years of sleep research, it is disappointing that so little is known about its specific physiological importance to the organism. It is believed to serve an anabolic function, as indicated by the general restorative value of a good night's sleep. Many attempts at delineating function have centered around sleep deprivation experiments, either total sleep deprivation, or selective deprivation of certain sleep stages. The consensus of results indicates that the total sleep process is necessary for normal waking function, but one stage of sleep has not proved to be more important than any other (Hartmann 1973).

CNS neurotransmitter regulation of sleep staging

The aforementioned open-loop CNS control mechanisms that regulate the parvocellular neurons of the hypothalamus, which produce the releasing and inhibiting factors for the anterior pituitary hormones, and the magnocellular neurons, which produce the posterior pituitary hormones (Hayward 1977), appear to have as a functional neurochemical substrate, inter alia, the synaptic amine neurotransmitters that are in high concentration in the hypothalamus and limbic system (Reichlin et al. 1977). Sleep–wake cycles and sleep staging during the hours of sleep appear to be influenced by these same neurotransmitters. There is considerable evidence, primarily from work with the cat (Jouvet 1972; Jouvet and Pujol 1974; Jouvet 1975), that a serotonergic mechanism in the median raphe nuclei of the brain stem triggers the normal progression from wakefulness into sleep and further progression into stages 3 and 4 sleep (SWS). The periodic appearance of REM sleep is believed to be triggered by serotonergic mechanisms and maintained by cholinergic and noradrenergic

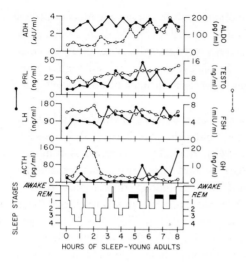

Fig. 9.3. Composite representation of the typical secretion patterns (plasma levels) of eight hormones during a normal 8-h sleep period in a young adult man. REM = rapid eye movement sleep; ACTH = adrenocorticotropic hormone; GH = growth hormone; LH = luteinizing hormone; FSH = follicle stimulating hormone; PRL = prolactin; TESTO = testosterone; ADH = antidiuretic hormone; ALDO = aldosterone. Hormones named on the left side of the figure are depicted by dots and a solid line; those named on the right side are depicted by open circles and a dashed line.

mechanisms in the brain stem. However, there is conflicting evidence from pharmacologic studies about which neurotransmitters are important in the various stages of sleep in the human (Wyatt 1972; Solis et al. 1979). The pharmacologic reduction of brain serotonin can decrease REM sleep without affecting other sleep stages, and the administration of a serotonin precursor can reverse this REM sleep reduction. The pharmacologic decrease of brain catecholamines increases REM sleep, and the administration of a catecholamine precursor decreases REM sleep. Thus, from pharmacologic studies in humans it appears that CNS serotonin concentrations are directly correlated with REM sleep, and CNS catecholamine concentrations are inversely correlated with this sleep stage; these findings in man are at some variance with studies of the neurotransmitter regulation of sleep in the cat. Nevertheless, the role of these transmitters in the orderly progression of sleep staging in the human, as well as in experimental animals, is generally accepted (Drucker-Colin and Spanis 1976).

The endocrinology of sleep in normal subjects

As mentioned above, it has been known for several years that in humans most hormones are secreted episodically; several have prominent circadian rhythms; and some of these rhythms are linked to the sleep–wake cycle (Rubin et al. 1974; Rubin 1975; Rubin and Poland 1976; Sassin 1977; Boyar 1978; Copinschi et al. 1978; Aschoff 1979; Krieger and Aschoff 1979; Wagner and Weitzman 1980; Rubin 1980). As a preface to the discussion of the dynamics of specific hormones in endogenously depressed patients, the following is an overview of normal sleep–endocrine relations (cf. Krieger 1979a for more detailed discussions). Fig. 9.3 shows a composite of five anterior pituitary hormones, adrenocorticotropic hormone (ACTH), growth hormone (GH), luteinizing hormone (LH), follicle stimulating hormone (FSH), and prolactin (PRL), as well as antidiuretic hormone (ADH), aldosterone

(ALDO), and testosterone (TESTO), in a typical young adult man (Rubin 1975).

ACTH has a prominent circadian rhythm, as does its target hormone cortisol, with lowest blood levels of both hormones occurring in the early hours of the sleep period and then rapidly increasing in the latter few hours of sleep to reach a maximum about the time of awakening. Once established, this rhythm appears to have considerable inertia, persisting when sleep is forced into a three-hour ultradian cycle and taking several weeks to readjust when the sleep–wake cycle is reversed. The individual secretory episodes of ACTH and cortisol do not correlate well with REM sleep episodes, but they do occur most frequently during the hours when REM sleep is maximal. GH, in contrast to ACTH, is released soon after sleep onset and is closely linked to SWS. Factors which alter GH secretion during waking hours have much less effect on the SWS-related release of GH. In contrast to the inertia of the ACTH rhythm following the alteration of sleep, GH immediately responds to a shifted sleep schedule, being released at the new time of onset of SWS.

The gonadotropins, LH and FSH, show very little circadian rhythm in adult humans (in contrast to their higher plasma levels during sleep in pubertal subjects). The individual secretory episodes of LH are prominent and randomly distributed throughout both day and night. FSH also is secreted episodically throughout the 24-h period, apparently independently from LH. Circulating FSH levels are generally more stable than those of LH. In some women the midcycle ovulatory surge of LH may begin in the latter hours of sleep or at the time of awakening. PRL has a prominent circadian rhythm, with blood levels beginning to increase shortly after sleep onset and reaching maximum values in the last hour or two of sleep.

The PRL rhythm, like that of GH, is quite dependent on sleep. Early awakening foreshortens the sleep-related PRL increase; partial or complete reversal of the sleep–wake cycle causes an immediate shift of PRL secretion to the new sleep schedule; and daytime naps result in PRL release. The individual secretory episodes of PRL may be entrained to sleep staging, with nadirs of PRL occurring during REM and peaks occuring during non-REM sleep. TSH, while not depicted in Fig. 9.3, also appears to be released episodically, although blood levels are normally quite stable. There is a circadian rhythm to TSH secretion, with highest circulating levels occurring in the late evening hours, usually prior to the time of sleep onset. Sleep itself appears to inhibit TSH secretion somewhat, as sleep deprivation can prolong the nocturnal TSH increase.

The posterior pituitary hormone vasopressin, or antidiuretic hormone, like the anterior pituitary hormones, is secreted episodically throughout the night in humans. These secretory pulses occur randomly, in no apparent relationship to sleep stages, and without any observable changes in sodium concentration, which is a reasonable reflection of plasma osmolality under normal conditions. ADH increases are generally short-lived, consistent with the 6–9 min half-life of this hormone.

The mineralocorticoid aldosterone, like the glucocorticoid cortisol, is secreted episodically both at night and during the day in normal subjects. There is a prominent nocturnal increase in plasma aldosterone levels, its circadian rhythm being similar both to those of ACTH and cortisol and to those of plasma renin activity and angiotensin II. The renin–angiotensin system appears to be the most potent influence on aldosterone secretion under a wide range of physiologic conditions, but ACTH also appears to be an important regulator of aldosterone secretion under normal circumstances. There also may be a 90-min ultradian rhythm of nocturnal aldosterone secretory episodes, but this has not been found in all studies.

The final hormone shown in Fig. 9.3, testosterone, also is secreted episodically and has a circadian rhythm, with highest levels occurring in the last hour or so of sleep. The circadian rhythm of testosterone accounts for about 20% of the total variance in its circulating levels throughout the day and night. The similarity of the testosterone circadian rhythm to that of PRL, with testosterone lagging behind PRL by 60–90 min, has led to the hypothesis that PRL may play a role in the nocturnal increase of testosterone. However, manipulation of nocturnal PRL levels by drugs (Jacobs et al. 1978) or by sleep–wake reversal (Miyatake et al. 1980) has little immediate effect on testosterone, so the relationship between the two hormones remains moot.

All the aforementioned hormones have been studied, to a greater or lesser extent, in depression. Other hormones not depicted in Fig. 9.3 also have been studied in this illness, and as background information their secretion patterns also will be mentioned.

Beta-lipotropin (β-LPH) appears to be derived from the same precursor molecule as ACTH. Their circadian rhythms are similar, but β-LPH has a longer plasma half-life than ACTH (Mullen et al. 1979; Krieger et al. 1980; Donald 1980). β-LPH may be a prohormone for the endorphins and methionine enkephalin. Because human β-endorphin assays only recently have become sensitive enough to measure circulating plasma levels (Krieger et al. 1980), and because most β-endorphin antisera have an appreciable cross-reactivity with β-LPH, the 24-h patterns of the endorphins and enkephalins in blood have not been elucidated completely. However, β-endorphin appears to have a circadian rhythm in the plasma of normal subjects very much like those of ACTH and cortisol, with little direct relationship of plasma β-endorphin fluctuations to sleep staging (Dent et al. 1981).

Finally, attention recently has been given to the pineal hormone melatonin, since assay refinements now permit fairly reliable measurement of its circulating levels in plasma. In man, melatonin is secreted episodically and has a clear circadian rhythm, with highest levels occurring during the lights off–sleep period, usually prior to the ACTH/cortisol rise (Wetterberg 1978; Wurtman and Ozaki 1978; Weinberg et al. 1979). The nocturnal secretory episodes of melatonin appear to be unrelated to sleep staging (Vaughan et al. 1978), and its circadian rhythm persists for several days following altered light–dark and sleep–wake cycles (Akerstedt et al. 1979; Vaughan et al. 1979). Melatonin is the putative releasing hormone for pineal arginine vasotocin (AVT), which appears to be secreted into the cerebrospinal fluid (CSF) with a circadian rhythm similar to that of melatonin (Pavel 1978). The release of AVT may be linked to sleep stages in normal subjects, in that CSF levels of AVT have been detectable following REM sleep, but not following non-REM sleep (Pavel et al. 1979).

The above overview of the endocrinology of sleep in normal subjects certainly is not exhaustive, but rather is meant to highlight those hormones that already have been studied, or have been hypothesized to play some role, in depression. On this background of normal sleep–endocrine relations, findings in depressive illness will be presented and discussed.

SLEEP–ENDOCRINE RELATIONS IN ENDOGENOUS DEPRESSION

In the preceding sections the basic structure, or architecture, of sleep and its regulation by CNS amine neurotransmitters have been presented, and the relationships of the secretion patterns of several hormones, as reflected by their plasma concentrations, to the sleep–wake cycle and sleep staging have been discussed. Changes in the structure of sleep and in the secretion patterns of many hormones occur in endogenous depression. These changes may be the result of alterations in the aforementioned CNS neurotransmitters, which also are believed to underlie the affect disturbances in this illness (Usdin et al. 1977; Lipton et al. 1978). In the following sections the sleep disturbances in depression will be outlined, the sleep-related and circadian secretion patterns of individual hormone axes will be considered, and relevant aspects of CNS neurotransmitter dysfunction will be linked theoretically to the endocrine changes in depression.

Sleep architecture in endogenous depression

As pointed out in the section on the typology of depression, one of the characteristic complaints of depressed patients is that they sleep poorly. Electrophysiologic studies of sleep have shown that depression is almost always accompanied by alterations in sleep staging, including increased sleep discontinuity (disruption of sleep architecture), reduced SWS, shortened REM latency (the interval from the onset of sleep until the onset of the first REM period), and increased REM activity (the sum of eye movement scores during REM sleep) (Kupfer 1977). The most prominent finding in depression is the decrease in REM latency. In normal subjects, the first REM period occurs 70–90 min after sleep onset, while in depressed patients the first REM period occurs in about half that time (Kupfer et al. 1978; Gillin et al. 1979). A positive correlation has been found between the severity of depression and the shortening of REM sleep latency (Spiker et al. 1978). These changes in sleep stage patterns occurring in endogenously depressed patients are not a transient phenomenon; they can persist for weeks in untreated patients and for months in patients who do not respond to treatment (Kupfer 1976; Coble et al. 1979).

Based upon sleep electrophysiology, endogenously depressed patients can be differentiated easily from normal control subjects. Of greater clinical relevance is whether endogenously depressed patients can be discriminated from other psychiatric patients, such as those with secondary depressions, schizophrenia, alcoholism, or drug addiction, and from patients with other medical disorders without psychiatric symptoms. While thorough sleep electrophysiology studies for all these groups of patients have not yet been performed, recent studies indicate that endogenously depressed patients do have unique sleep abnormalities that distinguish them from some of the other patient populations.

Kupfer et al. (1978), comparing the sleep parameters of 47 patients with primary depression and 48 patients with secondary depression (depressions following major psychiatric or medical illnesses), found that the primary depressives had significantly (1) shorter mean REM latency, (2) greater mean REM sleep percentage, (3) higher mean REM activity, (4) greater mean REM density, (5) more early morning awakening, (6) more intermittent wakefulness, (7) less time spent asleep, and (8) lower sleep efficiency than secondary depressives. Using discriminant function analysis, these investigators showed that the primary and secondary depressives could be distinguished with an 81% accuracy. The two variables that made the greatest contribution to the discriminant function were REM latency and REM activity. Further discriminant function analysis indicated that psychotic and non-psychotic subgroups of patients with primary depression could be distinguished with 75% accuracy, by using the variables of SWS percentage, sleep efficiency, and REM sleep percentage. Also, a similar analysis, using the variables of REM activity and intermittent nocturnal awakenings, discriminated with an 81% accuracy two subgroups of patients with secondary depression, those with and without major medical illness.

Similarly, Gillin et al. (1979) compared the sleep electrophysiology of three groups of subjects: 41 normal controls, 56 depressed patients, and 18 insomniacs. A discriminant function analysis incorporating eight sleep variables (sleep latency, sleep efficiency, REM time, REM %, early morning awake time, awake time, total recording period, and total sleep time) correctly classified 82% of the subjects. All of the normal controls, 72% of the depressives, and 77% of the insomniacs were accurately identified. In a prospective study, Gillin et al. (1979) applied their previously determined discriminant function equation to the sleep patterns of an additional 18 endogenously depressed patients; 82% of these patients were correctly classified. The studies of Kupfer et al. (1978) and Gillin et al. (1979) indicate that endogenously depressed patients have unique sleep abnormalities, the identification of which has potential usefulness for the differential diagnosis of endogenous depression.

Sleep studies in depression also may be useful for the prediction of clinical response to various treatment regimens. Kupfer et al. (1976) determined if the immediate post-treatment EEG sleep changes of 18 depressed patients were predictive of a later positive clinical response to antidepressant treatment. The seven good responders to 150–200 mg of amitriptyline showed significantly decreased REM sleep percentage, decreased REM sleep time, decreased REM activity, and increased REM latency, compared to the 11 non-responders after only two nights of amitriptyline treatment. The responders could not be distinguished from the non-responders by their pre-drug baseline sleep measures, but the responders and non-responders were discriminated with an 80% accuracy after the first two nights of drug treatment. Since it normally takes 1–2 weeks for antidepressant medication to effect a reduction in core clinical symptoms, a test to predict eventual responders to treatment would have considerable practical importance.

One variable that must be controlled in treatment response studies is possible inter-individual differences in absorption, distribution, and metabolism of antidepressant drugs between responders and non-responders. Kupfer et al. (1979) determined the relationship between blood levels of amitriptyline and nortriptyline and the early changes in sleep patterns associated with a clinical response to treatment in 25 primary depressives. The persistent reduction in REM percentage and prolongation of REM latency correlated significantly positively with plasma amitriptyline and nortriptyline levels, indicating that pharmacokinetic parameters may be important in the early EEG changes and eventual clinical response. These findings need further study.

Sleep deprivation therapy in depression

Acute sleep deprivation has a mild to moderate antidepressant effect in some endogenously depressed patients (Gerner et al. 1979), in contrast to its mild dysphoric effect in normal volunteers. The antidepressant effect of one night's sleep deprivation lasts only 24–48 h and has been reported to occur in approximately 50% of medication-free patients. No difference in the response of unipolar versus bipolar patients and no correlation with sex or length of illness have been found. However, an antidepressant response has been found more often in endogenous than in non-endogenous depressives, and also more frequently in patients with more severe depressions. Selective REM deprivation and partial sleep deprivation (forced early awakening) have produced results similar to those of all-night sleep deprivation (Vogel 1975; Vogel et al. 1975; Gerner et al 1979; Schilgen and Tölle 1980).

In contrast to the short-term effects of total or partial sleep deprivation, Vogel et al. (1975) reported the effects of selective sleep-stage deprivation chronically maintained. Thirty-four endogenously depressed patients were treated in a double-blind cross-over study in which they were deprived of REM sleep for three to nine weeks but were allowed one night of uninterrupted sleep every four to five nights. The overall antidepressant effect of this REM sleep reduction was similar to the reported efficacy of imipramine treatment of depression and was greater than the effect of selective non-REM sleep deprivation.

The mechanism by which sleep deprivation produces its antidepressant effect is unknown. Sleep deprivation may resynchronize the circadian rhythms involved in the pathophysiology of depression (Pflug and Tölle 1971). In support of this hypothesis, Wehr et al. (1979) reported that, in one patient, progressively advancing the sleep period by 6-h increments also had an antidepressant effect.

Although acute sleep deprivation does not appear to be clinically useful, because of its transient effect, the acute antidepressant response may be predictive of whether a patient will respond to other, more conventional types of therapy. Wirz-Justice et al. (1979) studied the relationship between the antidepressant effects of acute sleep deprivation and the long-term response to tricyclic antidepressant treatment in 52 depressed patients, not further clinically described. Thirty-four of these patients showed an antidepressant response to acute sleep deprivation, and, of this group, 24 also improved after tricyclic antidepressant treatment. In contrast, of the 18 patients who did not respond to sleep deprivation, only six improved with long-term antidepressant therapy. The difference between these two groups was statistically significant. Phillip and Werner (1979), in a study of 15 patients with endogenous and neurotic depressions, found that those patients who showed an antidepressant response to one night of partial sleep deprivation (forced early awakening) also showed a good clinical response to lofepramine treatment. This test could be particularly useful for outpatients, as they could deprive themselves of sleep at home for one night, or part of one night, and then be evaluated clinically the next day. The endocrine effects of sleep deprivation therapy in depression will be considered in a later section.

ACTH and cortisol rhythms in depression

As noted earlier, circulating ACTH and cortisol have a prominent circadian variation, with lowest levels occuring in the first few hours of sleep and peak levels occurring in the morning around the time of awakening (Krieger 1979b). Because of the impetus given to psychoendocrine research by Selye's formulation of the general adaptation syndrome (Selye 1973), and because colorimetric blood and urine corticosteroid measurement techniques were available 25 years ago, early endocrine studies of depression focused on this endocrine axis (Rubin and Mandell 1966; Mason 1968). Many studies showed that adrenal cortical activity was increased in depression compared to mania or normalcy. Some investigators believed that the subjectively experienced anxiety and dysphoria of the depressed patient resulted in an adrenal cortical stress response according to the Selye model (Sachar et al. 1970), while others postulated that both the depressed effect and the increased corticosteroid secretion could be secondary to an underlying disturbance of brain function (Rubin and Mandell 1966; Carroll 1976). Studies of the circadian pattern of corticosteroid secretion and its response to pharmacologic suppression support the latter hypothesis, that a CNS mechanism more fundamental than subjectively felt anxiety appears to underlie the increased corticosteroid production in endogenous depression.

Increased adrenal cortical activity occurs in apathetic as well as in anxious depressives, and it occurs throughout the entire 24 h, especially during the sleep period (Sachar et al. 1973a; Carroll et al. 1976; Rubin et al. 1980). Fig. 9.4 portrays mean hourly plasma cortisol concentrations over a 24-h period in seven unipolar depressed patients and 54 normal subjects (Sachar 1975). While the composite curves of the hourly means obliterated the episodic secretion patterns of individual subjects, it is apparent that the mean cortisol

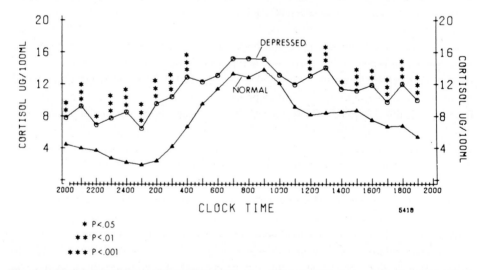

Fig. 9.4. Mean hourly plasma cortisol concentrations over a 24-h period for seven unipolar depressed patients and 54 normal subjects, with between-group significance levels for each time point. Figure reproduced, with permission, from Sachar (1975).

concentration for the depressed patients was higher at all times of the day and night. Fig. 9.4 further indicates that the greatest relative increase in cortisol concentration in the patients occurred at night, when cortisol levels normally are low; during these hours the patients had a two- to three-fold higher mean plasma cortisol level than the controls, The significance levels shown in Fig. 9.4 highlight the magnitudes of the hourly differences, although the p values appear not to have been corrected for the 24 separate statistical tests performed (Jacobs 1976). The p values do indicate that sampling only at certain times of the day, e.g. in the first hours after awakening (0600–1000), could fail to reveal statistically significant differences in plasma cortisol between patients and controls, whereas sampling during the first hours of sleep, in the late evening–early morning period, should detect these differences.

Fig. 9.4 also indicates an attenuation of the amplitude of the circadian cortisol rhythm in the depressed patients. For the 54 normal subjects there was a 75–90% deviation of the average peak and trough cortisol values from the overall 24 h mean, whereas for the seven patients the average peak and trough cortisol values deviated only 40% from the 24 h mean.

Fig. 9.5 portrays similar data for 15 primary endogenous depressives (six men, nine women) and eight normal age, sex, race, and menstrual status-matched control subjects studied by our research group (Rubin et al. 1980). The half-hourly blood sampling gave a better indication of the episodically fluctuating levels of cortisol in serum. Again, the patients had higher serum cortisol levels during most of the night and day, the difference being particularly evident between 2400 and 0300, when the mean cortisol level of the depressed patients was twice that of the control subjects. While in our study the amplitude

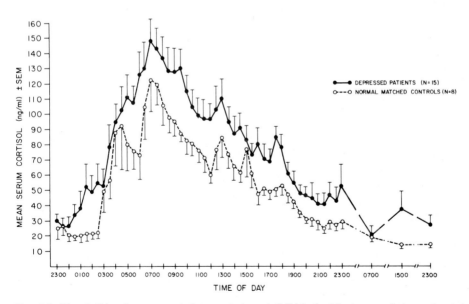

Fig. 9.5. Mean half-hourly serum cortisol concentrations, ± S.E.M., for 15 primary endogenous depressives and 8 normal control subjects matched to the patients on age, sex, race, and menstrual status. Figure reproduced from Rubin et al. (1980).

318

of the circadian cortisol rhythm was not blunted in the patients compared to the controls, in contrast to the data shown in Fig. 9.4, the circadian increase in cortisol appeared to begin several hours earlier in the patients (about midnight) compared to the control subjects (about 0300). This phase advance in cortisol secretion may be related to the circadian advance in the sleep–wake cycle (early morning awakening) that many endogenously depressed patients experience, but no studies that address this possibility have yet been published. It is of interest that following successful treatment of depressed patients, both their sleep architecture and their cortisol secretory patterns usually return to normal.

A specific indicator of the hyperactivity of the ACTH/cortisol axis in depression is the early escape of these hormones from dexamethasone suppression. Dexamethasone (1.0 or 2.0 mg p.o.) given at midnight normally suppresses ACTH and cortisol for a full 24 h. However, endogenously depressed patients often show an inappropriate increase in serum cortisol between 16 and 24 h after dexamethasone. Both the normal controls and the depressed patients shown in Fig. 9.5 were given the drug (1.0 mg p.o.) at 2300 on the second night, and serum cortisol was measured every 8 h for the next 24 h. The control subjects suppressed normally, whereas the depressed patients showed a typical pattern of cortisol escape at 16 and 24 h after administration. The dexamethasone suppression test has

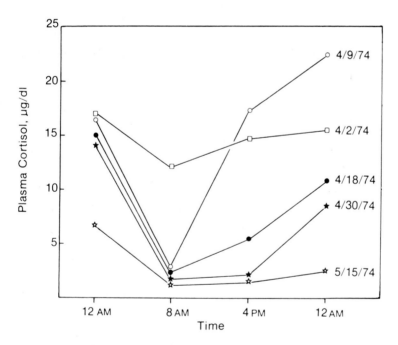

Fig. 9.6. Serial dexamethasone (DEX) suppression tests in a 49-year-old depressed woman before (2 and 9 April 1974) and during antidepressant drug treatment. DEX (1.0 mg p.o.) was given immediately after the first midnight plasma cortisol sample was drawn. The initial early cortisol escape from DEX suppression gradually converted to a normal, full 24-h suppression with symptomatic improvement. Figure reproduced, with permission, from Carroll et al. (1976). Copyright 1976 by the American Medical Association.

a high specificity for endogenous depression (few false positives in non-endogenously depressed patients and other types of psychiatric disorders), but its sensitivity is only 60–70% (30–40% false negatives in definitely endogenous depressives). It has a high construct validity, in that a positive dexamethasone suppression test is associated with familial depression (Schlesser et al. 1980); it is more frequently positive in suicidal compared to non-suicidal depressives; and it normalizes gradually with treatment (Carroll et al. 1976). Fig. 9.6 depicts typical dexamethasone suppression responses during illness and recovery in a 49-year-old, agitated, unipolar depressed woman with a strong family history of depression (Carroll et al. 1976). The first test (2 April) was carried out three days after hospital admission, and the second (9 April) was carried out a week later, when the patient was receiving placebo medication. High levels of pre–dexamethasone plasma cortisol at 2300 and obvious cortisol escape from dexamethasone suppression characterized the first two tests. The patient was then treated with antidepressant medication, and over the next five weeks her dexamethasone suppression tests gradually normalized as her illness remitted. At the time of her last test, which showed complete 24-h cortisol suppression, her pre-dexamethasone midnight cortisol level had decreased to the normal range.

The cortisol escape from dexamethasone suppression in depressed patients does not appear to be a result of altered pharmacokinetics of dexamethasone metabolism (Carroll et al. 1980; Rubin et al. 1980), and thus it most likely reflects enhanced limbic–hypothalamic driving of the pituitary–adrenal cortical axis. While different doses of dexamethasone have been tried in order to discriminate endogenous from non-endogenous depressives (Carroll et al. 1981), 2300 to midnight has been the time of dexamethasone administration used in all studies.

GH rhythms in depression

As mentioned earlier, the major secretory episode of GH in adults during the entire 24-h period occurs shortly after the onset of SWS, in the first hour or two of the sleep period, and is closely linked to this sleep stage (Quabbe 1979; Takahashi 1979; Parker et al. 1979; Mendelson et al. 1979). Elderly patients, in whom a normal reduction or loss of SWS occurs (Kales 1968), also may have reduced nocturnal GH secretion (Murri et al. 1980). Because GH secretion is enhanced by a variety of stimuli, GH provocation tests in depression have been performed with L-dopa, insulin-provoked hypoglycemia, 5-hydroxytryptophan, amphetamine, the α-adrenergic agonist clonidine, and the tricyclic antidepressant desmethylimipramine. While the GH response to L-dopa typically has been normal in depression, many of these other stimuli have revealed a blunted GH response (Rubin and Kendler 1977; Carroll et al. 1978; Rubin et al. 1979; Checkley 1980). Taken together, the data suggest that the defect resulting in the blunted GH response in depression is at the hypothalamic and not at the pituitary level, although some investigators have reported an inappropriate GH response to TRH in depression (Takahashi et al. 1975; Maeda et al. 1975).

Only one study of the 24-h secretion pattern of GH in depression has been published to date. Schilkrut et al. (1975) measured half-hourly plasma GH concentrations during sleep in six endogenously depressed patients, five bipolar and one unipolar, following one adaptation night in the sleep laboratory. Only one patient showed normal GH secretion in relation to his first SWS episode. Another patient, age 36, had a normal GH elevation but no SWS evident in her sleep recordings. Two patients showed only minimal nocturnal GH secretion, although they both had SWS, albeit reduced. The final two patients had delayed GH elevations, which were related only to their second SWS episodes of the night. As a group, the six depressives showed a shortened total sleep period, prolonged sleep latency (time between lights out and sleep onset), increased wake time, and reduced amounts of both SWS and REM sleep – the usual pattern of sleep disturbance in depression, as detailed earlier. Schilkrut et al. (1975) interpreted these data to indicate that the reduced nocturnal GH release in their depressed patients was probably related to their sleep disturbances. GH data from our laboratory are quite consistent with the findings of Schilkrut et al. (1975), and our interpretation of the link between disrupted sleep architecture and reduced nocturnal GH secretion in endogenous depression is similar (Rubin et al. unpublished observations).

Gonadotropin and gonadal steroid rhythms in depression

As noted earlier, in normal adults the gonadotropins (LH and FSH) are secreted episodically, with no apparent circadian rhythms, while testosterone has a circadian rhythm of modest amplitude, higher circulating levels occurring at night (Rebar and Yen 1979; Judd 1979). The gonadal steroid hormones (testosterone and the estrogens) have been implicated in the modulation of sexual and perhaps even aggressive behavior in adulthood (Schiavi and White 1976; Brown 1980; Rubin et al. 1981a). Since, as noted above, decreased energy in general and decreased sexual drive in particular are part of the symptom cluster of endogenous depression, the secretion patterns of the pituitary gonadotropins and their peripheral target hormones, the gonadal steroids, may have relevance in this illness (Rubin 1981).

Only a few studies of LH and FSH patterns in depression have been reported, and their results differ. Benkert (1975) measured plasma LH concentrations serially every 15 min for 4 h in seven unipolar endogenously depressed men and five bipolar manic men. Six of the depressed men and four of the manic men had plasma LH levels within the normal range, whereas one depressed and one manic patient had abnormally high, spiking levels. Following treatment and recovery from the affective illness episode, both men had LH values within the normal range. Unfortunately, Benkert (1975) gave no clinical, demographic, or treatment data about his patients. Neither FSH nor testosterone were measured in the plasma samples.

In a study of women, Altman et al. (1975) measured plasma LH concentrations serially every 15 min between 0900 and 1100 in 12 primary, unipolar, postmenopausal depressives and in 13 normal age-matched postmenopausal controls. The mean plasma LH concentration of the depressed women was about 30% less than that of the matched control group, a statistically significant difference. Neither FSH nor gonadal steroids were determined in these subjects.

We recently reported a preliminary study of plasma LH and FSH measured in samples taken every 30 min during sleep (2300–0700), during the day (0730–1500), and for $4\,^1/_2$ h (1530–2000) following an intravenous infusion of 100 μg LH-RH, in nine primary endogenously depressed men, eight unipolar and one bipolar, and in six age- and race-matched normal male control subjects (Rubin et al. 1981b). Average levels of both gonadotropins were 15–30% lower in the depressed men than in the controls both at night and during the day. However, this was a statistically non-significant difference, in part due to the small sample size. The increases of mean LH after LH-RH administration in the patients and controls were equivalent, whereas the mean post-LH-RH FSH increase in the patients was about half that of the controls. We also measured testosterone in our patients, as detailed below.

These few reports of plasma gonadotropin concentrations suggest reduced diurnal and nocturnal circulating LH, and perhaps FSH, levels in depressed patients compared to matched control subjects. This difference is evident in those studies (Altman et al. 1975; Rubin et al. 1981b) that utilized serial blood sampling over time to obtain an integrated measure of normally rapidly fluctuating LH levels as a result of episodic hormone secretion. Replication studies are needed to confirm or refute these findings.

There have been similarly few reported studies of gonadal steroid regulation in depression. Sachar et al. (1973b) measured plasma testosterone concentrations once, at 0800, in 15 severely depressed men, five bipolar and 10 unipolar, during illness and shortly after recovery. The mean pre-treatment plasma testosterone level in the 15 patients was not significantly different from their mean post-treatment level, and both were within the range of values for normal men in the investigator's laboratory. There was a high correlation between pre- and post-treatment levels of testosterone across subjects (+0.85) and a moderate negative correlation between age and the hormone (−0.62), but a weak, non-significant correlation between the degree of loss of libido and testosterone levels (+0.41) (our calculations of rank-order correlations). Gonadotropin levels were not measured in these patients.

Vogel et al. (1978) determined plasma testosterone once at 0900 in 27 primary, unipolar depressed men and in 13 age-matched normal male volunteers. Both total and free mean levels were about 30% lower in the patients than in the controls; these were statistically significant differences. In contrast, in a subset of 15 depressives and 12 controls, the mean plasma estradiol (E_2) level was 50% higher in the patients than in the control subjects, again a statistically significant difference. Unfortunately, Vogel et al. (1978) did not measure gonadotropin levels to complement their extensive gonadal steroid data.

In our aforementioned study of LH and FSH (Rubin et al. 1981b), we also measured plasma testosterone in the half-hourly nocturnal and diurnal plasma samples taken from the nine primary endogenously depressed men and six matched controls. The mean plasma testosterone concentrations both at night and during the day were about 20% lower in the patients than in the controls. The testosterone values in this study were based on multiple plasma samples and thus represented accurate estimations of testosterone concentrations. This finding of reduced circulating testosterone in depressed men accorded with the same finding in the study of Vogel et al. (1978); however, the smaller sample size as well as the smaller magnitude of the hormone difference obviated statistical significance in our study

(Rubin et al. 1981b), in contrast to the significant findings of Vogel et al. (1978).

Vogel et al. (1978) also studied women, measuring plasma E_2 and testosterone con-centrations at 0900 twice weekly in 22 primary, unipolar premenopausal depressives and in 10 normal age-matched premenopausal controls. The weekly mean plasma E_2 concentra-tions in the depressed women were 60–80 % higher than those in the matched control group; these were statistically significant differences. The weekly mean plasma testosterone concentrations in the patients similarly were 90–180% higher than those in the matched control group; again, these were statistically significant differences. Because of decreased testosterone binding to plasma protein in the depressed women, their mean free testosterone level was 300 % higher than that of the control subjects. Gonadotropins were not measured in these women.

These few reports of plasma gonadal steroid concentrations suggest reduced circulating testosterone, by 20–30%, both at night and during the day in depressed men compared to matched controls. However, the one study of testosterone before and shortly after treatment showed no difference (Sachar et al. 1973b), raising the question of whether reduced circulating testosterone in depressed men is a state-dependent phenomenon. There are no other data available at present to corroborate the findings of Vogel et al. (1978) of increased circulating E_2 in depressed men and of increased circulating E_2, and testosterone as well, in depressed women.

Taken together, these data on hypothalamo–pituitary–gonadal function in endogenously depressed patients suggest a dysfunction of this endocrine axis, as reflected by reduced circulating levels of LH, testosterone, and possibly FSH and increased circulating levels of E_2 in depressed men, and reduced LH but increased E_2 and testosterone in depressed women. As both gonadotropins and gonadal steroids were measured in the same blood samples in only a few studies, the findings become even more tenuous. Clearly, more detailed and comprehensive replication studies must be performed.

PRL rhythms in depression

As mentioned earlier, PRL secretion, like GH secretion, is sleep dependent, with progressively increasing circulating levels during the night (Frantz 1979). In contrast to GH, sleep-related PRL secretion usually is maintained in the elderly (Murri et al. 1980). Only a few studies of plasma PRL patterns in depression have been conducted. The PRL response to TRH has been reported as both augmented and reduced in depressed patients compared to normal controls. More consistent has been the finding, albeit in very few studies, that basal PRL levels in endogenously depressed patients are reduced. Mendlewicz et al. (1980a) measured plasma PRL concentrations twice, 15 minutes apart, at 0900 in five premenopausal and 19 postmenopausal depressed bipolar women and in 31 premenopausal and 11 postmenopausal normal women. Mean basal PRL levels in both the premenopausal and the postmenopausal depressives were significantly lower, by 50–80%, than in their corresponding controls. Both groups of depressed women also had significantly reduced PRL responses to TRH, by 50–60%, compared to their controls.

Asnis et al. (1980) measured plasma PRL levels three times, between 0900 and 0930, in

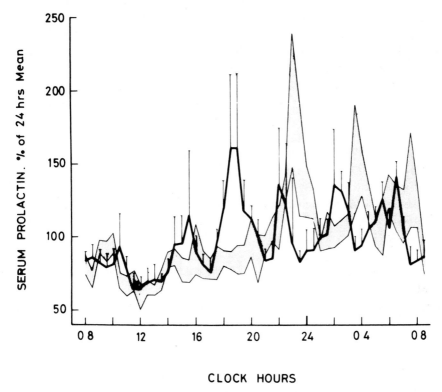

Fig. 9.7. Mean half-hourly serum PRL concentrations, ± S.E.M., for seven endogenous depressives and five normal control subjects. Shaded area represents ±1 S.E.M. for the controls. Figure reproduced, with permission, from Halbreich et al. (1979). Copyright 1979 by the American Medical Association.

15 female and four male endogenous depressives, both before treatment and after full recovery about six weeks later. The mean PRL concentration in the patients was significantly lower, by one-third, during their illness than after recovery.

Nielsen (1980) measured plasma PRL levels at 0800 and at 1400 in five female and 12 male endogenous depressives, both before treatment and during the third week of treatment with a tricyclic antidepressant. The mean pre-treatment PRL level in the patients was within the normal range. Following treatment there was a moderate, statistically significant increase of about 25 % in plasma PRL, probably related to drug therapy. PRL values at the two times of day were not different and were within the normal range.

Only two studies of circadian PRL patterns in depression, based on serial blood sampling, have been published to date. Halbreich et al. (1979) measured half-hourly serum PRL concentrations for 24 h in seven endogenously depressed patients, one of whom was bipolar, and in five normal control subjects. As shown in Fig. 9.7, the circadian PRL rhythm of the patients differed from that of the controls only insofar as the patients had an elevated mean PRL level at 1900, during which time they were fully alert. Nocturnal sleep-related PRL secretion appeared to be similar in the two groups of subjects. Halbreich et al. (1979) did not have a ready explanation for the increased PRL levels in their patients at this particular time of evening. PRL data from our laboratory are at variance with the findings of Halbreich et al. (1979), in that they do not replicate the PRL increase at 1900, and they reveal reduced nocturnal sleep-related PRL secretion, in depressed patients compared to matched normal controls (Rubin et al., unpublished observations). Our explanation for the latter finding is the same as that for the reduced nocturnal sleep-related GH secretion seen in depression, i.e. disruption of sleep architecture with consequent disturbance in the sleep-related secretion patterns of both hormones.

Mendlewicz et al. (1980b) measured half-hourly to hourly plasma PRL concentrations for 24 h in 10 unipolar and eight bipolar primary depressives and in 10 normal control subjects. The two groups of patients were similar to each other, being mostly women, and about 50% pre- and 50% post-menopausal, but the normal controls were young men. Fig. 9.8 summarizes the PRL data; the mean 24 h PRL levels in the bipolar and unipolar patients were 64% and 136%, respectively, of the mean 24 h PRL of the control subjects. The lower mean level of the bipolars apparently was due to a blunted nocturnal PRL increase, whereas the higher mean level in the unipolars appeared to result from increased daytime PRL secretion. These clearly different plasma PRL profiles between unipolar and bipolar depressives may prove to be a diagnostically useful differentiating feature, and replication studies are warranted.

TSH rhythms in depression

As mentioned earlier, there is a normal circadian rhythm of TSH secretion, with highest circulating levels occurring in the late evening hours, usually prior to the time of sleep onset (Weeke 1973; Parker et al. 1976; Azukizawa et al. 1976). Many studies of serum and plasma TSH patterns in depression have been performed, but these have dealt almost exclusively with the TSH response to exogenously administered TRH (Prange 1977; Hollister et al. 1977; Kirkegaard et al. 1978). In 40–50% of endogenously depressed patients the TSH response to TRH is blunted compared to control subjects. This response

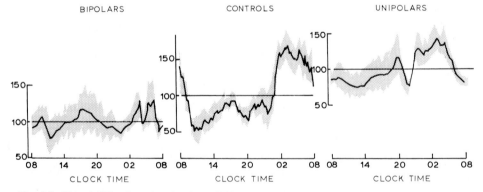

Fig. 9.8. Mean half-hourly to hourly plasma PRL concentrations for eight bipolar depressives, 10 normal controls, and 10 unipolar depressives. Shaded areas represent ± S.E.M. Figure reproduced, with permission, from Mendlewicz et al. (1980b).

generally reverts to normal with successful treatment of the depressive episode, but a persistently blunted TSH response in spite of clinical improvement may predict a relapse when antidepressant treatment is discontinued. The reduced TSH response to TRH in depression is not easily explained, as it occurs at the pituitary level, and there is no clear disturbance of overall thyroid function in this illness (Dewhurst et al. 1969; Kolakowska et al. 1977; Rinieris et al. 1978). One possibility is that CSF TRH may be elevated in depression (Kirkegaard et al. 1979), leading to down-regulation of the TRH receptors on the pituitary thyrotrophs. However, the failure of CSF TRH levels to decline in treated patients, in the face of clinical improvement and normalization of the TSH response to administered TRH, argues against this explanation.

Only two studies of circadian TSH patterns in depression have been published to date. Weeke and Weeke (1978) determined serum TSH concentrations at midnight, prior to sleep onset, and at 1400 in 13 female and six male endogenously depressed patients. There was a diminution or absence of the normal nocturnal increase of serum TSH, which was significantly correlated with the severity of depression as assessed by a rating scale. No gross disturbances of thyroid function were evident in these patients. Weeke and Weeke (1980) extended their studies by measuring serum TSH levels hourly for 24 h in one female and three male patients with severe endogenous depression. Fig. 9.9 portrays the four individual TSH profiles and indicates that, in general, the patients showed a pattern similar to that of normal subjects, with lowest serum TSH levels during the day and highest levels at night. Weeke and Weeke (1980) concluded that a phase shift of the TSH circadian rhythm could not account for their earlier finding of a significant correlation between the severity of depressive symptomatology and the blunting of the TSH rhythm.

Other hormone rhythms in depression

A deficiency of CNS vasopressin activity has been hypothesized as a neuroendocrine substrate of depression, and conversely, CNS vasopressin has been postulated to be hyperactive in mania (Gold et al. 1978). Preliminary data suggest an approximately 25%

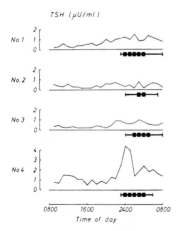

Fig. 9.9. Hourly serum TSH concentrations in four endogenous depressives. Horizontal lines indicate supine position at the time of blood sampling, and filled squares indicate sleep. Figure reproduced, with permission, from Weeke and Weeke (1980). Copyright 1980 by Munksgaard International Publishers, Copenhagen.

reduction of CSF vasopressin levels in drug-free unipolar and bipolar depressives compared to control subjects (Gold et al. personal communication). To date, there have been no studies reported of plasma vasopressin rhythms in depression.

Studies of opioid compounds and their precursors in plasma and CSF have been hindered by the non-specificity of most assay techniques. Jeffcoate et al. (1978) implied that plasma and CSF levels of β-LPH were normal in depression, although these investigators presented no data. Lindström et al. (1978) found a small elevation of two CSF endorphin-like compounds in four manic patients during their manic phases, but these compounds were not reduced when the patients were depressed. Pickar et al. (1980), using a radioreceptor assay sensitive primarily to opioid peptides (enkephalins and endorphins) and less so to opiate alkaloids (morphine, etc.), studied a 57-year-old manic-depressive woman and found higher plasma opioid peptide activity during a manic phase than during a depressive episode. No more detailed studies of plasma or CSF endorphin or enkephalin levels in depression have yet been reported.

Finally, as mentioned earlier, melatonin has a circadian rhythm in plasma, with highest levels occurring during sleep. Jimerson et al. (1977) found similar patterns of urine melatonin excretion in six patients with severe primary depression and in eight healthy controls; in both groups, increased melatonin excretion occurred at night. Two studies of plasma melatonin rhythms in depression have been published to date, and the results are at some variance with these urine melatonin data. Mendlewicz et al. (1980c) measured hourly plasma melatonin concentrations for 24 h in one bipolar and three unipolar depressed women. The patients were studied while ill, and again 4–6 weeks later, following successful treatment with tricyclic antidepressant medication. As indicated in Fig. 9.10, three of the four patients failed to show a normal nocturnal increase in plasma melatonin. These patterns persisted after treatment, suggesting a persistent disturbance of the factors controlling plasma melatonin levels, but this disturbance remains to be elucidated.

Wetterberg et al. (1981) measured serum cortisol and melatonin concentrations every 4 h before and after a dexamethasone suppression test in 12 patients with major depression. These patients did show a nocturnal increase in serum melatonin, which was inversely proportional to the degree of cortisol escape from dexamethasone suppression. These investigators proposed a pineal involvement in ACTH and cortisol regulation in depression, i.e. reduced melatonin suggests decreased pineal release of a putative corticotropin-releasing factor inhibiting factor, with consequent enhanced production of ACTH and escape from dexamethasone suppression. In future studies of depressed patients, it would be of interest to study both plasma melatonin and CSF AVT, since, as described earlier, the former also may be a releasing hormone for the latter.

Endocrine effects of sleep deprivation therapy in depression

As indicated above, short-term sleep deprivation has been used as a treatment for endogenous depression, with short-term positive results. A few studies have shown that acute sleep deprivation in depression also has an effect on some of the aforementioned hormone profiles. With reference to the hypothalamo–pituitary–adrenal cortical axis,

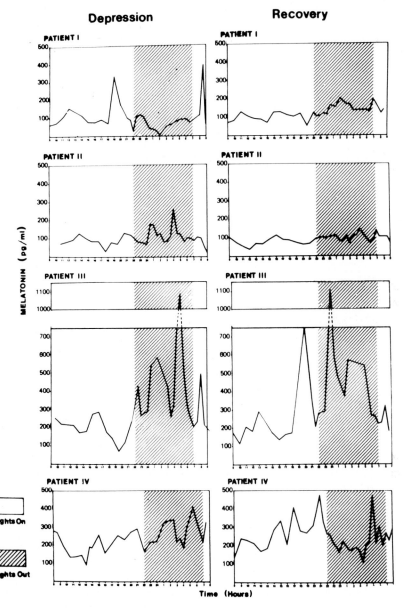

Fig. 9.10. Hourly plasma melatonin concentrations in four depressed women, three unipolar (I–III) and one bipolar (IV), before and after successful antidepressant treatment. Figure reproduced, with permission, from Mendlewicz et al. (1980c).

Yamaguchi et al. (1978) performed a single-night sleep deprivation trial on 17 male and three female endogenous depressives, 13 unipolar and seven bipolar. Ten normal control subjects also were studied. Plasma cortisol was measured every 4 h from 0800 the day

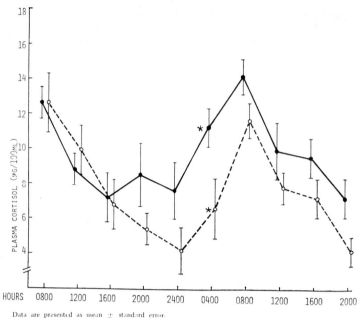

HOURS 0800 1200 1600 2000 2400 0400 0800 1200 1600 2000

Data are presented as mean ± standard error.
* The difference between the two groups was significant at 04.00 (P<0.02) (Mann-Whitney U test).

Fig. 9.11. Mean four-hourly plasma cortisol concentrations, ± S.E.M., for 20 endogenous depressives (solid line) and 10 normal controls (dashed line), before, during, and after one night of total sleep deprivation. Figure reproduced, with permission, from Yamaguchi et al. (1978).

before until 2000 the evening after the sleep-deprived night. As is portrayed in Fig. 9.11, on the day after sleep deprivation the mean cortisol concentrations of the depressed patients were higher than those of the controls and also were higher than their own levels on the day before sleep deprivation. The 12 patients who showed a clinical response to the deprivation therapy had a slightly more pronounced circadian cortisol rhythm than the eight non-responders. Similarly, Gerner et al. (1979) found a higher mean level of morning serum cortisol, after one night of sleep deprivation, in five depressed patients who showed a clinical response to the deprivation, compared to four depressed patients who were non-responders. Nasrallah et al. (1980) treated one recurrent, unipolar, psychomotor-retarded, primary, endogenously depressed man, first with total sleep deprivation three times per week for two weeks, and then by a course of electroconvulsive therapy (ECT). After the second sleep deprivation night his clinical state was mildly improved, and his overnight dexamethasone suppression test reverted from cortisol non-suppression to suppression (one 0800 post-dexamethasone sample only). Continued sleep deprivation did not produce further clinical improvement, and his dexamethasone test again showed cortisol escape. After eight subsequent sessions of ECT, both his clinical state and his dexamethasone test became normal.

With reference to other hormones, Vestergaard et al. (1979) measured serum PRL in seven women with primary endogenous depression and found their morning serum PRL levels lower after sleep deprivation than before it. This is not surprising, since PRL secretion is sleep related. Kvist and Kirkegaard (1980) determined the TSH response to TRH in 14 unipolar, four bipolar, and 10 unclassified endogenous depressives before and after a series of total sleep deprivations (two per week until recovery or clinical improvement ceased). Long-term follow up was accomplished on all patients. The eight patients in whom recovery occurred following the course of sleep deprivation were considered responders. Of these eight, five failed to normalize their TSH responses to TRH after treatment, and all five relapsed within a few weeks. The three responders who did show a normal TSH response after sleep deprivation remained free of symptoms for at least 6 months. This study amplifies and supports these investigators' earlier work on the predictive value of the post-treatment TSH response to TRH (Kirkegaard et al. 1975).

DISCUSSION

This review suggests that disturbances in the secretion patterns of several polypeptide and steroid hormones form a regular part of the syndrome of endogenous depression. Because the same putative CNS neurotransmitters appear to be involved both in the modulation of effects and in the regulation of the hypothalamic releasing and inhibiting factors, it is tempting to suggest, as mentioned earlier, that a common CNS neurotransmitter dysfunction underlies both the depressive state and the altered endocrine dynamics. Reduced norepinephrine neurotransmission has been the prime candidate in this regard (Rubin et al. 1973; Rubin and Kendler 1977; Checkley 1980), but proposing this hypothesis has been considerably easier than demonstrating it. There have been some suggestive studies, such as the finding by Garver et al. (1975), in 12 depressed patients, of a positive correlation between urine methoxyhydroxyphenylglycol (MHPG) excretion and the GH response to insulin hypoglycemia. MHPG has been considered the major urinary metabolite of CNS norepinephrine, and thus a reduction in MHPG excretion might indicate a reduced adrenergic stimulation of GH secretion in response to hypoglycemia in depression. However, not only is quantitation of urine MHPG somewhat difficult (Hollister et al. 1980), but also this compound in urine in fact may not come primarily from the CNS (Blombery et al. 1980). Thus, while attractive and of considerable heuristic value, the catecholamine deficiency hypothesis of depression is not yet supported by sufficient evidence.

Another explanation for the several endocrine changes in depression is that cortisol hypersecretion may be the primary disturbance, and the other changes (reduced GH response to various stimuli, blunted TSH response to TRH, etc.) all may be secondary to the hypercortisolemia, similar to the endocrine changes that occur in Cushing's syndrome (Kendler and Davis 1977). If this were so, the panoply of endocrine changes in depression should occur in the same individuals, i.e. the changes should be positively correlated in their severities. Again there have been some suggestive studies, such as the finding by Loosen et al. (1978), in seven unipolar depressed women, of an inverse relationship between 0900 serum cortisol levels and peak serum TSH responses to TRH. Detailed

330

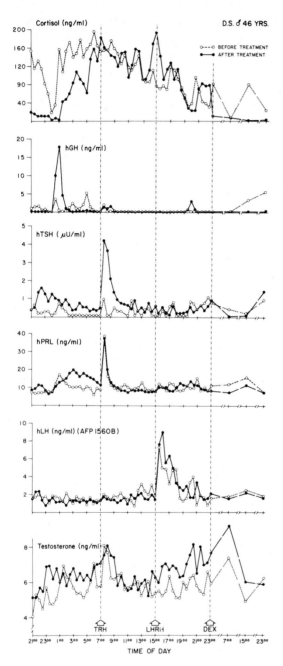

Fig. 9.12. Multiple half-hourly serum pituitary and steroid hormone concentrations in a 46-year-old endogenously depressed man before and after treatment. Arrows near bottom of figure indicate administration of TRH (100 µg i.v.), LH-RH (100 µg i.v.), and dexamethasone (1.0 mg p.o.). Figure reproduced from Rubin et al. (1980).

testing of this hypothesis requires multiple hormone measures, on multiple blood samples taken from each patient, before and after several endocrine perturbation tests. And, to achieve stability in the multivariate statistical analyses required to interrelate data on many hormones, a large sample size is required. Nevertheless, such studies are being undertaken, utilizing radioimmunoassay techniques to process thousands of blood samples. Fig. 9.12 portrays multiple serum hormone concentrations in an endogenously depressed man participating in our current study (Rubin et al. 1980, 1981a). Hormone profiles are shown both before and after antidepressant treatment. Several of the aforementioned hormone changes were apparent in this patient while he was ill, including nocturnal cortisol hypersecretion and escape from dexamethasone suppression, reduced nocturnal GH and PRL secretion, blunted TSH response to TRH, etc. While these endocrine disturbances did occur together in this particular man, we will need to study 40–50 patients both before and after treament to determine the interrelations of these changes across subjects, in order to support or refute the hypothesis of cortisol-induced secondary endocrine changes in depression.

SUMMARY

Several changes in hormone dynamics occur in patients with endogenous depression. These include hypersecretion and blunted circadian rhythms of ACTH and cortisol; early cortisol escape from dexamethasone suppression; reduced slow wave sleep-related GH secretion; reduced GH response to insulin hypoglycemia, amphetamine, clonidine and desmethylimipramine; blunted TSH circadian rhythm and blunted TSH response to TRH; reduced secretion of LH, and perhaps also of testosterone in male depressives; reduced sleep-related PRL secretion; and possible disturbances of other hormones as well. Some of these hormone changes may prove useful as aids in the differential diagnosis of the endogenous subtype of major depression and in the prediction of treatment response. Both the affect disturbance and the endocrine changes may be sequelae of common CNS amine neurotransmitter dysfunctions, but this attractive hypothesis remains to be verified.

AKNOWLEDGMENTS

Supported by National Institute of Mental Health (NIMH) Grants MH 28380 and MH 34471, by NIMH Research Scientist Development Award MH 47363 (to R.T.R.), and by NIH General Clinical Research Center Grant RR 00425.

REFERENCES

Akerstedt, T., Froberg, J.E., Friberg, Y. and Wetterberg, L. (1979) Melatonin excretion, body temperature and subjective arousal during 64 hours of sleep deprivation. Psychoneuroendocrinology 4, 219-225.

Altman, N., Sachar, E.J., Gruen, P.H., Halpern, F.S. and Eto, S. (1975) Reduced plasma LH concentrations in postmenopausal depressed women. Psychosom. Med. 37, 274-276.

American Psychiatric Association (1980) Diagnostic and Statistical Manual of Mental Disorders (Third Edition), Washington, D.C.

Anders, T., Emde, R. and Parmelee, A. (eds) (1971) A Manual of Standardized Terminology, Techniques and Criteria for Scoring of States of Sleep and Wakefulness in Newborn Infants. UCLA Brain Information Service,

NINDS Neurological Information Network, Los Angeles.

Aschoff, J. (1979) Circadian rhythms: general features and endocrinological aspects. In: Endocrine Rhythms (Krieger, D.T. ed.), pp. 1-61, Raven Press; New York.

Asnis, G.M., Nathan, R.S., Halbreich, U., Halpern, F.S. and Sachar, E.J. (1980) Prolactin changes in major depressive disorders. Am. J. Psychiat. 137, 1117-1118.

Avery, D. and Winokur, G. (1978) Suicide, attempted suicide, and relapse rates in depression: occurrence after ECT and antidepressant therapy. Arch. Gen. Psychiat. 35, 749-753.

Azukizawa, M., Pekary, A.E., Hershman, J.M. and Parker, D.C. (1976) Plasma thyrotropin, thyroxine, and triiodothyronine relationships in man. J. Clin. Endocrinol. Metab. 43, 533-542.

Benkert, O. (1975) Studies on pituitary hormone and releasing hormones in depression and sexual impotence. Prog. Brain Res. 42, 25-36.

Bergland, R.M. and Page, R.B. (1978) Can the pituitary secrete directly to the brain? (affirmative anatomical evidence). Endocrinology 102, 1325-1338.

Bergland, R.M. and Page, R.B. (1979) Pituitary-brain vascular relations: a new paradigm. Science 204, 18-24.

Blombery, P.A., Kopin, I.J., Gordon, E.K., Markey, S.P. and Ebert, M.H. (1980) Conversion of MHPG to vanillylmandelic acid: implications for the importance of urinary MHPG. Arch. Gen. Psychiat. 37, 1095-1098.

Boyar, R.M. (1978) Sleep-related endocrine rhythms. In: The Hypothalamus (Reichlin, S., Baldessarini, R.J. and Martin, J.B. eds), pp. 373-386, Raven Press, New York.

Brown, W.A. (1980) Testosterone and human behavior. Internat. J. Ment. Health, 9, 46-66.

Carroll, B.J. (1976) Limbic system-adrenal cortex regulation in depression and schizophrenia. Psychosom. Med. 38, 106-121.

Carroll, B.J. (1978) Neuroendocrine dysfunction in psychiatric disorders. In: Psychopharmacology: A Generation of Progress (Lipton, M.A., DiMascio, A. and Killam, K.F. eds), pp. 487-497, Raven Press, New York.

Carroll, B.J., Fielding, J.M. and Blashki, T.G. (1973) Depression rating scales: a critical review. Arch. Gen. Psychiat. 28, 361-366.

Carroll, B.J., Curtis, G.C. and Mendels, J. (1976) Neuroendocrine regulation in depression I. Limbic system-adrenocortical dysfunction. Arch. Gen. Psychiat. 33, 1039-1044.

Carroll, B.J., Schroeder, K., Mukhopadhyay, S., Greden, J.F., Feinberg, M., Ritchie, J. and Tarika, J. (1980) Plasma dexamethasone concentrations and cortisol suppression response in patients with endogenous depression. J. Clin. Endocrinol. Metab. 51, 433-437.

Carroll, B.J., Feinberg, M., Greden, J.F., Tarika, J., Albala, A.A., Haskett, R.F., James, N.McI., Kronfol, Z., Lohr, N., Steiner, M., de Vigne, J.P. and Young, E. (1981) A specific laboratory test for the diagnosis of melancholia: standardization, validation, and clinical utility. Arch. Gen. Psychiat. 38, 15-22.

Checkley, S.A. (1980) Neuroendocrine tests of monoamine function in man: a review of basic theory and its application to the study of depressive illness. Psychol. Med. 10, 35-53.

Coble, P.A., Kupfer, D.J., Spiker, D.G., Neil, J.F. and McPartland, R.J. (1979) EEG sleep in primary depression. J. Affect. Disorders 1, 131-138.

Copinschi, G., L'Hermite, M., Golstein, J., Leclercq, R., Desir, D., Vanhaelst, L., Virasoro, E., Robyn, C. and Van Cauter, E. (1978) Interrelations between circadian and ultradian variations of PRL, ACTH, cortisol, β-MSH and TSH in normal man. In: Progress in Prolactin Physiology and Pathology (Robyn, C. and Harter, M. eds), pp. 165-172, Elsevier, Amsterdam.

Dent, R.R.M., Guilleminault, C., Albert, L.H., Posner, B.I., Cox, B.M. and Goldstein, A. (1981) Diurnal rhythm of plasma immunoreactive β-endorphin and its relationship to sleep stages and plasma rhythms of cortisol and prolactin. J. Clin. Endocrinol. Metab. 52, 942-947.

Dewhurst, K.E., El Kabir, D.J., Harris, G.W. and Mandelbrote, B.M. (1969) Observations on the blood concentration of thyrotrophic hormone (T.S.H.) in schizophrenia and the affective states. Brit. J. Psychiat. 115, 1003-1011.

Doerr, P. and Pirke, K.M. (1976) Cortisol-induced suppression of plasma testosterone in normal adult males. J. Clin. Endocrinol. Metab. 43, 622-629.

Donald, R.A. (1980) ACTH and related peptides. Clin. Endocrinol. 12, 491-524.

Drucker-Colin, R.R. and Spanis, C.W. (1976) Is there a sleep transmitter? Prog. Neurobiol. 6, 1-22.

Feinberg, M., Carroll, B.J., Steiner, M. and Commorato, A.J. (1979) Misdiagnoses of endogenous depression with research diagnostic criteria. Lancet i, 267.

Frantz, A.G. (1979) Rhythms in prolactin secretion. In: Endocrine Rhythms (Krieger, D.T. ed.), pp. 175-186, Raven, New York.

Garver, D.L., Pandey, G.N., Dekirmenjian, H. and Deleon-Jones, F. (1975) Growth hormone and catecholamines in affective disease. Am. J. Psychiat. 132, 1149-1154.

Gerner, R.H., Post, R.M., Gillin, C. and Bunney Jr, W.E. (1979) Biological and behavioral effects of one night's sleep deprivation in depressed patients and normals. J. Psychiat. Res. 15, 21-40.

Gillin, J.C., Duncan, W., Pettigrew, K.D., Frankel, B.L. and Snyder, F. (1979) Successful separation of depressed, normal, and insomniac subjects by EEG sleep data. Arch. Gen. Psychiat. 36, 85-89.

Gold, P.W., Goodwin, F.K. and Reus, V.I. (1978) Vasopressin in affective illness. Lancet i, 1233-1236.

Halbreich, U., Grunhaus, L. and Ben-David, M. (1979) Twenty-four-hour rhythm of prolactin in depressive patients. Arch. Gen. Psychiat. 36, 1183-1186.

Hartmann, E. (1973) The Functions of Sleep, Yale University Press, New Haven.

Hayward, J.N. (1977) Functional and morphological aspects of hypothalamic neurons. Physiol. Rev. 57, 574-658.

Hollister, L.E., Davis, K.L. and Berger, P.A. (1977) Thyrotropin-releasing hormone and psychiatric disorders. In: Neuroregulators and Psychiatric Disorders (Usdin, E., Hamburg, D.A. and Barchas, J.D. eds), pp. 250-257, Oxford, New York.

Hollister, L.E., Davis, K.L. and Berger, P.A. (1980) Subtypes of depression based on excretion of MHPG and response to nortriptyline. Arch. Gen. Psychiat. 37, 1107-1110.

Jacobs, K.W. (1976) A table for the determination of experimentwise error rate (alpha) from independent observations. Educ. Psychol. Meas. 36, 899-903.

Jacobs, L.S., Mendelson, W.B., Rubin, R.T. and Bauman, J.E. (1978) Failure of nocturnal prolactin suppression by methysergide to entrain changes in testosterone in normal men. J. Clin. Endocrinol. Metab. 46, 561-566.

Jeffcoate, W.J., Lowry, P.J., Rees, L.H.., Hope, J. and Besser, G.M. (1978) β-Lipotropin and β-endorphin in human plasma and CSF. Endocrinology. 102, A142.

Jimerson, D.C., Lynch, H.L., Post, R.M., Wurtman, R.J. and Bunney, W.E. (1977) Urinary melatonin rhythms during sleep deprivation in depressed patients and normals. Life Sci. 20, 1501-1508.

Jouvet, M. (1972) The role of monoamines and acetylcholine-containing neurons in the regulation of the sleep-waking cycle. Ergebn. Physiol. 64, 166-307.

Jouvet, M. (1975) Cholinergic mechanisms and sleep. In: Cholinergic Mechanisms (Waser, P.G. ed.), pp. 455-476, Raven Press, New York.

Jouvet, M. and Pujol, J.-F. (1974) Effects of central alterations of serotoninergic neurons upon the sleep-waking cycle. Adv. Biochem. Pharmacol. 11, 199-209.

Judd, H.L. (1979) Biorhythms of gonadotropins and testicular hormone secretion. In: Endocrine Rhythms (Krieger, D.T. ed.), pp. 299-324, Raven, New York.

Kales, A. (1968) Sleep and dreams. Ann. Intern. Med. 68, 1078-1104.

Kendell, R.E. (1976) The classification of depressions: a review of contemporary confusion. Br. J. Psychiat. 129, 15-28.

Kendler, K.S. and Davis, K.L. (1977) Elevated corticosteroids as a possible cause of abnormal neuroendocrine function in depressive illness. Commun. Psychopharmacol. 1, 183-194.

Kirkegaard, C., Nørlem, N., Lauridsen, U.B. and Bjørum, N. (1975) Prognostic value of thyrotropin-releasing hormone stimulation test in endogenous depression. Acta Psychiat. Scand. 52, 170-177.

Kirkegaard, C., Bjørum, N., Cohn, D. and Lauridsen U.B. (1978) Thyrotropin-releasing hormone (TRH) stimulation test in manic-depressive illness. Arch. Gen. Psychiat. 35, 1017-1021.

Kirkegaard, C., Faber, J., Hummer, L. and Rogowski, P. (1979) Increased levels of TRH in cerebrospinal fluid from patients with endogenous depression. Psychoneuroendocrinology 4, 227-235.

Klein, D.F. (1974) Endogenomorphic depression: a conceptual and terminological revision. Arch. Gen. Psychiat. 31, 447-454.

Kolakowska, T. and Swigar, M.E. (1977) Thyroid function in depression and alcohol abuse. Arch. Gen. Psychiat. 34, 984-988.

Krieger, D.T. (ed.) (1979a) Endocrine Rhythms (Comprehensive Endocrinology, Vol. 1), Raven, New York.

Krieger, D.T. (1979b) Rhythms in CRF, ACTH, and corticosteroids. In: Endocrine Rhythms (Krieger, D.T. ed.), pp. 123-142, Raven, New York.

Krieger, D.T. and Aschoff, J. (1979) Endocrine and other biological rhythms. In: Endocrinology, Vol. 3 (DeGroot, L.J., Cahill, G.F., Odell, W.D., Martini, L., Nelson, D.H., Potts, J.T., Steinberger, E. and Winegrad, A. eds), pp. 2079-2109, Grune and Stratton, New York.

Krieger, D.T., Liotta, A.S., Brownstein, M.J. and Zimmerman, E.A. (1980) ACTH, β-lipotropin, and related peptides in brain, pituitary, and blood. Rec. Prog. Horm. Res. 36, 277-344.

Kupfer, D.J. (1976) REM latency: a psychobiologic marker for primary depressive disease. Biol. Psychiat. 11, 159-174.

Kupfer, D.J. (1977) EEG sleep correlates of depression in man. In: Animal Models in Psychiatry and Neurology (Hanin, I. and Usdin, E. eds), pp. 181-188, Pergamon, Oxford.

Kupfer, D.J., Foster, F.G., Reich, L., Thompson, K.S. and Weiss, B. (1976) EEG sleep changes as predictors in depression. Am. J. Psychiat. 133, 622-626.

Kupfer, D.J., Foster, F.G., Coble, P., McPartland, R.J. and Ulrich, R.F. (1978) The application of EEG sleep for the differential diagnosis of affective disorders. Am. J. Psychiat. 135, 69-74.

Kupfer, D.J., Hanin, I. and Spiker, D. (1979) EEG sleep and tricyclic plasma levels in primary depression. Commun. Psychopharmacol. 3, 73-80.

Kvist, J. and Kirkegaard, C. (1980) Effect of repeated sleep deprivation on clinical symptoms and the TRH test in endogenous depression. Acta Psychiat. Scand. 62, 494-502.

Lindström, L.H., Widerlöv, E., Gunne, L.-M., Wahlström, A. and Terenius, L. (1978) Endorphins in human cerebrospinal fluid: clinical correlations to some psychotic states. Acta Psychiat. Scand. 57, 153-164.

Lipton, M.A., DiMascio, A. and Killam, K.F. (eds) (1978) Psychopharmacology: A Generation of Progress, Raven, New York.

Loosen, P.T., Prange, A.J. and Wilson, I.C. (1978) Influence of cortisol on TRH-induced TSH response in depression. Am. J. Psychiat. 135, 244-246.

Maeda, K., Kato, Y., Ohgo, S., Chihara, K., Yoshimoto, Y., Yamaguchi, N., Kuromaru, S. and Imura, H. (1975) Growth hormone and prolactin release after injection of thyrotropin-releasing hormone in patients with depression. J. Clin. Endocrinol. Metab. 40, 501-505.

Mason, J.W. (1968) A review of psychoendocrine research on the pituitary-adrenal cortical system. Psychosom. Med. 30, 576-607.

Mendelson, W.B., Jacobs, L.S., Gillin, J.C. and Wyatt, R.J. (1979) The regulation of insulin-induced and sleep-related human growth hormone secretion: a review. Psychoneuroendocrinology 4, 341-349.

Mendlewicz, J., Linkowski, P. and Brauman, H. (1980a) Reduced prolactin release after thyrotropin-releasing hormone in manic depression. New Engl. J. Med. 302, 1091-1092.

Mendlewicz, J., van Cauter, E., Linkowski, P., L'Hermite, M. and Robyn, C. (1980b) The 24-hour profile of prolactin in depression. Life Sci. 27, 2015-2024.

Mendlewicz, J., Branchey, L., Weinberg, U., Branchey, M., Linkowski, P. and Weitzman, E.D. (1980c) The 24 hour pattern of plasma melatonin in depressed patients before and after treatment, Commun. Psychopharmacol. 4, 49-55.

Miyatake, A., Morimoto, Y., Oishi, T., Hanasaki, N., Sugita, Y., Iijima, S., Teshima, Y., Hishikawa, Y. and Yamamura, Y., (1980) Circadian rhythm of serum testosterone and its relation to sleep: comparison with the variation in serum luteinizing hormone, prolactin, and cortisol in normal men. J. Clin. Endocrinol. Metab. 51, 1365-1371.

Mullen, P.E., Jeffcoate, W.J., Linsell, C., Howard, R. and Rees, L.H. (1979) The circadian variation of immunoreactive lipotrophin and its relationship to ACTH and growth hormone in man. Clin. Endocrinol. 11, 533-539.

Murri, L., Barreca, T., Cerone, G., Massetani, R., Gallamini, A. and Baldassarre, M. (1980) The 24-h pattern of human prolactin and growth hormone in healthy elderly subjects. Chronobiologia 7, 87-92.

Nasrallah, H.A., Kuperman, S. and Coryell, W. (1980) Reversal of dexamethasone nonsuppression with sleep deprivation in primary depression. Am. J. Psychiat. 137, 1463-1464.

Nelson, J.C., Charney, D.S. and Vingiano, A.W. (1978) False-positive diagnosis with primary-affective-disorder criteria. Lancet ii, 1252-1253.

Nielsen, J.L. (1980) Plasma prolactin during treatment with nortriptyline. Neuropsychobiol. 6, 52-55.

Parker, D.C. Pekary, A.E. and Hershman, J.M. (1976) Effect of normal and reversed sleep-wake cycles upon nyctohemeral rhythmicity of plasma thyrotropin: evidence suggestive of an inhibitory influence in sleep. J. Clin. Endocrinol. Metab. 43, 318-329.

Parker, D.C., Rossman, L.G., Kripke, D.F., Gibson, W. and Wilson, K. (1979) Rhythmicities in human growth hormone concentrations in plasma. In: Endocrine Rhythms (Krieger, D.T. ed.), pp. 143-173, Raven, New York.

Pavel, S. (1978) Arginine vasotocin as a pineal hormone. J. Neural Transmission (Suppl.) 13, 135-155.

Pavel, S., Goldstein, R., Popoviciu, L., Corfariu, O., Foldes, A. and Farkas, E. (1979) Pineal vasotocin: REM sleep dependent release into cerebrospinal fluid of man. Waking Sleeping 3, 347-352.

Pflug, B. and Tölle, R. (1971) Therapie endogener Depressionen durch Schlafentzug. Nervenarzt 42, 117-124.

Philipp, M. and Werner, C. (1979) Prediction of lofepramine-response in depression based on response to partial sleep deprivation. Pharmakopsychiatrie 12, 346-348.

Pickar, D., Cutter, N.R., Naber, D., Post, R.M., Pert, C.B. and Bunney, W.E. (1980) Plasma opioid activity in manic-depressive illness. Lancet i, 937.

Poland, R.E. and Rubin, R.T. (1981) Contemporary neuroendocrine research strategies and methodologies in psychiatry. In: Neuroendocrine Regulation and Altered Behaviour (Hrdina, P.D. and Singhal, R.L. eds), pp. 363-379, Croom Helm, London.

Prange, A.J. (1977) Patterns of pituitary responses to thyrotropin–releasing hormone in depressed patients: a review. In: Phenomenology and Treatment of Depression (Fann, W.E., Karacan, I., Pokorny, A.D. and Williams, R.L. eds), pp. 1-15, Spectrum, New York.

Quabbe, H.J. (1977) Chronobiology of growth hormone secretion. Chronobiologia 4, 217-246.

Rebar, R.W. and Yen, S.S.C. (1979) Endocrine rhythms in gonadotropins and ovarian steroids with reference to reproductive processes. In: Endocrine Rhythms (Krieger, D.T. ed.), pp. 259-298, Raven, New York.

Rechtschaffen, A. and Kales, A. (eds) (1968) A Manual of Standardized Terminology, Techniques and Scoring System for Sleep Stages of Human Subjects. Public Health Service, U.S. Government Printing Office, Washington, D.C.

Reichlin, S., Baldessarini, R.J. and Martin, J.P. (eds) (1977) The Hypothalamus, Raven, New York.

Rinieris, P.M., Christodoulou, G.N., Souvatzoglou, A.M., Koutras, D.A., and Stefanis, C.N. (1978) Free-thyroxine index in psychotic and neurotic depression. Acta Psychiat. Scand. 58, 56-60.

Rubin, R.T. (1975) Sleep-endocrinology studies in man. In: Hormones, Homeostasis, and the Brain, Prog. Brain Res., Vol. 42 (Gispen, W.H., van Wimersma Greidanus, Tj.B., Bohus, B. and deWied, D. eds), pp. 73-80, Elsevier, Amsterdam.

Rubin, R.T. (1977) Strategies of neuroendocrine research in psychiatry. In: Neuroregulators and Psychiatric Disorders (Usdin, E., Hamburg, D.A. and Barchas, J.D. eds), pp. 233-241, Oxford, New York.

Rubin, R.T. (1980) Hormonal regulation of renal function during sleep. In: Physiology in Sleep (Orem, J. and Barnes, C.D. eds), pp. 181-201, Academic Press, New York.

Rubin, R.T. (1981) Sex steroid hormone dynamics in endogenous depression: a review. Int. J. Ment. Health, in press.

Rubin, R.T. and Kendler, K.S. (1977) Psychoneuroendocrinology: fundamental concepts and correlates in depression. In: Depression: Clinical, Biological, and Psychological Perspectives (Usdin, G. ed.), pp. 122-138, Brunner/Mazel, New York.

Rubin, R.T. and Mandell, A.J. (1966) Adrenal cortical activity in pathological emotional states: a review. Am. J. Psychiat. 123, 387-400.

Rubin, R.T. and Poland, R.E. (1976) Synchronies between sleep and endocrine rhythms in man and their statistical evaluation. Psychoneuroendocrinology 1, 281-290.

Rubin, R.T., Gouin, P.R. and Poland, R.E. (1973) Biogenic amine metabolism and neuroendocrine function in affective disorders. In: Psychiatry: Proceedings of the V World Congress of Psychiatry (de la Fuente, R. and Weisman, M.N. eds), pp. 1036-1039, Excerpta Medica, Amsterdam.

Rubin, R.T., Poland, R.E., Rubin, L.E. and Gouin, P.R. (1974) The neuroendocrinology of human sleep. Life Sci. 14, 1041-1052.

Rubin, R.T., Poland, R.E. and Hays, S.E. (1979) Psychoneuroendocrine research in endogenous depression: a review. In: Biological Psychiatry Today (Obiols, J., Ballus, C., Gonzalez-Monclus, E. and Pujol, J. eds), pp. 684-688, Elsevier/North Holland, Amsterdam.

Rubin, R.T., Poland, R.E., Blodgett, A.L.N., Winston, R.A., Forster, B. and Carroll, B.J. (1980) Cortisol dynamics and dexamethasone pharmacokinetics in primary endogenous depression: preliminary findings. In: Progress in Psychoneuroendocrinology (Brambilla, F., Racagni, G. and deWied, D. eds), pp. 223-234, Elsevier/North Holland, Amsterdam.

Rubin, R.T., Reinisch, J.R. and Haskett, R.F. (1981a) Postnatal gonadal steroid effects on human sexually dimorphic behavior: a paradigm of hormone-environment interaction. Science, 211, 1318-1324.

Rubin, R.T., Poland, R.E., Tower, B.B., Hart, P.A., Blodgett, A.L.N. and Forster, B. (1981b) Hypothalamo-pituitary-gonadal function in primary endogenously depressed men: preliminary findings. In: Steroid Hormone Regulation of the Brain (Fuxe, K., Gustafsson, J.-A. and Wetterberg, L. eds), pp. 387-396, Pergamon, Oxford.

Sachar, E.J. (1975) Neuroendocrine abnormalities in depressive illness. In: Topics in Psychoendocrinology (Sachar, E.J. ed.), pp. 135-156, Grune and Stratton, New York.

Sachar, E.J., Hellman, L., Fukushima, D.K. and Gallagher, T.F. (1970) Cortisol production in depressive illness. Arch. Gen. Psychiat. 23, 289-298.

Sachar, E.J., Hellman, L., Roffwarg, H.P., Halpern, F.S., Fukushima, D.K. and Gallagher, T.F. (1973a) Disrupted 24-hour patterns of cortisol secretion in psychotic depression. Arch. Gen. Psychiat. 28, 19-24.

Sachar, E.J., Halpern, F., Rosenfeld, R.S., Gallagher, T.F. and Hellman, L. (1973b) Plasma and urinary testosterone levels in depressed men. Arch. Gen. Psychiat. 28, 15-18.

Sassin, J.F. (1977) Sleep-related hormones. In: Neurobiology of Sleep and Memory (Drucker-Colin, R.R. and McGaugh, J.L. eds), pp. 361-372, Academic, New York.

Selye, H. (1973) The evolution of the stress concept. Am. Sci. 61, 692-699.

Schiavi, R.C. and White, D. (1976) Androgens and male sexual function: a review of human studies. J. Sex Marital Ther. 2, 214-228.

Schilgen, B. and Tölle, R. (1980) Partial sleep deprivation as therapy for depression. Arch. Gen Psychiat. 37, 267-271.

Schilkrut, R., Chandra, O., Osswald, M., Rüther, E., Baarfüsser, B. and Matussek, N. (1975) Growth hormone release during sleep and with thermal stimulation in depressed patients. Neuropsychobiology 1, 70-79.

Schlesser, M.A., Winokur, G. and Sherman, B.M. (1980) Hypothalamic–pituitary-adrenal axis activity in depressive illness: its relationship to classification. Arch. Gen. Psychiat. 37, 737-743.

Solis, H., Fernandez-Guardiola, A. and Valverde, R.C. (1979) Neuropharmacologic and neuroendocrine interrelations of human sleep. In: The Functions of Sleep (Drucker-Colin, R., Shkurovich, M. and Sterman, M.B. eds), pp. 147-170, Academic, New York.

Spiker, D.G., Coble, P., Cofsky, J., Foster, F.G. and Kupfer, D.J. (1978) EEG sleep and severity of depression. Biol. Psychiat. 13, 485-488.

Spitzer, R.L., Endicott, J. and Robins, E. (1978) Research diagnostic criteria: rationale and reliability. Arch. Gen. Psychiat. 35, 773-782.

Takahashi, Y. (1979) Growth hormone secretion related to the sleep and waking rhythm. In: The Functions of sleep (Drucker-Colin, R., Shkurovich, M. and Sterman, M.B. eds), pp. 113-145, Academic, New York.

Takahashi, S., Kondo, H. and Yoshimura, M. (1975) Enhanced growth hormone responses to TRH injection in bipolar depressed patients. Folia Psychiat. Neurol. Jpn 29, 215-220.

Tower, B.B., Clark, B.R. and Rubin, R.T. (1977) Preparation of ^{125}I polypeptide hormones for radioimmunoassay using glucose oxidase with lactoperoxidase. Life Sci. 21, 959-966.

Tower, B.B., Sigel, M.B., Rubin, R.T., Poland, R.E. and VanderLaan, W.P. (1978) The talc-resin-TCA test: rapid screening of radioiodinated polypeptide hormones for radioimmunoassay. Life Sci. 23, 2183-2192.

Tower, B.B., Sigel, M.B., Poland, R.E., VanderLaan, W.P. and Rubin, R.T. (1980) The talc-resin-TCA test for screening radioiodinated polypeptide hormones. In: Immunological Techniques (Vol. A), Methods in Enzymology (Van Vunakis, H. and Langone, J.J. eds), pp. 322-334, Academic Press, New York.

Usdin, E., Hamburg, D.A. and Barchas, J.A. (eds) (1977) Neuroregulators and Psychiatric Disorders, Oxford University Press, New York.

Vaughan, G.M., Allen, J.P., Tullis, W., Siler-Khodr, T.M., de la Pena, A. and Sackman, J.W. (1978) Overnight plasma profiles of melatonin and certain adenohypophyseal hormones in men. J. Clin. Endocrinol. Metab. 47, 566-571.

Vaughan, G.M., McDonald, S.D., Jordan, R.M., Allen, J.P., Bell, R. and Stevens, E.A. (1979) Melatonin, pituitary function and stress in humans. Psychoneuroendocrinology 4, 351-362.

Vestergaard, P., Bojer, B. and Kleist, N. (1979) Prolactin response to sleep deprivation. In: Origin, Prevention and Treatment of Affective Disorders (Schou, M. and Stromgren, E. eds), pp. 179-183, Academic, London.

Vogel, G.W. (1975) A review of REM sleep deprivation. Arch. Gen. Psychiat. 32, 749-761.

Vogel, G.W., Thurmond, A., Gibbons, P., Sloan, K., Boyd, M. and Walker, M. (1975) REM sleep reduction effects on depression syndromes. Arch. Gen. Psychiat. 32, 765-777.

Vogel, W., Klaiber, E.L. and Broverman, D.M. (1978) Roles of the gonadal steroid hormones in psychiatric depression in men and women. Prog. Neuro-Psychopharmacol. 2, 487-503.

Wagner, D.R. and Weitzman, E.D. (1980) Neuroendocrine secretion and biological rhythms in man. Psychiat. Clin. North Am. 3, 223-250.

Weeke, J. (1973) Circadian variation of serum thyrotropin level in normal subjects. Scand. J. Clin. Lab. Invest. 31, 337-342.

Weeke, A. and Weeke, J. (1978) Disturbed circadian variation of serum thyrotropin in patients with endogenous depression. Acta Psychiat. Scand. 57, 281-289.

Weeke, A. and Weeke, J. (1980) The 24-hour pattern of serum TSH in patients with endogenous depression. Acta Psychiat. Scand. 62, 69-74.

Wehr, T.A., Wirz-Justice, A., Goodwin, F.K., Duncan, W. and Gillin, J.C. (1979) Phase advance of the circadian sleep-wake cycle as an antidepressant. Science 206, 710-713.

Weinberg, U., D'Eletto, R.D., Weitzman, E.D., Erlich, S. and Hollander, C.S. (1979) Circulating melatonin in man: episodic secretion throughout the light-dark cycle. J. Clin. Endocrinol. Metab. 48, 114-118.

Wetterberg, L. (1978) Melatonin in humans: physiological and clinical studies. J. Neural Transmission (Suppl.) 13, 289-310.

Wetterberg, L., Aperia, B., Beck-Friis, J., Kjellman, B.F., Ljunggren, J.-G., Petterson, U., Sjölin, Å., Tham, A. and Unden, F. (1981) Pineal-hypothalamic-pituitary function in patients with depressive illness. In: Steroid Hormone Regulation of the Brain (Fuxe, K., Gustaffson, J.-A. and Wetterberg, L. eds), pp. 397-403, Pergamon, Oxford.

Wirz-Justice, A., Pühringer, W. and Hole, G. (1979) Response to sleep deprivation as a predictor of therapeutic results with antidepressant drugs. Am. J. Psychiat. 136, 1222-1223.

Wurtman, R.J. and Ozaki, Y. (1978) Physiological control of melatonin synthesis and secretion: mechanisms generating rhythms in melatonin, methoxytryptophol, and arginine vasotocin levels and effects on the pineal of endogenous catecholamines, the estrous cycle, and environmental lighting, J. Neural Transmission (Suppl.) 13, 59-70.

Wyatt, R.J. (1972) The serotonin-catecholamine-dream bicycle: a clinical study. Biol. Psychiat. 5, 33-64.

Yalow, R.S. (1978) Radioimmunoassay: a probe for the fine structure of biologic systems. Science 200, 1236-1245.

Yamaguchi, N., Maeda, K. and Kuromaru, S. (1978) The effects of sleep deprivation on the circadian rhythm of plasma cortisol levels in depressive patients. Folia Psychiat. Neurol. Jpn 32, 479-487.

E.E. Müller and R.M. MacLeod (eds) Neuroendocrine Perspectives Vol. 1
339

Chapter 10

Gonadotropic and antigonadotropic actions of LH-RH analogues

J. Sandow

INTRODUCTION

The hypothalamic–pituitary–gonadal system has a highly complex organization. Extensive studies on regulation of fertility and its mechanisms have been performed with synthetic luteinizing hormone-releasing hormone (LH-RH) and its analogues. The isolation and synthesis of the structure of LH-RH (see reviews by Schally et al. 1968; McCann and Porter 1969; Schally et al. 1972a,b, 1980) provided the basis from which to study the physiological effects of the LH-RH decapeptide, to define its anatomical localization in central nervous system and extrapituitary tissues, to study its receptor interaction and the enzymatic systems controlling the duration of hormone action, and to measure LH-RH concentrations in serum and biological fluids. Initial studies assumed a linear dose–response relationship between LH-RH stimulation and gonadotropin release. It was expected that one could use LH-RH in a manner similar to therapeutic injections of luteinizing hormone (LH) or human chorionic gonadotropin (hCG). Contrary to expectation, the therapeutic efficacy of LH-RH given by single or multiple daily injections was not satisfactory in infertility. An insufficient duration of action of the LH-RH decapeptide was suspected to be the cause. Synthetic modifications of the LH-RH molecule resulted in peptides of enhanced and prolonged biological activity (agonists), and peptides blocking the LH-RH effect (antagonists). It was hoped that increased potency and duration of action of agonists would achieve better stimulation of fertility, and that competitive LH-RH antagonists would have contraceptive activity by blocking the LH release in a manner similar to an active LH-RH immunization. This concept soon required extensive modification. High doses of agonists and LH-RH were found to exert 'paradoxical' antifertility effects, by mechanisms which only now are becoming clear.

The presently available agonists of the LH-RH (1–9) nonapeptide-ethylamide type release LH and FSH at considerably lower doses than LH-RH. They are active by nasal administration, and their contraceptive potential is under clinical investigation. Inhibitory analogues (antagonists) block the action of endogenous and exogenous LH-RH in rodents, primates and in the human, but despite impressive increases in potency still require doses in excess of the LH-RH dose (Saffran 1974; Sandow et al. 1978a). In this review, a critical examination of the concepts for stimulation of fertility and contraceptive application will be attempted, with due consideration of the rapid progress in this field. The rapid growth of the literature precludes comprehensiveness. In some instances, reviews are quoted, to which the reader is referred for the original publications.

The gonadotropic or antigonadotropic actions of LH-RH and its highly active agonists on the male and female reproductive tract depend on dose and frequency of administration. In low doses, LH-RH and agonists enhance fertility. At higher doses, after frequent administration or constant infusion, agonists act as contraceptive peptides in the same way and by the same mechanisms as high doses of LH-RH (Sandow et al. 1980c). The biological effects are primarily exerted via the pituitary, and the following definition is used for analysis: gonadotropic effects are caused by gonadotropin release, and can be mimicked by gonadotropin injections. Anti-gonadotropic effects are caused by reduced gonadotropin secretion, or impaired responsiveness of the target organ to gonadotropins. These effects cannot be mimicked directly by high doses of gonadotropins, because gonadotropin injections compensate only in part for reduced pituitary or target organ responsiveness. At very high doses, agonists have extrapituitary (direct) effects on the target organs for gonadotropins and gonadal steroids (ovary, uterus, placenta, testis, prostate). The physiological role of these direct gonadal effects is under investigation. There is evidence for gonadal LH-RH binding proteins (receptors), and for LH-RH-like peptides in gonadal tissue. These receptors may account for the direct effects of agonists on steroidogenesis by modulation of gonadotropin receptor function.

Table 10.1

HYPOTHALAMIC–PITUITARY–GONADAL RESPONSE TO LH-RH OR LH-RH AGONIST TREATMENT

Site of action	Conditioning factor
Hypothalamus	exposure to LH-RH or agonists (can affect endogenous LH-RH content and/or pulsatile secretion) enzyme activity (regulation of turnover) steroid exposure (long feedback)
Pituitary	pulse frequency and dose of LH-RH (priming by low doses, desensitization by high doses or constant infusion) LH-RH receptor (desensitization and/or depletion) enzyme activity (rate of LH-RH degradation) exposure to extracellular or intracellular LH increase (auto-feedback) steroid exposure (long feedback)
Gonad	amount of LH bound to receptors (acute changes in steroid biosynthesis = steroidogenic lesion, depletion of gonadal LH/FSH/prolactin receptors = down-regulation) gonadal peptide receptors (direct effect of agonists or LH-RH-like endogenous peptides) enzyme activity (LH-RH degradation).

Acute administration of LH-RH and agonists stimulates release of gonadotropins with concomitant or subsequent de novo synthesis. The released gonadotropins activate gonadal steroidogenesis. Hypothalamic–pituitary sensitivity to further stimulation is regulated by feedback signals from the pituitary and the gonads (Table 10.1). The systems involved will be discussed as hypothalamic–pituitary interaction in the absence of the gonads, pituitary–gonadal interaction (comparing induced gonadotropin release with exogenous gonadotropin stimulation), and hypothalamic–gonadal interaction (the classical feedback of gonadal steroids, gonadal LH-RH receptors and/or LH-RH-like peptides in the testis, ovary and placenta).

In experimental endocrinology, LH-RH has been studied with classical bioassays, where the expression of LH-RH action is a target organ response to gonadotropins released within a defined time period, and utilized by the target organ. When the target organ response is impaired after chronic LH-RH stimulation, the causes may be a temporary reduction in gonadotropin secretion after supraphysiological LH release, an imbalance of steroid production after hyperstimulation, or a temporary block of gonadotropin action by a reduction of target organ receptors. Paradoxical inhibition of fertility in experimental animals has greatly stimulated research on the mechanisms of pituitary desensitization and gonadotropin receptor regulation. In initial studies on chronic administration of LH-RH at high doses, we found a sex-specific response of ovarian stimulation and testicular inhibition (Fig. 10.1), when rats were treated with 1 mg kg^{-1}LH-RH once daily subcutaneously (s.c.) for 30 days. The suspected mechanism, activation of target organ feedback by excessive steroid production, was refuted by steroid profiles in serum and tissue. It became necessary to study multiple parameters of the hypothalamic–pituitary–gonadal function, to find an explanation for causes and effects. Chronic studies with agonists provided evidence that the contraceptive action is due to a complex interaction of different processes leading to pituitary and gonadal refractoriness during continuous or intermittent peptide administration.

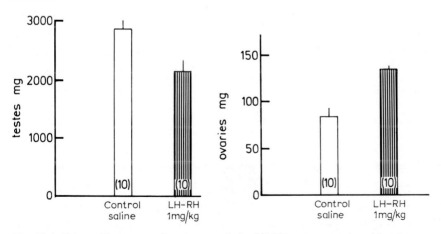

Fig. 10.1. Sex-specific response of target organs during LH-RH treatment: male and female rats treated with LH-RH 1 mg kg^{-1} s.c. once daily×30 days. Note decrease in testes weight but increase in ovarian weight (number of animals in parentheses).

342

In contrast to the gonadotropin-mediated mechanisms, direct gonadal action of LH-RH and agonists is not clearly understood. These antigonadotropic effects may be related to the modulation of function of the target organ receptor, by interference of heterologous ligands (LH-RH) with the homologous hormone receptors (LH and FSH). Direct gonadal effects have been studied in hypophysectomized rats or in vitro systems, but to be manifest they usually require the presence of gonadotropins.

LH-RH AGONISTS

The primary objective in the synthesis of LH-RH agonists was to produce substances that acted over a long period. Attempts to prolong the biological effect of LH-RH by depot preparations were partially successful, but the depot carriers increased the risk of antigenicity. Chemical modifications of the LH-RH decapeptide concentrated on amino acids 6 and 7 (Gly–Leu) and amino acids 9 and 10 (Pro–GlyNH$_2$). At the present time, all potent agonists (Fig. 10.2) are LH-RH (1–9) nonapeptide-ethylamide compounds with additional substitutions in position 6 (e.g. D-Ala^6, D-Leu^6, D-Trp^6, D-Ser (TBU)^6) or position 7 (N-MeLeu^7). Other modifications do not increase the biological potency (Saffran 1974, Schally et al. 1978, Sandow et al. 1978a). In this review, the abbreviation EA for LH-RH (1–9) nonapeptide-ethylamide derivatives will be used, indicating the respective changes in position 6. In our structure–activity studies, we found that substitution of position 6 with D-amino acids bearing a protective group in the side chain was more effective than simultaneous substitution of positions 6 and 7 by protected amino acids (König et al. 1978).

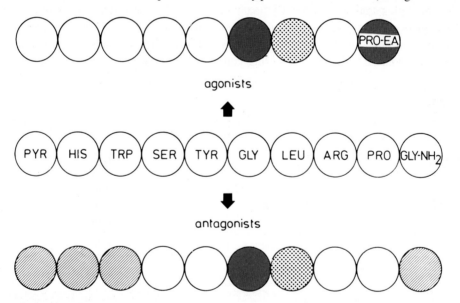

Fig. 10.2. Structure of LH-RH agonists and antagonists: agonists of increased biological activity are obtained by substitutions of Gly^6 and Pro-GlyNH$_2$. Antagonists of high inhibitory activity are obtained by substitutions in positions 1, 2, 3, 6 and 10 of the LH-RH decapeptide. Modification of Leu^7, e.g. by NMe-Leu^7 is permissible both in agonists and antagonists.

Exact potencies of agonists have to be calculated from direct comparisons with a standard compound in biological test systems. Suitable test-systems have been reviewed in Sandow et al. (1981a).

Agonistic potency is influenced by two separate components, increased receptor affinity and enhanced enzyme stability. Receptor affinity is tested in radioligand assays using the supernatant fraction of pituitary homogenates, or purified pituitary membranes (Clayton et al. 1979b; Perrin et al. 1980), or by pituitary uptake in vivo. Radioligand assays measure the initial hormone-binding step. The subsequent chain of effect is controversial; both the cAMP system (Labrie et al. 1978b, 1979) and cGMP systems (Naor et al. 1980) have been implicated. Enzyme stability of agonists is tested in vitro by competition with LH-RH for LH-RH-degrading enzymes (Kuhl et al. 1979; Sandow et al. 1980d), or measuring degradation by hypothalamic–pituitary enzymes (Marks and Stern 1974; Koch et al. 1977; Griffiths and Hopkinson 1979; Swift and Crighton, 1979). Enzyme resistance is of relevance both for decreased inactivation by liver and kidney, and for termination of hormone action at the receptor site by membrane-bound enzymes.

LH-RH ANTAGONISTS

Antagonists of LH-RH bind to the pituitary receptor and block the action of endogenous and exogenous LH-RH. Potent antagonists selectively block secretion of LH and FSH without an initial stimulation phase. Antigonadotropic effects of agonists require a transitory phase of supraphysiological LH release to induce pituitary inhibition and down-regu-

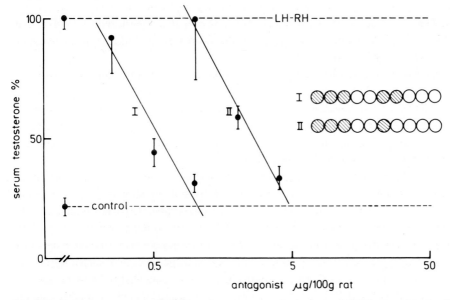

Fig. 10.3. Dose–response curve of inhibition of testosterone production by two LH-RH antagonists: the effect of 400 ng LH-RH per 4 h on testosterone production is dose — dependently reduced by peptide I and peptide II. Substitution of amino acids in the two inhibitors indicated by hatched circles. Antagonists were injected s.c. 5 min before onset of LH-RH infusion.

lation of LH receptors, whereas antagonists block LH release immediately. The structural development of LH-RH antagonists has been very interesting (Fig. 10.2). The initial modifications were based on changes in positions 2 and 3 (His–Trp). Substitution by D-amino acids, or elimination of His[2] produced antagonistic activity, which was enhanced by additional substitution of position 6 (Gly) by D-amino acids (Sandow et al. 1978a; Coy et al. 1979). Recent antagonists incorporate multiple substitutions in position 1, 2, 3, 6 and 10, either in the form of D-amino acids or halogenated D-amino acids. Antagonistic potency is expressed by the molar ratio of antagonist to LH-RH required to inhibit LH release or an LH-dependent biological event, e.g. ovulation or ascorbic acid depletion in rats. Highly potent antagonists block LH-RH action in vitro at a molar ratio of less than 10:1 (Rivier and Vale 1978), but are less effective in vivo.

Test systems for antagonistic potency in male rats are based on the inhibition of LH release and testosterone production. In our laboratory, we have evaluated the potency of antagonists by measuring inhibition of testosterone production induced by LH-RH infusion in rats of 100 g body weight (Sandow et al. 1980d). Antagonists were injected subcutaneously 5 min before the onset of an LH-RH infusion of 40 ng over 2 h. In control animals, serum testosterone increases about ten-fold under LH-RH infusion, an effect which is blocked by antagonists in a dose-dependent fashion (Fig. 10.3). There is also a reduction of LH, FSH and testosterone in serum, as well as testicular testosterone content. Antagonists also suppress corticosterone in serum and adrenals, but the dose required for corticosterone reduction is 100 times as high as the dose that blocks testosterone production (Sandow et al. 1980d, 1981a). Test systems for LH-RH antagonists measuring a target organ response are based on a gonadotropin-dependent event. Antigonadotropic potency can be expressed in terms of inhibition of ovulation (Coy et al. 1979; Bowers et al. 1980), reduction of ovarian ascorbic acid in pseudopregnant animals, or weight decrease of androgen-dependent organs after testosterone suppression.

Receptor affinity of LH-RH antagonists is not directly related to biological antigonadotropic potency. In radioligand assays, using pituitary receptors (Pedroza-Garcia et al. 1977; Heber and Odell 1978; Clayton and Catt 1979) or testicular Leydig cell receptors (Sharpe and Fraser 1980a), antagonists have a binding affinity similar to LH-RH. This is surprising, because in vivo such antagonists have to be injected with much higher doses to competitively block the effect of a given dose of LH-RH.

There are three components which determine antagonistic potency: binding affinity to pituitary (or extrapituitary) receptors, metabolic inactivation (in pituitary, liver, kidney and other tissues), and changes in receptor sensitivity to subsequent LH-RH stimulation. The first component, receptor affinity (binding) in vitro does not correlate with the antagonistic potency. The second component (metabolic inactivation) has not been studied in detail for any of the presently available highly active antagonists. In the absence of such information, an explanation may be based on the third component, antagonist-induced changes in receptor sensitivity to LH-RH. Since antagonists contain a large number of modified amino acids impairing enzyme degradation, and act for an extensive time in vivo, prolonged receptor interaction or occupancy can be assumed. However, LH-RH antagonists have relatively low biological potencies in terms of the doses required to block LH-RH action.

These observations could be explained by the following concept: pituitary cells have two different types of binding sites, one for triggering LH release (the 'true' receptor), and the second for termination of hormone stimulation (an 'enzyme-like' receptor). The two types of binding sites represent transitional stages of one large receptor molecule, or could be located in different structural elements of the cell membrane. Antagonists bind to the LH-RH receptor in vivo, as shown by pituitary accumulation in organ distribution studies with ^{125}I-labelled D-Phe^2, Phe^3, D-Phe^6-LH-RH and competitive displacement of a ^{125}I-labelled agonist by unlabelled antagonist in rats (Sandow et al. 1980d). After initial binding, antagonists block the LH-RH receptor by inducing a conformational change which makes LH-RH stimulation impossible, and/or by occupying the enzyme degradation site which is a prerequisite for receptor function.

One strong argument in favor of this hypothesis is the large number of modifications permissible in LH-RH antagonists. In a structure–activity study of the LH-RH molecule we found that changes in amino acids 1, 2, 3 and 10 were compatible with antagonism. There are probably two areas of interaction with the receptor (Fig. 10.4). The binding sequence is located in amino acids 4–9, corresponding to the LH-RH (4–9) hexapeptide. In this area the structure must be preserved and only substitution of position 6 (Gly) is permissible. In contrast to this stringent requirement, the inhibitor sequences in the N-terminal and C-terminal parts of the molecule may be substituted by numerous amino acids incompatible with receptor stimulation, and highly resistant to enzyme degradation. We suggest that these inhibitor sequences induce refractoriness of the LH-RH receptor, by blocking the LH-RH-degrading enzymes associated with the receptor protein (Kuhl and Baumann 1981; Sandow et al. 1981b). Prolonged antagonistic action in vivo is explained by the high enzyme resistance of such molecules, which retain the essential binding sequence for LH-RH (Schally et al. 1978; Sandow and König 1979).

The biological potential of LH-RH antagonists in the control of fertility has been explored in rodents and primates (Corbin et al. 1978b). Inhibition of ovulation in rats is

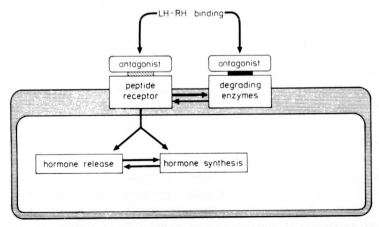

Fig. 10.4. LH-RH antagonists and their interaction with the pituitary LH-RH receptor: antagonists bind to peptide receptor with their binding sequence. Simultaneously they block LH-RH degrading enzymes by their inhibitor sequences. The receptor becomes refractory to exogenous and endogenous LH-RH.

used extensively for determining antagonistic potencies (Bowers et al. 1980). Ovulation is also blocked in rabbits (Phelps et al. 1977) and in hamsters, although here higher doses are required (de la Cruz et al. 1976; Nishi et al. 1976). The role of LH-RH for ovulation in primates and the usefulness of primate studies for evaluation of antagonists is less clear. In rhesus monkeys, an estradiol challenge can induce ovulation despite acute pituitary stalk section (Ferin et al. 1979). It has been suggested that the pre-ovulatory LH surge and ovulation can occur independently of an endogenous LH-RH increase, and postulated that antagonists would be ineffective in blocking ovulation in primates. However, LH secretion and ovulation are blocked by passive transfer of LH-RH antisera, in primates (McCormack et al. 1977) as well as in rodents (see review by Fraser 1980a). Long-term stalk section leads to pituitary refractoriness to estradiol stimulation, establishing the obligatory role of LH-RH. In chimpanzees, LH-RH antagonists inhibit the LH surge induced by injection of estradiol benzoate. There is a significant blunting of the LH response to estradiol after 5 mg s.c. of D-Pyr^1, D-Phe^2, D-Trp^3, D-Trp^6-LH-RH (Gosselin et al. 1979b). In subhuman primates, inhibition of ovulation by agonists requires higher doses than in the human (Fraser et al. (1980), although the chimpanzee responds normally to LH-RH or D-Trp^6-EA (Graham et al. 1979). It is difficult to decrease serum testosterone in rhesus monkeys even using very high doses of D-Ser (TBU)^6-EA (Wickings et al. 1980). It is conceivable that sensitivity to antagonists in monkeys is also lower than in rodents and in humans, so that testing in this species does not predict the antigonadotropic activity in the human. The inhibitory potency of an antagonist in monkeys and in the human can be expressed by the dose required to neutralize the effect of a test dose of LH-RH. In chimpanzees, 35 mg D-Phe^2, D-Trp^3, D-Phe^6-LH-RH blocked significantly the response to 10 µg LH-RH, and in baboons 40–50 mg D-Phe^2, Phe^3, D-Phe^6-LH-RH partially blocked the effect of 100 µg LH-RH (Hagino et al. 1977; Gosselin et al. 1979a). In rhesus monkeys, D-Phe^2, Pro^3, D-Phe^6-LH-RH 50 mg every 8 h, s.c. (total dose 300 mg per monkey), only partially prevented LH and FSH surges, and temporarily suppressed estradiol levels. Luteal progesterone increased, although at laparoscopy, corpora lutea were not identified (Wilks et al. 1980). The authors suggest that ovulation was prevented, but that follicular tissue was inappropriately luteinized. In postmenopausal women, elevated LH levels are reduced by 10 mg D-p-F-Phe^1, D-p-Cl-Phe^2, D-Trp^{3,6}, D-Ala^{10}-LH-RH for 4–6 h, whereas FSH levels are not lowered to the same extent. The delayed response of FSH to LH-RH suppression is also observed in sheep, where passive transfer of antisera readily suppressed LH pulsatility, but not FSH secretion (Fraser 1980a).

BIOLOGICAL TARGET SYSTEMS

The biological action of LH-RH is expressed by stimulation of tissues producing gonadal steroids, or reacting to gonadal steroids. In the male reproductive system, the testes, seminal vesicles, prostate and other androgen-dependent tissues manifest changes in androgen production. In the female reproductive system, the ovaries and uterus are the main markers of estrogen and progesterone production. The response of these target organs depends on gonadotropin utilization, and can be dissociated from the pituitary response when gonadotropin receptors are depleted. Changes in pituitary responsiveness can be detected by measuring the daily LH serum profile, which is the best indicator of agonist suppression. The pituitary response to LH-RH depends on exposure to steroids (reviewed by Fink 1979), which determine the LH/FSH ratio of the adult pituitary, and also the response of the fetal pituitary (Norman and Spies 1979). Suppressive effects of LH-RH agonists at the pituitary level are also exerted when gonadal steroids are low. There is a marked sex difference in the suppression of the pituitary by agonists. In the adult male, much higher daily doses of agonists are required to reduce tonic LH secretion than to block the cyclic LH discharge in the adult female. The state of the target organ after chronic LH-RH agonist treatment reflects gonadotropin utilization by available gonadotropin receptors. The divergent changes in pituitary sensitivity and target organ responsiveness must be monitored separately by LH release profiles and LH receptor determination. In the absence of data on daily LH release, pituitary LH/FSH content and gonadal LH/FSH/prolactin receptors, the antifertility effects of chronic treatment with high doses of LH-RH and agonists were thought previously to be paradoxical effects, based on a concept of unlimited positive pituitary-gonadal response to LH-RH stimulation. However, marked antifertility effects are also observed after high doses of pregnant mare's serum gonadotropin (PMSG) or hCG (Rothchild 1965; Yang and Chang 1968; Banik 1975; Friedrich et al. 1975; Pal et al. 1976). The gonadal reaction to excessive gonadotropin stimulation is restricted by temporary pituitary suppression (Hirono et al. 1972), desensitization of the target organ during the immediate post-stimulation phase (steroidogenic lesion) (Cigorraga et al. 1978), and subsequent down-regulation of gonadotropin receptors (Auclair et al. 1977). The biological response of the target organ is self-limiting; pituitary desensitization and gonadotropin receptor depletion protect against hyperstimulation by gonadotropin-producing adenomas as effectively as against hyperstimulation by pharmacological doses of LH-RH or agonists (Dufau et al. 1979).

The antifertility effects of agonists are more readily understood when subdivided into a time-dependent sequence of effects on pituitary responsiveness, steroid biosynthesis, and target organ responsiveness (see Table 10.4).

Hypothalamic–pituitary interaction (pituitary responsiveness)

The pituitary responds to a pulsatile pattern of LH-RH stimulation, but LH release is blocked upon continuous exposure (Shareha et al. 1976; Belchetz et al. 1978; De Koning et al. 1978; Ferin et al. 1978) or multiple high-dose injections (Sandow 1975). The requirement for pulsatile stimulation is also observed in dispersed pituitary cells (Smith and Vale 1980). Pituitary responsiveness of castrate animals can be studied as a model system for hypothalamic LH-RH control and the desensitization induced by agonists. In castrate animals and in menopausal women, there is a pronounced LH pulsatility (Gay and Sheth 1972; Neill et al. 1976; Knobil 1980; Gallo 1980). In the presence of steroid feedback, LH pulsatility varies with the stage of the cycle (Yen et al. 1972), and is modulated by steroid administration (Goodman and Karsch 1980). LH-RH pulses are mandatory for pituitary stimulation, in intact animals; by interacting with estrogens they permit the establishment of a normal menstrual cycle (Knobil 1980). There is a constant coupling between exogenous LH-RH pulses and LH peaks in rhesus monkeys with lesions of the arcuate nucleus, which eliminate endogenous LH-RH secretion.

Two factors determine pituitary responsiveness in gonadectomized animals: the frequency of LH-RH administration and the dose of LH-RH. Pituitary LH secretion is activated by regular pulses of a low LH-RH dose (Knobil et al. 1980), while injection of LH-RH antiserum abolishes LH pulsatility (Fraser 1980a).

In contrast, pituitary responsiveness is gradually reduced or abolished by high agonist doses. During clinical trials with agonists, doses were often applied which reduced LH release within days (Hanker et al. 1978; Happ et al. 1978b). These observations formed the basis for subsequent studies on peptide contraception (Dericks-Tan et al. 1977; Nillius et al. 1978; Bergquist et al. 1979c; Baumann et al. 1980).

In the castrate adrenalectomized rat, pituitary desensitization is characterized by low serum LH and FSH levels associated with greatly reduced pituitary LH and FSH content (Table 10.2). In the human, reduced tissue reserve can only be inferred indirectly from the impaired LH release after multiple agonist injections.

The appropriate pulse frequency for therapeutic LH-RH substitution during the follicular phase is one pulse at 2-hourly intervals. (Crowley and McArthur 1980b). In Kallman's syndrome, pulsatile infusion of LH-RH induces a normal menstrual cycle with an adequate luteal phase. In men with hypothalamic hypogonadism, pituitary LH and FSH secretion and testosterone production are activated by long-term pulsatile LH-RH infusion, and pubertal development is completed (Crowley and McArthur 1980a). Gonadal steroids are not required during the early stages of pituitary LH-RH activation, because puberty can be induced in sexually immature monkeys by pulsatile LH-RH administration (Wildt et al. 1980).

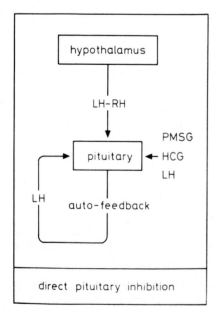

Fig. 10.5. Direct pituitary inhibition by endogenous or exogenous LH stimulation: endogenous inhibition is induced by supraphysiological LH-RH/agonist stimulation. Exogenous inhibition is induced by high doses of PMSG, hCG or LH. Pituitary auto-feedback reduces LH release after hyperstimulation. Reproduced from Sandow et al. (1978c, 1979c).

Table 10.2

PITUITARY INHIBITION BY CHRONIC TREATMENT WITH AN LH-RH AGONIST, D-Ser (TBU)⁶-ETHYLAMIDE (BUSERELIN), IN CASTRATE-ADRENA-LECTOMIZED RATS (CX/ADX): EFFECT ON GONADOTROPIN SECRETION AND STORAGE, AND HYPOTHALAMIC LH-RH CONTENT

Group No.	Duration of treatment	Treatment[A]	Daily dose per rat	Serum levels (ng ml^{-1})		Tissue content (μg per pituitary)		LH-RH (pg per hypothalamus)
				LH	FSH	LH	FSH	
1	14 days	CX/ADX Controls	0	356 ± 67.7[B]	882 ± 98.6	152 ± 13.6	14.9 ± 1.6	742 ± 89.5
2	14 days	CX/ADX Buserelin	50 ng	97 ± 29.7[C]	825 ± 35.4	88 ± 6.2[C]	5.8 ± 0.8[C]	493 ± 36.3[C]
3	28 days	CX/ADX Controls	0	1102 ± 339.7	2178 ± 264.1	215 ± 16.9	29.9 ± 4.2	1145 ± 198.2
4	28 days	CX/ADX Buserelin	50 ng	84 ± 21.2[C]	1294 ± 177.9[C]	80 ± 7.2[C]	6.7 ± 0.8[C]	796 ± 87.6

[A] Treatment for 14–28 days by one daily subcutaneous injection.
[B] Each point is the mean ±SEM of 8 determinations (groups 1, 2, 4) or 6 determinations (group 3).
[C] Significant difference vs controls by analysis of variance (ANOVA) at 95% level.

The ratio of LH to FSH release depends on the LH-RH pulse frequency. Pulses of increased frequency (30 min) decrease LH but not FSH release, and more frequent pulses (10 – 15 min), or constant infusion cause rapid pituitary desensitization. In contrast, a reduced frequency (3 h) results in increased FSH and low LH secretion (prepubertal pattern).

High doses of LH-RH inhibit LH secretion in the agonadal animal by reducing LH release and LH synthesis, probably at different LH-RH concentrations. The pituitary LH-RH receptors mediate acute LH release (Naor et al. 1980), and subsequent de novo synthesis could be either a consequence of LH depletion, or occur independently. Increasing LH concentrations in serum or in incubation media reduce subsequent LH release (auto-feedback). This mechanism is also activated by endogenous LH-RH stimulation (Fig. 10.5), and may operate via an intracellular LH-dependent feedback system. When LH-RH induces supraphysiological LH release, LH synthesis is simultaneously activated. If the rate of synthesis exceeds the rate of release, an increased intracellular LH concentration would amplify the temporary blocking of release, by pituitary auto-feedback. Induction of increased intracellular LH concentration may be inferred from the priming effect observed after repeated stimulation with small doses of LH-RH (Aiyer et al. 1974; Faure and Olivier 1978). A small LH-RH dose primes the pituitary by enhancing the response to subsequent LH-RH stimulation. Unfortunately, there are no conclusive data available on short-term changes in pituitary LH content, and the existence of two separate, but convertible pools for LH release and storage precludes conclusions based on total pituitary content (tissue reserve).

In studies on agonists, we have defined the concept of a 'physiological' dose maintaining regular LH pulsatility and a 'supraphysiological' dose reducing LH release and pituitary LH content, when given repeatedly on consecutive days (Sandow et al. 1978b). In the intact male rat, the physiological dose was related to the dose response after acute LH-RH or agonist injection (Sandow et al. 1980a). A minimal FSH-releasing dose (physiological dose) can be injected once daily, inducing reproducible LH increases, without pituitary desensitization. In castrate male rats, inhibition of LH release is observed within 4 – 5 days, if a dose 10 times as high as the physiological dose of LH-RH (1 µg s.c.) or an equivalent dose of an agonist (e.g. D-Ser (TBU)[6]-EA 50 ng s.c.) is injected once daily (Sandow et al. 1978c, 1979c). The extent of pituitary inhibition is proportional to the daily quantum of LH released, but independent of either gonadal or adrenal steroids. Inhibition of LH secretion by administration of supraphysiological doses of LH of hCG has been observed after infusion of hLH and hCG in the rabbit (Molitch et al. 1976), and after treatment of postmenopausal women with hCG (Miyake et al. 1976). It was also found after endogenous supraphysiological LH release induced by agonists in postmenopausal women (Bergquist et al. 1979d), amenorrheic women (Nillius and Wide 1977), normal cyclic women (Dericks-Tan et al. 1977) and normal men (Bergquist et al. 1979a). Pituitary auto-feedback could operate via pituitary LH receptors measuring extracellular LH concentrations (like a gonadal LH receptor), or via an intracellular mechanism sensitive to increased intracellular LH content (Fig. 10.5).

Pituitary inhibition by agonists in castrate animals requires daily injections to maintain inhibition. When the same daily dose is given by constant infusion of LH-RH or agonists, desensitization and pituitary inhibition is rapidly induced and maintained over prolonged time periods. Pituitary responsiveness is suppressed independently of gonadal steroid secretion in women with premature ovarian failure (Rabin and McNeill 1980). Target organ responsiveness may recover independent of pituitary inhibition. LH pulsatility in monkeys ceases during constant infusion of LH-RH (Belchetz et al. 1978). Delivery of LH-RH by osmotic minipumps leads to pituitary desensitization resulting in inhibition of implantation (Bowers and Folkers 1976) or reduced serum LH levels in sheep (Amundson and Wheaton 1979), or temporary decrease of androgen production (Sandow et al. 1981a). In male monkeys, implantation of agonists in pellets inhibits reproductive function (Vickery and MacRae 1980), but D-Trp[6]- LH-RH infusion (7 days) fails to induce luteolysis in baboons (Hagino et al. 1979).

During long-term agonist infusion by minipumps, desensitization is initiated by a phase of supraphysiological LH release. In castrate rats, pituitary inhibition is caused by LH release alone. In intact male rats, LH release and greatly stimulated testosterone secretion rapidly inhibit further LH secretion.

Is it the total dose of peptide infused per day that determines the extent of pituitary inhibition, or does pituitary inhibition require acute increments in LH secretion after daily

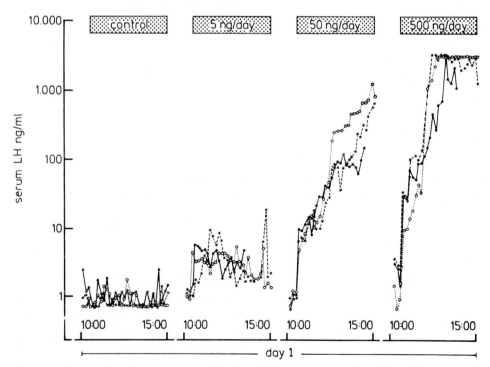

Fig. 10.6. Dose–response curve to acute minipump infusion of an LH-RH agonist: dose-dependent release of LH immediately after implantation of minipumps delivering a daily dose of 5, 50 or 500 ng D-Ser(TBU)[6]-EA (buserelin). LH measured in individual animals sampled from a jugular catheter.

injections? We administered a 1 to 100-fold physiological doses of an agonist by constant infusion for 7 or 14 days, and tested the changes induced in pituitary-testicular responsiveness. Daily doses of 5, 50 or 500 ng D-Ser (TBU)[6]-EA (buserelin), which were identical with those previously administered by s.c. injection were infused by osmotic minipump. (Sandow et al. 1980a). The initial phase of agonist action was characterized by rapidly increasing and greatly elevated levels of LH (Fig. 10.6) and testosterone. During the subsequent stage of peptide-induced pituitary desensitization, LH levels declined progressively towards basal levels, and the agonist acted directly on the pituitary cell without LH mediation. When minipumps were removed at the end of the 1- or 2-week infusion period and transplanted into male recipient rats, there was a dose-dependent testosterone increase, as in short-term infusion studies with LH-RH and buserelin in male rats (Sandow et al. 1978b), confirming that the pumps still contained biologically active buserelin. This was done because in previous studies with LH-RH given by minipump infusions in sheep a loss in LH responsiveness was noted, but ascribed to degradation of LH-RH in subcutaneous tissue (Amundson and Wheaton 1979). Acutely reduced pituitary responsiveness during LH-RH infusion also accounts for the failure to find elevated LH levels 16 h after minipump implantation (Catt et al. 1980; Harwood et al. 1980a). LH profiles in individual rats confirmed that the initially high LH release declined rapidly, and LH levels remained low

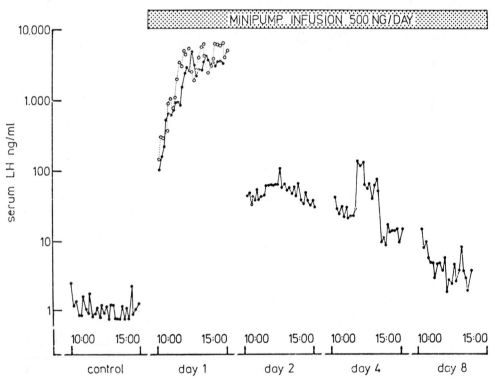

Fig. 10.7. Desensitization of pituitary LH secretion under long-term infusion: a dose of 500 ng D-Ser(TBU)[6]-EA (buserelin) per day elicits maximal LH release on day 1; levels decline rapidly until day 8 despite persistent infusion. LH sampled in individual animals from a jugular catheter for 5 h per day.

during the subsequent infusion period (Fig. 10.7). On day 12, pituitary responsiveness to an LH-RH injection was tested under continuing infusion. In all groups (control and buserelin-infused rats) basal LH levels were low; the response of control animals to LH-RH injection was rapid and sustained for 2 h. In the group receiving 5 ng buserelin per day, there was a smaller biphasic LH response to LH-RH, and the LH response was further reduced in the 50 ng buserelin group. At 500 ng buserelin per day, the LH-RH response was completely absent (Fig. 10.8). This dose-dependent reduction in LH-RH responsiveness confirms that under continuous agonist infusion pituitary responsiveness is blocked directly at a pituitary site of action. Pituitary desensitization is induced by LH release, but maintained by the agonist alone, without the participation of short or long feedback mechanisms. A detailed analysis of the multiple parameters of hypothalamic–pituitary–gonadal function revealed the pituitary as the primary site of agonist suppression, and excluded direct gonadal inhibition (Sandow 1979). At autopsy, after 7 or 14 days of continuous infusion, pituitary LH-RH receptors were determined by binding of [^{125}I]buserelin to a pituitary homogenate (Clayton et al. 1979b; Sandow et al. 1980a), LH and FSH in serum and pituitary were determined by RIA, and testicular function was monitored by measuring LH and prolactin receptors, testosterone in serum and testicular tissue. There was a clear dissociation between pituitary sensitivity and target organ responsiveness at the end of the infusion

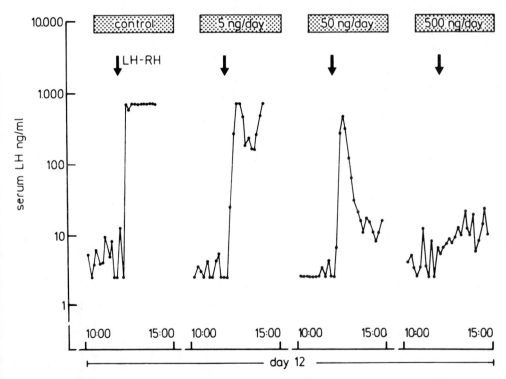

Fig. 10.8. Pituitary inhibition after a 12-day treatment with an LH-RH agonist: pituitary responsiveness was tested by injection of LH-RH 100 ng s.c. Note dose-dependent suppression of the pituitary response to LH-RH stimulation.

Table 10.3

DISSOCIATION OF PITUITARY AND TARGET ORGAN RESPONSIVENESS IN RATS RECEIVING CONSTANT DOSE INFUSIONS OF THE AGONIST D-Ser (TBU)^6-EA (BUSERELIN)

Group No.	Treatment[A]	Duration[A] of infusion	Daily dose per rat (ng)	Pituitary hormone content (µg per pituitary)		Testicular receptors (fmol per g)		Testosterone (ng per g testis)
				LH	FSH	LH	FSH	
1	Controls	7 days	0	116 ± 10.4[B]	129 ± 9.8	8.73 ± 0.4	1.95 ± 0.09	15.2 ± 1.5
2	Buserelin	7 days	5	117 ± 6.6	107 ± 6.1	8.44 ± 0.4	2.76 ± 0.12[C]	21.4 ± 2.7
3	Buserelin	7 days	50	100 ± 11.5	122 ± 7.0	8.45 ± 0.3	2.28 ± 0.12	25.6 ± 3.9[C]
4	Buserelin	7 days	500	9.5 ± 1.7[C]	25 ± 4.0[C]	7.20 ± 0.2[C]	3.15 ± 0.43[C]	26.7 ± 1.1[C]
5	Controls	14 days	0	174 ± 19.4	110 ± 9.6	5.74 ± 0.3	2.24 ± 0.02	28.7 ± 3.3
6	Buserelin	14 days	5	116 ± 16.2	95 ± 11	7.20 ± 0.6[C]	2.20 ± 0.04	42.6 ± 3.2[C]
7	Buserelin	14 days	50	135 ± 15.6	119 ± 8.2	6.77 ± 0.2	2.38 ± 0.04[C]	33.0 ± 1.9
8	Buserelin	14 days	500	11 ± 1.5[C]	25 ± 2.3[C]	6.97 ± 0.3	2.43 ± 0.03[C]	28.8 ± 2.5

[A] Subcutaneous implantation of minipumps delivering a daily dose of 5–500 ng.

[B] Each point is the mean ±SEM of 8 determinations (hormone content), or 4 determinations on pooled tissues (receptor levels).

[C] Significant difference vs controls by ANOVA at 95% level.

period. Transiently elevated LH levels had declined to low basal values after 7 and 14 days of infusion. Low LH secretion was associated with highly significant pituitary LH-FSH depletion (Table 10.3). Testicular receptors for LH and FSH had returned to normal values after 7 and 14 days of infusion, although marked changes are initially induced by LH-RH or agonists (Catt et al. 1980). The recovery of LH-FSH receptors despite pituitary inhibition, is in contrast to the marked receptor depletion after daily injections of the same doses (Sandow et al. 1980b), but finds its explanation in the sustained block of LH release during long-term infusion. When testicular function after 14 days of infusion was assessed by testosterone production in vitro (stimulated with 200 mU hCG), there was no impairment. It is clear that target organ responsiveness had recovered independently of persisting pituitary inhibition during prolonged, constant-dose infusion.

In contrast to target organ recovery, marked changes are observed at the hypothalamic and pituitary level after long-term agonist infusion. The endogenous hypothalamic LH-RH content was increased after 7 and 14 days of infusion, at the daily dose of 500 ng buserelin. This represents in vivo confirmation of previous results on in vitro inhibition of LH-RH degradation by hypothalamic–pituitary arylamidase preparations, in the presence of ago- nists with enhanced enzyme resistance (Sandow et al. 1979b). Endogenous hypothalamic LH-RH content increased progressively with the time of infusion. Pituitary LH-RH recep- tors decreased with duration of treatment, indicating that depletion (down-regulation) of LH-RH receptors can occur after prolonged periods of pituitary exposure to agonists. In contrast, the same doses injected once daily decreased pituitary sensitivity without a concomitant reduction in LH-RH receptors, indicating that acute pituitary desensitization does not involve the primary binding step at the pituitary membrane, but the uncoupling of

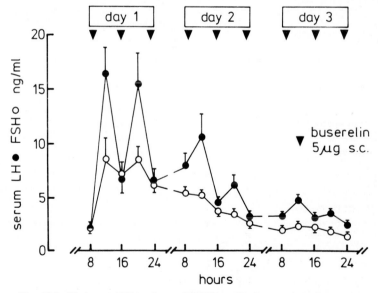

Fig. 10.9. Pituitary inhibition by an LH-RH agonist in normal cyclic women: daily injection of 5 μg D- Ser(TBU)[6]-EA (buserelin) s.c. at 8-h intervals causes a progressive decrease in LH and FSH release. Reproduced from Dericks-Tan et al. (1978).

356

the effector system (Sandow et al. 1980a, 1980b). The dramatic reduction in pituitary LH and FSH content after 7 and 14 days (Table 10.3) is only observed at the highest daily dose of buserelin; lower doses did not reduce gonadotropin content. Since LH and FSH levels in serum decline progressively during infusion (Fig. 10.9), the decrease in pituitary content can only be due to the direct inhibition of LH-FSH synthesis under constant infusion of the agonist. The marked reduction in gonadotropin content agrees well with observations in pseudopregnant rats, where agonists given between days 6 and 9 of pseudopregnancy greatly reduced pituitary LH content (Sandow et al. 1981a), and with the effect of minipump infusions of LH-RH in sheep (Amundson and Wheaton 1979).

Pituitary–gonadal interactions (target organ responsiveness and steroid regulation)

Agonists induce changes in gonadotropic receptors, which control in turn the synthesis of gonadal steroids. Gonadal stimulation depends on gonadotropin utilization, which is not equivalent to the amount of gonadotropin released. LH-FSH and prolactin receptors determine the gonadal response, and modulate the effect of pituitary stimulation (Catt et al. 1980). Changes in the sensitivity and quantity of gonadotropin receptors are critical for the biological effect of the huge amounts of LH and FSH released after agonist stimulation. During puberty, the incipient secretion of FSH and LH induces gonadal FSH and LH

Table 10.4

MECHANISM OF AGONIST-INDUCED ANTIFERTILITY EFFECTS

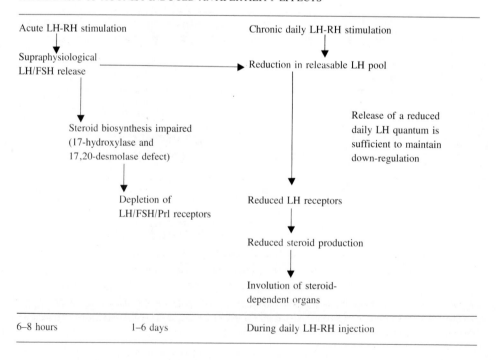

| 6–8 hours | 1–6 days | During daily LH-RH injection |

receptors (Catt and Dufau 1977; Catt et al. 1979a). Injection of pharmacological doses of hCG induces depletion of LH receptors (down-regulation) and desensitization of adenyl cyclase in the ovary (Conti et al. 1976) and testis (Hsueh et al. 1976). This mechanism is also activated by release of large quantities of endogenous LH by agonists (Auclair et al. 1977; Kledzik et al. 1978b). The short-term effect of acute injection of high LH-RH doses (1–100 μg i.v.) is identical with the effect of intravenous hCG injection, in that it induces defects in steroid biosynthesis (Table 10.4). The steroidogenic lesion is a partial defect in 17α-hydroxylase and 17,20-desmolase (Belanger et al. 1979; Dufau et al. 1979). In the long term, agonist injections deplete gonadotropin receptors (Table 10.4).

In contrast to gonadotropin receptor regulation, steroid feedback has only a minor role in agonist-induced antifertility. During physiological LH-RH stimulation, steroid feedback controls the differential release of LH and FSH. Follicular estrogen secretion induces the large releasable LH pool in the preovulatory phase of the cycle. The size of this pool determines the susceptibility of the female pituitary to agonist suppression. Androgens keep the releasable LH pool relatively small in the male, so that higher doses of agonists are required for suppression. During chronic agonist administration, steroid feedback is progressively eliminated by depletion of gonadotropin receptors after supraphysiological LH release. In consequence, uncoupling of gonadotropin secretion and steroid production by impaired gonadotropin utilization is a major determinant for the contraceptive, antiestrogenic and antiandrogenic activities of agonists observed in experimental animals (Johnson et al. 1976; Labrie et al. 1980a).

Hypothalamic–gonadal–interaction (extrapituitary effects)

There is increasing evidence for a direct interaction of agonists or functionally related endogenous LH-RH peptides with gonadal binding sites. This evidence comes from studies in hypophysectomized animals, demonstrating an inhibitory effect on LH-hCG receptors and testicular weight (Hsueh and Erickson 1979a; Bambino et al. 1980), and by analogous observations in female hypophysectomized rats (Hsueh and Erickson 1979b), and inhibition of steroid production in granulosa cell cultures (Clayton et al. 1979a; Hsueh and Ling 1979). The functional significance of these mechanisms in intact animals is not clear (Badger et al. 1980). Much higher agonist doses are required in hypophysectomized animals to counteract the effect of exogenous gonadotropins than to inhibit gonadal function in animals with an intact pituitary. It has been suggested that gonadal LH-RH like peptides may serve as feedback regulators of target organ and hypothalamic sensitivity (Sharpe and Fraser 1980b). The presence of agonist receptors in Leydig cells and granulosa cells has been established, but their functional role is still under investigation. Many antigonadotropic effects of agonists have been ascribed to extrapituitary mechanisms, whereas they can be explained equally well by reduced pituitary and target organ responsiveness after supraphysiological LH release. In this review, such observations will be discussed critically with regard to the question of whether the evidence for extrapituitary effects is compelling.

FEMALE REPRODUCTIVE TRACT

Numerous observations on the antigonadotropic and contraceptive effects of high doses of LH-RH and agonists in rodents and rabbits have supported the idea of an intrinsic antifertility effect of agonists (Corbin et al. 1978a). The value of such studies for prediction in the human is severely limited by species-specific differences in luteal function and the role of the ovary during pregnancy. LH-RH affects ovarian function (follicular maturation, ovulation and luteal function), the function of steroid-dependent organs (uterine growth, implantation and induction of parturition), and placental function. Both pro- and anti-fertility effects are directly or indirectly gonadotropin dependent, and paradoxical changes in target organ responsiveness are due to receptor regulation by circulating gonadotropins (Conti et al. 1976; Auclair et al. 1977; Catt et al. 1979).

Follicular maturation

LH-RH is essential for follicular maturation. In rats and rabbits actively immunized against LH-RH, estrogen levels are low and follicular maturation is absent (Fraser 1980a). Development of ovarian follicles requires adequate quantitative FSH stimulation (Richards 1979). The endogenous LH-RH pulse frequency in puberty can be estimated from the increasingly frequent peaks of FSH and LH. To mimic this pattern, infrequent small LH-RH doses have been used to induce follicular maturation. In the rhesus monkey, low LH-RH frequency favors FSH release, whereas LH release is relatively low. Stimulation of follicular maturation by LH-RH was demonstrated in rabbits, sheep and in the human. In the rabbit, the follicle-stimulating dose (once daily for 8 days s.c.) is 8 times lower than the ovulatory dose (Sandow 1975). The incidence of ovulation is significantly increased after follicle stimulating pretreatment (Sandow 1977), and the formation of functional luteal tissue was confirmed in ovarian homogenates by decreased estradiol content with a concomitant progesterone increase. Induction of follicular maturation in anestrous animals is of great importance for veterinary medicine. The fertility of ewes can be increased if follicular maturation is started during late anestrous, but daily LH-RH injections for this purpose have failed (Crighton et al. 1975). Ovulatory LH peaks of physiological magnitude were not followed by a luteal progesterone increase due to insufficient follicular maturation. If ewes are pretreated with low dose intermittent infusions of LH-RH (3 µg every 6 h for several days), adequate progesterone responses can be obtained during anoestrous (Domanski et al. 1977). A continuous stimulus of LH-RH by minipump infusions is unsuitable, because the pituitary is rapidly desensitized (Amundson and Wheaton 1979). The pituitary LH content is reduced by 95 % after 4 weeks of infusion (240 µg LH-RH per day). This study was still performed under the erroneous assumption that small LH-RH doses given continuously do not interfere with pituitary LH-RH responsiveness (for discussion see Belchetz et al. 1978). When LH-RH is given by multiple (pulsatile) injections (250–1000 ng at 2 h intervals for 8 days), a normal preovulatory LH increase with luteal progesterone increase is elicited in anoestrous sheep (McLeod and Haresign 1980; Haresign and McLeod 1980).

In the human, follicular maturation is arrested in a variety of conditions. One classical syndrome is secondary amenorrhea associated with anorexia nervosa. LH-RH (500 µg at 8 h intervals) successfully induced follicular maturation in women with anorexia nervosa (Mortimer et al. 1975; Nillius et al. 1975; Nillius 1976). Pulsatile LH-RH infusion also reinitiated follicular maturation and estrogen secretion in anorexia nervosa (LH-RH pulses, 25 ng per kg at 2-h intervals) (Marshall and Kelch 1979).

Primary or secondary amenorrhea of presumed hypothalamic origin can be corrected by pulsatile therapy with LH-RH, or in less severe LH-RH deficiency, by nasal administration of agonists. Pulsatile LH-RH treatment of primary amenorrhea in Kallman's syndrome resulted in normal follicular development. The infusion induced an intial high surge of LH and FSH, followed by ovulation with an adequate luteal progesterone increase between days 17 and 27 (Crowley and McArthur 1980b). The dose of LH-RH (25 ng per kg or about 1.2 µg per patient) was given s.c. at 2 h intervals for 27 days. Treatment of secondary amenorrhea with a pulsatile portable infusion pump (LH-RH 10–20 µg i.v. every 90 min) was followed by ovulation after 9–19 days (Leyendecker 1979; Leyendecker et al. 1980). A lower dose of LH-RH (1.2 µg s.c.) was also effective.

Hypothalamic amenorrhea can be visualized as an endocrine imbalance of variable severity. In more severe cases, hypothalamic secretion has to be fully substituted by synthetic LH-RH. In less severe deficiencies, LH-RH treatment may serve as a synchronizing or supportive stimulus. This concept can account both for the absolute LH-RH requirement in severe hypothalamic hypogonadism, and for the therapeutic efficacy of nasal agonist treatment, which requires the presence of a partially functioning pituitary system. Agonist treatment in low doses presumably increases pituitary LH content (Sandow et al. 1980a) and endogenous LH-RH secretion is regularized. The therapeutic effect of inducing regular menstrual cycles is often preserved for some time after stopping agonist administration (Brandau et al. 1980a,b).

An important consideration for the dosage to be used in pulsatile LH-RH therapy is the critical effect of follicular maturation on the luteal phase. A defective luteal phase observed after pulsatile LH-RH therapy in women with secondary amenorrhea may be the consequence of an underlying disturbance of follicular development. If a supraphysiological dose of LH-RH is used for substitution during the follicular phase, FSH levels may remain relatively low and cause a defective corpus luteum. In the human, the granulosa cells are the most important source of estradiol (McNatty and Baird 1978). The follicular levels of estradiol are high in follicles containing FSH, hence, reduced FSH stimulation during the follicular phase prevents the formation of a sufficient number of granulosa cells and subsequently results in a defective luteal phase. Reduced FSH release after high dose LH-RH pulses during the follicular phase would cause impaired luteal function through this mechanism.

In veterinary medicine, a disorder of follicular maturation e.g. bovine cystic ovarian disease, has been successfully treated with LH-RH (Dobson et al. 1977), and similarly anestric-acyclic cows respond positively to an agonist (Humke and Zuber 1977).

Higher doses of agonists inhibit follicular maturation in prepubertal animals, and block the hCG effect on ovarian weight in hypophysectomized rats (Rippel and Johnson 1976b;

Ying and Guillemin 1979). It was difficult to understand and explain why the expected stimulatory (gonadotropic) effects were not observed during chronic agonist treatment. The pituitary of the immature rat responds to LH-RH stimulation, and antigonadotropic effects are easily induced in immature and prepubertal female rats by pituitary hyperstimulation. Rats of 22–25 days respond to nonapeptide agonists (D-Ala[6], D-Leu[6], D-Ser (TBU)[6]-EA) with a sustained supraphysiological FSH and LH release, lasting 6–8 h (Vilchez-Martinez et al. 1974; Sandow et al. 1978b). After a single dose of agonist, FSH and LH receptors in the ovary decline within 6–8 h (Kledzik et al. 1978b); in this respect multiple consecutive injections are even more detrimental. Receptor depletion explains the failure of immature rats to respond in the hCG-augmentation assay of Steelman and Pohley, when agonists were substituted for FSH (Rippel and Johnson 1976b). The target organ response, viz. augmentation of ovarian weight by formation of multiple corpora lutea, is blocked by an induced deficiency of FSH receptors. Follicular development is arrested and there is no target for the additional hCG injection. The complex biological situation can only be analyzed by the simultaneous application of multiple techniques which correlate hormone levels in serum and tissue with the corresponding receptor concentrations (for discussion see Brenner and West 1975; Sandow 1979).

We consistently failed to induce follicular maturation by single injections of agonists in immature rats in the superovulation model (Zarrow et al. 1958; Sandow et al. 1976b), when trying to substitute PMSG priming with agonists. However, multiple small doses are likely to be effective. Supraphysiological doses of agonists delay pubertal development in female rats by inhibiting the onset of follicular estrogen secretion. The inhibition of pubertal changes in the ovary depends on the age of immature rats. When treatment starts at 22 days of age (D-Leu[6]-EA, 0.5 or 3 μg s.c. twice daily), vaginal opening is delayed and estrous cycles are absent, due to lack of appropriate gonadotropin secretion. Maturation of the ovaries and the uterus is retarded (Johnson et al. 1976), but weight developments is normalized within 30 days after treatment. In rats of 25 days, daily injection of D-Trp[6]-LH-RH (1 μg s.c. for 10 days) increases ovarian weight, but reduces uterine weight. There is a delay in vaginal opening (delayed follicular maturation), impaired pituitary responsiveness to LH-RH and decreased pituitary LH content. Hypothalamic LH-RH content is increased, possibly by inhibition of endogenous LH-RH degradation (Vilchez-Martinez et al. 1979). As in other studies of this design, no hormone receptor measurements were included, so that intercurrent changes in gonadotropin responsiveness are uncertain. In prepubertal rats of 35 days, daily injection of D-Ser (TBU)[6]-EA (50 ng s.c. for 28 days) also increases ovarian weight, whereas uterine weight is reduced. This divergence is due to an increased rate of ovulation which deprives the uterus of follicular estrogen stimulation. The ovaries consist mainly of luteinized tissue, and progesterone content is elevated (Sandow et al. 1978b). We have found similar changes in prepubertal rats of 35 days treated with very high agonist doses (50–200 μg per kg, D-Ser (TBU)[6]-EA, once daily) for 30 days.

In mature animals, the effect of chronic agonist treatment on follicular function depends on the dose administered. In stump-tailed macaques *(Macaca arctoides)*, 5 μg D-Ser(TBU)[6]-EA daily s.c. suppressed ovulation in the majority of animals, but did not prevent intermittent estradiol increases (Fig. 10.10; Fraser et al. 1980; Fraser 1980b).

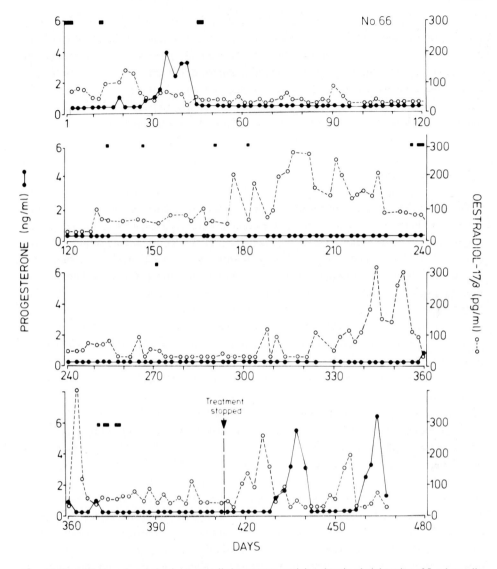

Fig. 10.10. Inhibition of ovulation in stump-tailed macaques receiving chronic administration of 5 μg buserelin per day s.c. Note absence of luteal progesterone increases from days 50 to 400, but intercurrent increases in estradiol-17β. After treatment, follicular maturation is resumed and ovulation is confirmed by normal luteal progesterone increases (H.M. Fraser, unpublished observations).

In a human contraceptive study, during 6 months of nasal administration of 200–400 μg D-Ser(TBU)[6]-EA, spontaneous estradiol increases were found despite daily agonist administration (Schmidt-Gollwitzer et al. 1981). In some women estradiol levels remained low, whereas in others normal increases were recorded. The individual response may reflect differences in pituitary sensitivity to agonist suppression. In precocious puberty, daily s.c. injection of 4 μg per kg D-Trp[6]-EA blocked the previously elevated LH and FSH levels within 8 weeks of therapy (Crowley et al. 1981). Estradiol levels fell below 20 pg ml[-1] during treatment, and proliferation of the vaginal epithelium was prevented. In precocious puberty, suppression of follicular maturation was temporary and ceased when agonist injections were stopped. In the rat, prepubertal animals undergo normal maturational events, and in adult rats, regular estrous cycles are re-established when agonist inhibition is withdrawn. Repletion of pituitary LH and FSH stores in the rat only takes 5–7 days.

Induction of ovulation

Ovulation with subsequent fertilization requires the presence of adequately matured Graafian follicles and oocytes. LH-RH injection has induced ovulation in all mammalian and nonmammalian species tested so far (Schally et al. 1978). In immature follicles, high doses of LH-RH can induce inappropriate ovulation. Since ovulation simply requires the release of an ovulatory quantum of LH, it is a very reliable bioassay for LH-RH activity; in immature rats it is convenient to synchronize follicular maturation by injecting 10 IU of PMSG. Spontaneous ovulation is blocked by pentobarbital (Sandow et al. 1976b), and the ovulatory response to LH-RH can be calculated both from the LH and FSH release 1 h after injection, or from the occurrence of ovulation. In this test, the ED_{50} of LH-RH by subcutaneous route is about 500 ng and the peptide is effective after intravenous, intramuscular or intraperitoneal injection and at higher doses after vaginal, rectal, nasal, or oral administration. Ovulation has also been induced by cutaneous application of very high doses of LH-RH in a suitable solvent (dimethylsulfoxide).

Inappropriate ovulation can be induced by LH-RH and agonists, during stages of follicular development which do not permit formation of a functional corpus luteum, or during implantation and pregnancy (Banik and Givner 1975, 1976; Jones 1979a). Early studies by Ying (1973) established an antiovulatory effect of high doses of LH-RH. The strong imbalance in steroid secretion may significantly affect tubal ovum transport, so that no ova are found in the oviducts at autopsy, even though ovulation has occurred. In adult rats, 20–120 ng D-Ala[6]-EA s.c. can induce ovulation at any stage of the cycle, and a rhythmic antifertility effect of this agonist, injected every third day in cyclic rats, has been described (Banik and Givner 1976). In pregnant rats, rabbits and guinea pigs, high doses of LH-RH or agonists can induce ovulation. In the rabbit, such inappropriate ovulations cause luteinization of all available follicles, depriving the rabbit of its physiological luteotropic estrogen secretion, and resulting in luteolysis (Rippel and Johnson 1976a). In the rat, inappropriate ovulations are induced at any time from day 6 to 21 of pregnancy (Jones 1979a), resulting in an increased ratio of progesterone/estrogen secretion (Bercu et al. 1980). Reduced estrogen secretion causes insufficient formation of myometrial oxytocin receptors and delay of parturition. It is known from studies with gonadotropin induced ovulation that insufficient follicular maturation will prevent the ovum upon ovulation from being released from the Graafian follicle, resulting in its entrapment, with subsequent luteinization of the unruptured follicle containing the trapped ovum. A similar mechanism has been discussed for the action of LH-RH antagonists in monkeys (Wilks et al. 1980).

The precoital contraceptive effect of LH-RH (Corbin et al. 1978a) and agonists may be due to a long-lasting gonadotropin receptor depletion, associated with reduced progesterone and decreased uterine weight (Kledzik et al. 1978b), or to release of the ovum into a milieu unsuitable for ovum transport and implantation.

Inhibition of ovulation

LH-RH agonists or antagonists prevent ovulation by different mechanisms. If follicular maturation is impaired or suppressed by chronic agonist treatment, lack of a preovulatory estrogen peak results in an inability to ovulate. The preovulatory LH increase is also impaired or prevented by reduction of the releasable LH pool. Antagonists prevent the preovulatory LH increase due to competitive occupancy of pituitary LH-RH receptors. Agonists block ovulation at considerably lower doses than antagonists.

The mechanisms leading to anovulation can be deduced from changes in pituitary hormone content and receptor concentrations. These tissue indices are not directly accessible in clinical studies, and have to be inferred from animal experiments. The predictive value of such complementary investigation for planning and interpretation of clinical studies is considerable. Clinical development of a contraceptive peptide requires an intimate understanding of the pharmacological effects of high doses of agonists. In the human, practical application by a self-administered method, e.g. nasal spray or suppositories, is preferable to injections. The doses required for precoital contraception (inhibition of ovulation) and postcoital contraception (luteolysis) can be predicted from animal experiments.

Maturational changes in the immature rat ovary are postponed by early agonist treatment. In adult rats, agonists suppress follicular maturation but do not prevent luteinization (Table 10.5). In rats receiving D-Ser-(TBU)^6-EA (0.05–125 µg kg^{-1} once daily) for 6 months, there is increased luteinization producing a temporary block of ovulation and lengthening estrous cycles. The ovary is constantly stimulated, and pituitary LH release is confirmed by the presence of functional luteal tissue. In contrast, antagonists block the preovulatory LH increase in cyclic rats, and in immature rats primed with PMSG (Beattie et al. 1976; de la Cruz et al. 1976; Coy et al. 1979), but have no effect on luteal function. Inhibition of ovulation by antagonists requires precise knowledge of the expected time of ovulation. Administration throughout the follicular phase is impractical because of the high doses required for LH inhibition. The obligatory requirement for LH-RH in ovulation has been disputed: in rhesus monkeys acute pituitary stalk section does not prevent ovulation, and an estradiol challenge is sufficient to induce ovulation (Ferin et al. 1979). However, this special experimental situation cannot be interpreted as evidence for independence of ovulation from LH-RH. Passive transfer of LH-RH antisera before ovulation effectively blocks ovulation in several species, including the rhesus monkey (see reviews by Fraser 1980a, 1981).

Inhibition of ovulation by agonists begins with pituitary desensitization. A timed block of ovulation is not practical due to a lack of rapid, sensitive and economical methods of

Table 10.5

OVARIAN FUNCTION IN RATS AFTER LONG-TERM TREATMENT WITH AN LH-RH AGONIST, D-Ser (TBU)[6]-EA (BUSERELIN)

Group No.	Treatment[A]	Daily dose	Ovarian weight (mg)	Tertiary follicles	Corporea lutea	Progesterone (µg per ovary)
1	Controls, saline	0.2 ml	112 ± 22^B	3.2 ± 0.4	12.3 ± 3.5	0.92 ± 0.7
2	Buserelin	0.05 µg kg^{-1}	132 ± 24	1.0 ± 0.0^C	28.4 ± 6.6^C	1.73 ± 0.8^C
3	Buserelin	2.5 µg kg^{-1}	120 ± 34	1.0 ± 0.0^C	27.5 ± 6.4^C	1.74 ± 0.9^C
4	Buserelin	125 µg kg^{-1}	70 ± 14^C	1.0 ± 0.0^C	25.1 ± 6.0^C	1.15 ± 0.5

Under long-term treatment, there is no ovarian involution, but increased formation of corpora lutea due to inappropriate ovulations.
[A] One daily subcutaneous injection for 6 months.
[B] Each point is the mean ±SEM of 20 determinations.
[C] Significant difference vs controls by ANOVA at 95% level.

predicting the expected time of ovulation. Agonist contraception relies on the onset of menstrual bleeding, as the natural index for ovarian cyclicity. Treatment with low doses of the agonist (D-Ser(TBU)^6-EA, 5 µg thrice daily s.c.) during the follicular phase of the menstrual cycle (Fig. 10.9) reduces pituitary sensitivity within 3–4 days (Dericks-Tan et al. 1977). Reduced pituitary responsiveness is probably associated with depletion of pituitary gonadotropin content, since pituitary LH and FSH content is reduced in animals under daily agonist injections (Sandow et al. 1979a; von Rechenberg et al. 1979). In the human, pituitary responsiveness may depend on the releasable LH pool as a function of total pituitary LH content. After agonist desensitization, the pituitary releases a small daily quantum of LH under agonist stimulation, but it cannot provide the large LH quantum required for ovulation. At higher doses of agonist, reduced estradiol levels may also impair the LH surge. This concept explains why follicular estradiol increases are neither abolished in cyclic women taking agonists by nasal spray (Bergquist et al. 1979b, 1979c; Schmidt-Gollwitzer et al. 1981), nor in stump-tailed macaques receiving daily injections of agonists (Fraser et al. 1980). The nasal route is a practical way for chronic administration of oligopeptides; nasal resorption of LH-RH in the human is 1–2% (Fink et al. 1974; Bourguignon et al. 1974), and LH-RH agonists have similar resorption rates. After oral or buccal administration, resorption is not sufficient for practical application, but agonists are resorbed in small quantities by the vaginal and rectal routes (Saito et al. 1977).

Effects on corpus luteum function

Therapeutic administration of hCG stimulates luteal progesterone production and supports a defective corpus luteum (Leyendecker 1979). In contrast to hCG, neither LH-RH injections nor infusions have been of therapeutic value in rescuing a defective corpus luteum. On the contrary, several consecutive high doses of LH-RH agonists reduce in vivo luteal progesterone production by LH receptor down-regulation, and in vitro by a direct action on granulosa cell function (Clayton et al. 1979a).

The human corpus luteum requires only minimal LH support, because the physiological frequency of LH pulses during the luteal phase in the human is reduced to one pulse at 4 hourly intervals (Yen et al. 1972). The release of an unphysiological amount of LH by substitution with frequent LH-RH pulses may reduce luteal sensitivity and cause insufficient gonadotropin utilization by the newly formed corpus luteum.

Experimental studies in rats and rabbits (Yoshinaga and Fujino 1979, Corbin et al. 1978a, Bex and Corbin 1980), monkeys (Raynaud et al. 1979; Hagino et al. 1979) and in the human (Koyama et al. 1978; Lemay et al. 1979a,b; Casper and Yen 1979) support the luteolytic action of LH-RH and its potent agonists. Injection of LH-RH in pseudopregnant rats (Table 10.6) or LH-RH agonists in pregnant rats (Rivier et al. 1978) induces a transient progesterone rise; repeated injections cause luteal down-regulation. The postcoital contraceptive effect in the rat (Corbin et al. 1977) is due to luteal deficiency caused by reduction of LH receptors (Bex and Corbin 1979), and possibly magnified by a reduction in estradiol secretion (Lee and Ryan 1974), and prolactin receptors. LH-RH treatment in the rat before and during implantation (200 µg s.c. days 1–7 after mating) and after implanta-

Table 10.6

EFFECT OF LH-RH ON OVARIAN ASCORBIC ACID DEPLETION IN INTACT AND HYPOPHYSECTOMIZED PSEUDOPREGNANT RATS

Group No.		Treatment i.m.	Dose per rat	Ovarian ascorbic acid[A] (μg per 100 mg)	Serum progesterone[A] (ng ml^{-1})
1	Intact	Saline	0.2 ml	95.1 ± 2.91	355 ± 29.6
2	Intact	LH-RH	0.3 μg	68.4 ± 1.41[B]	498 ± 28.9[B]
3	Intact	LH-RH	0.6 μg	52.7 ± 3.81[B]	506 ± 40.0[B]
4	Intact	LH-RH	1.2 μg	47.2 ± 2.41[B]	601 ± 26.2[B]
5	Hypophysectomized	Saline	0.2 ml	27.8 ± 5.02	47 ± 10.0
6	Hypophysectomized	LH-RH	1.2 μg	21.5 ± 2.89	80 ± 25.0

Sprague-Dawley rats, 22-day-old received on day 1 at 9:00 a.m. 50IU PMSG and on day 3 at 3:00 p.m. 25IU HCG; hypophysectomy was performed on day 2. LH-RH injected on day 6 and autopsy performed 1 h later.

[A] Ovarian ascorbic acid determined by photometry and serum progesterone by RIA.

[B] Significant difference vs respective controls by ANOVA at 95% level.

tion (days 7–12 of pregnancy) reduces ovarian LH binding within 24 h of the first dose, and receptor depletion is maintained by further injections. The resulting decrease in progesterone terminates pregnancy, similarly to ovariectomy (Yochim and Zarrow 1961). A marked decrease in LH and FSH receptors was also found after D-Ala[6]-EA (100 µg, once daily) administered from days 7 to 12 of pregnancy, resulting in termination of the pregnancy (Kledzik et al. 1978a). Progesterone substitution therapy protects against the postimplantational contragestational effect of high LH-RH doses (Humphrey et al. 1977).

The antigonadotropic action of agonists on the corpus luteum has two alternative explanations: a pituitary-dependent effect, and an LH-independent, direct effect on ovarian steroidogenesis. These mechanisms are not mutually exclusive; they could operate under different doses or simultaneously in intact animals. Studies on LH regulation of the luteal LH receptor (see reviews by Dufau and Catt 1978; Catt et al. 1979a; Catt et al. 1980) have confirmed that acute LH hyperstimulation has negative effects on the subsequent gonadal response to LH stimulation. The initial effect is desensitization of the steroid-producing granulosa cell to LH stimulation, with subsequent down-regulation of the number of luteal LH receptors. It is clearly acute supraphysiological LH release which activates the luteolytic mechanism, because antagonists even in high doses fail to induce luteolysis. Subsequently, prolonged treatment reduces LH secretion (Rivier et al. 1978) and depletes pituitary LH content, eliminating LH support to corpus luteum. LH-dependent luteolysis is characterized by reduced gonadotropin utilization after uncoupling of the LH effector mechanism (luteal adenyl cyclase system), despite high levels of circulating LH.

Luteolysis in nonpregnant animals is monitored by progesterone production of an established corpus luteum; treatment starts several days after ovulation. We have studied luteolysis in pseudopregnant rats, where placental progesterone production does not interfere with the evaluation. Immature rats were primed with PMSG/hCG (von Rechenberg et al. 1979; Sandow et al. 1981a), and received daily injections of the peptide from days 6-9 of pseudopregnancy. LH-RH and the agonist buserelin significantly lowered serum progesterone and ovarian ascorbic acid content (Sandow et al. 1979a). The luteolytic potency of LH-RH analogues of increasing potency was strictly related to their LH-releasing activity. The LH-RH antagonist D-Phe[2], D-Phe[3], D-Phe[6]-LH-RH (200 µg s.c. for 4 days) was ineffective because it does not stimulate LH-release.

An analysis of hypothalamic–pituitary–gonadal function at the end of treatment confirmed pituitary hyperstimulation as the mechanism of action in luteolysis.

Endogenous LH-RH content was reduced by treatment with LH-RH or buserelin, but pituitary LH-RH receptors did not decline, a finding which is in accordance with studies in male rats (Sandow et al. 1980b). LH-RH (100 µg s.c. × 4 days) significantly lowered ovarian LH receptors, and buserelin was highly effective at a lower dose (5 ng s.c. for 4 days) (Table 10.7). The FSH receptors in ovarian homogenates were also down-regulated. Ovarian prolactin receptors were increased after treatment, although they usually decrease after agonist hyperstimulation in adult rats. Serum LH and FSH levels were still elevated 24 h after the last buserelin injection, confirming supraphysiological release. The agonist induced extensive dose-dependent depletion of pituitary LH content, whereas LH-RH itself was much less effective in this respect. The importance of supraphysiological LH release

Table 10.7

LUTEOLYSIS IN PSEUDOPREGNANT RATS, INDUCED BY A 3-DAY TREATMENT WITH LH-RH OR THE AGONIST D-Ser (TBU)^6-ETHYLAMIDE (BUSERELIN): EFFECT ON HYPOTHALAMIC-PITUITARY FUNCTION AND OVARIAN RECEPTORS

Group No.	Treatment days 6–9 of pseudopregnancy	Daily dose per rat	Hypothalamic-pituitary function		Ovarian function (receptors fmol per g tissue)		
			LH-RH content (ng per hypothalamus)	LH-RH receptors (fmol buserelin per pituitary)	LH	FSH	PRL
1	Controls	0	2.67 ± 0.29	0.79 ± 0.01	81.1 ± 2.8	18.5 ± 0.2	2.4 ± 0.6
2	LH-RH	0.1 µg	1.75 ± 0.19^A	0.93 ± 0.03	83.1 ± 1.0	18.5 ± 1.8	7.1 ± 0.5^A
3	LH-RH	1 µg	1.46 ± 0.13^A	0.92 ± 0.02	66.9 ± 0.9^A	15.8 ± 0.2	11.3 ± 0.8^A
4	LH-RH	10 µg	1.69 ± 0.12^A	0.52 ± 0.03	70.2 ± 0.9^A	16.9 ± 0.6	4.0 ± 0.9
5	LH-RH	100 µg	1.51 ± 0.19^A	0.78 ± 0.12	63.4 ± 1.6^A	14.1 ± 0.5^A	9.6 ± 0.4^A
6	Buserelin	5 ng	1.58 ± 0.14^A	0.79 ± 0.12	53.7 ± 1.2^A	14.1 ± 0.2^A	5.9 ± 0.2^A
7	Buserelin	50 ng	1.36 ± 0.09^A	1.06 ± 0.01	53.4 ± 1.0^A	16.2 ± 1.6	10.7 ± 0.4^A
8	Buserelin	500 ng	1.33 ± 0.12^A	1.18 ± 0.04^A	44.7 ± 1.2^A	13.8 ± 0.9^A	12.9 ± 0.8^A
9	Buserelin	5000 ng	1.62 ± 0.16^A	1.06 ± 0.01	38.6 ± 0.7^A	12.5 ± 0.4^A	6.9 ± 0.5^A

Hypothalamic LH-RH content determined by RIA (mean ± SEM of 8 determinations), pituitary LH-RH receptors determined by [^{125}I]buserelin binding, LH receptors by ^{125}I-labelled hCG binding, FSH receptors by ^{125}I-labelled hFSH, and prolactin receptors by ^{125}I-labelled hPRL binding (mean ± SEM of 4 determinations on pooled tissues per group).

^{A} Significant difference vs controls by ANOVA at 95% level.

was also confirmed by comparing the effect of frequent or infrequent injections of the same total dose of the peptide on progesterone levels in pseudopregnancy. Multiple daily injections (which release a large amount of LH) reduced progesterone more effectively than injections made every second day (Sandow et al. 1981a).

A second mechanism which may participate in the luteolytic effect of agonists was established by in vitro studies on agonist binding to luteal LH-RH receptors and the effect on hCG-stimulated progesterone production by granulosa cells (Clayton et al. 1979a; Hsueh et al. 1980). The stimulatory effect of low concentrations of hCG on progesterone production was completely inhibited by buserelin. A maximum progesterone response was elicited by stimulation with high hCG concentrations despite addition of the agonist (Clayton et al. 1979a,b). A reduced number of LH binding sites after the down-regulation effect of LH-RH or hCG in vivo may be compensated by the strong stimulatory effect of hCG, because full steroid production can still be elicited after depletion of spare receptors (Catt and Dufau 1977). The protective effect of hCG on luteal progesterone production in early pregnancy may be due to hCG's ability to act despite the presence of reduced LH receptors. Specific high-affinity binding sites for LH-RH agonists on luteal cells were also found by Harwood et al. (1980a,b), though ovarian uptake of ^{125}I labelled D-Leu^6-EA in rats is low in comparison with pituitary uptake (Mayar et al. 1979).

The exact mechanism of agonist modulation of granulosa cell function is not known (Behrmann et al. 1980). Agonists do not inhibit binding of labelled LH or FSH to the ovary (Hsueh and Erickosn 1979a), but they reduce LH-induced activation of the adenyl cyclase system by blocking stimulus–secretion coupling. LH-RH antagonists can neutralize the inhibition of steroid production resulting from addition of LH-RH (Hsueh and Ling 1979).

Effects on the uterus and on implantation

Two types of gonadotropic and antigonadotropic interactions of LH-RH and its agonists with the uterus have been discussed. The classical mechanism is related to dependence of estradiol production by gonadotropins in pubertal and adult animals, causing uterine growth or involution. A second mechanism has been proposed, which comprises a direct uterine site of action of LH-RH peptides.

In immature animals, inhibition of uterine growth by agonists is related to delayed onset of puberty and temporary suppression of estradiol production. Normal uterine development begins when peptide administration is stopped. In the adult animal, ovarian estrogen production can be largely suppressed. In rats with hormone-dependent tumors, D-Leu^6-EA (5 µg s.c., twice daily) reduces tumor size significantly, similar to ovariectomy (Johnson et al. 1976; De Sombre et al. 1976). In adult rats, high doses of agonists cause ovarian and uterine involution, whereas lower doses only reduce estrogen production by favoring luteinization, without causing ovarian involution (Table 10.5), and do not suppress uterine growth. In hypophysectomized pseudopregnant rats, we have failed to observe a suppressive effect on ovarian ascorbic acid content and luteal progesterone production, despite priming of follicular/luteal development with PMSG-hCG (Table 10.6). It is not clear whether this failure is due to the absence of prolactin after hypophysectomy or reflects instead the lack of a direct gonadal effect of agonists. In intact immature mice, LH-RH stimulates uterine development (Corbin et al. 1978a), but the peptide also increases uterine weight in hypophysectomized rats (Corbin and Beattie 1975). However, the latter findings were probably artifacts due to incomplete hypophysectomy. In the human, the pars tuberalis contains a high proportion of gonadotropic cells (Baker 1977). In the rat, residual LH cells in the supradiaphragmatic pars tuberalis after parapharyngeal hypophysectomy (Gross and Page 1979) undergo marked hyperplasia and are a source of error in studies with hypophysectomized animals. In our own studies, we have not been able to stimulate uterine growth with LH-RH or agonists in ovariectomized rats, or in immature rats treated with LH-RH (Schröder et al. 1973). The lack of a direct action on the uterus of LH-RH and two agonists (D-Ala[6], NMe-Leu[7]-EA and D-Trp[6], NMe-Leu[7]-EA) has been confirmed by Jones (1979b).

Unequivocal demonstration of an extrapituitary effect in vivo would require hypophysectomy with simultaneous blockage of the remaining LH cells by passive transfer of an LH antiserum. Unfortunately, this procedure also eliminates ovarian-testicular stimulation. The remaining LH cells can also be suppressed by high doses of agonists, a finding which would be interpreted as an extrapituitary (direct gonadal) effect.

Inhibition of implantation by LH-RH and agonists (postcoital contraception) is related to the severe imbalance in steroid production caused by pituitary hyperstimulation (Bex and Corbin 1979). Implantation depends on adequate preparation of the uterine milieu for the blastocyst, and any disturbance of the local factors (estrogens, progesterone, prostaglandins) endangers or prevents implantation (Psychoyos 1973; Brenner and West 1975). Prenidatory treatment with LH-RH (500 μg, twice daily from days 1 to 3) reduced fetal size at autopsy (day 15) by delayed implantation, and terminated pregnancy (150 μg, twice daily from days 1 to 7) in rats (Humphrey et al. 1978). Similar results were obtained by us with an agonist in rats and rabbits (Sandow 1977).

Effects on pregnancy

The effects of LH-RH during pregnancy in rats and rabbits are related to the different role of the pituitary in pregnancy of rodents, or in man. During pregnancy, the human pituitary becomes increasingly refractory to LH-RH stimulation. Gonadotropin release is blocked by high estrogen and chorionic gonadotropin levels (Rubinstein et al. 1978; Sowers et al. 1978). In contrast, in the rat ovulation can be induced by LH-RH (250 μg s.c. twice daily administered from days 6 to 22 of pregnancy) (Jones 1979c). The experimental evidence for effects on pregnancy relies on the administration of high doses of agonists in rats and rabbits, and on in vitro findings of LH-RH and LH-RH-like peptides in the placenta. Since placental function and the contribution of the ovaries to maintenance of pregnancy are different between species, the effects observed in the rat and in the rabbit cannot be extrapolated to primates.

In the rat, pregnancy depends on ovarian progesterone production until day 12, and can be terminated by hypophysectomy or passive transfer of LH antiserum (Madhwa Raj and Mougdal 1970). After day 12, pregnancy is partly maintained after hypophysectomy by placental progesterone production via a placental LH-like chorionic gonadotropin (Haour et al. 1976; MacDonald and Beattie 1979; Bex and Corbin 1980). Treatment of hypophysectomized rats with LH-RH (200 μg s.c. twice daily) on days 12 to 16 of pregnancy results in fetal resorption and decreased plasma progesterone by day 18. This may indicate a placental site of action for LH-RH suppression, but it could also be due to the LH cells remaining in the pars tuberalis after hypophysectomy which are inhibited by LH-RH treatment. Suppression of this residual LH secretion (Gross and Page 1979) would deprive the rat of its ovarian progesterone, which is important for maintenance of pregnancy. Both in hypophysectomized control rats and hypophysectomized LH-RH treated rats, ovarian weight was greatly reduced on day 18 when fetal resorption had occurred, but was only slightly reduced by LH-RH in rats maintaining their pregnancies (McDonald and Beattie 1979). A direct action of LH-RH on the pregnant uterus has been postulated, because local injections of LH-RH into one uterine horn result in fetal resorption (Jones 1979b). In this study the LH increase in plasma after local LH-RH injection was not measured, but it may have contributed significantly to the termination of pregnancy by down-regulation of luteal LH receptors, since LH-RH is resorbed from the uterus in, e.g., the sheep. Administration of LH-RH by the intravenous route or intra-vaginally was without effect on pregnancy, but no other oligopeptides were injected locally for comparison. A direct local effect of LH-RH may involve e.g. an antihistaminic effect on implantation (Shelesnyak 1957), because many substances interfere with implantation when injected into the uterus. Measurement of luteal LH, FSH and prolactin receptors after local LH-RH injection would facilitate determination of a local or general site of action.

Evidence for an LH-RH-like peptide in the placenta was provided by extraction of LH-RH-like immunoreactive material from placental tissue, and the demonstration of stimulation of hCG production by LH-RH in cultured placental tissue (Siler-Khodr and Khodr 1978; Khodr and Siler-Khodr 1978, 1979). In the human, injection of LH-RH or agonists during pregnancy does not stimulate hCG secretion (Tamada et al. 1976; Casper et al. 1980). One would expect that, if the placenta were under LH-RH control, it should react to single doses of agonists with hCG release, even though the pituitary is inhibited by circulating estrogens. On the other hand, it is surprising that incubation of placental tissue in vitro with LH-RH results in a suppression of progesterone production rather than stimulation (Wilson and Jaward 1980). Intriguing questions are left open for physiological studies. Does LH-RH pulsatility cease in pregnancy, is hCG release under the control of a placental LH-RH or do agonists affect placental progesterone production either directly or indirectly? These questions can only be answered unambiguously in species where ovarian progesterone production can be eliminated without termination of pregnancy.

In rats, the effects of LH-RH and agonists on pregnancy are not mediated by the placenta, but by LH-induced stimulation of the ovary during pregnancy. In pregnant rats treated with LH-RH a dose-related reduction in litter size and an increase in neonatal mortality was noted in our own studies. This finding was attributed to a prolongation of gestation due to delayed induction of labor. Studies on myometrial estrogen and oxytocin receptors (Bercu et al. 1980) have explained the difficulty in induction of labor by a pituitary dependent effect of LH-RH. Treatment of pregnant rats with LH-RH (0.5 μg s.c. per 100 g, twice daily) from day 13 of pregnancy until delivery results in a reduced estradiol/progesterone ratio in serum, probably due to inappropriate ovulations with luteinization of additional follicles, and a decrease in ovarian estradiol production. There is a reduction of nuclear and cytosolic estradiol receptors, and a concomitant decrease in myometrial oxytocin receptors. The change in uterine contractility impairs or prevents timely induction of labor. We have consistently observed a decrease in estradiol and an increase in progesterone in nonpregnant rats under high dose treatment with LH-RH or D-Ser (TBU)^6-EA (Sandow et al. 1978b). D-Ser(TBU)^6-EA (200 μg s.c. per kg for 30 days) in prepubertal rats augments ovarian weight with a higher incidence of corpora lutea, whereas uterine weight (an index of estradiol production) is decreased. In contrast to other investigators, we have not observed ovarian atrophy after long-term administration (Table 10.5). Inhibition of parturition in rats treated with LH-RH or agonists during pregnancy is due to a hormone-dependent change in myometrial contractility; this is induced by increased progesterone production by additional corpora lutea formed following inappropriate ovulations.

In extensive studies, fetal and neonatal developments have been studied in LH-RH and agonist-treated rats receiving injections from days 1 to 16 of pregnancy. There was no effect of LH-RH or agonists on postnatal development, pubertal changes or visual and auditory functions in the offspring. However, slight changes were noted in skeletal development of the fetuses due to the imbalance in steroid production (reduced estradiol/progesterone ratio) of the dams treated during pregnancy.

MALE REPRODUCTIVE SYSTEM

LH-RH has found an important therapeutic application in the treatment of cryptorchidism, and in hypogonadotropic hypogonadism. In cryptorchidism, administration of a nasal spray several times daily for two to four weeks is followed by testicular descent, without undesirable androgenic symptoms (Illig et al. 1977; Happ et al. 1978a). In prepubertal boys, the pituitary responds predominantly with an FSH release (prepubertal release pattern), and LH only increases after several days of LH-RH administration. Therefore, the therapeutic effect of LH-RH in cryptorchidism must be attributed to initial FSH release, subsequently supplemented by an LH release of relatively smaller magnitude. In hypogonadotropic hypogonadism, attempts to raise plasma testosterone by three or four daily injections (Mortimer et al. 1974) have not been very successful. The experimental results of pulsatile LH-RH substitution (Knobil 1980) provided a rational therapeutic concept for pulsatile substitution in hypogonadal men (Crowley and McArthur 1980b). Pulsatile infusion of 25 ng kg^{-1} LH-RH s.c. at 2 h intervals over periods of several months resulted in a progressive testosterone increase followed by initiation of spermatogenesis. In contrast, daily injections of LH-RH in men with Kallman's syndrome do not maintain prolonged testosterone increases but gradually decrease pituitary–testicular responsiveness, and agonist injections become progressively ineffective in hypogonadal men because of pituitary desensitization at higher doses (Crowley et al. 1980c). The hypogonadal state is characterized by decreased pituitary sensitivity to agonists, but with progessive activation of LH synthesis, it becomes susceptible to suppression. A dose of 5 μg D-Ser(TBU)^6-EA

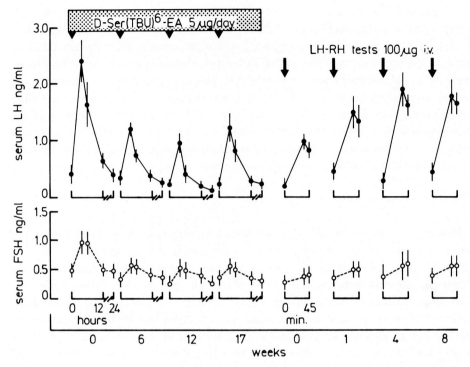

Fig. 10.11. Pituitary inhibition by an LH-RH agonist in normal men: daily injections of 5 μg D-Ser(TBU)[6]-EA (buserelin) s.c. progressively reduce the LH and FSH response. There is a long-lasting response to each individual injection, even after 17 weeks. Recovery of pituitary responsiveness tested by LH-RH injections, 100 μg i.v. A normal response is reestablished 4 weeks after treatment.

s.c. every second day is compatible with reproducible LH release in normal men (Wiegelmann et al. 1977). In hypogonadal men, pituitary LH release is increased during 7 days of treatment with a daily dose of 5 μg D-Ser(TBU)[6]-EA, whereas this dose progressively reduces pituitary sensitivity in normal men (Smith et al. 1979).

Injecting 5 μg D-Ser(TBU)[6]-EA into normal men (Bergquist et al. 1979a) consistently decreases serum testosterone but the pituitary response to daily injections is preserved over a period of 17 weeks. The magnitude of daily LH release is reduced, but appears to be sufficient to maintain down-regulation of the testicular LH receptors. Within 4 weeks after treatment, a normal pituitary response to LH-RH is reestablished (Fig. 10.11), and testosterone returns to pretreatment levels.

Pubertal development

Pulsatile LH-RH substitution has a beneficial effect on pubertal development, and intermittent agonist stimulation with minimal effective doses avoiding decreased pituitary responsiveness is also therapeutically effective (Mies 1980). The suppressive effect of supraphysiological agonist doses on testosterone secretion and development of accessory sex organs in the rat and dog formed the ground for detailed studies on hypothalamic–pituitary–gonadal interaction (Sandow et al. 1976a, Sandow et al. 1978a,b, Tcholakian et al. 1978a). In immature rats of 30 days, maturational processes in the testes are inhibited during a 7 day-treatment with 50 ng D-Ser(TBU)^6-EA, a 10-fold physiological dose (Sharpe et al. 1979). LH and FSH release were inhibited, pituitary gonadotropin content reduced, and the response of the testis to hCG in vitro was impaired by a reduction in testicular LH–hCG receptors. During prolonged treatment (28 days), reversible involution of the androgen-dependent organs was observed (Sandow et al. 1978c). The effects on testicular function in adult rats resemble those in prepubertal animals, together with additional effects on the germinal epithelium and Leydig cell function.

Effect on androgen-dependent organs

Hypophysectomy and/or castration is followed by atrophy of the androgen-dependent organs (ventral prostate, seminal vesicles, levator ani muscle) and testicular involution. These effects are also observed after prolonged agonist treatment, but the mechanism is not simply gonadotropin withdrawal, but a lack of testicular gonadotropin responsiveness. In early chronic tolerance studies with high doses of LH-RH in rats and dogs, a reduction in the weight of the testes and accessory sex organs was noted (Fig. 10.1). These changes were ascribed to activation of a strong androgen feedback from the hyperstimulated testes with ensuing inhibition of pituitary LH secretion. However, it was soon found that testosterone in serum decreased after chronic treatment with LH-RH or agonists (Sandow 1977; Sandow et al. 1978b). In therapeutic studies with LH-RH, decreased pituitary responsiveness and reduced testosterone secretion had also been noted in prepubertal bulls (Mongkonpunya et al. 1975, Haynes et al. 1977), and in men with psychogenic impotence (Davies et al. 1977). In rats, the weight of androgen-dependent organs is reduced both after daily injections of LH-RH (Oshima et al. 1975; Sandow et al. 1979c), and agonists (Sandow et al. 1976a, Rivier et al. 1979; Sharpe et al. 1979; Labrie et al. 1980a; Sandow et al. 1980d), or after intermittent injections (Pelletier et al. 1978; Cusan et al. 1979; Rivier et al. 1979; Sandow et al. 1980d). Reduced androgen production after supraphysiological LH-RH stimulation is due to a decrease in pituitary sensitivity (Fig. 10.12) and a decrease in target organ sensitivity (loss of LH receptors in the testes and decreased hCG responsiveness). Both mechanisms are clearly linked, but pituitary and testicular responsiveness can be regulated to some extent independently by varying the dose and frequency of pituitary stimulation. After intermittent agonist injections (twice weekly), testicular responsiveness is greatly reduced but pituitary responsiveness is not affected, because pituitary LH release recovers more rapidly than the testicular LH receptor concentration. After daily injections, pituitary responsiveness is gradually suppressed, together with the occurrence of testicular receptor down-regulation. Under constant dose infusion of agonists, target organ responsiveness recovers independently of prevailing pituitary suppression (Table 10.3).

In dogs, involution of the testes and prostate (Sandow et al. 1976a, 1978b) and reduced testosterone levels are found after 6 month's treatment with D-Ser(TBU)^6-EA (125 µg per kg s.c. once daily) (Table 10.8), but testosterone returns to normal within 8 weeks of treatment

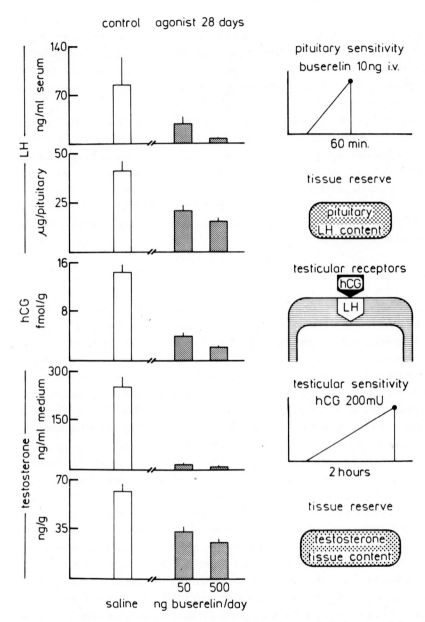

Fig. 10.12. Effect of chronic LH-RH agonist treatment on pituitary-testicular function: pituitary function tested by sensitivity to injection of 10 ng buserelin i.v., and pituitary LH content (tissue reserve). Testicular function tested by hCG binding, testosterone production after incubation with hCG 200 mU in vitro for 2 h and testicular testosterone content (tissue reserve). Note dose-dependent reduction in pituitary-testicular sensitivity, pituitary LH content and testicular testosterone content.

withdrawal, LH secretion is greatly reduced, with subsequent testosterone decrease, but prolactin secretion is unaffected. In the male rat, reduction in prolactin secretion and pituitary content has been frequently reported during agonist-induced suppression (Sandow et al. 1978b; Rivier et al. 1979). The role of prolactin suppression is not clear, because prolactin receptors in the testis are acutely down-regulated after agonist injection, without increases in prolactin release.

A promising therapeutic approach has been proposed (Labrie et al. 1980a) for the treatment of hormone-dependent prostate cancer; it comprises a combination of agonist inhibition of the pituitary with peripheral androgen blockage by an anti-androgen. During tumor therapy with a 'pure' anti-androgen, the negative feedback inhibition of the pituitary by testosterone is gradually released, resulting in unrestrained LH secretion with progressive increases of peripheral androgen production. However, when pituitary LH secretion is suppressed by an agonist, the remaining low levels of circulating androgens can be effectively blocked by the anti-androgen.

Effects on testicular function

There are two separate lines of evidence for pituitary–testicular interaction and hypothalamic–testicular interaction. In immature animals, reduction of testicular weight by agonists is a consequence of delayed maturation. In adult animals, testicular weight decreases as a result of reduced androgen production. Both mechanisms are pituitary dependent. There is a marked sex difference in the proclivity of the male and female pituitary to be suppressed by agonists. Considerably higher doses are required for half-maximal inhibition of androgen production in rats (Sandow et al. 1978b), dogs (Sandow et al. 1980a) and monkeys (Fraser et al. 1980; Wickings et al. 1980) than for blocking ovulation by preovulatory pituitary desensitization in the respective species. In men, there is also a higher dose requirement for suppression of testosterone production (Bergquist et al. 1979a; Labrie et al. 1980a) than for inhibition of ovulation in women (Bergquist et al. 1979c). The higher dose requirement may be a reflection of a smaller releasable LH pool in the male pituitary, which is less readily affected by LH depletion. This would agree with the reduced pituitary suppression occurring in hypogonadal men (Smith et al. 1979).

Male fertility requires sufficient sperm production, adequate sperm maturation, intact function of the epididymis and accessory sex organs. Agonists reduce fertility by a pituitary-dependent block of testosterone production, with Leydig cell function as the final common pathway. Reduced testosterone production affects libido, mating behavior and sperm maturation. In the dog, loss of libido may be a crucial factor in limiting fertility. In rats, agonists can lower serum testosterone to 5–10 % of the control values without affecting fertility (Tcholakian et al. 1978a; Sandow et al. 1980a). However, spermatogenesis in the rat is maintained despite low intratesticular testosterone concentrations (Cunningham and Huckins 1979), and other species may be more predictive for the human. If pituitary–testicular function is suppressed by estradiol benzoate pretreatment (50 μg s.c. for 21 days), it cannot be restored to normal by subsequent agonist administration (D-Leu[6]-EA, 200 ng s.c. for 30 days). This is not surprising, because testosterone production previously inhibited by

Table 10.8

TESTICULAR FUNCTION IN MALE DOGS AFTER LONG-TERM TREATMENT WITH AN LH-RH AGONIST, D-Ser (TBU)⁶-EA (BUSERELIN)

Group No.	Treatment[A]	Daily dose ($\mu g\ kg^{-1}$)	Hormones (ng per ml serum)			Organ weights (g)	
			LH	PRL	Testosterone	Testis	Prostate
1	Saline	0	81.0 ± 9.8[B]	2.12 ± 0.51	0.89 ± 0.65	17.3 ± 4.1	6.0 ± 0.6
2	Buserelin	0.05	24.8 ± 11.8	1.57 ± 0.14	0.81 ± 0.47	12.3 ± 6.1	3.1 ± 1.3
3	Buserelin	2.5	9.6 ± 3.7[C]	2.00 ± 0.69	0.06 ± 0.02	4.1 ± 1.2[C]	1.3 ± 0.4[C]
4	Buserelin	125	6.8 ± 2.3[C]	2.09 ± 0.26	0.05 ± 0.02	2.9 ± 0.7[C]	1.7 ± 0.3[C]

Under long-term treatment, there is reversible involution of testis and prostate due to pituitary desensitization and reduced androgen production.

[A] One daily subcutaneous injection for 6 months.
[B] Each point is the mean ±SEM of 5 determinations.
[C] Significant difference vs controls by ANOVA at 95% level.

378

estradiol administration cannot recover during persistent receptor down-regulation under agonist administration (Tcholakian et al. 1978b).

Pharmacological doses of agonists inhibit gonadal function in hypophysectomized animals and in vitro (Hsueh and Erickson 1979b). A direct action via gonadal LH-RH receptors has been inferred from these experiments (Arimura et al. 1979; Clayton et al. 1980b). There is strong evidence for hypothalamic–testicular interaction, supported by in vitro findings of testicular LH-RH/agonist receptors (Fig. 10.13) and LH-RH-like peptides which are secreted by the testes. Receptors for buserelin have been identified in Leydig cells isolated from adult rat testes (Sharpe and Fraser 1980a; Lefebvre et al. 1981). After stimulation with hCG, LH-RH like activity in the rat testes is increased (Sharpe and Fraser 1980b). The role of such LH-RH-like peptides in the testes could be to regulate testis function by an intratesticular loop, as well as to exert a feedback action on hypothalamic–pituitary receptors. Accumulation in Leydig cells was confirmed in perfused human testes by autoradiography with [^{125}I]buserelin (A. Isidori, personal communication). In our

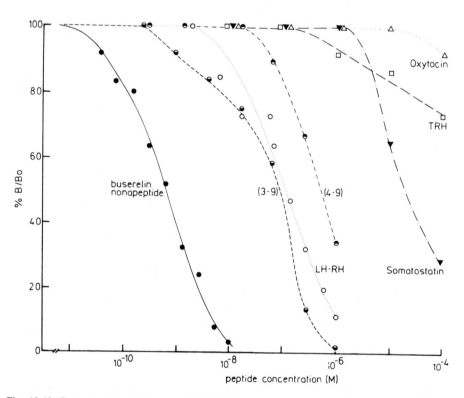

Fig. 10.13. Presence of gonadal receptors for LH-RH and agonists in Leydig cells of rats: radioligand assay using [^{125}I]buserelin. Competitive displacement by unlabelled buserelin-nonapeptide and its (3–9)heptapeptide and (4–9)hexapeptide, and synthetic LH-RH. Somatostatin, TRH and oxytocin have low receptor affinity. These gonadal binding sites may mediate a direct gonadal action of LH-RH agonists. Reproduced from Sharpe and Fraser (1980).

own organ distribution studies, we have not found accumulation of [^{125}I]buserelin in rat testis in contrast to the pituitary, which may be due to the small population of Leydig cells. The functional role of LH-RH-like peptides in the testes, also tentatively named gonado-crinins, can only be established after elucidation of their chemical structure.

Sertoli cell function

There are few reports on the effect of LH-RH on Sertoli cell function. Estradiol production by Sertoli cells of immature rat testes in vitro is not stimulated by addition of LH-RH (van Damme et al. 1979). In cryptorchid testes, LH-RH may have a regulatory effect on Sertoli cell function via FSH release, or by suppressing a peptide factor which inhibits testicular descent. Acid ethanol extracts of rat and macaque seminiferous tubules contain an oligopeptide active in the Leydig cell LH-RH radioreceptor assay, but not in LH-RH radioimmunoassay. This peptide may be a feedback inhibitor of Leydig cell function, secreted by the Sertoli cell (Sharpe et al. 1981).

Leydig cell function

There is evidence both for LH-dependent and direct regulation of Leydig cell function by LH-RH and agonists. The Leydig cell receptor for LH-RH, identified by binding of buserelin (Sharpe and Fraser 1980a) has high affinity for the agonist, and recognizes agonist fragments of decreased biological activity with lower affinity. The cell has some affinity for somatostatin at high concentrations (Fig. 10.13). An unequivocal identification of endogenous LH-RH-like peptides in radioligand or radioimmunoassays is not possible, due to limited specificity, and their chemical isolation is required.

The functional regulation of testicular LH-RH receptors is unknown. Pretreatment of intact or hypophysectomized rats with LH-RH (6.6 μg at 8-h intervals for 3 days) increases testicular LH-RH-receptors, in accordance with findings at the pituitary level (Bourne et al. 1980). The testicular binding proteins measured in radioligand assays may be in part LH-RH degrading enzymes; LH-RH and agonists are inactivated by enzymes in testicular homogenates (Sandow 1975). An evaluation of the enzyme components in Leydig cell preparations is required to establish the proposed functional role of a receptor protein and to exclude the possibility of an interaction with enzyme proteins, binding agonists and LH-RH with high affinity.

Is there evidence for direct inhibition of testicular function by agonists or LH-RH hypersecretion in vivo? The low LH-RH concentrations in serum certainly do not preclude a direct gonadal effect, because vasopressin also regulates kidney function in the absence of detectable serum levels, except in certain experimentally induced elevations. In intact rats receiving high daily doses of agonists, there is a striking reduction in target organ sensitivity, as assessed by testosterone production in vitro after hCG-stimulation. Reduced sensitivity is caused by a loss of LH receptors (Sandow et al. 1980b). In hypophysectomized rats treated with increasing doses of buserelin, there is also a suppression of LH receptors, and of the hCG-stimulated testosterone production by Leydig cells (Table 10.9).

Table 10.9

EFFECT OF D-Ser (TBU)[6]-EA (BUSERELIN) ON GONADAL FUNCTION IN HYPOPHYSECTOMIZED MALE RATS

Group No.	Treatment[A]		Daily dose per rat	Testicular receptors[B] (fmol per g testis)		Incubation with 250 mU hCG (ng testosterone per testis[D])		
				LH	PRL	Controls	2 h	4 h
1	Intact		0	9.5 (8)[C]	2.91	30.9	225	519
2	Hypophysectomized	controls	0	17.0 (5)	3.72	4.98	177	487
3	Hypophysectomized	buserelin	5 ng	12.6 (9)	3.33	0.28	5.52	9.6
4	Hypophysectomized	buserelin	50 ng	11.9 (8)	3.83	0.22	5.57	11.7
5	Hypophysectomized	buserelin	500 ng	11.6 (6)	4.22	0.37	6.24	11.8

Buserelin treatment of hypophysectomized rats reduces testicular LH but not PRL receptors; the hCG-stimulated testosterone production is also reduced by agonist treatment.

A Sprague-Dawley rats, initial body weight 80 g, were treated 20 days after hypophysectomy with buserelin, one daily subcutaneous injection for 14 days.
B Determined by binding of ^{125}I-labelled hCG and ^{125}I-labelled hPRL in pooled tissues (4 determinations per pool).
C Number of rats in parentheses.
D Testosterone in media determined by RIA.

This effect could be due either to direct gonadal inhibition (modulation of LH receptor function by a testicular, LH-RH, receptor) or to suppression of residual LH cells in the pars tuberalis (Gross and Page 1979).

Under continuous infusion of LH-RH agonists, we have not found gonadal inhibition in intact rats receiving minipump infusions of buserelin for 7–14 days (Table 10.3), LH declines to basal levels, but there is no direct testicular inhibition reducing testis weight, target organ receptors or testosterone tissue reserve. This may indicate the need in vivo of much higher agonist doses for inhibition or desensitization of a direct gonadal site of action.

Germinal epithelium and sperm maturation

In early studies on the stimulation of fertility by LH-RH we found that reactivation of spermatogenesis in blinded hamsters or hamsters under a short photoperiod was dose dependent. In a low dose range (50–100 ng LH-RH daily), tubular diameter was increased and spermatogenesis was reactivated. In a high dose range (500–1000 ng LH-RH daily), tubular diameter was also increased, but spermatogenesis was arrested at the primary spermatocyte stage (Sandow 1975; Sandow and Hahn 1978). Decreased pituitary sensitivity and reduced testosterone levels were associated with higher inhibitory doses of LH-RH.

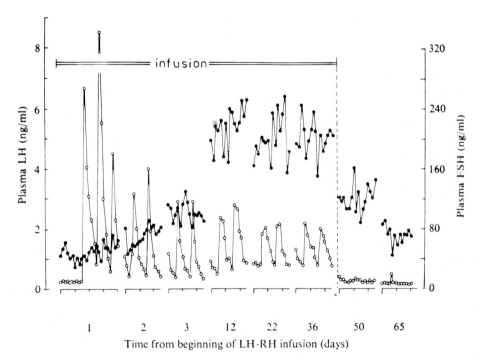

Fig. 10.14. Pituitary activation by regular LH-RH pulses: in rams during the spring nonmating season, pulses of 500 ng LH-RH at 2-h intervals induce progressive spiking of LH (○), followed by steadily rising FSH pulses (●). LH and FSH levels decline immediately when the infusion is stopped. Reproduced from Lincoln (1979).

Testicular function is also reactivated in the ram during the spring non-mating season by pulsatile infusion of LH-RH (Fig. 10.14). Frequent LH-RH injections stimulate testosterone more than infrequent pulses (Lincoln 1979b; Lincoln and Short 1980).

In the rat, daily or intermittent agonist injections inhibit spermatogenesis at the primary spermatocyte stage. The histological changes are disseminated, and vary greatly from animal to animal, and even between different sections of one testis. During the initial stages, polynucleated giant cells are observed, indicating resorption of elements of the germinal epithelium. At later stages, there are focal lesions consisting of tubules depopulated of germinal epithelium except for the primary spermatocytes and spermatogonia (Rivier et al. 1979; Cusan et al. 1979; Labrie et al. 1980b). Concomitantly, there is an inhibitory effect on the epididymis, which is devoid of sperm and contains necrotic cellular elements. The histological findings are due to suppressed androgen production (Sandow et al. 1980a). When agonist administration is stopped, pituitary LH secretion rapidly returns to normal, gonadal LH receptors are restored, and so is androgen production. The regressive changes of the germinal epithelium are fully reversed (Labrie et al. 1980b). Despite long-term suppression, the testicular changes in dogs are also fully reversible within 8 to 10 weeks after treatment (Sandow et al. 1980a).

LH-RH RECEPTORS AND MECHANISM OF ACTION

The gonadotropic effect of endogenous LH-RH is exerted via pulsatile secretion into the hypophyseal portal vessels, binding to oligopeptide receptors on pituitary cell membranes, and subsequent activation of an intracellular effector chain (Labrie et al. 1978a). Duration of hormone action is limited by enzyme degradation. Which steps in this process are involved in the antigonadotropic effects? Receptors for LH-RH and agonists are found in the anterior pituitary (Clayton et al. 1976b; Perrin et al. 1980); hypothalamus (Kuhl and Baumann 1980), testes (Lefebvre et al. 1981; Sharpe and Fraser 1980a; Clayton et al. 1980b), ovary (Harwood et al. 1980a,b), and in other tissues (Marshall et al. 1977). Pituitary LH-RH receptors can be measured in radioligand assays or by pituitary accumulation of agonists in vivo (Mayar et al. 1979; Sandow et al. 1980b).

These studies indicate that pituitary receptor regulation is in some respects different from gonadal receptor regulation. There is no change in pituitary uptake of [^{125}I]buserelin in male rats pretreated for 28 days with 50–500 ng buserelin (Sandow et al. 1980b), or of ^{125}I-labelled D-Leu^6-EA in female rats pretreated with estradiol-17β (Becker et al. 1979). Gonadotropin receptors in the ovary and testis are depleted after supraphysiological LH stimulation (Catt et al. 1980). In contrast, stimulation of the anterior pituitary with supraphysiological doses of LH-RH–agonists does not readily induce a depletion in LH-RH receptors, but rather an increase in receptor number (Sandow et al. 1979c, 1980d, 1981b; Clayton et al. 1980a). Only upon prolonged exposure by peptide infusion is there a pronounced decrease in pituitary LH-RH receptors (Clayton et al.; Sandow et al. unpublished observations). The LH-RH effector system is controversial; stimulation of adenyl cyclase activity has been reported by some authors (Labrie et al. 1978a), but disputed by others (Baumann and Kuhl 1980; Naor et al. 1980). It is interesting to compare the effector system for angiotensin stimulation of adrenal steroid production, which is also not mediated by adenyl cyclase (Catt et. al. 1979b). Enzymes inactivating angiotensin and LH-RH are functionally related, there is a strong inhibition of LH-RH degradation by angiotensin in vitro (Kuhl et al. 1979), and by fragments of an angiotensin antagonist (Sandow et al. 1979b). Neuronal activity of angiotensin cells in the brain is inhibited by iontophoretic application of LH-RH (Phillips 1980). The adrenal angiotensin receptor has substantial binding affinity for LH-RH, whereas adrenal steroidogenesis is not affected by LH-RH (Capponi and Catt 1979). We suggest that receptor recognition and degradative mechanisms of oligopeptide hormones are overlapping, so that one peptide may control the degradation and hence the duration of hormone action of another peptide.

The receptor interaction of antagonists and synthetic enzyme substrates with pituitary LH-RH receptors is of particular interest. In pituitary and testicular radioligand assays, LH-RH antagonists devoid of LH-releasing activity have higher affinity than LH-RH, despite their relatively low biological potency in terms of the molar ratio of antagonist required to block LH-RH action (Heber and Odell 1978; Perrin et al. 1980; Clayton and Catt 1979). Pituitary receptors also have significant affinity for biologically inactive synthetic enzyme substrates like L-leucine-4-nitroanilide and L-cystine-4-bis-nitroanilide (Kuhl and Baumann 1980; Sandow et al. 1981b). This interaction of biologically inactive molecules with a receptor protein is intriguing. In view of the extensive substitution of antagonists with D-amino acids enhancing their enzyme resistance, the binding of antagonists and enzyme substrates may be due to an enzyme component forming an integral part of the LH-RH receptor. One consequence of receptor occupancy by antagonists would be induction of a conformational change, which makes the receptor unresponsive to LH-RH.

The concept of a dual nature of the LH-RH receptor also provides an attractive hypothesis for the termination of hormone action at the pituitary receptor site. LH-RH receptor and LH-RH degrading enzyme may be two conformational states of one protein or associated proteins. If the hormone–receptor complex formed during recognition of LH-RH subsequently becomes a hormone-enzyme complex engaged in LH-RH degradation, this would explain temporary desensitization observed after high doses of LH-RH or agonists. In the nonreceptive state, the desensitized pituitary receptor binds the labelled ligand when tested in vitro, but cannot recognize and translate the signal in vivo. The conformational change could also account for the lack of LH-RH receptor depletion after high doses of agonists, despite desensitization of the LH response.

CLINICAL APPLICATIONS

When the structure of LH-RH was elucidated in 1971, Schally made a number of predictions for the therapeutic applications of agonists and antagonists. Physiological control of pituitary gonadotropin secretion by pulsatile LH-RH stimulation was then unknown. With the knowledge now at hand (see Knobil 1980), a more certain outcome can be reached for future clinical applications.

384

Stimulation of fertility

In clinical conditions characterized by a lack or insufficiency of hypothalamic LH-RH secretion, pulsatile LH-RH or agonist substitution will be the method of choice. This therapy requires the use of suitable programmed infusion pumps. For practical reasons, in less severe LH-RH deficiency, regulation or support of pituitary function by intermittent pulses of LH-RH or agonists delivered by nasal spray or another self administered method would be preferable. Such treatment has been successful in secondary amenorrhea (Katzorke et al. 1980; Brandau et al. 1980b). A good example for substitution of a partial LH-RH deficiency is the therapeutic effect of LH-RH in cryptorchidism (Illig et al. 1977; Happ et al. 1978a).

Contraceptive applications

When LH-RH agonists are injected daily in supraphysiological doses or given by a nasal spray, pituitary gonadotropin release is temporarily inhibited, and pituitary LH and FSH content are reduced upon prolonged administration. This approach has been successfully used for inhibition of ovulation. In precocious puberty, relatively high doses of agonists are required for reducing gonadotropin secretion to prepubertal basal levels. In this situation, continuous infusion of agonists may reduce the time interval required for pituitary desensitization, and could also reduce the dose required for inhibition.

Control of ovulation is readily achieved with relatively low doses of agonists given by nasal spray. This method prevents the preovulatory LH surge by reducing the releasable LH pool required for induction of ovulation. Antagonists prevent the preovulatory LH surge by a different mechanism of action, making the pituitary refractory to the endogenous LH-RH stimulus, but their potency is not sufficient for nasal administration. In the control of male fertility, agonists reduce testosterone production and lead to loss of libido, unless supplementation with androgens is provided.

In the treatment of hormone-dependent tumors, agonists may find an important role for symptomatic therapy by suppressing gonadal steroid secretion. Suppression can be induced with high doses initially given by infusion or injection, and subsequently maintained by nasal spray. When ovarian/testicular steroid production is lowered, the doses of anti-estrogen or anti-androgen required to neutralize remaining endogenous steroids can be reduced considerably.

With respect to the newly found gonadal LH-RH-like peptides, and their receptors, a more detailed knowledge of the chemical structure is required for an assessment of the biological significance of such peptides and their presumptive mechanisms of action.

ACKNOWLEDGMENTS

Research on LH-RH control of reproduction entered a very active and fruitful period with the disclosure of the structure of LH-RH in June 1971, ten years ago. This review is therefore respectfully dedicated to the pioneering work and continuing initiative in analogue development of Prof. A.V. Schally and his group. The author would like to thank Drs H.M. Fraser, R.N. Clayton and H. Kuhl for scientific discussion of specific topics covered in this review, and Drs S. Nillius, G. Lincoln and R.M. Sharpe for permission to use illustrations taken from their work. The experimental contributions of Miss B. Krauss and Mr S. Kille have been of special importance for the work reported here. Studies in the author's laboratory were supported with RIA-reagents kindly made available by the National Institute of Health, National Pituitary Agency, and Drs A.F. Parlow and G.D. Niswender.

REFERENCES

Aiyer, M.S., Chiappa, S.A. and Fink, G. (1974) A priming effect of luteinizing hormone-releasing factor on the anterior pituitary gland in the female rat. J. Endocrinol. 62, 573-588.

Amundson, B.C. and Wheaton, J.E. (1979) Effects of chronic LH-RH treatment on brain LH-RH content, pituitary and plasma LH and ovarian follicular activity in the anestrous ewe. Biol. Reprod. 20, 633-638.

Arimura, A., Serafini, P., Talbot, S. and Schally, A.V. (1979) Reduction of testicular luteinizing hormone/human chorionic gonadotrophin receptors by (D-Trp[6])-luteinizing hormone releasing hormone in hypophysectomized rats. Biochem. Biophys. Res. Commun. 90, 687-693.

Auclair, C., Kelly, P.A., Labrie, F., Coy, D.H. and Schally, A.V. (1977) Inhibition of testicular luteinizing hormone receptor level by treatment with a potent luteinizing hormone-releasing hormone agonist or human chorionic gonadotropin. Biochem. Biophys. Res. Commun. 76, 855-862.

Badger, T.M., Beitins, Z., Ostrea, T., Crisafulli, J.M., Little, R. and Saidel, M.E. (1980) Luteinizing hormone-releasing hormone does not inhibit testosterone production in rat interstitial cells in vitro. Endocrinology 106, 1149-1153.

Baker, B.L. (1977) Cellular composition of the human pituitary pars tuberalis as revealed by immunocytochemistry. Cell Tissue Res. 182, 151-163.

Bambino, T.H., Schreiber, J.R. and Hsueh, A.J.W. (1980) Gonadotropin-releasing hormone and its agonist inhibit testicular luteinizing hormone receptor and steroidogenesis in immature and adult hypophysectomized rats. Endocrinology 107, 908-917.

Banik, U.K. (1975) Pregnancy-terminating effect of human chorionic gonadotrophin in rats. J. Reprod. Fert. 42, 67-76.

Banik, U.K. and Givner, M.L. (1975) Ovulation induction and antifertility effects of an LH-RH analogue (AY-25,205) in cyclic rats. J. Reprod. Fert. 44, 87-94.

Banik, U.K. and Givner, M.L. (1976) Effects of luteinizing hormone-releasing hormone analog on mating and fertility in rats. Fertil. Steril. 27, 1078-1084.

Baumann, R. and Kuhl, H. (1980) Effect of LH-RH and a highly potent LH-RH analog upon pituitary adenyl cyclase activity. Horm. Metab. Res. 12, 128-130.

Baumann, R., Kuhl, H., Taubert, H.D. and Sandow, J. (1980): Ovulation inhibition by daily i.m. administration of a highly active LH-RH analog (D-Ser(TBU)[6]-LH-RH(1-9)-nonapeptide-ethylamide). Contraception 21, 191-197.

Beattie, C.W., Corbin, A., Foell, T.J., Garsky, V., Rees, R.W.A. and Yardley, J. (1976) Anti-ovulatory/anti-pregnancy effects of D-Phe[2]-LH-RH analogs administered early in the rat estrous cycle. Contraception 13, 341.

Becker, S.R., Gaskins, C.T. and Reeves, J.J. (1979) Pituitary uptake of ^{125}I-D-Leu[6], Des-Gly NH$_2$[10]LH-RH-ethylamide in ovariectomized rats pretreated with oestradiol-17β J. Reprod. Fert. 57, 295-300.

Behrman, H.R., Preston, S.L. and Hall, A.K. (1980) Cellular mechanism of the antigonadotropic action of luteinizing hormone-releasing hormone in the corpus luteum. Endocrinology 107, 656-664.

Belanger, A., Auclair, C., Seguin, C., Kelly, P.A. and Labrie, F. (1979) Down-regulation of testicular androgen biosynthesis and LH receptor levels by an LH-RH agonist: role of prolactin. Mol. Cell. Endocrinol. 13, 47.

Belchetz, P.E., Plant, T.M., Nakai, Y., Keogh, E.J. and Knobil, E. (1978) Hypophysial responses to continuous and intermittent delivery of hypothalamic gonadotropin-releasing hormone. Science 202, 631-632.

Bercu, B.B., Hyashi, A., Poth, M., Alexandrova, M., Soloff, M.S. and Donahoe, P.K. (1980) LH-RH induced delay of parturition. Endocrinology 107, 504-508.

Bergquist, C., Nillius, S.J., Bergh, T., Skarin, G. and Wide, L. (1979a) Inhibitory effects on gonadotropin secretion and gonadal function in men during chronic treatment with a potent stimulatory luteinizing hormone-releasing hormone analogue. Acta. Endocrinol. (Copenhagen) 91, 601-608.

Bergquist, C., Nillius, S.J. and Wide, L. (1979b) Inhibition of ovulation in women by intranasal treatment with a luteinizing hormone-releasing hormone agonist. Contraception 19, 497-506.

Bergquist, C., Nillius, S.J. and Wide, L. (1979c) Intranasal gonadotropin-releasing hormone agonist as a contraceptive agent. Lancet ii, 215-217.

Bergquist, C., Nillius, S.J. and Wide, L. (1979d) Reduced gonadotropin secretion in postmenopausal women during treatment with a stimulatory LRH analogue. J. Clin. Endocrinol. Metab. 49, 472-474.

Bex, F.J. and Corbin, A. (1979) Mechanism of the postcoital contraceptive effect of luteinizing hormone-releasing hormone: ovarian luteinizing hormone receptor interactions. Endocrinology 105, 139-145.

Bex, F.J. and Corbin, A. (1980): Antifertility effects of LH-RH and its agonists. In: Reproductive Processes and Contraception (McKerns, K.W. ed), Plenum Press, New York, in press.

Bourguignon, J.P., Burger, H.G. and Franchimont, P. (1974) Radioimmunoassay of serum luteinizing hormone-releasing hormone (LH-RH) after intra-nasal administration and evaluation of the gonadotrophic response. Clin. Endocrinol. 3, 437-440.

Bourne, G.A., Regiani, S., Payne, A.H. and Marshall, J.C. (1980) Testicular GnRH receptors – characterization and localization on interstitial tissue. J. Clin. Endocrinol. Metab. 51, 407-409.

Bowers, C.Y. and Folkers, K. (1976) Contraception and inhibition of ovulation by minipump infusion of the luteinizing hormone releasing hormone, active analogs and antagonists. Biochem. Biophys. Res. Commun. 72, 1003-1007.

Bowers, C.Y., Humphries, J., Wasiak, T., Folkers, K., Reynolds, G.A. and Reichert, L.E. (1980) On the inhibitory effects of luteinizing hormone-releasing hormone analogs. Endocrinology 106, 674-683.

Brandau, H., Kellermann, W. and von der Ohe, M. (1980a) Ovulationsinduktion durch intranasale Therapie mit dem LH-RH Analogon Buserelin (D-Ser(Bu^t)^6-LH-RH(1-9)Nonapeptid-Ethylamid). 43. Tagung d. Deutschen Ges. f. Gynäk. u. Geburtsh., Hamburg, 29.9.-3.10.1980, Arch. Gynecol, in press.

Brandau, H., Sandow, J. and von der Ohe, M. (1980b): Induction of ovulation by intranasal application of the LH-RH analogue buserelin (D-Ser(TBU)^6 LH-RH(1-9)nonapeptide-ethylamide). 6th International Congress of Endocrinology, Abstr. No. 342.

Brenner, R.M. and West, N.B. (1975): Hormonal regulation of the reproductive tract in female mammals. Annu. Rev. Physiol. 37, 273-303.

Capponi, A.M. and Catt, K.J. (1979) Angiotensin II receptors in adrenal cortex and uterus: binding and activation properties of angiotensin analogues. J. Biol. Chem. 254, 5120-5127.

Casper, R.F. and Yen, S.S.C. (1979) Induction of luteolysis in the human with a long-acting analog of luteinzing hormone-releasing factor. Science 204, 408-410.

Casper, R.F., Sheehan, K., Erickson, G. and Yen, S.C.C. (1980) Neuropeptides and fertility control in the female. In: Proceedings of the P.A.R.F.R. Workshop on Fertility Regulation, Mexico 1980, Harper and Row, in press.

Catt, K.J. and Dufau, M.L. (1977) Peptide hormone receptors. Annu. Rev. Physiol. 39, 529-557.

Catt, K.J., Baukal, A.J., Davies, D.F. and Dufau, M.L. (1979a) Luteinizing hormone-releasing hormone-induced regulation of gonadotropin and prolactin receptors in the rat testis. Endocrinology 104, 17-25.

Catt, K.J., Harwood, J.P., Aguilera, G. and Dufau, M.L. (1979b) Hormonal regulation of peptide receptors and target cell responses. Nature 280, 109-116.

Catt, K.J., Harwood, J.P., Clayton, R.N., Davies, T.F., Chan, V., Kaitineni, M., Nozu, K. and Dufau, M.L. (1980) Regulation of peptide hormone receptors and gonadal steroidogenesis. Rec. Progr. Horm. Res. 36, 557-622.

Cigorraga, S.B., Dufau, M.L. and Catt, K.J. (1978) Regulation of luteinizing hormone receptors and steroidogenesis in gonadotropin-desensitized Leydig cells. J. Biol. Chem. 253, 4297-4304.

Clayton, R.N. and Catt, K.J. (1979) Receptor binding affinity of gonadotropin-releasing hormone analogs: Analysis by radioligand-receptor assay. Endocrinology 106, 1154-1159.

Clayton, R.N., Harwood, J.P. and Catt, K.J. (1979a) Gonadotropin-releasing hormone analogue binds to luteal cells and inhibits progesterone production. Nature 282, 90-91.

Clayton, R.N., Shakespear, R.A. and Marshall, J.C. (1979b) Radioiodinated nondegradable gonadotropin-releasing hormone analogs: new probes for the investigation of pituitary gonadotropin-releasing hormone receptors. Endocrinology 105, 1369-1381.

Clayton, R.N., Solano, A.R., Garcia-Vela, A., Dufau, M.L. and Catt, K.J. (1980a) Regulation of pituitary receptors for gonadotropin-releasing hormone during the rat estrous cycle. Endocrinology 107, 699-705.

Clayton, R.N., Katikineni, M., Chan, V., Dufau, M.L. and Catt, K.J. (1980b) Direct inhibition of testicular function by gonadotropin-releasing hormone: Mediation by specific gonadotropin-releasing hormone receptors in interstitial cells. Biochemistry 77, 4459-4463.

Conti, M., Harwood, J.P., Hsueh, A.J.W., Dufau, M.L. and Catt, K.J. (1976) Gonadotropin-induced loss of hormone receptors and desensitization of adenylate cyclase in the ovary. J. Biol. Chem. 251, 7729-7731.

Corbin, A., Beattie, C.W., Rees, R., Yardley, J., Foell, T.J., Chai, S.Y., McGregor, H., Garsky, V., Sarantakis, pregnancy with a peptide analogue of luteinizing hormone-releasing hormone. Endocrinol. Res. Commun. 2, 1-23.

Corbin, A., Beattie, C.W., Rees, R., Yardley, J., Foell, T.J., Chai, S.Y., McGregor, H., Gasky, V., Sarantakis, D. and McKinley, W.A. (1977) Postcoital contraceptive effects of agonist analogs of luteinizing hormone-releasing hormone. Fertil. Steril. 28, 471-475.

Corbin, A., Beattie, C.W., Tracy, J., Jones, R., Foell, T.J., Yardley, J. and Rees, R.W. (1978a) The anti-reproductive pharmacology of LH-RH and agonistic analogues. Int. J. Fertil. 23, 81-92.

Corbin, A., Jasczak, S., Peluso, J., Shandilya, N.L. and Hafez, E.S.E. (1978b) Effect of LH-RH peptide antagonist on serum LH, ovulation and menstrual cycle of crab-eating macaque. Contraception 18, 105-120.

Coy, D.H., Mezo, I., Pedroza, E., Nekola, M.V., Vilchez-Martinez, J.A., Piyachaturawat, P. and Schally, A.V. (1979) LH-RH antagonists with potent anovulatory activity. In Peptides: Structure and Biological Function (Gross, E. and Meienhofer, J. eds), pp. 775-779, Pierce Chemical Company.

Crighton, D.B., Foster, J.P., Haresign, W. and Scott, S.A. (1975) Plasma LH and progesterone levels after single or multiple injections of synthetic LH-RH in anestrous ewes and comparison with levels during the estrous cycle. J. Reprod. Fert. 44, 121-124.

Crowley Jr, W.F. and McArthur, J.W. (1980a) Induction of puberty in hypogonadotropic males: use of low-dose pulsatile luteinizing hormone-releasing hormone (LH-RH) administration. Endocrinology 106 (Suppl.), 260, Abstract 743.

Crowley Jr, W.F. and McArthur, J.W. (1980b) Stimulation of the normal menstrual cycle in Kallman's syndrome by pulsatile administration of luteinizing hormone-releasing hormone (LH-RH). J. Clin. Endocrinol Metab. 51, 173-175.

Crowley Jr, W.F., Beitins, I.Z., Vale, W., Kliman, B., Rivier, J., Rivier, C. and McArthur, J.W. (1980) The biological activity of a potent analogue of gonadotropin-releasing hormone in normal and hypogonadotropic men. New England J. Med. 302, 1052-1057.

Crowley Jr, W.F., Comite, F., Vale, W., Rivier, J., Loriaux, D.L. and Cutler, G.B. (1981) Therapeutic use of pituitary desensitization with a long-acting LH-RH agonist: A potential new treatment for idiopathic precocious puberty. J. Clin. Endocrinol. Metab. 52, 270-272.

Cunningham, G.R. and Huckins, C. (1979) Persistence of complete spermatogenesis in the presence of low intratesticular concentrations of testosterone. Endocrinology 105, 177-186.

Cusan, L., Auclair, C., Belanger, A., Ferland, L., Kelly, P.A., Seguin, C. and Labrie, F. (1979) Inhibitory effects of a long term treatment with a luteinizing hormone-releasing hormone agonist on the pituitary-gonadal axis in male and female rats. Endocrinology 104, 1369-1376.

Davies, T.F., Gomez-Pan, A., Watson, M.J., Mountjoy, C.Q., Hanaker, J.P., Besser, G.M. and Hall, R. (1977) Reduced gonadotrophin response to releasing hormone after chronic administration to impotent men. Clin. Endocrinol. 6, 213-218.

de la Cruz, A., Arimura, A., de la Cruz, K. and Schally, A.V. (1976) Effect of administration of antiserum to luteinizing hormone-releasing hormone on gonadal function during the estrous cycle in the hamster. Endocrinology 98, 490-497.

De Sombre, E.R., Johnson, E.S. and White, W.F. (1976) Regression of rat mammary tumors by a gonadoliberin analog. Cancer Res. 26, 3830-3833.

De Koning, J., Van Dieten, J.A.M. and Rees, G.P. (1978) Refractoriness of the pituitary gland after continuous exposure to LH-RH. J. Endocrinol. 79, 311-318.

Dericks-Tan, J.S.E., Hammer, E. and Taubert, H.D. (1977) The effect of D-Ser(TBU)[6]-LH-RH-EA[10] upon gonadotropin release in normally cyclic women. J. Clin. Endocr. Metab. 45, 597-600.

Dobson, H., Franklin, J.E.F. and Ward, W.R. (1977) Bovine cystic ovarian disease: plasma hormone concentrations and treatment. Vet. Rec. 101, 459-461.

Domanski, E., Prekop, F., Skubiszewski, B., Wrobleska, B. and Stupnicka, E. (1977) Effect of prolonged infusion of small doses of LH-RH on the release of LH and ovulation in ewes during mid-anestrous. J. Reprod. Fertil. 51, 457-460.

Dufau, M.L. and Catt, K.J. (1978) Gonadotropin receptors and regulation of steroidogenesis in the testis and ovary. Vitam. Horm. 36, 461-592.

Dufau, M.L., Cigorraga, S., Baukal, A.J., Sorrel, S., Bator, J.M., Neubauer, J.F. and Catt, K.J. (1979) Androgen biosysnthesis in Leydig cells after testicular desensitization by luteinizing hormone-releasing hormone and human chorionic gonadotropin. Endocrinology 105, 1314-1321.

Faure, N. and Olivier, G.C. (1978) Hypersensitivity of the human gonadotrophs to the repeated administration of small doses of LH-RH. Horm. Res. 9, 12-21.

Ferin, M., Bogumil, J., Drewes, J., Durenfurth, I., Jewelewicz R. and Vande Wiele, R.L. (1978) Pituitary and ovarian hormone responses to 48 h gonadotropin-releasing hormone (GnRH) infusion in female rhesus monkeys. Acta Endocrinol. (Copenhagen) 89, 48-59.

Ferin, H., Rosenblatt, H., Carmel, P.W., Antunes, J.L. and Vande Wiele, R.L. (1979) Estrogen-induced gonadotropin surges in female rhesus monkeys after pituitary stalk section. Endocrinology 104, 50-52.

Fink, G. (1979) Feedback actions of target hormones on hypothalamus and pituitary with special reference to gonadal steroids. Annu. Rev. Physiol. 41, 571-585.

Fink, G., Gennser, G., Liedholm, P., Thorell, J. and Moulder, J. (1974) Comparison of plasma levels of luteinizing hormone-releasing hormone in men after intravenous or intranasal administration. J. Endocrinol. 63, 351-360.

Fraser, H.M. (1980a) Inhibition of reproductive function by antibodies to luteinizing hormone-releasing hormone. In Immunological Aspects of Reproduction and Fertility Control. (Hearn, J.P. ed), pp. 143-170. MTP Press Ltd, London.

Fraser, H.M. (1980b) Contraceptive effects of an agonist of luteinizing hormone-releasing hormone: a long-term study on the female stumptailed monkey (Macaca arctoides). J. Endocrinol. 85, 13P.

Fraser, H.M. (1981) Luteinizing hormone-releasing hormone and fertility control. In: Oxford Reviews of Reproductive Biology (Finn, C.A. ed), Oxford University Press, Oxford, in press.

Fraser, H.M., Laird, N.C. and Blakeley, D.M. (1980) Decreased pituitary responsiveness and inhibition of the luteinizing hormone surge and ovulation in the stumptailed monkey (Macaca arctoides) by chronic treatment with an agonist of luteinizing hormone-releasing hormone. Endocrinology 106, 452-457.

Friedrich, F., Kemeter, P., Salzer, H. and Breitenecker, G. (1975) Ovulation inhibition with human chorionic gonadotrophin. Acta Endocrinol. (Copenhagen) 78, 332-342.

Gallo, R.V. (1980) Neuroendocrine regulation of pulsatile luteinizing hormone release in the rat. Neuroendocrinology 30, 122-131.

Gay, V.L. and Sheth, N.A. (1972) Evidence for a periodic release of LH in castrated male and female rats. Endocrinology 90, 158-162.

Goodman, R.L. and Karsch, F.J. (1980) Pulsatile secretion of luteinizing hormone: Differential suppression by ovarian steroids. Endocrinology 107, 1286-1290.

Gosselin, R.E., Fuller, G.B., Coy, D.H., Schally, A.V. and Hobson, W.C. (1979a) Inhibition of gonadotrophin release in chimpanzees by the LH-RH antagonist (D-Phe[2], D-Trp[3], D-Phe[6])-LH-RH (40480). Proc. Soc. Exp. Biol. Med. 161, 21-24.

Gosselin, R.E., Hobson, W.C. and Vale, W. (1979b) Inhibition of LH-RH or estrogen-induced gonadotrophin surges by an LH-RH analog in chimpanzees. Society for the Study of Reproduction, Annual Meeting, Abstract.

Graham, C.E., Gould, K.G., Collins, D.C. and Preedy, R.K. (1979) Regulation of gonadotropin release by luteinizing hormone-releasing hormone and estrogen in chimpanzees. Endocrinology 105, 269-275.

Griffiths, E.C. and Hopkinson, R.C.N. (1979) Inactivation of two hyperactive LH-RH analogues by rat hypothalamic peptidases. Horm. Res. 10, 223-242.

Gross, D.S. and Page, R.B. (1979) Luteinizing hormone and follicle-stimulating hormone production in the pars tuberalis of hypophysectomized rats. Am. J. Anat. 156, 285-291.

Hagino, N., Coy, D.H., Schally, A.V. and Arimura, A. (1977) Inhibition of release in the baboon by inhibitory analogs of luteinizing hormone-releasing hormone. Horm. Metab. Res. 9, 247-248.

Hagino, N., Nakamoto, O., Kunz, Y., Arimura, A., Coy, D.H. and Schally, A.V. (1979) Effect of D-Trp[6]-LH-RH on the pituitary-gonadal axis during the luteal phase in the baboon. Acta Endocrinol (Copenhagen) 91, 217-223.

Hanker, J.P., Bohnet, H.G., Mühlenstedt, D., Nowack, C. and Schneider, H.P.G. (1978) Gonadotrophin release during chronic administration of D-Ser(TBU)[6]-LH-RH-EA in functional amenorrhea. Acta Endocrinol. (Copenhagen) 89, 625-631.

Haour, F., Tell, G. and Sanchez, P. (1976) Mise en évidence et dosage d'une gonadotrophine chorionique chez le rat (rCG). C.R. Acad. Sci. 282, Ser. D-86, 1183-1186.

Happ, J., Kollmann, F., Krawehl, C., Neubauer, M., Krause, U., Demisch, K., Sandow, J., von Rechenberg, W. and Beyer, J. (1978a) Treatment of cryptorchidism with pernasal gonadotropin-releasing hormone therapy. Fertil. Steril. 29, 546-551.

Happ, J., Scholz, P., Weber, T., Cordes, U., Schramm, P., Neubauer, M. and Beyer, J. (1978b) Gonadotropin secretion in eugonadotropic human males and postmenopausal females under long-term application of a potent analog of gonadotropin-releasing hormone. Fertil. Steril. 30, 674-678.

Haresign, W. and McLeod, B.J. (1980) LH release and luteal function in Gn-RH treated anoestrous ewes pretreated with PMSG. Soc. Study of Fertility, Annual Conference, Oxford, Abstract No.5.

Harwood, J.P., Clayton, R.N. and Catt, K.J. (1980a) Ovarian gonadotropin-releasing hormone receptors. I. Properties and inhibition of luteal cell function. Endocrinology 107, 407-413.

Harwood, J.P., Clayton, R.N., Chen, T.T., Knox, G. and Catt, K.J. (1980b) Ovarian gonadotropin-releasing hormone receptors. II. Regulation and effects on ovarian development. Endocrinology 107, 414-421.

Haynes, N.M., Hafs, H.D. and Manns, J.G. (1977) Effect of chronic administration of gonadotrophin releasing hormone and thyrotrophin releasing hormone to pubertal bulls on plasma luteinizing hormone, prolactin and testosterone concentrations, the number of epididymal sperm and body weight. J. Endocrinol. 73, 227-234.

Heber, D. and Odell, W.D. (1978) Pituitary receptor binding activity of active, inactive, superactive and inhibitory analogs of gonadotropin-releasing hormone. Biochem. Biophys. Res. Commun. 82, 67-73.

Hirono, M., Igarashi, M. and Matsumoto, S. (1972) The direct effect of hCG upon pituitary gonadotrophin secretion. Endocrinology 90, 1214-1219.

Hsueh, A.J.W. and Erickson, G.F. (1979a) Extrapituitary action of gonadotrophin-releasing hormone: direct inhibition of ovarian steroidogenesis. Science 204, 854-855.

Hsueh, A.J.W. and Erickson, G.F. (1979b) Extra-pituitary inhibition of testicular function by luteinizing hormone-releasing hormone. Nature, Lond. 281, 66-67.

Hsueh, A.J.W. and Ling, N.C. (1979) Effect of an antagonist analogue of gonadotropin releasing hormone upon ovarian granulosa cell function. Life Sci. 25, 1223-1230.

Hsueh, A.J.W., Dufau, M.L. and Catt, K.J. (1976) Regulation of luteinizing hormone receptors in testicular interstitial cells by gonadotropin. Biochem. Biophys. Res. Commun. 72, 1145-1152.

Hsueh, A.J.W., Wang, C. and Erickson, G.F. (1980) Direct inhibitory effect of gonadotropin-releasing hormone upon follicle-stimulating hormone induction of luteinizing hormone receptor and aromatase activity in rat granulosa cells. Endocrinology 106, 1697-1705.

Humke, R. and Zuber, H. (1977) Die Behandlung von Anöstrie und Azyklie des Rindes durch ein LH-RH Analog. Berl. Münch. Tierärztl. Wschr. 90, 229-234.

Humphrey, R.R., Windsor, B.L., Reel, J.R. and Edgren, R.A. (1977) The effect of luteinizing hormone-releasing hormone (LH-RH) in pregnant rats. 1. Postnidatory effects, Biol. Reprod. 16, 614-621.

Humphrey, R.R., Windsor, B.L., Jones, D.C., Reel. J.R. and Edgren, R.A. (1978) The effects of luteinizing hormone-releasing hormone (LH-RH) in pregnant rats. 2. Prenidatory effects and delayed parturition. Biol. Reprod. 19, 84-91.

Illig, R., Kollmann, F., Borkenstein, M., Kuber, W., Exner, G.U., Kellerer, K., Lunglmayer, L. and Prader, A.

(1977) Treatment of cryptorchidism by intranasal synthetic luteinizing hormone-releasing hormone. Lancet 2, 518-520.

Johnson, E.S., Gendrich, B.S. and White, W.F. (1976) Delay of puberty and inhibition of reproductive processes in the rat by a gonadotropin-releasing hormone agonist analog. Fertil. Steril. 27, 853-860.

Jones, R.C. (1979a) Local antifertility effect of luteinizing hormone-releasing hormone (LRH). Contraception 20, 569-577.

Jones, R.C. (1979b) The effect of luteinizing releasing hormone (LRH) and two agonist analogues on uterine growth in hypophysectomized, ovariectomized and intact rats. Int. J. Fertil. 24, 188-192.

Jones, R.C. (1979c) Induction of ovulation in the pregnant rat with luteinizing hormone releasing hormone (LRH). Contraception 19, 233-237.

Katzorke, T., Propping, D., von der Ohe, M. and Taubert, H.D. (1980) Clinical evaluation of the effects of a new long-acting superactive luteinizing hormone-releasing hormone (LH-RH) analog, D-Ser (TBU)[6]-desGly[10]-ethylamide-LH-RH in women with secondary amenorrhea. Fertil. Steril. 33, 35-42.

Khodr, G. and Siler-Khodr, T.M. (1978) The effect of luteinizing hormone-releasing factor on human chorionic gonadotrophin secretion. Fertil. Steril. 30, 301-304.

Khodr, G. and Siler-Khodr, T.M. (1979) Placental luteinizing hormone-releasing factor and its synthesis. Science 207, 315-317.

Kledzik, G.S., Cusan, L., Auclair, C., Kelly, P.A. and Labrie, F. (1978a) Inhibitory effect of a luteinizing hormone (LH)-releasing hormone agonist on rat ovarian LH and follicle-stimulating hormone receptor levels during pregnancy. Fertil. Steril. 29, 560-564.

Kledzik, G.S., Cusan, L., Auclair, C., Kelly, P.A. and Labrie, F. (1978b) Inhibition of ovarian luteinizing hormone (LH) and follicle-stimulating hormone receptor levels with an LH-releasing hormone agonist during the oestrous cycle in the rat. Fertil. Steril. 30, 348-353.

Knobil, E. (1980) The neuroendocrine control of the menstrual cycle. Rec. Progr. Horm. Res. 36, 53-88.

Knobil, E., Plant, T.M., Wildt, L., Belchetz, P.E. and Marshall, G. (1980) Control of the rhesus monkey menstrual cycle: Permissive role of hypothalamic gonadotropin-releasing hormone. Science 207, 1371-1372.

Koch, Y., Baram, T., Hazum, E. and Friedkin, M. (1977) Resistance to enzymic degradation of LH-RH analogs possessing increased biological activity. Biochem. Biophys. Res. Commun. 74, 488-491.

König, W., Sandow, J. and Geiger, R. (1978) LH-RH analogues containing glutamine and glutamic acid. In: Hypothalamic Hormones – Chemistry, Physiology and Clinical Applications (Gupta, D. and Voelter, W., eds) pp. 13-20. Verlag Chemie, Weinheim.

Koyama, T., Ohkura, T., Kumasaka, T. and Saito, M. (1978) Effect of postovulatory treatment with luteinizing hormone-releasing hormone analog on the plasma level of progesterone in women. Fertil. Steril. 30, 549-552.

Kuhl, H. and Baumann, R. (1981) New aspects on the physiological significance of LRH receptors of pituitary plasma membranes. Acta Endocrinol. (Copenhagen) 96, 36-45.

Kuhl, H., Sandow, J., Krauss, B. and Taubert, H.D. (1979) Enzyme kinetic studies and inhibition by oligopeptides of LH-RH degradation in rat hypothalamus and pituitary. Neuroendocrinology 28, 339-348.

Labrie, F., Auclair, C., Cusan, L., Kelly, P.A., Pelletier, G. and Ferland, L. (1978a) Inhibitory effect of LH-RH and its agonists on testicular gonadotrophin receptors and spermatogenesis in the rat. Internat J. Androl. Suppl. 2, 303-318.

Labrie, F., Drouin, J., Ferland, L., Lagace, L., Beaulieu, M., Lean, A. de, Kelly, P.A., Caron, M.G. and Raymond, V. (1978b) Mechanisms of action of hypothalamic hormones in the anterior pituitary gland and specific modulation of their activity by sex steroids and thyroid hormones. Rec. Progr. Horm. Res. 34, 25-93.

Labrie, F., Borgeat, P., Drouin, J., Beaulieu, M., Lagace, L., Ferland, L. and Raymond, V. (1979) Mechanism of action of hypothalamic hormones in the adenohypophysis. Annu. Rev. Physiol. 41, 555-569.

Labrie, F., Belanger, A., Cusan, L., Seguin, C., Pelletier, G., Kelly, P.A., Reeves, J.J., Lefebvre, F.A., Lemay, A., Gourdeau, Y. and Raynaud, J.P. (1980a) Antifertility effects of LH-RH agonists in the male. J. Androl. 1, 209-227.

Labrie, F., Cusan, L., Seguin, C., Belanger, A., Pelletier, G., Reeves, J., Lefebvre, F.A., Kelly, P.A., Lemay, A. and Raynaud, J.P. (1980b) Antifertility effects of LH-RH agonists in the male rat and inhibition of testicular steroidogenesis in man. Internat J. Fertil. 25, 157-170.

Lee, C.Y. and Ryan, R.J. (1974) Estrogen stimulation of human chorionic gonadotropin binding by luteinized rat ovarian slices. Endocrinology 95, 1691-1693.

Lefebvre, R.A., Reeves, J.J., Seguin C., Massicotte, J. and Labrie, F. (1981) Specific binding of a potent LH-RH agonist in rat testis. Mol. Cell. Endocrinol., in press.

Lemay, A., Labrie, F., Ferland, L. and Raynaud, J.P. (1979a) Possible luteolytic effects of luteinizing hormone-releasing hormone in normal women. Fertil. Steril. 31, 29-34.

Lemay, A., Labrie, F., Belanger, A. and Raynaud, J.P. (1979b) Luteolytic effect of intranasal administration of (D-Ser(TBU)[6], des-Gly-NH$_2$[10])-luteinizing hormone-releasing hormone ethylamide in normal women. Fertil. Steril. 32, 646-651.

Leyendecker, G. (1979) The pathophysiology of hypothalamic ovarian failure; diagnostic and therapeutical considerations. Eur. J. Obstet. Gynec. Repr. Biol. 9, 175.

Leyendecker, G., Wildt, L. and Hansmann, M. (1980) Pregnancies following chronic intermittent (pulsatile) administration of GnRH by means of a portable pump (Zyklomat). A new approach in the treatment of infertility in hypothalamic amenorrhea. J. Clin. Endocrinol. Metab. 51, 1214-1216.

Lincoln, G.A. (1979a) Use of a pulsed infusion of luteinizing hormone releasing hormone to mimic seasonally induced endocrine changes in the ram. J. Endocrinol. 83, 251-260.

Lincoln, G.A. (1979b) Differential control of luteinizing hormone and follicle-stimulating hormone by luteinizing hormone releasing hormone in the ram. J. Endocrinol. 80, 133-140.

Lincoln, G.A. and Short, R.V. (1980) Seasonal breeding: Nature's contraceptive. Rec. Progr. Horm. Res. 36, 1-52.

MacDonald, G.J. and Beattie, C.W. (1979) Pregnancy failure in hypophysectomized rats following LH-RH administration. Life Sci. 24, 1103-1110.

Madhwra, Raj, H.G. and Mougdal, N.R. (1970) Hormonal control of gestation in the intact rat. Endocrinology 86, 874-889.

Marks, N. and Stern, F. (1974) Enzymatic mechanisms for the inactivation of luteinizing hormone-releasing hormone (LH-RH). Biochem. Biophys. Res. Commun. 61, 1458-1463.

Marshall, J.C. and Kelch, R.P. (1979) Low dose pulsatile gonadotropin-releasing hormone in anorexia nervosa: A model of human pubertal development. J. Clin. Endocrinol. Metab. 49, 712-718.

Marshall, J.C., Shakespear, R.A. and Odell, W.D. (1977) LH-RH pituitary plasma membrane binding: The presence of specific binding sites in other tissues. Clin. Endocrinol. 5, 671-677.

Mayar, M.Q., Tarnavsky, G.K. and Reeves, J.J. (1979) Ovarian growth and uptake of iodinated D-Leu[6], des Gly NH$_2$[10]-LH-RH-ethylamide in hCG treated rats. Proc. Soc. Exp. Biol. Med. 161, 216-219.

McCann, S.M. and Porter, J.C. (1969) Hypothalamic pituitary stimulating and inhibiting hormones. Physiol. Rev. 49, 240-284.

McCormack, J.T., Plant, T.M., Hess, D.L. and Knobil, E. (1977) The effect of luteinizing hormone releasing hormone (LH-RH) antiserum administration on gonadotrophin secretion in the rhesus monkey. Endocrinology 100, 663-667.

McLeod, B.J. and Haresign, W. (1980) The induction of ovulation and luteal function in anoestrous ewes treated with small dose multiple injections of Gn-RH. Soc. Study of Fertility, Annual Conference, Oxford, Abstract No. 6.

McNatty, C.P. and Baird, D.T. (1978) Relationship between follicle-stimulating hormone, androstenedione and oestradiol in human follicular fluid. J. Endocr. 76, 527-531.

Mies, R. (1980) Effects of the LH-RH analogue D-Ser(TBU)[6]-EA[10] in delayed puberty. Acta Endocrinol. (Copenhagen) Suppl. 234, 77-78.

Miyake, A., Tanizawa, O., Aono, T., Yasuda, M. and Kurachi, K. (1976) Suppression of luteinizing hormone in castrated women by the administration of human chorionic gonadotropin. J. Clin. Endocrinol. Metab. 43, 928-932.

Molitch, M., Edmonds, M., Jones, E.E. and Odell, W.D. (1976) Short-loop feedback control of luteinizing hormone in the rabbit. Am. J. Physiol. 203, 907-910.

Mongkonpunya, K., Hafs, H.D., Convey, E.M. and Tucker, H.A. (1975) Serum LH and testosterone and sperm numbers in pubertal bulls chronically treated with gonadotropin releasing hormone. J. Anim. Sci. 41, 160-165.

Mortimer, C.H., McNeilly, A.S., Fisher, R.A., Murray, M.A.F. and Besser, G.M. (1974) Gonadotrophin-releasing hormone therapy in hypogonadal males with hypothalamic or pituitary dysfunction. Brit. Med. J. 4,

617-621.

Mortimer, C.H., Besser, G.M. and McNeilly, A.S. (1975) Gonadotrophin-releasing hormone therapy in the induction of puberty, potency, spermatogenesis and ovulation in patients with hypothalamic-pituitary-gonadal dysfunction. In: Hypothalamic Hormones (Motta, M., Crosignani, P.G. and Martini, L. eds), pp. 325-335, Academic Press, London.

Naor, Z., Clayton, R.N. and Catt, K.J. (1980) Characterization of gonadotropin-releasing hormone receptors in cultured rat pituitary cells. Endocrinology 107, 1144-1152.

Neill, J.D., Dailey, R.A., Tsou, R.C., Patton, J. and Tindall, G. (1976) Control of the ovarian cycle in the monkey. In: Control of Ovulation in the Human (Crosignani, P.G. and Mishell, D.R. eds), pp. 115-125, Academic Press, London.

Nillius, S.J. (1976): Therapeutic use of luteinizing hormone-releasing hormone in the human female. In: The Hypothalamus and Endocrine Functions, Vol. 3, Topics in Molecular Endocrinology (Labrie, F., Meites, J. and Pelletier, G. eds), Plenum Press, New York.

Nillius, S.J. and Wide, L. (1977) Acute and chronic effects of the stimulatory luteinizing hormone-releasing hormone analogue D-Ser(TBU)^6-EA^{10}-LH-RH on the gonadotrophin and gonadal steroid secretion in women with amenorrhea. Acta Endocrinol. (Copenhagen) Suppl. 212, 138.

Nillius, S.J., Fries, H. and Wide, L. (1975) Successful induction of follicular maturation and ovulation by prolonged treatment with luteinizing hormone-releasing hormone (LH-RH) in women with anorexia nervosa. Am. J. Obstet. Gynecol 122, 921-928.

Nillius, S.J., Bergquist, C. and Wide, L. (1978) Inhibition of ovulation in women by chronic treatment with a stimulatory LRH analogue – a new approach to birth control? Contraception 17, 537-545.

Nishi, N., Coy, D.H., Coy, E.J., Arimura, A. and Schally, A.V. (1976) Suppression of LH-RH-induced ovulation in hamsters and rats by synthetic analogues of LH-RH. J. Reprod. Fertil. 48, 119-124.

Norman, R.L. and Spies, H.G. (1979) Effect of luteinizing hormone-releasing hormone on the pituitary-gonadal axis in fetal and intact rhesus monkeys. Endocrinology 105, 655-659.

Oshima, H., Nankin, H.R., Fan, D.F., Treon, P.H., Yanaihara, T., Nijzato, N., Yoshida, K.I. and Ochiai, K.I. (1975) Delay in sexual maturation of rats caused by synthetic LH-releasing hormone: enhancement of steroid-Δ 4-5α-dehydrogenase in testes. Biol. Reprod. 12, 491-497.

Pal, A.K., Gupta, T. and Chatterjee, A. (1976) Pregnant mare's serum gonadotrophin. Acta Endocrinol. (Copenhagen) 83, 506-511.

Pedroza-Garcia, E., Vilchez-Martinez, J.A., Fishback, J., Arimura, A. and Schally, A.V. (1977) Binding capacity of luteinizing hormone-releasing hormone and its analogues for pituitary receptor sites. Biochem. Biophys. Res. Commun. 79, 234-238.

Pelletier, G., Cusan, L., Auclair, C., Kelly, P.A., Desy, L. and Labrie, F. (1978) Inhibition of spermatogenesis in the rat by treatment with (D-Ala^6, des-Gly-NH$_2$^{10})LH-RH-ethylamide. Endocrinology 103, 641-643.

Perrin, M.H., Rivier, J.E. and Vale, W.V. (1980): Radioligand assay for gonadotropin-releasing hormone: relative potencies of agonists and antagonists. Endocrinology 106, 1289-1296.

Phelps, C.P., Coy, D.H., Schally, A.V. and Saywer, C.H. (1977) Blockade of LH release and ovulation in the rabbit with inhibitory analogues of luteinizing hormone releasing hormone. Endocrinology 100, 1526-1532.

Phillips, M.J. (1980) Biological effects of angiotensin in the brain. In Enzymatic Release of Vasoactive Peptides (Gross, F. and Vogel, G. eds) pp. 335-381, Raven Press, New York.

Psychoyos, A. (1973) Endocrine control of egg implantation. In: Handbook of Physiology, Section 7, Vol. II/2 (Greep, R.O. and Astwood, E.B. eds), pp. 187-215, American Physiological Society, Washington.

Rabin, D. and McNeill, L.W. (1980) Pituitary and gonadal desensitization after continuous luteinizing hormone-releasing hormone infusion in normal females. J. Clin. Endocrinol. Metab. 51, 873-876.

Raynaud, J.P., Azadian-Boulanger, G., Mary, J., Mouren, M., Lemay, A., Ferland, L., Auclair, C. and Labrie, F. (1979) Action luteolytique de la LH-RH chez la rate, la guenon et la femme. In: L'implantation de l'Oeuf (Du Mesnil Du Buisson, F., Psychoyos, A. and Thomas, K. eds), p. 273-284, Masson, Paris.

Rechenberg, W.v., Sandow, J., Baeder, C. and Stoll, W. (1979) Luteolysis by LH-RH analogues and prostaglandins: a comparison. Acta Endocrinol. (Copenhagen) Suppl. 225, 105.

Richards, J.S. (1979) Hormonal control of ovarian follicular development: a 1978 perspective. Rec. Progr. Horm. Res. 35, 343-373.

Rippel, R.H. and Johnson, E.S. (1976a) Regression of corpora lutea in the rabbit after injection of a gonadotropin-releasing peptide. Proc. Soc. Exp. Biol. Med. 152, 29-32.

Rippel, R.H. and Johnson, E.S. (1976b) Inhibition of hCG-induced ovarian and uterine augmentation in the immature rat by analogs of GnRH. Proc. Soc. Exp. Biol. Med. 152, 432-436.

Rivier, J.E. and Vale, W.W. (1978) (D-pGlu^1, D-Phe^2, D-Trp^{3,6})-LRF. A potent luteinizing hormone-releasing factor antagonist in vitro and inhibitor of ovulation in the rat. Life Sci. 23, 869-876.

Rivier, C., Rivier, J. and Vale, W. (1978) Chronic effects of (D-Trp^6-Pro^9-NEt) luteinizing hormone-releasing factor on reproductive processes in the female rat. Endocrinology 103, 2299-2305.

Rivier, C., Rivier, J. and Vale, W. (1979) Chronic effects of (D-Trp^6, Pro^9-NET) luteinizing hormone-releasing factor on reproductive processes in the male rat. Endocrinology 105, 1191-1201.

Rothchild, J. (1965) The corpus luteum-hypophysis relationship. The luteolytic effect of luteinizing hormone (LH) in the rat. Acta Endocrinol. (Copenhagen) 49, 107-119.

Rubinstein, L.M., Parlow, A.F., Derzko, C. and Hershman, J. (1978) Pituitary gonadotropin response to LH-RH in human pregnancy. Obstetr. Gynecol. 52, 172-175.

Saffran, M. (1974) Chemistry of hypothalamic hypophysiotropic factors. In: Handbook of Physiology: Endocrinology, Vol. IV, Part 2, pp. 575-586, American Physiological Society, Washington, D.C.

Saito, M., Kumasaki, T., Yaoi, Y., Nishi, N., Arimura, A., Coy, D.H. and Schally, A.V. (1977) Stimulation of luteinizing hormone (LH) and follicle-stimulating hormone by D-Leu^6, des-Gly^{10}-NH$_2$/LH-releasing hormone ethylamide after subcutaneous, intravaginal, and intrarectal administration to women. Fertil. Steril. 28, 240-245.

Sandow, J. (1975) Hypothalamic control of anterior pituitary hormone secretion: physiological aspects. In: Basic Applications and Clinical Uses of Hypothalamic Hormones, (Charro-Salgado, A., Fernandez-Durango, R. and Lopez del Campo, G. eds). pp. 113-123, Excerpta Medica, Amsterdam.

Sandow, J. (1977) Risultati clinici e sperimentali sugli ormoni ipotalamici per il controllo della sterilità e della fertilità. In: Il Controllo della Fecondità (Pescetto, G., Martini, L. and De Cecco, L. eds), pp. 205-225, Cofese Edizioni, Palermo.

Sandow, J. (1979) Toxicological evaluation of drugs affecting the hypothalamic-pituitary system. Pharmac. Ther. 5, 297-304.

Sandow, J. and Hahn, M. (1978) Chronic treatment with LH-RH in golden hamsters. Acta Endocr. (Copenhagen) 88, 601-610.

Sandow, J. and König, W. (1979) Studies with fragments of a highly active analogue of luteinizing hormone-releasing hormone. J. Endocrinol 81, 175-182.

Sandow, J., Rechenberg, W.v., König, W. and Hahn, M. (1976a) Physiological studies with highly active analogues of LH-RH. Chemiker-Zeitung 100, 537.

Sandow, J., Rechenberg, W.v., and Jerzabek, G. (1976b) The effect of LH-RH, prostaglandins and synthetic analogues of LH-RH on ovarian metabolism. Eur. J. Obstetr. Gynecol. Biol. 6, 185-190.

Sandow, J., König, W., Geiger, R., Uhmann, R. and Rechenberg, W.v. (1978a) Structure-activity relationships in the LH-RH molecule. In: Control of Ovulation (Crighton, O.B., Haynes, N.B., Foxcroft, G.R. and Lamming, G.E. eds), pp. 46-49, Butterworths, London.

Sandow, J., Rechenberg, W.v., König, W., Hahn, M., Jerzabek, G. and Fraser, H.M. (1978) Physiological studies with highly active analogues of LH-RH. In: Hypothalamic Hormones: Chemistry, Physiology and Clinical Applications, (Gupta, D. and Voelter, W. eds), pp. 307-325. Verlag Chemie, Weinheim.

Sandow, J., Rechenberg, W.v., Jerzabek, G. and Stoll, W. (1978c) Pituitary gonadotropin inhibition by a highly active analogue of LH-RH. Fertil. Steril. 30, 205-209.

Sandow, J., Rechenberg, W.v. and Engelbart, K. (1979a) Hormonal and pharmacological action of buserelin (Receptal^R), a potent form of gonadotropin-releasing hormone. The Blue Book for the Veterinary Profession 29, 363-372.

Sandow, J., Kuhl, H. and Krauss, B. (1979b) Studies on enzyme stability of luteinizing hormone-releasing hormone analogues. J. Endocrinol. 81, 157P-158P.

Sandow, J., Rechenberg, W.v., Kuhl, H., Baumann, R., Krauss, B., Jerzabek, G. and Kille, S. (1979c) Inhibitory control of the pituitary LH secretion by LH-RH in male rats. Horm. Res. 11, 303-317.

Sandow, J., Rechenberg, W.v., Baeder, C. and Engelbart, K. (1980a) Antifertility effects of an LH-RH analogue in male rats and dogs. Int. J. Fertil. 25, 213-221.

Sandow, J., Rechenberg, W.v., Jerzabek, G., Engelbart, K., Kuhl, H. and Fraser, H.M. (1980b) Hypothalamic-pituitary-testicular function in rats after supraphysiological doses of a highly active LRH analogue (buserelin). Acta Endocrinol. (Copenhagen) 94, 489-496.

Sandow, J., Ohe, M.v.d. and Kuhl, H. (1980c). LH-RH and its analogues in contraception. In: Endocrinology 1980, 6th. Internat. Congr. Endocrinol., Melbourne, pp. 528-531, Australian Academy of Sciences, Canberra.

Sandow, J., Geiger, R., Schally, A.V. and Coy, D.H. (1980d). Inhibition of testosterone production and pituitary LH-RH binding in rats by LH-RH antagonists. Acta Endocrinol. (Copenhagen) Suppl. 234, 79.

Sandow, J., Clayton, R.N. and Kuhl, H. (1981a). Pharmacology of LH-RH and its analogues. In: Endocrinology of Human Infertility: New Aspects (Crosignani, P.G. and Rubin, B.L. eds) pp. 221-246, Academic Press, London.

Sandow, J., Kuhl, H., Jerzabek, G., Kille, S. and Rechenberg, W.v. (1981b). The reproductive pharmacology and contraceptive application of LH-RH and its analogues. In: The Gonadotropins: Basic Science and Clinical Aspects in Females (Flamigni, C. and Givens, J.R. eds), Academic Press, London, in press.

Schally, A.V., Arimura, A., Bowers, C.Y., Kastin, A.J., Sawano, S. and Redding, T.W. (1968) Hypothalamic neurohormones regulating anterior pituitary function. Recent Progr. Horm. Res. 24, 497-588.

Schally, A.V., Kastin, A.J. and Arimura, A. (1972a) FSH-releasing hormone and LH-releasing hormone. Vitam. Horm. 30, 83-164.

Schally, A.V., Kastin, A.J. and Arimura, A. (1972b) The hypothalamus and reproduction. Am. J. Obstet. Gynecol. 114, 423-442.

Schally, A.V., Coy, D.H. and Meyers, C.A. (1978) Hypothalamic regulatory hormones. Annu. Rev. Biochem. 47, 89-128.

Schally, A.V., Arimura, A. and Coy, D.H. (1980). Recent approaches to fertility control based on derivatives of LH-RH. Vitam. Horm. 38, 258-314.

Schmidt-Gollwitzer, M., Hardt, W., Schmidt-Gollwitzer, K. and Nevenny-Stickel, J. (1981). Influence of the LH-RH analogue buserelin on cyclic ovarian function and on endometrium. A new approach to fertility control? Contraception 23, 187-196.

Schneider, H.P.G. and Dahlen, H.G. (1975). Influence of iterative iv injection of LRH in women. In: Some Aspects of Hypothalamic Regulation of Endocrine Functions, (Franchimont, P. ed), pp. 163-171, Schattauer Verlag, Stuttgard.

Schröder, H.G., Sandow, J., Seeger, K., Engelbart, K. and Vogel, H.G. (1973). The effect of synthetic LH-RH on induction of ovulation near puberty. In: Hypothalamic Hypophysiotropic Hormones: Physiological and Clinical Studies, (Gual, C. and Rosemberg, E.M. eds), pp. 48-52, Excerpta Medica, Amsterdam.

Shareha, A.M., Ward, W.R. and Birchall, K. (1976) Effect of continuous infusion of gonadotropin-releasing hormone in ewes at different times of the year. J. Reprod. Fertil. 46, 331-340.

Sharpe, R.M. and Fraser, H.M. (1980a) Leydig cell receptors for luteinizing hormone-releasing hormone and its agonists and their modulation by administration or deprivation of the releasing hormone. Biochem. Biophys. Res. Commun. 95, 256-262.

Sharpe, R.M. and Fraser, H.M. (1980b) hCG-stimulation of testicular LH-RH-like activity. Nature 287, 642-643.

Sharpe, R.M., Fraser, H.M. and Sandow, J. (1979) Effect of treatment with an agonist of luteinizing hormone-releasing hormone on early maturational changes in pituitary and testicular function in the rat. J. Endocrinol 80, 249-257.

Sharpe, R.M., Fraser, H.M., Cooper, I. and Rommerts, F.F.G. (1981) Sertoli cell –Leydig cell communication via an LH-RH-like factor. Nature 290, 785-787.

Shelesnyak, M.C. (1957) Some experimental studies on the mechanism of ova-implantation in the rat. Recent Progr. Horm. Res. 13, 269-322.

Siler-Khodr, T.M. and Khodr, G. (1978) Luteinizing hormone releasing factor content of the human placenta. Am. J. Obstet. Gynecol. 130, 216-219.

Smith, M.A. and Vale, W.W. (1980) Superfusion of rat anterior pituitary cells attached to cytodex beads: validation of a technique. Endocrinology 107, 1425-1431.

Smith, R., Donald, R.A., Espiner, E.A., Stronach, S.G. and Edwards, I.A. (1979) Normal adults and subjects with hypogonadotropic hypogonadism respond differently to D-Ser-(TBU)[6], des-Gly[10]-NH$_2$-LH-RH-EA. J. Clin. Endocrinol. Metab. 48, 167-170.

Sowers, J.R., Colantino, M., Fayez, J. and Jonas, H. (1978) Pituitary response to LH-RH in midtrimester pregnancy. Obstet. Gynecol. 52, 685-688.

Swift, A.D. and Crighton, D.B. (1979) Relative activity, plasma elimination and tissue degradation of synthetic luteinizing hormone-releasing hormone and certain of its analogues. J. Endocrinol. 80, 141-152.

Tamada, T., Akabori, A., Konuma, S. and Araki, S. (1976) Lack of release of human chorionic gonadotropin by gonadotropin releasing hormone. Endocrinol. Jpn 23, 531-533.

Tcholakian, R.K., De la Cruz, A., Chowdhury, M., Steinberger, A., Coy, D.C. and Schally, A.V. (1978a) Unusual anti-reproductive properties of the analog (D-Leu[6], desGlyNH$_2$[10])-luteinizing hormone-releasing hormone ethylamide in male rats. Fertil. Steril. 30, 600-603.

Tcholakian, R.K., De la Cruz, A., Chowdhury, M., Schally, A.V. and Steinberger, A. (1978b) Effects of an LH-RH analogue in male rats pretreated with estradiol benzoate. J. Reprod. Fertil. 54, 441-445.

Van Damme, M.P., Robertson, D.M., Marena, R., Ritzen, E.M. and Diczfaluzy, M. (1979) A sensitive and specific in vitro bioassay method for the measurement of the follicle-stimulating activity. Acta Endocrinol. (Copenhagen) 91, 224-237.

Vickery, B.H. and McRae, G.I. (1980) Effects of continuous treatment of male baboons with superagonists of LH-RH. Int. J. Fertil. 25, 179-184.

Vilchez-Martinez, J.A., Coy, D.H., Arimura, A., Coy, E.J., Hirotsu, Y. and Schally, A.V. (1974) Synthesis and biological properties of Leu[6]-LH-RH and D-Leu[6], desGly-NH$_2$[10]-LH-RH ethylamide. Biochem. Biophys. Res. Commun. 59, 1226-1232.

Vilchez-Martinez, J.A., Pedroza, E., Arimura, A. and Schally, A.V. (1979) Paradoxical effects of D-Trp[6]-luteinizing hormone-releasing hormone on the hypothalamic-pituitary-gonadal axis in immature female rats. Fertil. Steril. 31, 677-682.

Wickings, E.J., Zaidi, P. and Nieschlag, E. (1980) Effects of chronic, high dose luteinizing hormone-releasing hormone agonist treatment on pituitary and testicular function in rhesus monkeys. Acta Endocrinol. (Copenhagen) Suppl. 234, 78.

Wiegelmann, W., Solbach, H.G., Kiley, H.K. and Kruskemper, H.L. (1977) LH and FSH response to long-term application of LH-RH analogue in normal males. Horm. Metab . Res. 9, 521-522.

Wildt, L., Marshall, G. and Knobil, E. (1980) Experimental induction of puberty in the infantile female rhesus monkey. Science 207, 1373-1375.

Wilks, J.W., Folkers, K., Humphries, J. and Bowers, C.Y. (1980) Effect of D-Phe[2], Pro[3], D-Phe[6]/luteinizing hormone-releasing hormone, an antagonist, on prevulatory gonadotropin secretion in the rhesus monkey. Biol. Reprod. 23, 1-9.

Wilson, E.A. and Jawad, M.J. (1980) Luteinizing hormone-releasing hormone suppression of human placental progesterone production. Fertil. Steril. 33, 91-93.

Yang, W.H. and Chang, M.C. (1968) Interruption of pregnancy in the rat and hamster by administration of PMS or hCG. Endocrinology 83, 217-224.

Yen, S.S.C., Tsai, C.C., Naftolin, F., Vandenberg, G. and Ajabor, L. (1972) Pulsatile patterns of gonadotropin release in subjects with and without ovarian function. J. Clin. Endocrinol. Metab. 34, 671-675.

Ying, S.Y. (1973) Inhibitory effect of luteinizing hormone releasing hormone (LHRH) on the process of ovulation in the rat. Endocrinology 92, A-142.

Ying, S.Y. and Guillemin, R. (1979) D-Trp[6]-Pro[9]-Net-luteinizing hormone-releasing factor inhibits follicular development in hypophysectomized rats. Nature Lond. 280, 593-595.

Yochim, J.M. and Zarrow, M.X. (1961) Action of estradiol, progesterone and relaxin in the maintenance of gestation in the castrated pregnant rat. Fertil. Steril. 12, 263-276.

Yoshinaga, K. and Fujino, M. (1979) Hormonal control of implantation in the rat: inhibition by luteinizing hormone-releasing hormone and its analogues. In: Maternal Recognition of Pregnancy, pp. 85-110, Excerpta Medica, Amsterdam.

Zarrow, W.X., Caldwell, A.L., Hafez, E.S.E. and Pincus, G. (1958) Superovulation in the immature rat as a possible assay for LH and hCG. Endocrinology 63, 748-758.

Author index

Subject index